Pathophysiology of Heart Disease

A Collaborative Project
of Medical Students
and Faculty

FIFTH EDITION

Edition

5

Pathophysiology of Heart Disease

A Collaborative Project of Medical Students and Faculty

Editor

Leonard S. Lilly, MD

Professor of Medicine
Harvard Medical School
Chief, Brigham and Women's/Faulkner Cardiology
Brigham and Women's Hospital
Boston, Massachusetts

Wolters Kluwer | Lippincott Williams & Wilkins
Health

Philadelphia · Baltimore · New York · London
Buenos Aires · Hong Kong · Sydney · Tokyo

Acquisitions Editor: Crystal Taylor
Product Manager: Julie Montalbano
Design and Art Direction: Doug Smock, Jennifer Clements
Production & Composition: MPS Limited, A Macmillan Company

5th Edition

351 West Camden Street   Two Commerce Square
Baltimore, MD 21201   2001 Market Street
                              Philadelphia, PA 19103

Printed in China.

9 8 7 6 5 4 3 2 1

Library of Congress Cataloging-in-Publication Data

Pathophysiology of heart disease : a collaborative project of medical students and faculty / editor Leonard S. Lilly.—5th ed.
  p. ; cm.
Includes bibliographical references and index.
ISBN 978-1-60547-723-7
1. Heart—Pathophysiology. I. Lilly, Leonard S. II. Harvard Medical School.

[DNLM: 1. Heart Diseases—physiopathology. WG 210]
RC682.9.P255 2011
616.1'207—dc22

2010029159

DISCLAIMER

Care has been taken to confirm the accuracy of the information present and to describe generally accepted practices. However, the authors, editors, and publisher are not responsible for errors or omissions or for any consequences from application of the information in this book and make no warranty, expressed or implied, with respect to the currency, completeness, or accuracy of the contents of the publication. Application of this information in a particular situation remains the professional responsibility of the practitioner; the clinical treatments described and recommended may not be considered absolute and universal recommendations.

The authors, editors, and publisher have exerted every effort to ensure that drug selection and dosage set forth in this text are in accordance with the current recommendations and practice at the time of publication. However, in view of ongoing research, changes in government regulations, and the constant flow of information relating to drug therapy and drug reactions, the reader is urged to check the package insert for each drug for any change in indications and dosage and for added warnings and precautions. This is particularly important when the recommended agent is a new or infrequently employed drug.

Some drugs and medical devices presented in this publication have Food and Drug Administration (FDA) clearance for limited use in restricted research settings. It is the responsibility of the health care provider to ascertain the FDA status of each drug or device planned for use in their clinical practice.

To purchase additional copies of this book, call our customer service department at **(800) 638-3030** or fax orders to **(301) 223-2320**. International customers should call **(301) 223-2300**.

Visit Lippincott Williams & Wilkins on the Internet: http://www.lww.com. Lippincott Williams & Wilkins customer service representatives are available from 8:30 am to 6:00 pm, EST.

Dedicated in Loving Memory of My Father
DAVID LILLY
(1922–2009)

Foreword

It is axiomatic that when designing any product or service, the needs of the prospective user must receive primary consideration. Regrettably, this is rarely the case with medical textbooks, which play a vital role in the education of students, residents, fellows, practicing physicians, and paramedical professionals. Most books are written for anyone who will read—or preferably buy—them. As a consequence, they often provide a little for everyone but not enough for anyone. Many medical textbooks are reminiscent of the one-room schoolhouse, which included pupils ranging from the first to the twelfth grade. The need to deal with subject matter at enormously disparate levels of sophistication interfered with the educational process.

Medical educators appreciate that the needs of medical students exposed to a subject for the first time differ importantly from those of practicing physicians who wish to review an area learned previously or to be updated on new developments in a field with which they already have some familiarity. The lack of textbooks designed specifically for students leads faculty at schools around the country to spend countless hours preparing and duplicating voluminous lecture notes, and providing students with custom-designed "camels" (a camel is a cow created by a committee!).

Pathophysiology of Heart Disease: A Collaborative Project of Medical Students and Faculty, represents a refreshing and innovative departure in the preparation of a medical text. Students—that is, potential consumers—dissatisfied with currently available textbooks on cardiology, made their needs clear. Fortunately, their pleas fell on receptive ears. Dr. Leonard Lilly, a Professor of Medicine at Harvard Medical School, and a respected cardiologist at the Brigham and Women's and Faulkner Hospitals, has served as the leader of this project. He has brought together a group of talented Harvard medical students and faculty who have collaborated closely to produce this superb introductory text *specifically* designed to meet the needs of medical students during their initial encounters with patients with heart disease. While *Pathophysiology of Heart Disease* is not meant to be encyclopedic or all inclusive, it is remarkably thorough.

Quite appropriately, the first four editions of this fine book were received enthusiastically, and *Pathophysiology of Heart Disease* is now a required or recommended text at many medical schools not only in the United States, but also in other countries. It has been translated into other languages, has received two awards of excellence from the American Medical Writers Association, and has inspired several other student–faculty collaborative book projects. This fifth edition is not only an updated but also an expanded version of the fourth edition. Many of the figures have been redrawn and enhanced to display complex concepts in uncomplicated ways. As such, it will prove to be even more valuable than its predecessors.

Dr. Lilly and his colleagues—both faculty and students—have made a significant and unique contribution in preparing this important book. Future generations of medical educators and students, and ultimately the patients that they serve, will be indebted to them for this important contribution.

EUGENE BRAUNWALD, MD
Distinguished Hersey Professor of Medicine
Harvard Medical School
Boston, Massachusetts

Preface

This textbook is a comprehensive introduction to diseases of the cardiovascular system. Although excellent cardiology reference books are available, their encyclopedic content can overwhelm the beginning student. Therefore, this text was created to serve as a simplified bridge between courses in basic physiology and the care of patients in clinical settings. It is intended to help medical students and physicians-in-training form a solid foundation of knowledge of diseases of the heart and circulation, and is designed to be read in its entirety during standard courses in cardiovascular pathophysiology. Emphasis has been placed on the basic mechanisms by which cardiac illnesses develop, in order to facilitate the later in-depth study of clinical diagnosis and therapy.

The original motivation for writing this book was the need for such a text voiced by our medical students, as well as their desire to participate in its creation and direction. Consequently, the book's development is unusual in that it represents a close collaboration between Harvard medical students and cardiology faculty, who shared in the writing and editing of the manuscript. The goal of this pairing was to focus the subject matter on the needs of the student, while providing the expertise of our faculty members. In this updated and rewritten fifth edition of *Pathophysiology of Heart Disease*, the collaborative effort has continued, between a new generation of medical students and our cardiovascular faculty.

The introductory chapters of the book review basic cardiac anatomy and physiology, and describe the tools needed for understanding clinical aspects of subsequently presented material. The remainder of the text addresses the major groups of cardiovascular diseases. The chapters are designed and edited to be read in sequence but are sufficiently cross-referenced so that they can also be used out of order. The final chapter describes the major classes of cardiovascular drugs and explains the physiologic rationale for their uses.

It has been a great privilege for me to collaborate with the 92 talented, creative, and energetic medical students who have contributed to the five editions of this book. Their intellect, enthusiasm, and dedication have significantly facilitated the completion of each manuscript. I am also indebted to my faculty colleague coauthors for their time, their expertise, and their continued commitment to this project.

I deeply appreciate the thoughtful and constructive comments received from faculty and students around the globe pertaining to the previous editions of this book. These communications have been very helpful in directing the current revision, and the many warm remarks have been an important source of encouragement. I also acknowledge with gratitude several individuals who provided material, detailed comments and reviews, or other support to this edition: Behnood Bikdeli, Douglas Burtt, Sharmila Dorbala, Marcelo Di Carli, Raymond Kwong, Frank Rybicki, Frederick Schoen, and Pinak Shah. Additionally, I thank Jovette Auguste and Pamela Nettles for their invaluable administrative assistance.

It has been a pleasure to work with the editorial and production staffs of our publisher, Lippincott Williams & Wilkins. In particular, I thank Julie Montalbano, Crystal Taylor, Jennifer Clements, Jonathan Dimes and Arijit Biswas for their skill and professionalism in bringing this edition to completion.

Finally, a project of this magnitude could not be undertaken without the strong support and patience of my family, and for that I am very grateful.

On behalf of the contributors, I hope that this book enhances your understanding of cardiovascular diseases and provides a solid foundation for further learning and clinical care of your patients.

LEONARD S. LILLY, MD
Boston, Massachusetts

List of Contributors

Student Contributors

David D. Berg (MD 2011)

Neal A. Chatterjee (MD 2010)

Ranliang Hu (MD 2010)

Henry Jung (MD 2010)

Christopher T. Lee (MD 2011)

Fan Liang (MD 2010)

Ken Young Lin (MD, PhD 2010)

Christopher A. Miller (MD 2011)

Stephen R. Pomedli (MD 2011)

Yin Ren (MD 2014)

June-Wha Rhee (MD 2011)

Jordan B. Strom (MD 2011)

Cyrus K. Yamin (MD 2011)

Faculty Contributors

Elliott M. Antman, MD
Professor of Medicine
Harvard Medical School
Cardiovascular Division, Brigham and
Women's Hospital
Boston, Massachusetts

Eugene Braunwald, MD (Foreword)
Distinguished Hersey Professor of Medicine
Harvard Medical School
Chairman, TIMI Study Group, Brigham and
Women's Hospital
Boston, Massachusetts

David W. Brown, MD
Assistant Professor of Pediatrics
Harvard Medical School
Cardiology Division, Children's Hospital
Boston, Massachusetts

Patricia Challender Come, MD
Associate Professor of Medicine
Harvard Medical School
Cardiologist, Harvard Vanguard Medical
Associates
Associate Physician, Brigham and Women's
Hospital
Boston, Massachusetts

Mark A. Creager, MD
Professor of Medicine
Harvard Medical School
Director, Vascular Center
Simon C. Fireman Scholar in Cardiovascular
Medicine, Brigham and Women's Hospital
Boston, Massachusetts

G. William Dec, MD
Roman W. DeSanctis Professor of Medicine
Harvard Medical School
Chief, Cardiology Division, Massachusetts
General Hospital
Boston, Massachusetts

Elazer R. Edelman, MD, PhD
Thomas D. and Virginia W. Cabot Professor
of Health Sciences and Technology
Massachusetts Institute of Technology
Director, Harvard-MIT Biomedical
Engineering Center
Professor of Medicine
Harvard Medical School
Boston, Massachusetts

Michael A. Fifer, MD
Associate Professor of Medicine
Harvard Medical School
Director, Cardiac Catheterization
Laboratory
Massachusetts General Hospital
Boston, Massachusetts

Peter Libby, MD
Mallinckrodt Professor of Medicine
Harvard Medical School
Chief, Cardiovascular Division, Brigham and
Women's Hospital
Boston, Massachusetts

Leonard S. Lilly, MD
Professor of Medicine
Harvard Medical School
Chief, Brigham and Women's/Faulkner
Cardiology
Brigham and Women's Hospital
Boston, Massachusetts

Patrick T. O'Gara, MD
Associate Professor of Medicine
Harvard Medical School
Director of Clinical Cardiology
Brigham and Women's Hospital
Boston, Massachusetts

Marc S. Sabatine, MD, MPH
Associate Professor of Medicine
Harvard Medical School
Cardiovascular Division, Brigham and
Women's Hospital
Boston, Massachusetts

William G. Stevenson, MD
Professor of Medicine
Harvard Medical School
Director, Clinical Cardiac Electrophysiology
Program, Brigham and Women's Hospital
Boston, Massachusetts

Gary R. Strichartz, PhD
Professor of Anaesthesia (Pharmacology)
Harvard Medical School
Director, Pain Research Center
Vice Chairman of Research, Department of
Anesthesia, Brigham and Women's Hospital
Boston, Massachusetts

Gordon H. Williams, MD
Professor of Medicine
Harvard Medical School
Director, Specialized Center of Research in
Hypertension
Director, Center for Clinical Investigation
Brigham and Women's Hospital
Boston, Massachusetts

Table of Contents

Basic Cardiac Structure and Function

Ken Young Lin
Elazer R. Edelman
Gary Strichartz
Leonard S. Lilly

Knowledge of normal cardiac structure and function is crucial to understanding diseases that afflict the heart. This chapter reviews basic cardiac anatomy and electrophysiology as well as the events that lead to cardiac contraction.

CARDIAC ANATOMY AND HISTOLOGY

Although the study of cardiac anatomy dates back to ancient times, interest in this field has recently gained momentum. The development of sophisticated cardiac imaging procedures such as coronary angiography, echocardiography, computed tomography, and magnetic resonance imaging has made

essential an intimate knowledge of the spatial relationships of cardiac structures. Such information also proves helpful in understanding the pathophysiology of heart disease. This section emphasizes the aspects of cardiac anatomy that are important to the clinician— that is, the "functional" anatomy.

Pericardium

The heart and roots of the great vessels are enclosed by a fibroserous sac called the pericardium (Fig. 1.1). This structure consists of two layers: a strong outer fibrous layer and an inner serosal layer. The inner serosal layer adheres to the external wall of the heart and is

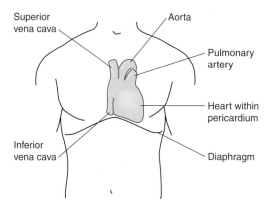

Superior vena cava

Aorta

Pulmonary artery

Heart within pericardium

Inferior vena cava

Diaphragm

Figure 1.1. **The position of the heart in the chest.** The superior vena cava, aorta, and pulmonary artery exit superiorly, whereas the inferior vena cava projects inferiorly.

called the **visceral pericardium**. The visceral pericardium reflects back on itself and lines the outer fibrous layer, forming the **parietal pericardium**. The space between the visceral and parietal layers contains a thin film of pericardial fluid that allows the heart to beat in a minimal-friction environment.

The pericardium is attached to the sternum and the mediastinal portions of the right and left pleurae. Its many connections to the surrounding structures keep the pericardial sac firmly anchored within the thorax and therefore help to maintain the heart in its normal position.

Emanating from the pericardium in a superior direction are the aorta, the pulmonary artery, and the superior vena cava (see Fig. 1.1). The inferior vena cava projects through the pericardium inferiorly.

Surface Anatomy of the Heart

The heart is shaped roughly like a cone and consists of four muscular chambers. The right and left ventricles are the main pumping chambers. The less muscular right and left atria deliver blood to their respective ventricles.

Several terms are used to describe the heart's surfaces and borders (Fig. 1.2). The **apex** is formed by the tip of the left ventricle, which points inferiorly, anteriorly, and to the left. The **base** or posterior surface of the heart is formed by the atria, mainly the left, and lies between the lung hila. The **anterior** surface of the heart is shaped by the right atrium and ventricle. Because the left atrium and ventricle lie

more posteriorly, they form only a small strip of this anterior surface. The **inferior** surface of the heart is formed by both ventricles, primarily the left. This surface of the heart lies along the diaphragm; hence, it is also referred to as the diaphragmatic surface.

Observing the chest from an anteroposterior view (as on a chest radiograph; see Chapter 3), four recognized borders of the heart are apparent. The right border is established by the right atrium and is almost in line with the superior and inferior venae cavae. The inferior border is nearly horizontal and is formed mainly by the right ventricle, with a slight contribution from the left ventricle near the apex. The left ventricle and a portion of the left atrium make up the left border of the heart, whereas the superior border is shaped by both atria. From this description of the surface of the heart emerge two basic "rules" of normal cardiac anatomy: (1) right-sided structures lie mostly anterior to their left-sided counterparts, and (2) atrial chambers are located mostly to the right of their corresponding ventricles.

Internal Structure of the Heart

Four major valves in the normal heart direct blood flow in a forward direction and prevent backward leakage. The atrioventricular valves (tricuspid and mitral) separate the atria and ventricles, whereas the semilunar valves (pulmonic and aortic) separate the ventricles from the great arteries (Fig. 1.3). All four heart valves are attached to the fibrous **cardiac skeleton**, which is composed of dense connective tissue. The cardiac skeleton also serves as a site of attachment for the ventricular and atrial muscles.

The surface of the heart valves and the interior surface of the chambers are lined by a single layer of endothelial cells, termed the **endocardium**. The subendocardial tissue contains fibroblasts, elastic and collagenous fibers, veins, nerves, and branches of the conducting system and is continuous with the connective tissue of the heart muscle layer, the myocardium. The **myocardium** is the thickest layer of the heart and consists of bundles of cardiac muscle cells, the histology of which is described later in the chapter. External to the myocardium is a layer of connective tissue and

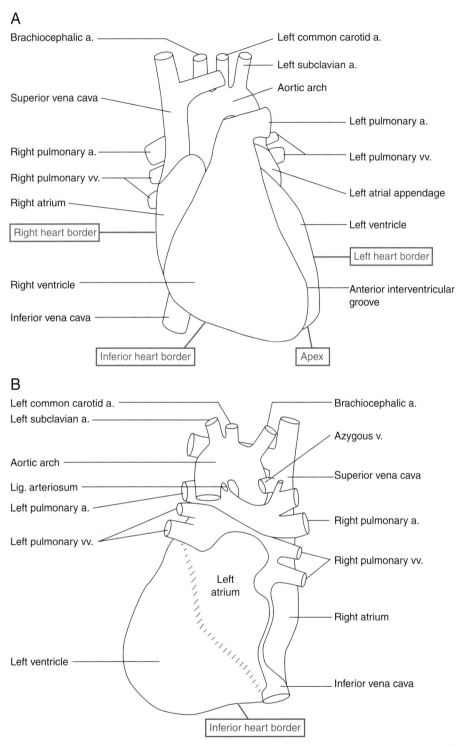

Figure 1.2. The heart and great vessels. A. The anterior view. **B.** The posterior aspect (or base), as viewed from the back. a, artery; lig, ligamentum; vv, veins.

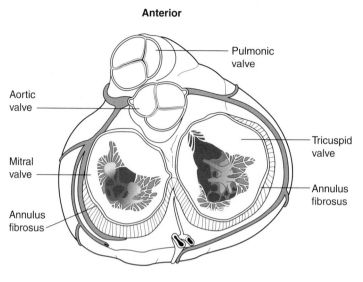

Anterior

Pulmonic valve

Aortic valve

Tricuspid valve

Mitral valve

Annulus fibrosus

Annulus fibrosus

Posterior

Figure 1.3. **The four heart valves viewed from above with atria removed.** The figure depicts the period of ventricular filling (diastole) during which the tricuspid and mitral valves are open and the semilunar valves (pulmonic and aortic) are closed. Each annulus fibrosus surrounding the mitral and tricuspid valves is thicker than those surrounding the pulmonic and aortic valves; all four contribute to the heart's fibrous skeleton, which is composed of dense connective tissue.

adipose tissue through which pass the larger blood vessels and nerves that supply the heart muscle. The **epicardium** is the outermost layer of the heart and is identical to, and just another term for, the visceral pericardium previously described.

Right Atrium and Ventricle

Opening into the **right atrium** are the superior and inferior venae cavae and the coronary sinus (Fig. 1.4). The venae cavae return deoxygenated blood from the systemic veins into the right atrium, whereas the coronary sinus carries venous return from the coronary arteries. The interatrial septum forms the posteromedial wall of the right atrium and separates it from the left atrium. The **tricuspid valve** is located in the floor of the atrium and opens into the right ventricle.

The **right ventricle** (see Fig. 1.4) is roughly triangular in shape, and its superior aspect forms a cone-shaped outflow tract, which leads to the pulmonary artery. Although the inner wall of the outflow tract is smooth, the rest of the ventricle is covered by a number of irregular bridges (termed **trabeculae carneae**) that give the right ventricular wall a sponge-like appearance. A large trabecula that crosses the ventricular cavity is called the **moderator band**. It carries a component of the right bundle branch of the conducting system to the ventricular muscle.

The right ventricle contains three **papillary muscles**, which project into the chamber and via their thin, stringlike **chordae tendineae** attach to the edges of the tricuspid valve leaflets. The leaflets, in turn, are attached to the fibrous ring that supports the valve between the right atrium and ventricle. Contraction of the papillary muscles prior to other regions of the ventricle tightens the chordae tendineae, helping to align and restrain the leaflets of the tricuspid valve as they are forced closed. This action prevents blood from regurgitating into the right atrium during ventricular contraction.

At the apex of the right ventricular outflow tract is the **pulmonic valve**, which leads to the pulmonary artery. This valve consists of three cusps attached to a fibrous ring. During relaxation of the ventricle, elastic recoil of the pulmonary

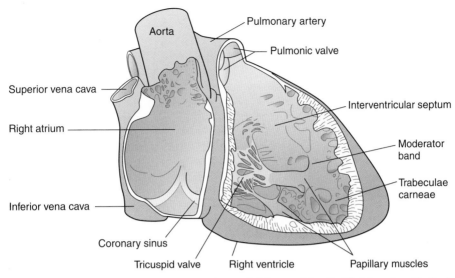

Figure 1.4. Interior structures of the right atrium and right ventricle. (Modified from Goss CM. *Gray's Anatomy*. 29th ed. Philadelphia, PA: Lea & Febiger; 1973:547.)

arteries forces blood back toward the heart, distending the valve cusps toward one another. This action closes the pulmonic valve and prevents regurgitation of blood back into the right ventricle.

Left Atrium and Ventricle

Entering the posterior half of the **left atrium** are the four pulmonary veins (Fig. 1.5). The wall of the left atrium is about 2 mm thick, being slightly greater than that of the right atrium. The mitral valve opens into the left ventricle through the inferior wall of the left atrium.

The cavity of the **left ventricle** is approximately cone shaped and longer than that of the right ventricle. In a healthy adult heart, the wall thickness is 9 to 11 mm, roughly three times that of the right ventricle. The aortic vestibule is a smooth-walled part of the left ventricular cavity located just inferior to the aortic valve. Inferior to this region, most of the ventricle is covered by trabeculae carneae, which are finer and more numerous than those in the right ventricle.

The left ventricular chamber (see Fig. 1.5B) contains two large papillary muscles. These are larger than their counterparts in the right ventricle, and their chordae tendineae are thicker but less numerous. The chordae tendineae of each papillary muscle distribute to both leaflets of the **mitral valve**. Similar to the case in the right ventricle, tensing of the chordae tendineae during left ventricular contraction helps restrain and align the mitral leaflets, enabling them to close properly and preventing the backward leakage of blood.

The **aortic valve** separates the left ventricle from the aorta. Surrounding the aortic valve opening is a fibrous ring to which is attached the three cusps of the valve. Just above the right and left aortic valve cusps in the aortic wall are the origins of the right and left coronary arteries (see Fig. 1.5B).

Interventricular Septum

The interventricular septum is the thick wall between the left and right ventricles. It is composed of a muscular and a membranous part (see Fig. 1.5B). The margins of this septum can be traced on the surface of the heart by following the anterior and posterior interventricular grooves. Owing to the greater hydrostatic pressure within the left ventricle, the large muscular portion of the septum bulges toward the right ventricle. The small, oval-shaped membranous part of the septum is thin and located just inferior to the cusps of the aortic valve.

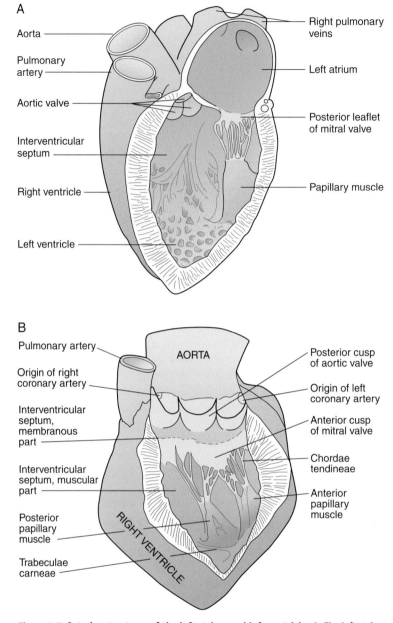

A

Aorta

Pulmonary artery

Aortic valve

Interventricular septum

Right ventricle

Left ventricle

Right pulmonary veins

Left atrium

Posterior leaflet of mitral valve

Papillary muscle

B

Pulmonary artery

Origin of right coronary artery

Interventricular septum, membranous part

Interventricular septum, muscular part

Posterior papillary muscle

Trabeculae carneae

AORTA

Posterior cusp of aortic valve

Origin of left coronary artery

Anterior cusp of mitral valve

Chordae tendineae

Anterior papillary muscle

RIGHT VENTRICLE

Figure 1.5. Interior structures of the left atrium and left ventricle. A. The left atrium and left ventricular (LV) inflow and outflow regions. **B.** Interior structures of the LV cavity. (Modified from Agur AMR, Lee MJ. *Grant's Atlas of Anatomy.* 9th ed. Baltimore, MD: Williams & Wilkins; 1991:59.)

To summarize the functional anatomic points presented in this section, the following is a review of the path of blood flow through the heart: Deoxygenated blood is delivered to the heart through the inferior and superior venae cavae, which enters into the right atrium. Flow continues through the tricuspid valve orifice into the right ventricle. Contraction of the right ventricle propels the blood across the pulmonic valve to the pulmonary artery and lungs, where carbon dioxide is released and oxygen is absorbed. The oxygen-rich blood returns to the heart through the pulmonary veins to the left atrium and then passes across the mitral valve into the left ventricle. Contraction of the left ventricle pumps the oxygenated blood across the aortic valve into the aorta, from which it is distributed to all other tissues of the body.

Impulse-Conducting System

The impulse-conducting system (Fig. 1.6) consists of specialized cells that initiate the heartbeat and electrically coordinate contractions of the heart chambers. The **sinoatrial (SA) node** is a small mass of specialized cardiac muscle fibers in the wall of the right atrium. It is located to the right of the superior vena cava entrance and normally initiates the electrical impulse for contraction. The **atrioventricular (AV) node** lies beneath the endocardium in the inferoposterior part of the interatrial septum.

Distal to the AV node is the **bundle of His**, which perforates the interventricular septum posteriorly. Within the septum, the bundle of His bifurcates into a broad sheet of fibers that continues over the left side of the septum, known as the **left bundle branch**, and a compact, cablelike structure on the right side, the **right bundle branch**.

The right bundle branch is thick and deeply buried in the muscle of the interventricular septum and continues toward the apex. Near the junction of the interventricular septum and the anterior wall of the right ventricle, the right bundle branch becomes subendocardial and bifurcates. One branch travels across the right ventricular cavity in the moderator band, whereas the other continues toward the tip of the ventricle. These branches eventually arborize into a finely divided anastomosing plexus that travels throughout the right ventricle.

Functionally, the left bundle branch is divided into an anterior and a posterior fascicle and a small branch to the septum. The anterior fascicle runs anteriorly toward the apex, forming a subendocardial plexus in the area of the anterior papillary muscle. The posterior fascicle travels to the area of the posterior papillary muscle; it then divides into a subendocardial plexus and spreads to the rest of the left ventricle.

The subendocardial plexuses of both ventricles send distributing **Purkinje fibers** to the ventricular muscle. Impulses within the His–Purkinje system are transmitted first to

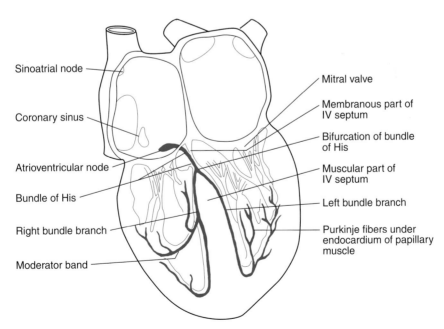

Figure 1.6. Main components of the cardiac conduction system. This system includes the sinoatrial node, atrioventricular node, bundle of His, right and left bundle branches, and the Purkinje fibers. The moderator band carries a large portion of the right bundle. IV, interventricular.

the papillary muscles and then throughout the walls of the ventricles, allowing papillary muscle contraction to precede that of the ventricles. This coordination prevents regurgitation of blood flow through the AV valves, as discussed earlier.

Cardiac Innervation

The heart is innervated by both parasympathetic and sympathetic afferent and efferent nerves. Preganglionic *sympathetic* neurons located within the upper five to six thoracic levels of the spinal cord synapse with second-order neurons in the cervical sympathetic ganglia. Traveling within the cardiac nerves, these fibers terminate in the heart and great vessels. Preganglionic *parasympathetic* fibers originate in the dorsal motor nucleus of the medulla and pass as branches of the vagus nerve to the heart and great vessels. Here the fibers synapse with second-order neurons located in ganglia within these structures. A rich supply of vagal afferents from the inferior and posterior aspects of the ventricles mediates important cardiac reflexes, whereas the abundant vagal efferent fibers to the SA and AV nodes are active in modulating electrical impulse initiation and conduction.

Cardiac Vessels

The cardiac vessels consist of the coronary arteries and veins and the lymphatics. The largest components of these structures lie within the loose connective tissue in the epicardial fat.

Coronary Arteries

The heart muscle is supplied with oxygen and nutrients by the right and left coronary arteries, which arise from the root of the aorta just above the aortic valve cusps (Fig. 1.7; see also Fig. 1.5B). After their origin, these vessels pass anteriorly, one on each side of the pulmonary artery (see Fig. 1.7).

The large **left main coronary artery** passes between the left atrium and the pulmonary trunk to reach the AV groove. There it divides into the **left anterior descending (LAD) coronary artery** and the circumflex artery.

The LAD travels within the anterior interventricular groove toward the cardiac apex. During its descent on the anterior surface, the LAD gives off septal branches that supply the anterior two thirds of the interventricular septum and the apical portion of the anterior papillary muscle. The LAD also gives off diagonal branches that supply the anterior surface of the left ventricle. The **circumflex artery** continues within the left AV groove and passes around the left border of the heart to reach the posterior surface. It gives off large obtuse marginal branches that supply the lateral and posterior wall of the left ventricle.

The **right coronary artery (RCA)** travels in the right AV groove, passing posteriorly between the right atrium and ventricle. It supplies blood to the right ventricle via acute marginal branches. In most people, the distal RCA gives rise to a large branch, the **posterior descending artery** (see Fig. 1.7C). This vessel travels from the inferoposterior aspect of the heart to the apex and supplies blood to the inferior and posterior walls of the ventricles and the posterior one third of the interventricular septum. Just before giving off the posterior descending branch, the RCA usually gives off the **AV nodal artery**.

The posterior descending and AV nodal arteries arise from the RCA in 85% of the population, and in such people, the coronary circulation is termed *right dominant*. In approximately 8%, the posterior descending artery arises from the circumflex artery instead, resulting in a *left dominant* circulation. In the remaining population, the heart's posterior blood supply is contributed to from branches of both the RCA and the circumflex, forming a *codominant* circulation.

The blood supply to the SA node is also most often (70% of the time) derived from the RCA. However, in 25% of normal hearts, the **SA nodal artery** arises from the circumflex artery, and in 5% of cases, both the RCA and the circumflex artery contribute to this vessel.

From their epicardial locations, the coronary arteries send perforating branches into the ventricular muscle, which form a richly branching and anastomosing vasculature in the walls of all the cardiac chambers. From this plexus arise a massive number of capillaries that form an elaborate network surrounding each cardiac muscle fiber. The muscle fibers located just

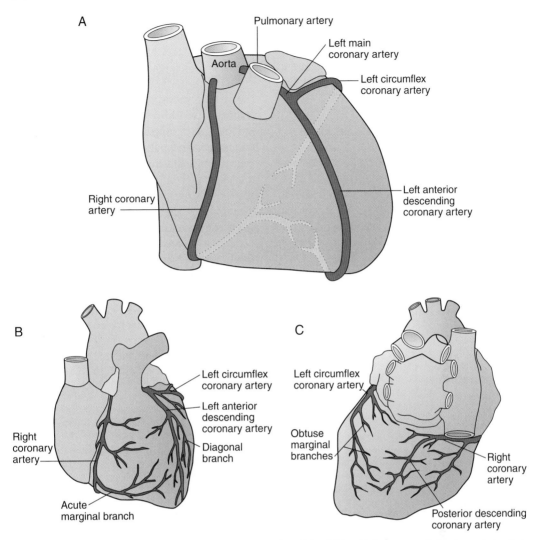

A

Pulmonary artery

Left main
coronary artery

Aorta

Left circumflex
coronary artery

Right coronary
artery

Left anterior
descending
coronary artery

B

Left circumflex
coronary artery

Left anterior
descending
coronary artery

Diagonal
branch

Right
coronary
artery

Acute
marginal branch

C

Left circumflex
coronary artery

Obtuse
marginal
branches

Right
coronary
artery

Posterior descending
coronary artery

Figure 1.7. Coronary artery anatomy. A. Schematic representation of the right and left coronary arteries demonstrates their orientation to one another. The left main artery bifurcates into the circumflex artery, which perfuses the lateral and posterior regions of the left ventricle (LV), and the anterior descending artery, which perfuses the LV anterior wall, the anterior portion of the intraventricular septum, and a portion of the anterior right ventricular (RV) wall. The right coronary artery (RCA) perfuses the right ventricle and variable portions of the posterior left ventricle through its terminal branches. The posterior descending artery most often arises from the RCA. **B.** Anterior view of the heart demonstrating the coronary arteries and their major branches. **C.** Posterior view of the heart demonstrating the terminal portions of the right and circumflex coronary arteries and their branches.

beneath the endocardium, particularly those of the papillary muscles and the thick left ventricle, are supplied either by the terminal branches of the coronary arteries or directly from the ventricular cavity through tiny vascular channels, known as **thebesian veins**.

Collateral connections, usually <200 μm in diameter, exist at the subarteriolar level between the coronary arteries. In the normal heart, few of these collateral vessels are visible. However, they may become larger and func-

tional when atherosclerotic disease obstructs a coronary artery, thereby providing blood flow to distal portions of the vessel from a nonobstructed neighbor.

Coronary Veins

The coronary veins follow a distribution similar to that of the major coronary arteries. These vessels return blood from the myocardial capillaries to the right atrium predominantly via the coronary sinus. The major veins lie in the epicardial fat, usually superficial to their arterial counterparts. The thebesian veins, described earlier, provide an additional potential route for a small amount of direct blood return to the cardiac chambers.

Lymphatic Vessels

The heart lymph is drained by an extensive plexus of valved vessels located in the subendocardial connective tissue of all four chambers. This lymph drains into an epicardial plexus from which are derived several larger lymphatic vessels that follow the distribution of the coronary arteries and veins. Each of these larger vessels then combines in the AV groove to form a single lymphatic conduit, which exits

the heart to reach the mediastinal lymphatic plexus and ultimately the thoracic duct.

Histology of Ventricular Myocardial Cells

The mature myocardial cell (also termed the **myocyte**) measures up to 25 μm in diameter and 100 μm in length. The cell shows a cross-striated banding pattern similar to that of the skeletal muscle. However, unlike the multinucleated skeletal myofibers, myocardial cells contain only one or two centrally located nuclei. Surrounding each myocardial cell is the connective tissue with a rich capillary network.

Each myocardial cell contains numerous **myofibrils**, which are long chains of individual **sarcomeres**, the fundamental contractile units of the cell (Fig. 1.8). Each sarcomere

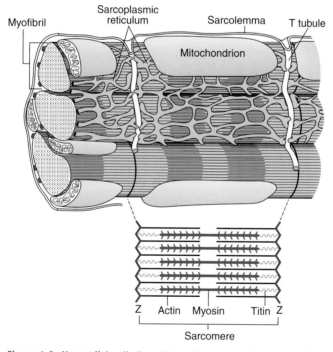

Figure 1.8. Myocardial cell. Top, Schematic representation of the ultrastructure of the myocardial cell. The cell consists of multiple parallel myofibrils surrounded by mitochondria. The T tubules are invaginations of the cell membrane (the sarcolemma) that increase the surface area for ion transport and transmission of electrical impulses. The intracellular sarcoplasmic reticulum houses most of the intracellular calcium and abuts the T tubules. (Modified from Katz AM. *Physiology of the Heart*. 2nd ed. New York, NY: Raven Press; 1992:21.) **Bottom,** Expanded view of a sarcomere, the basic unit of contraction. Each myofibril consists of serially connected sarcomeres that extend from one Z line to the next. The sarcomere is composed of alternating thin (actin) and thick (myosin) myofilaments. Titin is a protein that tethers myosin to the Z line and provides elasticity.

is made up of two groups of overlapping filaments of contractile proteins. Biochemical and biophysical interactions occurring between these myofilaments produce muscle contraction. Their structure and function are described later in the chapter.

Within each myocardial cell, the neighboring sarcomeres are all in register, producing the characteristic cross-striated banding pattern seen by light microscopy. The relative densities of the cross bands identify the location of the contractile proteins. Under physiologic conditions, the overall sarcomere length (Z-to-Z distance) varies between 2.2 and 1.5 μm during the cardiac cycle. The larger dimension reflects the fiber stretch during ventricular filling, whereas the smaller dimension represents the extent of fiber shortening during contraction.

The myocardial cell membrane is termed the **sarcolemma**. A specialized region of the membrane is the **intercalated disk**, a distinct characteristic of cardiac muscle tissue. Intercalated disks are seen on light microscopic study as darkly staining transverse lines that cross chains of cardiac cells at irregular intervals. They represent the gap junction complexes at the interface of adjacent cardiac fibers and establish structural and electrical continuity between the myocardial cells.

Another functional feature of the cell membrane is the **transverse tubular system** (or **T tubules**). This complex system is characterized by deep, fingerlike invaginations of the sarcolemma (Fig. 1.9; see also Fig. 1.8). Similar to the intercalated disks, transverse tubular membranes establish pathways for rapid transmission of the excitatory electrical impulses that initiate contraction. The T tubule system increases the surface area of the sarcolemma in contact with the extracellular environment, allowing the transmembrane ion transport accompanying excitation and relaxation to occur quickly and synchronously.

The **sarcoplasmic reticulum (SR)** is an extensive intracellular tubular membrane network that complements the T tubule system both structurally and functionally. The SR abuts the T tubules at right angles in lateral sacs, called the terminal cisternae (see Fig. 1.9). These sacs house most of intracellular calcium stores; the release of these stores is important in linking membrane excitation with activation of the contractile apparatus. Lateral sacs also abut the intercalated disks and the sarcolemma,

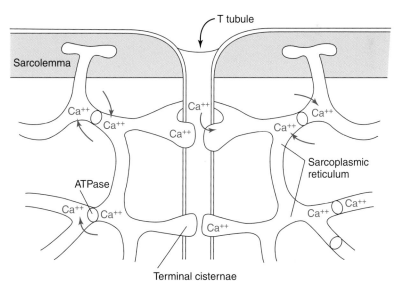

Figure 1.9. Schematic view of the tubular systems of the myocardial cell. The T tubules, invaginations of the sarcolemma, abut the sarcoplasmic reticulum at right angles at the terminal cisternae sacs. This relationship is important in linking membrane excitation with intracellular release of calcium from the sarcoplasmic reticulum.

providing each with a complete system for excitation–contraction coupling.

To serve the tremendous metabolic demand placed on the heart and the need for a constant supply of high-energy phosphates, the myocardial cell has an abundant concentration of mitochondria. These organelles are located between the individual myofibrils and constitute approximately 35% of cell volume (see Fig. 1.8).

BASIC ELECTROPHYSIOLOGY

Rhythmic contraction of the heart relies on the organized propagation of electrical impulses along its conduction pathway. The marker of electrical stimulation, the **action potential**, is created by a sequence of ion fluxes through specific channels in the sarcolemma. To provide a basis for understanding how electrical impulses lead to cardiac contraction, the process of cellular depolarization and repolariza-

tion is reviewed here. This material serves as an important foundation for topics addressed later in the book, including electrocardiography (see Chapter 4) and cardiac arrhythmias (see Chapters 11 and 12).

Cardiac cells capable of electrical excitation are of three electrophysiologic types, the properties of which have been studied by intracellular microelectrode and patch-clamp recordings:

1. Pacemaker cells (e.g., SA node, AV node)
2. Specialized rapidly conducting tissues (e.g., Purkinje fibers)
3. Ventricular and atrial muscle cells

The sarcolemma of each of these cardiac cell types is a phospholipid bilayer that is largely impermeable to ions. There are specialized proteins interspersed throughout the membrane that serve as ion channels, cotransporters, and active transporters (Fig. 1.10). These

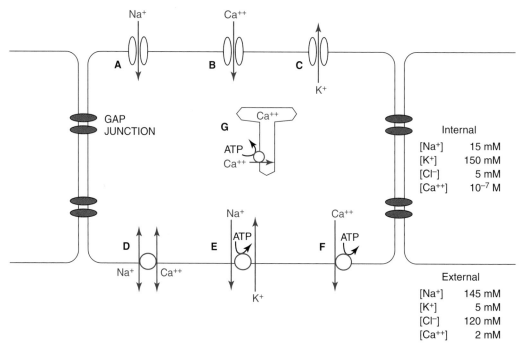

Figure 1.10. Ion channels, cotransporters, and active transporters of the myocyte. A. Sodium entry through the fast sodium channel is responsible for the rapid upstroke (phase 0) of the action potential (AP) in nonpacemaker cells. **B.** Calcium enters the cell through calcium channel during phase 2 of the Purkinje fiber and muscle cell AP and is the main channel responsible for depolarization of pacemaker cells. **C.** Potassium exits through a potassium channel to repolarize the cell during phase 3 of the AP, and open potassium channels contribute to the resting potential (phase 4) of nonpacemaker cells. **D.** Sodium–calcium exchanger helps maintain the low intracellular calcium concentration. **E.** Sodium–potassium ATPase pump maintains concentration gradients for these ions. **F, G.** Active calcium transporters aid removal of calcium to the external environment and sarcoplasmic reticulum, respectively.

help to maintain ionic concentration gradients and charge differentials between the inside and the outside of the cardiac cells. Note that normally, the Na^+ and Ca^{++} concentrations are much higher outside the cell and the K^+ concentration is much higher inside.

Ion Movement and Channels

The movement of specific ions across the cell membrane serves as the basis of the action potential. Ion transport depends on two major factors: (1) the energetic favorability and (2) the permeability of the membrane for the ion.

Energetics

The two major forces that drive the energetics of ion transport are the *concentration gradient* and the *transmembrane potential* (voltage). Molecules diffuse from areas of high concentration to areas of lower concentration—the gradient between these values is a determinant of the rate of ion flow. For example, the extracellular Na^+ concentration is normally 145 mM, while the concentration inside the myocyte is 15 mM. As a result, a strong force tends to drive Na^+ into the cell, down its concentration gradient.

The transmembrane potential of cells exerts an electrical force on ions (i.e., like charges repel one another, and opposite charges attract). The transmembrane potential of a myocyte at rest is about −90 mV (the inside of the cell is negative relative to the outside). Extracellular Na^+, a positively charged ion, is therefore attracted to the relatively negatively charged interior of the cell. Thus, there is a strong tendency for Na^+ to enter the cell because of both the steep concentration gradient and the electrical attraction.

Permeability

If there is such a strong force driving Na^+ into the cell, what keeps this ion from actually moving inside? The membrane of the cell at its resting potential is *not permeable* to sodium. The phospholipid bilayer of the cell membrane is composed of a hydrophobic core that does not allow simple passage of charged, hydrophilic particles. Instead, permeability of the membrane is dependent on the opening of specific **ion channels**, specialized proteins that span the cell membrane and contain hydrophilic pores through which certain charged atoms can pass under specific circumstances.

Most types of ion channels share similar protein sequences and structures, consisting of repeating transmembrane domains (Fig. 1.11). Each of these domains contains six membrane-spanning segments. The fourth segment (see S_4 in Fig. 1.11) includes a sequence of positively charged amino acids (lysine and arginine) that reacts to the membrane potential, and therefore that segment is thought to confer voltage sensitivity to the channel, as described below.

The several types of cardiac ion channels vary by two functional properties: selectivity and gating. Each type of channel is normally *selective* for a specific ion, which is a manifestation of the size and structure of its pore. For example, in cardiac cells, some channels permit the passage of sodium ions, some are specific for potassium, and others allow only calcium to pass through.

An ion can pass through its specific channel only at certain times. That is, the ion channel is *gated*—at any given moment, the channel is either open or closed. The more time a channel is in its open state, the larger the number of ions that pass through it and therefore, the greater the transmembrane current.

Cells contain a population of each type of ion channel, and each individual channel may be in the open or closed state; it is the voltage across the membrane that determines what fraction of these channels is open at a given time. Therefore, the gating of channels is said to be **voltage sensitive**. As the membrane voltage changes during depolarization and repolarization of the cell, specific channels open and close, with corresponding alterations in the ion fluxes across the sarcolemma.

An example of voltage-sensitive gating is apparent in the cardiac channel known as the **fast sodium channel**. The transmembrane protein that forms this channel assumes various conformations depending on the cell's membrane potential (Fig. 1.12). At a voltage of −90 mV (the typical resting voltage of a ventricular muscle cell), the channels are primarily in a closed, *resting state*, such that Na⁺ ions cannot pass through. In this resting state,

the channels are available for conversion to the open configuration.

A rapid wave of depolarization causes the membrane potential to become less negative and activates the resting channels to the *open state* (see Fig. 1.12B). Na⁺ ions readily permeate through the open channels, and an inward

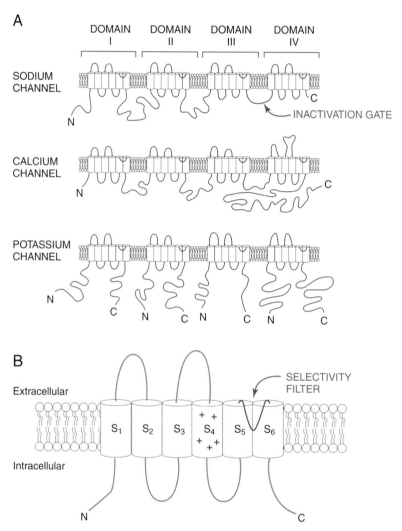

Figure 1.11. **Structure of ion channels. A.** Ion channels consist of glycosylated proteins arranged as repeating transmembrane domains. Each domain consists of six membrane-spanning segments. The potassium channel has four separate domains in a tetrameric structure, while the sodium and calcium channels contain four domains covalently linked as a single unit. In the case of the sodium channel, the loop connecting domains III and IV is believed to serve as the channel's inactivation gate. **B.** Enlarged view of a single domain of the sodium channel showing the six membrane-spanning segments. The S_4 segment of each domain contains a sequence of positively charged amino acids, which confers the channel's voltage sensitivity. The peptide loops connecting segments 5 and 6 in each domain form the selectivity filter for the channel's pore, which allows sodium, but not other ions, to pass through. (Parts **A** and **B** are reproduced in part from Katz AM. *Physiology of the Heart.* 2nd ed. New York, NY: Raven Press; 1992:427, 429, with permission.)

C

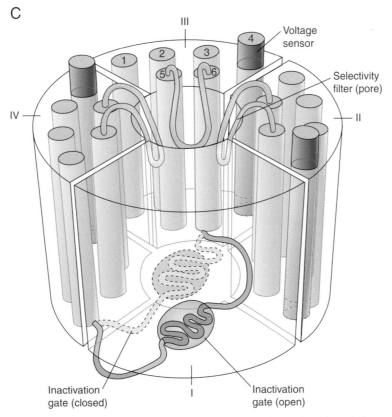

Figure 1.11. (Continued) C. A three-dimensional schematic of the sodium channel, showing how the four domains wrap around the channel's pore. The selectivity filter formed by the loops connecting segments 5 and 6 is shown near the extracellular opening of the channel, while the inactivation gate (the loop between domains III and IV) is displayed on the cytosolic side. (Reproduced from Nelson CL, Cox MM. *Lehninger's Principles of Biochemistry*. 3rd ed. New York, NY: Worth; 2000:428, with permission requested.)

Na^+ current ensues. However, the activated channels remain open for only a brief time, a few thousandths of a second, and then spontaneously close to an *inactive state* (see Fig. 1.12C). Channels in the inactivated conformation cannot be directly converted back to the open state.

The inactivated state persists until the membrane voltage has repolarized nearly back to its original resting level. Until it does so, the inactivated channel prevents any flow of sodium ions. Thus, during normal cellular depolarization, the voltage-dependent fast sodium channels conduct for a short period and then inactivate, unable to conduct current again until the cell membrane has nearly fully repolarized and the channels re-

cover from the inactivated to the closed resting state.

Another important attribute of cardiac fast sodium channels should be noted. If the transmembrane voltage of a cardiac cell is *slowly* depolarized and maintained chronically at levels less negative than the usual resting potential, inactivation of channels occurs *without* initial opening and current flow. Furthermore, as long as this partial depolarization exists, the closed, inactive channels cannot recover to the resting state. Thus, the fast sodium channels in such a cell are persistently unable to conduct Na^+ ions. This is the typical case in cardiac pacemaker cells (e.g., the SA and AV nodes) in which the membrane voltage is generally less negative

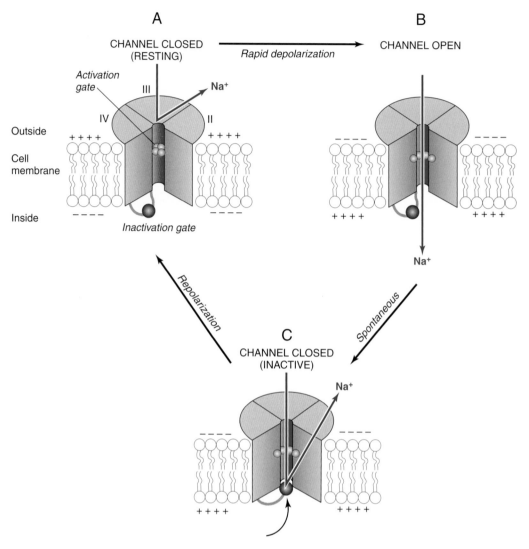

Figure 1.12. Schematic representation of gating of fast sodium channels. A. The four covalently linked transmembrane domains (I, II, III, IV) form the sodium channel, which is guarded by activation and inactivation gates. (Here, domain I is cut away to show the transmembrane pore.) In the resting membrane, most channels are in a closed state. Even though the inactivation gate is open, Na+ ions cannot easily pass through because the activation gate is closed. **B.** A rapid depolarization changes the cell membrane voltage and forces the activation gate to open, presumably mediated by translocation of the charged portions of segment 4 in each domain. With the channel in this conformation (in which both the activation and inactivation gates are open), Na+ ions permeate into the cell. **C.** As the inactivation gate spontaneously and quickly closes, the sodium current ceases. The inactivation gating function is thought to be achieved by the peptide loop that connects domains III and IV and swings into the intracellular opening of the channel pore *(black arrow)*. The channel cannot reopen directly from this closed, inactive state. Cellular repolarization returns the channel to the resting condition **(A)**. During repolarization, as high negative membrane voltages are reachieved, the activation gate closes and the inactivation gate reopens.

than −70 mV throughout the cardiac cycle. As a result, the fast sodium channels in pacemaker cells are persistently inactivated and do not play a role in the generation of the action potential in these cells (Box 1.1). Calcium and potassium channels in cardiac cells also act in voltage-dependent fashions, but they behave differently than the sodium channels, as described later.

Resting Potential

In cardiac cells at rest, prior to excitation, the electrical charge differential between

---

BOX *1.1* Mechanism of Fast Sodium Channels

A key characteristic of fast sodium channels is their ability to activate and then inactivate rapidly when the cell is depolarized. The mechanism by which this occurs has been investigated for many decades. In the mid-1900s, Hodgkin and Huxley studied the action potential in squid giant axons (*J Physiol.* [Lond] 1952; 117:500–544). They found that ion channels act as if they contain a series of "gates" that open and close in a specific pattern when the membrane potential is altered. In the case of the sodium channel, the researchers postulated the presence of *m* gates that are closed in the resting state and *h* gates that are open in the resting state. Depolarization of the membrane causes the *m* gates to open quickly, which allows Na^+ ions to pass through the channel (equivalent to the open channel in Fig. 1.12B). However, that same depolarization of the cell also causes the *h* gates to close, which blocks the passage of sodium ions (the closed, inactive state in Fig. 1.12C). Na^+ can flow through the channel only when both sets of gates are open. Since the *m* gates open faster than the *h* gates close, there is a brief period (about 1 msec) during which Na^+ can pass through. After the membrane repolarizes to voltages more negative than about –60 mV, the *m* gates shut, the *h* gates reopen, and the channel returns to the closed, resting state (see Fig. 1.12A), available for activation once again.

More recent research has demonstrated that ion channel activity is actually more complex than suggested by this model, but there are important correlates with current molecular concepts. For example, the cluster of positively charged amino acids on segment 4 (S_4) of the ion channel domain (see Fig. 1.11) is believed to be the voltage sensor for the *m* gates that cause the channel to open during depolarization. In the resting state, the strong positive charge on S_4 causes it to be pulled inward toward the negative membrane potential. During depolarization, as the membrane charge becomes less, S_4 can move outward, resulting in a conformational change in the protein that results in channel opening. Inactivation (the *h* gates) is thought to be achieved by the peptide loop that connects domains III and IV of the sodium channel (see Figs. 1.11 and 1.12) that swings into and occludes the channel during depolarization.

---

the inside and outside of a cell results in a **resting potential**. The magnitude of the resting potential of a cell depends on two main properties: (1) the concentration gradients for all the different ions between the inside and outside of the cell, and (2) the relative permeabilities of ion channels that are open at rest.

As in other tissues such as nerve cells and skeletal muscle, the potassium concentration is much greater inside cardiac cells compared with outside the cells. This is attributed to cell membrane transporters, the most important of which is Na^+K^+-ATPase. This protein "pump" couples the energy of ATP hydrolysis to export three Na^+ ions out of the cell in exchange for the inward movement of two K^+ ions. This acts to maintain intracellular Na^+ at low levels and intracellular K^+ at high levels.

Cardiac myocytes contain a set of potassium channels that are open in the resting state (termed *inward rectifier* potassium channels), at a time when other ionic channels

(i.e., sodium and calcium) are closed. Therefore, the resting cell membrane is much more permeable to potassium than to other ions. As a result, K^+ flows in an outward direction down its concentration gradient, removing positive charges from the cell. The predominant counter ions for potassium within the cell are large negatively charged proteins that are unable to diffuse outward along with K^+. Thus, as potassium ions exit the cell, the anions that are left behind cause the interior of the cell to become electrically negative with respect to the outside.

However, as the interior of the cell becomes more *negatively* charged by the outward flux of potassium, the *positively* charged K^+ ions are attracted back by the electrical potential toward the cellular interior, an effect that slows their net exit from the cell. Thus, the two opposing forces directing the flux of potassium ions through their open channels in the resting state are (1) the concentration gradient, which favors outward passage of potassium, and (2) the electrostatic

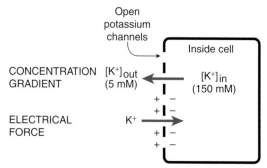

Equilibrium (Nernst) potential = $-26.7 \ln ([K^+]_{in}/[K^+]_{out}) = -91mV$

Figure 1.13. The resting potential of a cardiac muscle cell is determined by the balance between the concentration gradient and electrostatic forces for potassium, because only potassium channels are open at rest. The concentration gradient favors outward movement of K⁺, whereas the electrical force attracts the positively charged K⁺ ions inward. The equilibrium (resting) potential can be approximated by the Nernst equation for potassium, as shown here.

force, which attracts potassium back into the cell (Fig. 1.13). At equilibrium, these forces are balanced and there is zero net movement of K^+ across the membrane. The electrical potential at which that occurs is known as the *potassium equilibrium potential* and in ventricular myocytes is −91 mV, as calculated by the Nernst equation, shown in Figure 1.13. Since at rest the membrane is almost exclusively permeable to potassium ions alone, this value closely approximates the cell's resting potential.

The permeability of the cardiac myocyte cellular membrane for sodium is minimal in the resting state because the channels that conduct that ion are essentially closed. However, there is a slight leak of sodium ions into the cell at rest. This tiny inward current of positively charged ions explains why the actual resting potential is slightly less negative (−90 mV) than would be predicted if the cell membrane were truly only permeable to potassium. The sodium ions that slowly leak into the myocyte at rest (and the much larger amount that enters during the action potential) are continuously removed from the cell and returned to the extracellular environment by Na^+K^+-ATPase, as previously described.

Action Potential

When the cell membrane voltage is altered, its permeability to specific ions changes because of the voltage-gating characteristics of the ion channels. Each type of channel has a characteristic pattern of activation and inactivation that determines the progression of the electrical signal. This discussion begins by following the development of the action potential in a typical cardiac muscle cell (Fig. 1.14). The unique characteristics of action potentials in cardiac pacemaker cells are described thereafter.

Cardiac Muscle Cell

Until stimulated, the resting potential of a cardiac muscle cell remains stable, at approximately −90 mV. This resting state before depolarization is known as **phase 4** of the action potential. Following phase 4, four additional phases characterize depolarization and repolarization of the cell (see Fig. 1.14).

Phase 0

At the resting membrane voltage, sodium and calcium channels are closed. Any process that makes the membrane potential less negative than the resting value causes some sodium channels to open. As these channels open, sodium ions rapidly enter the cell, flowing down their concentration gradient, and toward the negatively charged cellular interior. The entry of Na^+ ions into the cell causes the transmembrane potential to become progressively less

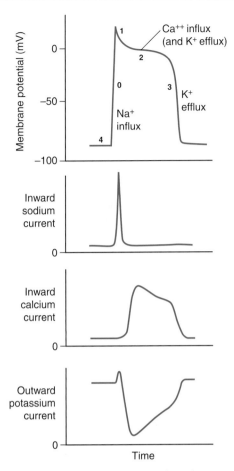

Figure 1.14. Schematic representation of a myocyte action potential (AP) and relative net ion currents for Na⁺, Ca⁺⁺, and K⁺. The resting potential is represented by phase 4 of the AP. Following depolarization, Na⁺ influx results in the rapid upstroke of phase 0; a transient outward potassium current is responsible for partial repolarization during phase 1; slow Ca⁺⁺ influx (and relatively low K⁺ efflux) results in the plateau of phase 2; and final rapid repolarization largely results from K⁺ efflux during phase 3.

negative, which in turn causes more sodium channels to open and promotes further sodium entry into the cell. When the membrane voltage approaches the **threshold potential** (approximately −70 mV in cardiac muscle cells), enough of these fast Na⁺ channels have opened to generate a self-sustaining inward Na⁺ current. The entry of positively charged Na⁺ ions exceeds the charge imbalance that was caused by K⁺ ion movement at rest, such that the cell depolarizes, transiently, to a net positive potential.

The prominent influx of sodium ions is responsible for the rapid upstroke, or phase 0, of the action potential. However, the Na⁺ channels remain open for only a few thousandths of a second and are then quickly inactivated, preventing further influx (see Fig. 1.14). Thus, while activation of these fast Na⁺ channels causes the rapid early depolarization of the cell, the rapid inactivation makes their major contribution to the action potential short lived.

Phase 1

Following rapid phase 0 depolarization into the positive voltage range, a brief current of repolarization returns the membrane potential to approximately 0 mV. The responsible current is carried by the outward flow of K⁺ ions through a type of transiently activated potassium channel.

Phase 2

This relatively long phase of the action potential is mediated by the balance of an outward K⁺ current in competition with an inward Ca⁺⁺ current, which flows through specific L-type calcium channels. The latter channels begin to open during phase 0, when the membrane voltage reaches approximately −40 mV, allowing Ca⁺⁺ ions to flow down their concentration gradient into the cell. Ca⁺⁺ entry proceeds in a more gradual fashion than the initial influx of sodium, because with calcium channels, activation is slower and the channels remain open much longer compared with sodium channels (see Fig. 1.14). During this phase, the Ca⁺⁺ influx is balanced by an approximately equal outward charge movement via K⁺ efflux, through another specific type of potassium channel (termed *delayed rectifier* potassium channels), such that there is no net current and the membrane potential does not change for a prolonged period, which is known as the **plateau**. Calcium ions that enter the cell during this phase play a critical role in triggering additional internal calcium release from the SR, which is important in initiating myocyte contraction, as discussed later in the chapter. As the Ca⁺⁺ channels gradually inactivate and the efflux of K⁺ begins to exceed the influx of calcium, phase 3 begins.

Phase 3

This is the final phase of repolarization that returns the transmembrane voltage back to the resting potential of approximately −90 mV. A continued outward potassium current and low membrane permeability for other cations are responsible for this period of rapid repolarization. Phase 3 completes the action potential cycle, with a return to resting phase 4, preparing the cell for the next stimulus for depolarization.

To preserve normal transmembrane ionic concentration gradients, sodium and calcium ions that enter the cell during depolarization must be returned to the extracellular environment, and potassium ions must return to the cell interior. As shown in Figure 1.10, Ca^{++} ions are removed by the sarcolemmal $Na^+–Ca^{++}$ exchanger and to a lesser extent by the ATP-consuming calcium pump (sarcolemmal Ca^{++}-ATPase). The corrective exchange of Na^+ and K^+ across the cell membrane is mediated by Na^+K^+-ATPase, as described earlier.

Specialized Conduction System

The process described in the previous sections applies to the action potential of cardiac muscle cells. The cells of the specialized conduction system (e.g., Purkinje fibers) behave similarly, although the resting potential is slightly more negative and the upstroke of phase 0 is even more rapid.

Pacemaker Cells

The upstroke of the action potential of cardiac muscle cells does not normally occur spontaneously. Rather, when a wave of depolarization reaches the myocyte from neighboring cells, its membrane potential becomes less negative and an action potential is triggered.

Certain heart cells do not require external provocation to initiate their action potential. Rather, they are capable of self-initiated depolarization in a rhythmic fashion and are known as **pacemaker cells**. They are endowed with the property of **automaticity**, by which the cells undergo spontaneous depolarization during phase 4. When the threshold voltage is reached in such cells, the action potential upstroke is triggered (Fig. 1.15).

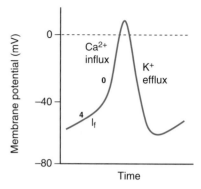

Figure 1.15. Action potential of a pacemaker cell. Phase 4 is characterized by gradual, spontaneous depolarization owing to the pacemaker current (I_f). When the threshold potential is reached, at about −40 mV, the upstroke of the action potential follows. The upstroke of phase 0 is less rapid than in nonpacemaker cells because the current represents Ca^{++} influx through the relatively slow calcium channels.

Cells that display pacemaker behavior include the SA node (the "natural pacemaker" of the heart) and the AV node. Although atrial and ventricular muscle cells do not normally display automaticity, they may do so under disease conditions such as ischemia.

The shape of the action potential of a pacemaker cell is different from that of a ventricular muscle cell in three ways:

1. The maximum negative voltage of pacemaker cells is approximately −60 mV, substantially less negative than the resting potential of ventricular muscle cells (−90 mV). *The persistently less negative membrane voltage of pacemaker cells causes the fast sodium channels within these cells to remain inactivated.*

2. Unlike that of cardiac muscle cells, phase 4 of the pacemaker cell action potential is not flat but has an upward slope, representing spontaneous gradual depolarization. This spontaneous depolarization is the result of an ionic flux known as the **pacemaker current** (denoted by I_f). Current evidence indicates that the pacemaker current is carried predominantly by Na^+ ions. The ion channel through which the pacemaker current passes is different from the fast sodium channel responsible for phase 0 of the action potential.

Rather, this pacemaker channel opens during *repolarization* of the cell, as the membrane potential approaches its most negative values. The inward flow of positively charged Na$^+$ ions through the pacemaker channel causes the membrane potential to become progressively less negative during phase 4, ultimately depolarizing the cell to its threshold voltage (see Fig. 1.15).

3. The phase 0 upstroke of the pacemaker cell action potential is less rapid and reaches a lower amplitude than that of a cardiac muscle cell. These characteristics result from the fast sodium channels of the pacemaker cells being inactivated and the upstroke of the action potential relying solely on Ca^{++} influx through the relatively slow calcium channels.

Repolarization of pacemaker cells occurs in a fashion similar to that of ventricular muscle cells and relies on inactivation of the calcium channels and increased activation of potassium channels with enhanced K$^+$ efflux from the cell.

Refractory Periods

Compared with electrical impulses in nerves and skeletal muscle, the cardiac action potential is much longer in duration. This results in a prolonged refractory period during which the muscle cannot be restimulated. Such a long period is physiologically necessary because it allows the ventricles sufficient time to empty their contents and refill before the next contraction.

There are different levels of refractoriness during the action potential, as illustrated in Figure 1.16. The degree of refractoriness primarily reflects the number of fast Na$^+$ channels that have recovered from their inactive state and are capable of reopening. As phase 3 of the action potential progresses, an increasing number of Na$^+$ channels recover and can respond to the next depolarization. This, in turn, corresponds to an increasing probability that a stimulus will trigger an action potential and result in a propagated impulse.

The *absolute* refractory period refers to the time during which the cell is completely unexcitable to a new stimulation. The *effective* refractory period includes the absolute refractory period but extends beyond it to include a short interval of phase 3, during which stimulation produces a localized action potential that is not strong enough to propagate further. The *relative* refractory period is the interval during which stimulation triggers an action potential

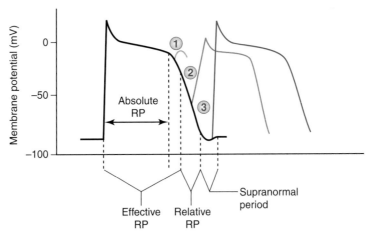

Figure 1.16. Refractory periods (RPs) of the myocyte. During the absolute refractory period (ARP), the cell is unexcitable to stimulation. The effective refractory period includes a brief time beyond the ARP during which stimulation produces a localized depolarization that does not propagate (curve 1). During the relative refractory period, stimulation produces a weak action potential (AP) that propagates, but more slowly than usual (curve 2). During the supranormal period, a weaker-than-normal stimulus can trigger an AP (curve 3).

that is conducted, but the rate of rise of the action potential is lower during this period because some of the Na$^+$ channels are inactivated and some of the delayed rectifier K$^+$ channels remain activated, thus reducing the available net inward current. Following the relative refractory period, a short "supranormal" period is present in which a less-than-normal stimulus can trigger an action potential.

The refractory period of atrial cells is shorter than that of ventricular muscle cells, such that atrial rates can generally exceed ventricular rates during rapid arrhythmias (see Chapter 11).

Impulse Conduction

During depolarization, the electrical impulse spreads along each cardiac cell, and rapidly from cell to cell, because each myocyte is connected to its neighbors through low-resistance gap junctions. The speed of tissue depolarization (phase 0) and the conduction velocity along the cell depend on the number of sodium channels and on the magnitude of the resting potential. Tissues with a high concentration of Na$^+$ channels, such as Purkinje fibers, have a large, fast inward current, which spreads quickly within and between cells to support rapid conduction. In contrast, the less negative the resting potential, the greater the number of inactivated fast sodium channels, and therefore the less rapid the upstroke velocity (Fig. 1.17). Thus, alterations in the resting potential greatly affect the upstroke and conduction velocity of the action potential.

Normal Sequence of Cardiac Depolarization

Electrical activation of the heartbeat is normally initiated at the SA node (see Fig. 1.6). The impulse spreads to the surrounding atrial muscle through intercellular gap junctions that provide electrical continuity between the cells. Ordinary atrial muscle fibers participate in the propagation of the impulse from the SA to the AV node, although in certain regions the fibers are more densely arranged, facilitating conduction.

Fibrous tissue surrounds the tricuspid and mitral valves, such that there is no direct electrical connection between the atrial and ventricular chambers other than through the AV node. As the electrical impulse reaches the AV node, a delay in conduction (approximately 0.1 sec) is encountered. This delay occurs because the small-diameter fibers in this region conduct slowly, and the action potential is of the "slow" pacemaker type (recall that the fast sodium channels are permanently inactivated in pacemaker tissues, such that the upstroke velocity relies on the slower calcium channels). The pause in conduction at the AV node is actually beneficial because it allows the atria time to contract and fully empty their contents before ventricular stimulation. In addition, the delay allows the AV node to serve as a "gatekeeper" of conduction from atria to ventricles, which is critical for limiting the rate of ventricular stimulation during abnormally rapid atrial rhythms.

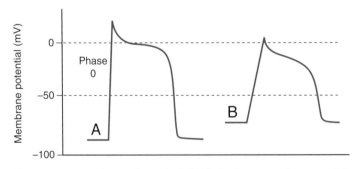

Figure 1.17. Dependence of speed of depolarization on resting potential. **A.** Normal resting potential (RP) and rapid rise of phase 0. **B.** Less negative RP results in slower rise of phase 0 and lower maximum amplitude of the action potential.

After traversing the AV node, the cardiac action potential spreads into the rapidly conducting bundle of His and Purkinje fibers, which distribute the electrical impulses to the bulk of the ventricular muscle cells. This allows for precisely timed stimulation and contraction of the ventricular myocytes.

EXCITATION–CONTRACTION COUPLING

This section reviews how the electrical action potential leads to physical contraction of cardiac muscle cells, a process known as excitation–contraction coupling. During this process, chemical energy in the form of high-energy phosphate compounds is translated into the mechanical energy of myocyte contraction.

Contractile Proteins in the Myocyte

Several distinct proteins are responsible for cardiac muscle cell contraction (Fig. 1.18). Two of the proteins, actin and myosin, are the chief contractile elements. Two other proteins, tropomyosin and troponin, serve regulatory functions.

Myosin is arranged in thick filaments, each composed of lengthwise stacks of approximately 300 molecules. The myosin filament exhibits globular heads that are evenly spaced along its length and contain myosin ATPase, an enzyme that is necessary for contraction to occur. **Actin**, a smaller molecule, is arranged in thin filaments as an α-helix consisting of two strands that interdigitate between the thick myosin filaments

(see Fig. 1.8). **Titin** (also termed connectin) is a protein that helps tether myosin to the Z line of the sarcomere and provides elasticity to the contractile process.

Tropomyosin is a double helix that lies in the grooves between the actin filaments and, in the resting state, inhibits the interaction between myosin heads and actin, thus preventing contraction. **Troponin** sits at regular intervals along the actin strands and is composed of three subunits. The troponin T (TnT) subunit links the troponin complex to the actin and tropomyosin molecules. The troponin I (TnI) subunit inhibits the ATPase activity of the actin–myosin interaction. The troponin C (TnC) subunit is responsible for binding calcium ions that regulate the contractile process.

Calcium-Induced Calcium Release and the Contractile Cycle

The sensitivity of TnC to calcium establishes a crucial role for intracellular Ca^{++} ions in cellular contraction. The cycling of calcium in and out of the cytosol during each action potential effectively couples electrical excitation to physical contraction.

Recall that during phase 2 of the action potential, activation of L-type Ca^{++} channels results in an influx of Ca^{++} ions into the myocyte. The small amount of calcium that enters the cell in this fashion is not sufficient to cause contraction of the myofibrils, but it triggers a much greater Ca^{++} release from the SR, as follows: The T tubule invaginations of

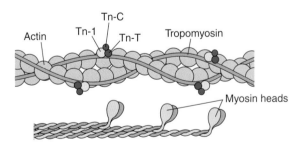

Figure 1.18. **Schematic diagram of the main contractile proteins of the myocyte, actin, and myosin.** Tropomyosin and troponin (components TnI, TnC, and TnT) are regulatory proteins.

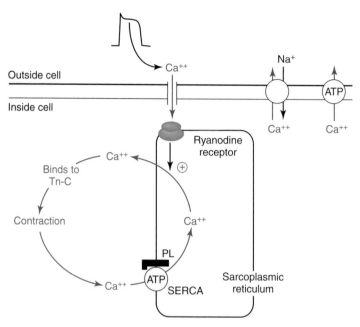

Figure 1.19. Calcium ion movements during excitation and contraction in cardiac muscle cells. Ca^{++} enters the cell through calcium channels during phase 2 of the action potential, triggering a much larger calcium release from the sarcoplasmic reticulum (SR) via the ryanodine receptor complex. The binding of cytosolic Ca^{++} to troponin C (TnC) allows contraction to ensue. Relaxation occurs as Ca^{++} is returned to the SR by sarco(endo)plasmic reticulum calcium ATPase (SERCA). Phospholamban (PL) is a major regulator of this pump, inhibiting Ca^{++} uptake in its dephosphorylated state. Excess intracellular calcium is returned to the extracellular environment by sodium–calcium exchange and to a smaller degree by the sarcolemmal Ca^{++}-ATPase.

the sarcolemmal membrane bring the L-type channels into close apposition with specialized Ca^{++} release receptors in the SR, known as **ryanodine receptors** (Fig. 1.19). When calcium enters the cell and binds to the ryanodine receptor, the receptor undergoes a conformational change, which results in a much greater release of Ca^{++} into the cytosol from the abundant stores in the terminal cisternae of the SR. Thus, the initial L-type Ca^{++} current signal is amplified by this mechanism, known as **calcium-induced calcium release (CICR)**, and the cytosolic calcium concentration dramatically increases.

As calcium ions bind to TnC, the activity of TnI is inhibited, which induces a conformational change in tropomyosin. The latter event exposes the active site between actin and myosin, enabling contraction to proceed.

Contraction ensues as myosin heads bind to actin filaments and "flex," thus causing the interdigitating thick and thin filaments to move past each other in an ATP-dependent reaction (Fig. 1.20). The first step in this process is activation of the myosin head by hydrolysis of ATP, following which the myosin head binds to actin and forms a cross bridge. The interaction between the myosin head and actin results in a conformational change in the head, causing it to pull the actin filament inward.

Next, while the myosin head and actin are still attached, ADP is released, and a new molecule of ATP then binds to the myosin head, causing it to release the actin filament. The cycle can then repeat. Progressive coupling and uncoupling of actin and myosin causes the muscle fiber to shorten by increasing the overlap between the myofilaments within each sarcomere. In the presence of ATP, this process continues for as long as the cytosolic calcium concentration remains sufficiently high to inhibit the troponin–tropomyosin blocking action.

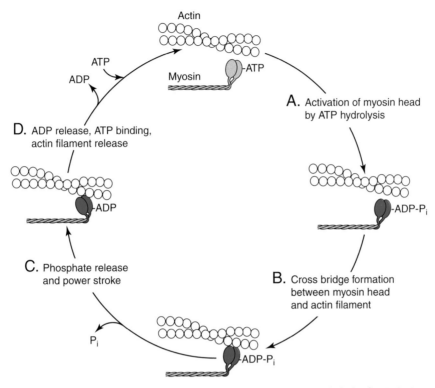

Actin

ATP

ADP

Myosin

-ATP

A. Activation of myosin head
by ATP hydrolysis

D. ADP release, ATP binding,
actin filament release

-ADP

-ADP-P$_i$

C. Phosphate release
and power stroke

P$_i$

B. Cross bridge formation
between myosin head
and actin filament

-ADP-P$_i$

Figure 1.20. **The contractile process. A.** Myosin head is activated by hydrolysis of ATP. **B.** During cellular depolarization, cytoplasmic calcium concentration increases and removes the troponin–tropomyosin inhibition, such that a cross bridge is formed between actin and myosin. **C.** Inorganic phosphate (P$_i$) is released and a conformational change in the myosin head draws the actin filament inward. **D.** ADP is released and replaced by ATP, causing the myosin head to dissociate from the actin filament. As the process repeats, the muscle fiber shortens. The cycle continues until cytosolic calcium concentration decreases at the end of phase 2 of the action potential.

Myocyte relaxation, like contraction, is synchronized with the electrical activity of the cell. Toward the end of phase 2 of the action potential, L-type channels inactivate, arresting the influx of Ca^{++} into the cell and abolishing the trigger for CICR. Concurrently, calcium is pumped back into the SR and out of the cell. Calcium is sequestered back into the SR primarily by **sarco(endo)plasmic reticulum Ca^{++} ATPase** (SERCA), as shown in Figure 1.19. The small amount of Ca^{++} that entered the cell through L-type calcium channels is removed via the sarcolemmal Na$^+$–Ca^{++} exchanger and to a lesser extent by the ATP-consuming calcium pump, sarcolemmal Ca^{++}-ATPase (see Fig. 1.10).

As cytosolic Ca^{++} concentrations fall and calcium ions dissociate from TnC, tropomyosin once again inhibits the actin–myosin interaction, leading to relaxation of the contracted cell. The contraction–relaxation cycle can then repeat with the next action potential.

β-Adrenergic and Cholinergic Signaling

There is substantial evidence that the concentration of Ca^{++} within the cytosol is the major determinant of the force of cardiac contraction with each heartbeat. Mechanisms that raise intracellular Ca^{++} concentration enhance force development, whereas factors that lower Ca^{++} concentration reduce the contractile force.

β-Adrenergic stimulation is one mechanism that enhances calcium fluxes in the myocyte and thereby strengthens the force of ventricular contraction (Fig. 1.21). Catecholamines (e.g., norepinephrine) bind to the myocyte β$_1$-adrenergic receptor, which is coupled to and activates the G protein system (G$_s$) attached

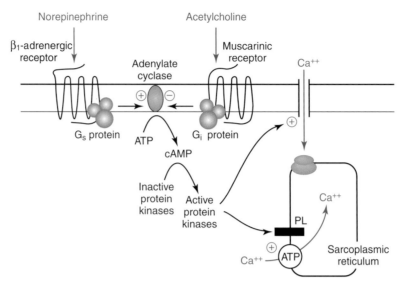

Figure 1.21. Effects of β-adrenergic and cholinergic stimulation on cardiac cellular signaling and calcium ion movement. The binding of a ligand (e.g., norepinephrine) to the β₁-adrenergic receptor induces G protein–mediated stimulation of adenylate cyclase and formation of cyclic AMP (cAMP). The latter activates protein kinases, which phosphorylate cellular proteins, including ion channels. Phosphorylation of the slow Ca^{++} channel enhances calcium movement into the cell and therefore strengthens the force of contraction. Protein kinases also phosphorylate phospholamban (PL), reducing the latter's inhibition of Ca^{++} uptake by the sarcoplasmic reticulum. The enhanced removal of Ca^{++} from the cytosol facilitates relaxation of the myocyte. Cholinergic signaling, triggered by acetylcholine binding to the muscarinic receptor, activates inhibitory G proteins that reduce adenylate cyclase activity and cAMP production, thus antagonizing the effects of β-adrenergic stimulation.

to the inner surface of the cell membrane. G_s in turn stimulates membrane-bound adenylate cyclase to produce cyclic AMP (cAMP) from ATP. cAMP then activates intracellular protein kinases, which phosphorylate cellular proteins, including the L-type calcium channels within the cell membrane. Phosphorylation of the calcium channel augments Ca^{++} influx, which triggers a corresponding increase in Ca^{++} release from the SR, thereby enhancing the force of contraction.

β-Adrenergic stimulation of the myocyte also enhances myocyte *relaxation*. The return of Ca^{++} from the cytosol to the SR is regulated by **phospholamban (PL)**, a low molecular weight protein in the SR membrane. In its dephosphorylated state, PL inhibits Ca^{++} uptake by SERCA (see Fig. 1.19). However, β-adrenergic activation of protein kinases (see Fig. 1.21) causes PL to become phosphorylated, an action that blunts PL's inhibitory effect. The subsequently greater uptake of calcium ions by the SR hastens Ca^{++} removal from the cytosol,

promoting myocyte relaxation. The increased cAMP activity also results in phosphorylation of TnI, an action that inhibits actin–myosin interactions and therefore further enhances relaxation of the cell.

Cholinergic signaling via parasympathetic inputs (mainly from the vagus nerve) opposes the effects of β-adrenergic stimulation (see Fig. 1.21). Acetylcholine released from parasympathetic nerve terminals binds to the muscarinic M_2 receptor on cardiac cells. This receptor also activates G proteins, but in distinction to the β-adrenergic receptor, it is coupled to G_i, an *inhibitory* G protein system. G_i associated with cholinergic stimulation inhibits adenylate cyclase activity and reduces cAMP formation. At the sinus node, these actions of cholinergic stimulation serve to reduce heart rate. In the myocardium, the effect is to counteract the force of contraction induced by β-adrenergic stimulation. It should be noted that ventricular cells are much less sensitive to this cholinergic effect than atrial cells, likely reflecting different degrees of G protein coupling.

Thus, physiologic or pharmacologic catecholamine stimulation of the myocyte β_1-adrenergic receptor enhances contraction of the cell, while cholinergic stimulation opposes that enhancement. We will return to these important properties in later chapters.

SUMMARY

The anatomic structure, cellular composition, and conduction pathways of the heart form an efficient system for repetitive, organized contractions. As a result, the heart is capable of purposeful stimulation billions of times during the life span of a normal person. With each contraction cycle, the heart receives and propagates blood through the circulation to provide nutrients to and remove waste products from the body's tissues.

The following chapters explore what can go wrong with this remarkable system.

Acknowledgments

Contributors to the previous editions of this chapter were Vivek Iyer, MD; Kirsten Greineder, MD; Stephanie Harper, MD; Scott Hyver, MD; Paul Kim, MD; Rajeev Malhotra, MD; Laurence Rhines, MD; James D. Marsh, MD; Gary R. Strichartz, MD; and Leonard S. Lilly, MD.

Additional Reading

Bers DM. Calcium cycling and signaling in cardiac myocytes. *Annu Rev Physiol.* 2008;70:23–49.

Katz AM. *Physiology of the Heart.* 4th ed. Philadelphia, PA: Lippincott Williams & Wilkins; 2006.

Opie LH. *Heart Physiology, from Cell to Circulation.* 4th ed. Philadelphia, PA: Lippincott Williams & Wilkins; 2004.

Rockman HA, Koch WJ, Lefkowitz RJ. Seven-transmembrane-spanning receptors and heart function. *Nature.* 2002;415:206.

Saucerman JJ, McCulloch AD. Cardiac beta-adrenergic signaling: from subcellular microdomains to heart failure. *Ann N Y Acad Sci.* 2006;1080:348–346.

vanBuren P, Palmer BM. Cooperative activation of the cardiac myofilament: the pivotal role of tropomyosin. *Circulation.* 2010;121:351–353.

Wilcox BR, Cook AC, Anderson RH. *Surgical Anatomy of the Heart.* Cambridge, MA: Cambridge University Press, 2005.

Zipes DP, Jalife J, eds. *Cardiac Electrophysiology: From Cell to Bedside.* 5th ed. Philadelphia, PA: Saunders; 2009.

The Cardiac Cycle: Mechanisms of Heart Sounds and Murmurs

Henry Jung
Leonard S. Lilly

CARDIAC CYCLE
HEART SOUNDS
First Heart Sound (S$_1$)
Second Heart Sound (S$_2$)
Extra Systolic Heart Sounds
Extra Diastolic Heart Sounds

MURMURS
Systolic Murmurs
Diastolic Murmurs
Continuous Murmurs

Cardiac diseases often cause abnormal findings on physical examination, including pathologic heart sounds and murmurs. These findings are clues to the underlying pathophysiology, and proper interpretation is essential for successful diagnosis and disease management. This chapter describes heart sounds in the context of the normal cardiac cycle and then focuses on the origins of pathologic heart sounds and murmurs.

Many cardiac diseases are mentioned briefly in this chapter as examples of abnormal heart sounds and murmurs. Because each of these conditions is described in greater detail later in the book, it is not necessary to memorize the examples presented here. Rather, the goal of this chapter is to explain the mechanisms by which the abnormal sounds are produced, so that their descriptions will make sense in later chapters.

CARDIAC CYCLE

The cardiac cycle consists of precisely timed electrical and mechanical events that are responsible for rhythmic atrial and ventricular contractions. Figure 2.1 displays the pressure relationships between the left-sided cardiac chambers during the normal cardiac cycle and serves as a platform for describing key events. Mechanical **systole** refers to the phase of ventricular contraction, and **diastole** refers to the phase of ventricular relaxation and filling. Throughout the cardiac cycle, the right and left atria accept blood returning to the heart from the systemic veins and from the pulmonary veins, respectively. During diastole, blood passes from the atria into the ventricles across the open tricuspid and mitral valves, causing a gradual increase in ventricular diastolic pressures. In late diastole, atrial contraction propels

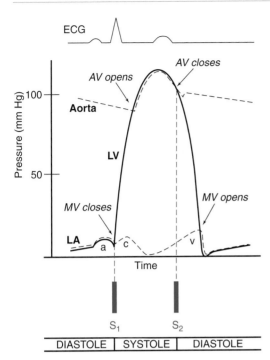

Figure 2.1. The normal cardiac cycle, showing pressure relationships between the left-sided heart chambers. During diastole, the mitral valve (MV) is open, so that the left atrial (LA) and left ventricular (LV) pressures are equal. In late diastole, LA contraction causes a small rise in pressure in both the LA and LV (the *a* wave). During systolic contraction, the LV pressure rises; when it exceeds the LA pressure, the MV closes, contributing to the first heart sound (S_1). As LV pressure rises above the aortic pressure, the aortic valve (AV) opens, which is a silent event. As the ventricle begins to relax and its pressure falls below that of the aorta, the AV closes, contributing to the second heart sound (S_2). As LV pressure falls further, below that of the LA, the MV opens, which is silent in the normal heart. In addition to the *a* wave, the LA pressure curve displays two positive deflections: the *c* wave represents a small rise in LA pressure as the MV closes and bulges toward the atrium, and the *v* wave is the result of passive filling of the LA from the pulmonary veins during systole, when the MV is closed.

a final bolus of blood into each ventricle, an action that produces a brief further rise in atrial and ventricle pressures, termed the *a* wave (see Fig. 2.1).

Contraction of the ventricles follows, signaling the onset of mechanical systole. As the ventricles start to contract, the pressures within them rapidly exceed atrial pressures. This results in the forced closure of the tricuspid and mitral valves, which produces the first heart sound, termed S_1. This sound has two

nearly superimposed components: the mitral component slightly precedes that of the tricuspid valve because of the earlier electrical activation of the left ventricle (see Chapter 4).

As the right and left ventricular pressures rapidly rise further, they soon exceed the diastolic pressures within the pulmonary artery and aorta, forcing the pulmonic and aortic valves to open, and blood is ejected into the pulmonary and systemic circulations. The ventricular pressures continue to increase during the initial portion of this ejection phase, and then decline as ventricular relaxation commences. Since the pulmonic and aortic valves are open during this phase, the aortic and pulmonary artery pressures rise and fall in parallel to those of the corresponding ventricles.

At the conclusion of ventricular ejection, the ventricular pressures decline below those of the pulmonary artery and aorta (the pulmonary artery and aorta are elastic structures that maintain their pressures longer), such that the pulmonic and aortic valves are forced to close, producing the second heart sound, S_2. Like the first heart sound (S_1), this sound consists of two parts: the aortic (A_2) component normally precedes the pulmonic (P_2) because the diastolic pressure gradient between the aorta and left ventricle is greater than that between the pulmonary artery and the right ventricle, forcing the aortic valve to shut more readily. The ventricular pressures fall rapidly during the subsequent relaxation phase. As they drop below the pressures in the right and left atria, the tricuspid and mitral valves open, followed by diastolic ventricular filling and then repetition of this cycle.

Notice in Figure 2.1 that in addition to the *a* wave, the atrial pressure curve displays two other positive deflections during the cardiac cycle: the *c* wave represents a small rise in atrial pressure as the tricuspid and mitral valves close and bulge into their respective atria. The *v* wave is the result of passive filling of the atria from the systemic and pulmonary veins during systole, a period during which blood accumulates in the atria because the tricuspid and mitral valves are closed.

BOX *2.1*   Jugular Venous Pulsations and Assessment of Right-Heart Function

Bedside observation of jugular venous pulsations in the neck is a vital part of the cardiovascular examination. With no structures impeding blood flow between the internal jugular (IJ) veins and the superior vena cava and right atrium (RA), the height of the IJ venous column (termed the "jugular venous pressure," or JVP) is an accurate representation of the RA pressure. Thus, the JVP provides an easily obtainable measure of right-heart function.

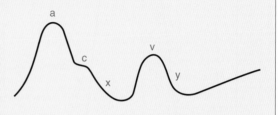

Typical fluctuations in the jugular venous pulse during the cardiac cycle, manifested by oscillations in the overlying skin, are shown in the figure (notice the similarity to the left atrial pressure tracing in Fig. 2.1). There are two major upward components, the *a* and *v* waves, followed by two descents, termed *x* and *y*. The *x* descent, which represents the pressure decline following the *a* wave, may be interrupted by a small upward deflection (the *c* wave) at the time of tricuspid valve closure, but that is usually not distinguishable in the JVP. The *a* wave represents transient venous distension caused by back pressure from RA contraction. The *v* wave corresponds to passive filling of the RA from the systemic veins during systole, when the tricuspid valve is closed. Opening of the tricuspid valve in early diastole allows blood to rapidly empty from the RA into the right ventricle; that fall in RA pressure corresponds to the *y* descent.

Conditions that abnormally raise right-sided cardiac pressures (e.g., heart failure, tricuspid valve disease, pulmonic stenosis, pericardial diseases) elevate the JVP, while reduced intravascular volume (e.g., dehydration) decreases it. In addition, specific disease states can influence the individual components of the JVP, examples of which are listed here for reference and explained in subsequent chapters:

> **Prominent *a*:** right ventricular hypertrophy, tricuspid stenosis
> **Prominent *v*:** tricuspid regurgitation
> **Prominent *y*:** constrictive pericarditis

Technique of Measurement

The JVP is measured as the maximum *vertical* height of the internal jugular vein (in cm) above the center of the right atrium, and in a normal person is ≤9 cm. Because the sternal angle is located approximately 5 cm above the center of the RA, the JVP is calculated at the bedside by adding 5 cm to the vertical height of the top of the IJ venous column above the sternal angle.

The right IJ vein is usually the easiest to evaluate because it extends directly upward from the RA and superior vena cava. First, observe the pulsations in the skin overlying the IJ with the patient supine and the head of the bed at about a 45° angle. Shining a light obliquely across the neck helps to visualize the pulsations. Be sure to examine the IJ, not the external jugular vein. The former is medial to, or behind, the sternocleidomastoid muscle, whereas the external jugular is usually more lateral. Although the external jugular is typically easier to see, it does not accurately reflect RA pressure because it contains valves that interfere with venous return to the heart.

If the top of the IJ column is not visible at 45°, the column of blood is either too low (below the clavicle) or too high (above the jaw) to be measured in that position. In such situations, the head of the bed must be lowered or raised, respectively, so that the top of the column becomes visible. As long as the top can be ascertained, the vertical height of the JVP above the sternal angle will accurately reflect RA pressure, no matter the angle of the head of the bed.

Sometimes it can be difficult to distinguish the jugular venous pulsations from the neighboring carotid artery. Unlike the carotid, the JVP is usually not pulsatile to palpation, it has a double rather than a single upstroke, and it declines in most patients by assuming the seated position or during inspiration.

At the bedside, systole can be approximated as the period from S_1 to S_2, and diastole from S_2 to the next S_1. Although the duration of systole remains constant from beat to beat, the length of diastole varies with the heart rate: the faster the heart rate, the shorter the diastolic phase. The main sounds, S_1 and S_2, provide a framework from which all other heart sounds and murmurs can be timed.

The pressure relationships and events depicted in Figure 2.1 are those that occur in the left side of the heart. Equivalent events occur simultaneously in the right side of the heart in the right atrium, right ventricle, and pulmonary artery. At the bedside, clues to right-heart function can be ascertained by examining the jugular venous pulse, which is representative of the right atrial pressure (see Box 2.1).

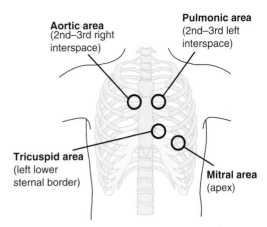

Figure 2.2. **Standard positions of stethoscope placement for cardiac auscultation.**

HEART SOUNDS

Commonly used stethoscopes contain two chest pieces for auscultation of the heart. The concave "bell" chest piece, meant to be applied lightly to the skin, accentuates low-frequency sounds. Conversely, the flat "diaphragm" chest piece is designed to be pressed firmly against the skin to eliminate low frequencies and therefore accentuate high-frequency sounds and murmurs. Some modern stethoscopes incorporate both the bell and diaphragm functions into a single chest piece; in these models, placing the piece lightly on the skin brings out the low-frequency sounds, while firm pressure accentuates the high-frequency ones. The sections below describe when, and where on the chest, to listen for high- versus low-frequency sounds.

First Heart Sound (S_1)

S_1 is produced by the closure of the mitral and tricuspid valves in early systole and is loudest near the apex of the heart (Fig. 2.2). It is a high-frequency sound, best heard with the diaphragm of the stethoscope. Although mitral closure usually precedes tricuspid closure, they are separated by only about 0.01 sec, such that the human ear appreciates only a single sound. An exception occurs in patients with right bundle branch block (see Chapter 4), in whom these components *may* be audibly split because of delayed right ventricular contraction and late closure of the tricuspid valve.

Three factors determine the intensity of S_1: (1) the distance separating the leaflets of the open valves at the onset of ventricular contraction; (2) the mobility of the leaflets (normal, or rigid because of stenosis); and (3) the rate of rise of ventricular pressure (Table 2.1).

The distance between the open valve leaflets at the onset of ventricular contraction relates to the electrocardiographic PR interval (see Chapter 4), the period between the onset of atrial and ventricular activation. Atrial contraction at the end of diastole forces the tricuspid and mitral valve leaflets apart. As they start to drift

Table 2.1. Causes of Altered Intensity of First Heart Sound (S_1)
Accentuated S_1
1. Shortened PR interval
2. Mild mitral stenosis
3. High cardiac output states or tachycardia (e.g., exercise or anemia)
Diminished S_1
1. Lengthened PR interval: first-degree AV nodal block
2. Mitral regurgitation
3. Severe mitral stenosis
4. "Stiff" left ventricle (e.g., systemic hypertension)

back together, ventricular contraction forces them shut, from whatever position they are at, as soon as the ventricular pressure exceeds that in the atrium. An *accentuated* S_1 results when the PR interval is shorter than normal because the valve leaflets do not have sufficient time to drift back together and are therefore forced shut from a relatively wide distance.

Similarly, in *mild* mitral stenosis (see Chapter 8), a prolonged diastolic pressure gradient exists between the left atrium and ventricle, which keeps the mobile portions of the mitral leaflets farther apart than normal during diastole. Because the leaflets are relatively wide apart at the onset of systole, they are forced shut loudly when the left ventricle contracts.

S_1 may also be accentuated when the heart rate is more rapid than normal (i.e., tachycardia) because diastole is shortened and the leaflets have insufficient time to drift back together before the ventricles contract.

Conditions that *reduce* the intensity of S_1 are also listed in Table 2.1. In first-degree atrioventricular (AV) block (see Chapter 12), a diminished S_1 results from an abnormally prolonged PR interval, which delays the onset of ventricular contraction. Consequently, following atrial contraction, the mitral and tricuspid valves have *additional* time to float back together so that the leaflets are forced closed from only a small distance apart and the sound is softened.

In patients with mitral regurgitation (see Chapter 8), S_1 is often diminished in intensity because the mitral leaflets may not come into full contact with one another as they close. In *severe* mitral stenosis, the leaflets are nearly fixed in position throughout the cardiac cycle, and that reduced movement lessens the intensity of S_1.

In patients with a "stiffened" left ventricle (e.g., a hypertrophied chamber), atrial contraction results in a higher-than-normal pressure at the end of diastole. This greater pressure causes the mitral leaflets to drift together more rapidly, so that they are forced closed from a smaller-than-normal distance when ventricular contraction begins, thus reducing the intensity of S_1.

Second Heart Sound (S_2)

The second heart sound results from the closure of the aortic and pulmonic valves and therefore has aortic (A_2) and pulmonic (P_2) components. Unlike S_1, which is usually heard only as a single sound, the components of S_2 vary with the respiratory cycle: they are normally fused as one sound during expiration but become audibly separated during inspiration, a situation termed normal or **physiologic splitting** (Fig. 2.3).

One explanation for normal splitting of S_2 is as follows. Expansion of the chest during inspiration causes the intrathoracic pressure to become more negative. The negative pressure transiently increases the capacitance (and reduces the impedance) of the intrathoracic pulmonary vessels. As a result, there is a temporary delay in the diastolic "back pressure" of the pulmonary artery responsible for the closure of the pulmonic valve. Thus, P_2 is delayed; that is, it occurs *later* during inspiration than during expiration.

Inspiration has the opposite effect on A_2. Because the capacity of the intrathoracic pulmonary veins is increased by the negative pressure generated by inspiration, the venous return to the left atrium and ventricle temporarily decreases. Reduced filling of the LV diminishes the stroke volume during the next systolic contraction and therefore shortens the time required for LV emptying. Therefore, aortic valve closure (A_2) occurs slightly *earlier* in inspiration than during expiration. The combination of an earlier A_2 and delayed P_2 during inspiration causes audible separation of the two components. Since these components are high-frequency sounds, they are best heard with the diaphragm of the stethoscope, and splitting of S_2 is usually most easily appreciated near the second left intercostal space next to the sternum (the pulmonic area in Fig. 2.2).

Abnormalities of S_2 include alterations in its intensity and changes in the pattern of splitting. The intensity of S_2 depends on the velocity of blood coursing back toward the valves from the aorta and pulmonary artery after the completion of ventricular contraction, and the suddenness with which that motion is arrested by the closing valves. In systemic hypertension or pulmonary arterial hypertension, the diastolic pressure in the respective great artery is higher than normal, such that the ve-

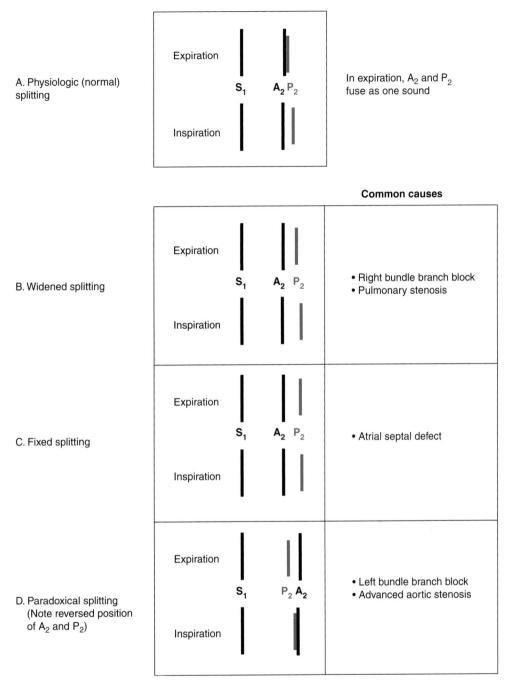

Common causes

A. Physiologic (normal) splitting

In expiration, A_2 and P_2 fuse as one sound

B. Widened splitting

• Right bundle branch block
• Pulmonary stenosis

C. Fixed splitting

• Atrial septal defect

D. Paradoxical splitting (Note reversed position of A_2 and P_2)

• Left bundle branch block
• Advanced aortic stenosis

Figure 2.3. Splitting patterns of the second heart sound (S_2). A_2, aortic component; P_2, pulmonic component of S_2; S_1, first heart sound.

locity of the blood surging toward the valve is augmented and S_2 is accentuated. Conversely, in *severe* aortic or pulmonic valve stenosis, the valve commissures are nearly fixed in position, such that the contribution of the stenotic valve to S_2 is diminished.

There are three types of abnormal splitting of S_2: widened, fixed, and paradoxical. **Widened splitting** of S_2 refers to an increase in the time interval between A_2 and P_2, such that the two components are audibly separated *even during expiration* and become more widely separated in inspiration (see Fig. 2.3). This pattern is usually the result of delayed closure of the pulmonic valve, which occurs in right bundle branch block (described in Chapter 4) and pulmonic valve stenosis (see Chapter 16).

Fixed splitting of S$_2$ is an abnormally widened interval between A$_2$ and P$_2$ that persists unchanged through the respiratory cycle (see Fig. 2.3). The most common abnormality that causes fixed splitting of S$_2$ is an atrial septal defect (see Chapter 16). In that condition, chronic volume overload of the right-sided circulation results in a high-capacitance, low-resistance pulmonary vascular system. This alteration in pulmonary artery hemodynamics delays the back pressure responsible for the closure of the pulmonic valve. Thus, P$_2$ occurs later than normal, even during expiration, such that there is wider-than-normal separation of A$_2$ and P$_2$. The pattern of splitting does not change (i.e., it is fixed) during the respiratory cycle because (1) inspiration does not substantially increase further the already elevated pulmonary vascular capacitance, and (2) augmented filling of the right atrium from the systemic veins during inspiration is counterbalanced by a reciprocal decrease in the left-to-right transatrial shunt, eliminating respiratory variations in right ventricular filling.

Paradoxical splitting (also termed "reversed" splitting) refers to audible separation of A$_2$ and P$_2$ during *expiration* that fuses into a single sound on *inspiration*, the opposite of the normal situation. It reflects an abnormal delay in the closure of the aortic valve such that P$_2$ *precedes* A$_2$. In adults, the most common cause is left bundle branch block (LBBB). In LBBB, described in Chapter 4, the spread of electrical activity through the left ventricle is impaired, resulting in delayed ventricular contraction and late closure of the aortic valve, causing A$_2$ to abnormally follow P$_2$. Then during inspiration, as in the normal case, the pulmonic valve closure sound becomes delayed and the aortic valve closure sound moves earlier. This results in *narrowing*, and often superimposition, of the two sounds; thus, there is no apparent split at the height of inspiration (see Fig. 2.3). In addition to LBBB, paradoxical splitting may be

observed under circumstances in which left ventricular ejection is greatly prolonged, such as aortic stenosis.

Extra Systolic Heart Sounds

Extra systolic heart sounds may occur in early, mid-, or late systole.

Early Extra Systolic Heart Sounds

Abnormal early systolic sounds, or *ejection clicks*, occur shortly after S$_1$ and coincide with the opening of the aortic or pulmonic valves (Fig. 2.4). These sounds have a sharp, high-pitched quality, so they are heard best with the diaphragm of the stethoscope placed over the aortic and pulmonic areas (see Fig. 2.2).

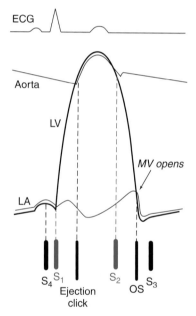

Figure 2.4. Timing of extra systolic and diastolic heart sounds. S$_4$ is produced by atrial contraction into a "stiff" left ventricle (LV). An ejection click follows the opening of the aortic or pulmonic valve in cases of valve stenosis or dilatation of the corresponding great artery. S$_3$ occurs during the period of rapid ventricular filling; it is normal in young people, but its presence in adults implies LV contractile dysfunction. The timing of an opening snap (OS) is placed for comparison, but it is not likely that all of these sounds would appear in the same person. LA, left atrium; MV, mitral valve.

Ejection clicks indicate the presence of aortic or pulmonic valve stenosis or dilatation of the pulmonary artery or aorta. In stenosis of the aortic or pulmonic valve, the sound occurs as the deformed valve leaflets reach their maximal level of ascent into the great artery, just prior to blood ejection. At that moment, the rapidly ascending valve reaches its elastic limit and decelerates abruptly, an action thought to result in the sound generation. In dilatation of the root of the aorta or pulmonary artery, the sound is associated with sudden tensing of the aortic or pulmonic root with the onset of blood flow into the vessel. The *aortic ejection click* is heard at both the base and the apex of the heart and does not vary with respiration. In contrast, the *pulmonic ejection click* is heard only at the base and its intensity diminishes during inspiration (see Chapter 16).

Mid- or Late Extra Systolic Heart Sounds

Clicks occurring in mid- or late systole are usually the result of systolic prolapse of the mitral or tricuspid valves, in which the leaflets bulge abnormally from the ventricular side of the AV junction into the atrium during ventricular contraction, often accompanied by valvular regurgitation (described in Chapter 8). They are loudest over the mitral or tricuspid auscultatory regions, respectively.

Extra Diastolic Heart Sounds

Extra heart sounds in diastole include the opening snap (OS), the third heart sound (S_3), the fourth heart sound (S_4), and the pericardial knock.

Opening Snap

Opening of the mitral and tricuspid valves is normally silent, but mitral or tricuspid valvular stenosis (usually the result of rheumatic heart disease; see Chapter 8) produces a sound, termed as *snap*, when the affected valve opens. It is a sharp, high-pitched sound, and its timing does not vary significantly with respiration. In mitral stenosis (which is much more common than tricuspid valve stenosis), the OS is heard best between the apex and the left sternal

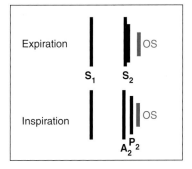

Figure 2.5. Timing of the opening snap (OS) in mitral stenosis does not change with respiration. On inspiration, normal splitting of the second heart sound (S_2) is observed so that three sounds are heard. A_2, aortic component; P_2, pulmonic component of S_2; S_1, first heart sound.

border, just after the aortic closure sound (A_2), when the left ventricular pressure falls below that of the left atrium (see Fig. 2.4).

Because of its proximity to A_2, the A_2–OS sequence can be confused with a widely split second heart sound. However, careful auscultation at the pulmonic area during inspiration reveals three sounds occurring in rapid succession (Fig. 2.5), which correspond to aortic closure (A_2), pulmonic closure (P_2), and then the OS. The three sounds become two on expiration because A_2 and P_2 normally fuse.

The severity of stenosis can be approximated by the time interval between A_2 and the OS: the more advanced the stenosis, the shorter the interval. This occurs because the degree of left atrial pressure elevation corresponds to the severity of mitral stenosis. When the ventricle relaxes in diastole, the greater the left atrial pressure, the earlier the mitral valve opens. Compared with severe stenosis, mild disease is marked by a less elevated left atrial pressure, lengthening the time it takes for the left ventricular pressure to fall below that of the atrium. Therefore, in mild mitral stenosis, the OS is widely separated from A_2, whereas in more severe stenosis, the A_2–OS interval is narrower.

Third Heart Sound (S_3)

When present, an S_3 occurs in early diastole, following the opening of the AV valves, during the ventricular rapid filling phase (see Fig. 2.4). It is a dull, low-pitched sound best heard with the bell of the stethoscope. A left-sided S_3 is typically loudest over the cardiac apex while the patient lies in the left lateral decubitus position. A right-sided S_3 is better appreciated at the lower-left sternal border. Production of the S_3 appears to result from tensing of the chordae tendineae during rapid filling and expansion of the ventricle.

An S_3 is a normal finding in children and young adults. In these groups, an S_3 implies the presence of a supple ventricle capable of normal rapid expansion in early diastole. Conversely, when heard in middle-aged or older adults, an S_3 is often a sign of disease, indicating volume overload owing to congestive heart failure, or the increased transvalvular flow that accompanies advanced mitral or tricuspid regurgitation (described in Chapter 8). A pathologic S_3 is sometimes referred to as a **ventricular gallop.**

Fourth Heart Sound (S_4)

When an S_4 is present, it occurs in late diastole and coincides with contraction of the atria (see Fig. 2.4). This sound is generated by the left (or right) atrium vigorously contracting against a stiffened ventricle. Thus, an S_4 usually indicates the presence of cardiac disease—specifically, a decrease in ventricular compliance typically resulting from ventricular hypertrophy or myocardial ischemia. Like an S_3, the S_4 is a dull, low-pitched sound and is best heard with the bell of the stethoscope. In the case of the more common left-sided S_4, the sound is loudest at the apex, with the patient lying in the left lateral decubitus position. S_4 is sometimes referred to as an **atrial gallop.**

Quadruple Rhythm or Summation Gallop

In a patient with both an S_3 and S_4, those sounds, in conjunction with S_1 and S_2, produce a quadruple beat. If a patient with a quadruple rhythm develops tachycardia, diastole becomes shorter in duration, the S_3 and S_4 coalesce, and a **summation gallop** results.

The summation of S_3 and S_4 is heard as a long middiastolic, low-pitched sound, often louder than S_1 and S_2.

Pericardial Knock

A pericardial knock is an uncommon, high-pitched sound that occurs in patients with severe constrictive pericarditis (see Chapter 14). It appears early in diastole soon after S_2 and can be confused with an OS or an S_3. However, the knock appears slightly later in diastole than the timing of an OS and is louder and occurs earlier than the ventricular gallop. It results from the abrupt cessation of ventricular filling in early diastole, which is the hallmark of constrictive pericarditis.

MURMURS

A murmur is the sound generated by turbulent blood flow. Under normal conditions, the movement of blood through the vascular bed is laminar, smooth, and silent. However, as a result of hemodynamic and/or structural changes, laminar flow can become disturbed and produce an audible noise. Murmurs result from any of the following mechanisms:

1. Flow across a partial obstruction (e.g., aortic stenosis)
2. Increased flow through normal structures (e.g., aortic systolic murmur associated with a high-output state, such as anemia)
3. Ejection into a dilated chamber (e.g., aortic systolic murmur associated with aneurysmal dilatation of the aorta)
4. Regurgitant flow across an incompetent valve (e.g., mitral regurgitation)
5. Abnormal shunting of blood from one vascular chamber to a lower-pressure chamber (e.g., ventricular septal defect [VSD])

Murmurs are described by their timing, intensity, pitch, shape, location, radiation, and response to maneuvers. *Timing* refers to whether the murmur occurs during systole or diastole, or is continuous (i.e., begins in systole and continues into diastole). The *intensity* of the murmur is typically quantified by a grading system. In the case of *systolic murmurs*:

Grade 1/6 (or I/VI):	Barely audible (i.e., medical students may not hear it!)
Grade 2/6 (or II/VI):	Faint but immediately audible
Grade 3/6 (or III/VI):	Easily heard
Grade 4/6 (or IV/VI):	Easily heard and associated with a palpable thrill
Grade 5/6 (or V/VI):	Very loud; heard with stethoscope lightly on chest
Grade 6/6 (or VI/VI):	Audible without the stethoscope directly on the chest wall

And in the case of *diastolic murmurs*:

Grade 1/4 (or I/IV):	Barely audible
Grade 2/4 (or II/IV):	Faint but immediately audible
Grade 3/4 (or III/IV):	Easily heard
Grade 4/4 (or IV/IV):	Very loud

Pitch refers to the frequency of the murmur, ranging from high to low. High-frequency murmurs are caused by large pressure gradients between chambers (e.g., aortic stenosis) and are best appreciated using the diaphragm chest piece of the stethoscope. Low-frequency murmurs imply less of a pressure gradient between chambers (e.g., mitral stenosis) and are best heard using the stethoscope's bell piece.

Shape describes how the murmur changes in intensity from its onset to its completion. For example, a *crescendo–decrescendo* (or "diamond-shaped") murmur first rises and then falls off in intensity. Other shapes include *decrescendo* (i.e., the murmur begins at its maximum intensity and grows softer) and *uniform* (the intensity of the murmur does not change).

Location refers to the murmur's region of maximum intensity and is usually described in terms of specific auscultatory areas (see Fig. 2.2):

Aortic area:	Second to third right intercostal spaces, next to sternum
Pulmonic area:	Second to third left intercostal spaces, next to sternum
Tricuspid area:	Lower-left sternal border
Mitral area:	Cardiac apex

From their primary locations, murmurs are often heard to *radiate* to other areas of the chest, and such patterns of transmission relate to the direction of the turbulent flow. Finally, similar types of murmurs can be distinguished from one another by simple bedside *maneuvers*, such as standing upright, Valsalva (forceful expiration against a closed airway), or clenching of the fists, each of which alters the heart's loading conditions and can affect the intensity of many murmurs. Examples of the effects of maneuvers on specific murmurs are presented in Chapter 8.

When reporting a murmur, some or all of these descriptors are mentioned. For example, you might describe a particular patient's murmur of aortic stenosis as "A grade III/VI high-pitched, crescendo–decrescendo systolic murmur, heard best at the upper-right sternal border, with radiation toward the neck."

Systolic Murmurs

Systolic murmurs are subdivided into systolic ejection murmurs, pansystolic murmurs, and late systolic murmurs (Fig. 2.6). A **systolic ejection murmur** is typical of aortic or pulmonic valve stenosis. It begins after the first heart sound and terminates before or during S_2, depending on its severity and whether the obstruction is of the aortic or pulmonic valve. The shape of the murmur is of the crescendo–decrescendo type (i.e., its intensity rises and then falls).

The ejection murmur of *aortic stenosis* begins in systole after S_1, from which it is separated by

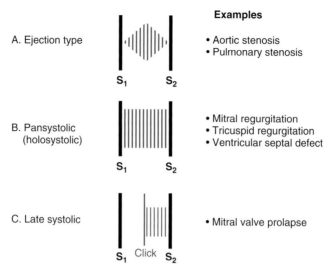

Examples

A. Ejection type
- Aortic stenosis
- Pulmonary stenosis

S_1 S_2

B. Pansystolic (holosystolic)
- Mitral regurgitation
- Tricuspid regurgitation
- Ventricular septal defect

S_1 S_2

C. Late systolic
- Mitral valve prolapse

S_1 Click S_2

Figure 2.6. **Classification of systolic murmurs.** Ejection murmurs are crescendo–decrescendo in configuration, whereas pansystolic murmurs are uniform throughout systole. A late systolic murmur often follows a midsystolic click and suggests mitral (or tricuspid) valve prolapse.

a short audible gap (Fig. 2.7). This gap corresponds to the period of isovolumetric contraction of the left ventricle (the period after the mitral valve has closed but before the

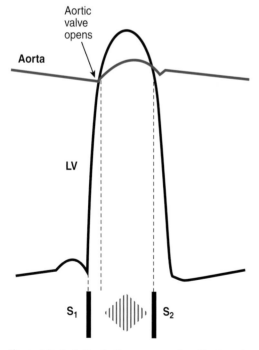

Aortic valve opens

Aorta

LV

S_1 S_2

Figure 2.7. **Systolic ejection murmur of aortic stenosis.** There is a short delay between the first heart sound (S_1) and the onset of the murmur. LV, left ventricle; S_2, second heart sound.

aortic valve has opened). The murmur becomes more intense as flow increases across the aortic valve during the rise in left ventricular pressure (crescendo). Then, as the ventricle relaxes, forward flow decreases, and the murmur lessens in intensity (decrescendo) and finally ends prior to the aortic component of S_2. The murmur may be immediately preceded by an ejection click, especially in mild forms of aortic stenosis.

Although the intensity of the murmur does *not* correlate well with the severity of aortic stenosis, other features do. For example, the more severe the stenosis, the longer it takes to force blood across the valve, and the later the murmur peaks in systole (Fig. 2.8). Also, as shown in Figure 2.8, as the severity of stenosis increases, the aortic component of S_2 softens because the leaflets become more rigidly fixed in place.

Aortic stenosis causes a high-frequency murmur, reflecting the sizable pressure gradient across the valve. It is best heard in the "aortic area" at the second and third intercostal spaces close to the sternum (see Fig. 2.2). The murmur typically radiates toward the neck (the direction of turbulent blood flow) but often can be heard in a wide distribution, including the cardiac apex.

The murmur of *pulmonic stenosis* also begins after S_1, it may be preceded by an ejection click,

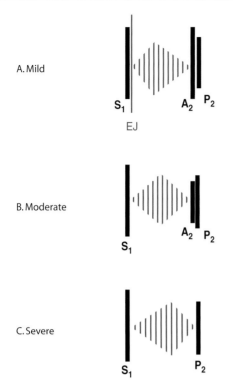

A. Mild

S$_1$ EJ A$_2$ P$_2$

B. Moderate

S$_1$ A$_2$ P$_2$

C. Severe

S$_1$ P$_2$

Figure 2.8. The severity of aortic stenosis affects the shape of the systolic murmur and the heart sounds. A. In mild stenosis, an ejection click (EJ) is often present, followed by an early peaking crescendo–decrescendo murmur and a normal aortic component of S$_2$ (A$_2$). **B.** As stenosis becomes more severe, the peak of the murmur becomes more delayed in systole and the intensity of A$_2$ lessens. The prolonged ventricular ejection time delays A$_2$ so that it merges with or occurs after the pulmonic component of S$_2$ (P$_2$); the ejection click may not be heard. **C.** In severe stenosis, the murmur peaks very late in systole, and A$_2$ is usually absent because of immobility of the valve leaflets. S$_1$, first heart sound; S$_2$, second heart sound.

but unlike aortic stenosis, it may extend beyond the A$_2$ sound. That is, if the stenosis is severe, it will result in a very prolonged right ventricular ejection time, elongating the murmur, which will continue beyond the closure of the aortic valve and end just before the closure of the pulmonic valve (P$_2$). Pulmonic stenosis is usually loudest at the second to third left intercostal spaces close to the sternum. It does not radiate as widely as aortic stenosis, but sometimes it is transmitted to the neck or left shoulder.

Young adults often have *benign systolic ejection murmurs* owing to increased systolic flow across normal aortic and pulmonic valves. This type of murmur often becomes softer or disappears when the patient sits upright.

Pansystolic (also termed **holosystolic**) murmurs are caused by regurgitation of blood across an incompetent mitral or tricuspid valve or through a VSD (see Chapter 16). These murmurs are characterized by a uniform intensity throughout systole (Fig. 2.6). In mitral and tricuspid valve regurgitation, as soon as ventricular pressure exceeds atrial pressure (i.e., when S$_1$ occurs), there is immediate retrograde flow across the regurgitant valve. Thus, there is no gap between S$_1$ and the onset of these pansystolic murmurs, in contrast to the systolic ejection murmurs discussed earlier. Similarly, there is no significant gap between S$_1$ and the onset of the systolic murmur of a VSD, because left ventricular systolic pressure exceeds right ventricular systolic pressure (and flow occurs) quickly after the onset of contraction.

The pansystolic murmur of advanced *mitral regurgitation* continues through the aortic closure sound because left ventricular pressure remains greater than that in the left atrium at the time of aortic closure. The murmur is heard best at the apex, is high pitched and "blowing" in quality, and often radiates toward the left axilla; its intensity does not change with respiration.

Tricuspid valve regurgitation is best heard along the left lower sternal border. It generally radiates to the right of the sternum and is high pitched and blowing in quality. The intensity of the murmur increases with inspiration because the negative intrathoracic pressure induced during inspiration enhances venous return to the heart. The latter augments right ventricular stroke volume, thereby increasing the amount of regurgitated blood.

The murmur of a *VSD* is heard best at the fourth to sixth left intercostal spaces, is high pitched, and may be associated with a palpable thrill. The intensity of the murmur does not increase with inspiration, nor does it radiate to the axilla, which helps distinguish it from tricuspid and mitral regurgitation, respectively. Of note, the *smaller* the VSD, the greater the turbulence of blood flow between the left and right ventricles and the *louder* the murmur. Some of the loudest murmurs ever heard are those associated with small VSDs.

Late systolic murmurs begin in mid-to-late systole and continue to the end of systole (see Fig. 2.6). The most common example is mitral regurgitation caused by *mitral valve prolapse*—bowing of abnormally redundant and elongated valve leaflets into the left atrium during ventricular contraction. This murmur is usually preceded by a midsystolic click and is described in Chapter 8.

Diastolic Murmurs

Diastolic murmurs are divided into early decrescendo murmurs and mid-to-late rumbling murmurs (Fig. 2.9). **Early diastolic murmurs** result from regurgitant flow through either the aortic or pulmonic valve, with the former being much more common in adults. If produced by *aortic valve regurgitation*, the murmur begins at A_2, has a decrescendo shape, and terminates before the next S_1. Because diastolic relaxation of the left ventricle is rapid, a pressure gradient develops immediately between the aorta and lower-pressured left ventricle in patients with aortic regurgitation, and the murmur therefore displays its

maximum intensity at its onset. Thereafter in diastole, as the aortic pressure falls and the LV pressure increases (as blood regurgitates into the ventricle), the gradient between the two chambers diminishes and the murmur decreases in intensity. Aortic regurgitation is a high-pitched murmur, best heard using the diaphragm of the stethoscope along the left sternal border with the patient sitting, leaning forward, and exhaling.

Pulmonic regurgitation in adults is usually due to pulmonary arterial hypertension. It is an early diastolic decrescendo murmur similar to that of aortic regurgitation, but it is best heard in the pulmonic area (Fig. 2.2) and its intensity may increase with inspiration.

Mid-to-late diastolic murmurs result from either turbulent flow across a *stenotic mitral or tricuspid valve* or less commonly from abnormally increased flow across a normal mitral or tricuspid valve (see Fig. 2.9). If resulting from stenosis, the murmur begins after S_2 and is preceded by an OS. The shape of this murmur is unique. Following valvular opening (and the OS), the murmur is at its loudest because the pressure gradient between the atrium and

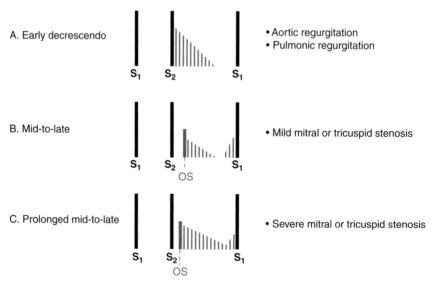

Figure 2.9. Classification of diastolic murmurs. A. An early diastolic decrescendo murmur is typical of aortic or pulmonic valve regurgitation. **B.** Mid-to-late low-frequency rumbling murmurs are usually the result of mitral or tricuspid valve stenosis, and follow a sharp opening snap (OS). Presystolic accentuation of the murmur occurs in patients in normal sinus rhythm because of the transient rise in atrial pressure during atrial contraction. **C.** In more severe mitral or tricuspid valve stenosis, the opening snap and diastolic murmur occur earlier and the murmur is prolonged. S_1, first heart sound; S_2, second heart sound.

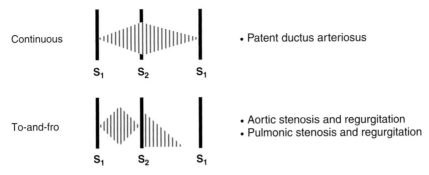

Figure 2.10. A continuous murmur peaks at, and extends through, the second heart sound (S₂). A to-and-fro murmur is not continuous; rather, there is a systolic component and a distinct diastolic component, separated by S₂. S₁, first heart sound.

ventricle is at its maximum. The murmur then decrescendos or disappears totally during diastole as the transvalvular gradient decreases. The degree to which the murmur fades depends on the severity of the stenosis. If the stenosis is severe, the murmur is prolonged; if the stenosis is mild, the murmur disappears in mid-to-late diastole. Whether the stenosis is mild or severe, the murmur intensifies at the end of diastole in patients in normal sinus rhythm, when atrial contraction augments flow (and turbulence) across the valve (see Fig. 2.9). Since the pressure gradient across a stenotic mitral valve tends to be fairly low, the murmur of mitral stenosis is low pitched and is heard best with the bell of the stethoscope at the apex, while the patient lies in the left lateral decubitus position. The much less common murmur of tricuspid stenosis is better auscultated at the lower sternum, near the xiphoid process.

Hyperdynamic states such as fever, anemia, hyperthyroidism, and exercise cause increased flow across the normal tricuspid and mitral valves and can therefore result in a diastolic murmur. Similarly, in patients with advanced mitral regurgitation, the expected systolic murmur can be accompanied by an additional diastolic murmur owing to the increased volume of blood that must return across the valve to the left ventricle in diastole. Likewise, patients with either tricuspid regurgitation or an atrial septal defect (see Chapter 16) have increased flow, and may therefore display a diastolic flow murmur, across the tricuspid valve.

Continuous Murmurs

Continuous murmurs are heard throughout the cardiac cycle. Such murmurs result from conditions in which there is a persistent pressure gradient between two structures during both systole and diastole. An example is the murmur of *patent ductus arteriosus*, in which there is an abnormal congenital communication between the aorta and the pulmonary artery (see Chapter 16). During systole, blood flows from the high-pressure ascending aorta through the ductus into the lower-pressure pulmonary artery. During diastole, the aortic pressure remains greater than that in the pulmonary artery and the flow continues across the ductus. This murmur begins in early systole, crescendos to its maximum at S₂, then decrescendos until the next S₁ (Fig. 2.10).

The "to-and-fro" combined murmur in a patient with both aortic stenosis and aortic regurgitation could be mistaken for a continuous murmur (see Fig. 2.10). During systole, there is a diamond-shaped ejection murmur, and during diastole a decrescendo murmur. However, in the case of a to-and-fro murmur, the sound does not extend through S₂ because it has discrete systolic and diastolic components.

SUMMARY

Abnormal heart sounds and murmurs are common in acquired and congenital heart disease and can be predicted by the underlying pathology. Although it may seem difficult to remember even the basic features presented here, it

Table 2.2. Common Heart Sounds

Sound	Location	Pitch	Significance
S_1	Apex	High	Normal closure of mitral and tricuspid valves
S_2	Base	High	Normal closure of aortic (A_2) and pulmonic (P_2) valves
Extra systolic sounds			
Ejection clicks	*Aortic:* apex and base	High	Aortic or pulmonic stenosis, or dilatation of aortic root or pulmonary artery
	Pulmonic: base	High	
Mid-to-late click	*Mitral:* apex	High	Mitral or tricuspid valve prolapse
	Tricuspid: LLSB	High	
Extra diastolic sounds			
Opening snap	Apex	High	Mitral stenosis
S_3	*Left-sided:* apex	Low	Normal in children
			Abnormal in adults: indicates heart failure or volume overload state
S_4	*Left-sided:* apex	Low	Reduced ventricular compliance

LLSB, lower-left sternal border.

Table 2.3. Common Murmurs

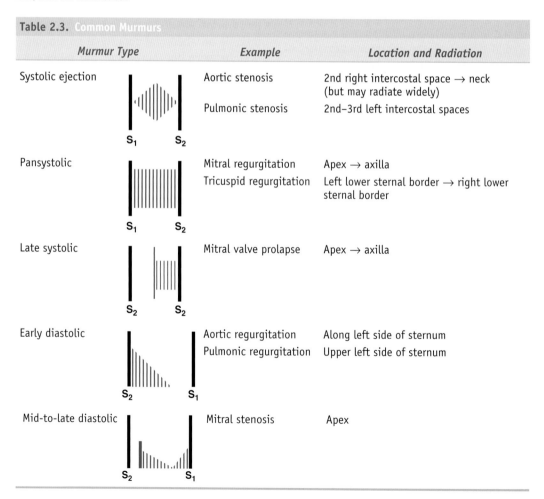

Murmur Type		Example	Location and Radiation
Systolic ejection		Aortic stenosis	2nd right intercostal space → neck (but may radiate widely)
		Pulmonic stenosis	2nd–3rd left intercostal spaces
Pansystolic		Mitral regurgitation	Apex → axilla
		Tricuspid regurgitation	Left lower sternal border → right lower sternal border
Late systolic		Mitral valve prolapse	Apex → axilla
Early diastolic		Aortic regurgitation	Along left side of sternum
		Pulmonic regurgitation	Upper left side of sternum
Mid-to-late diastolic		Mitral stenosis	Apex

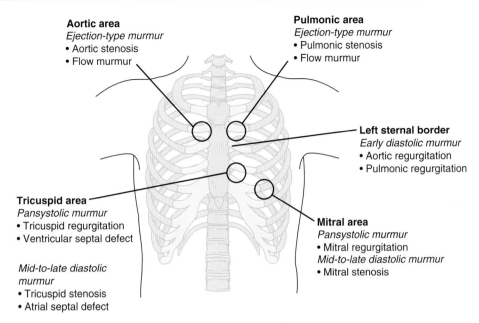

Aortic area
Ejection-type murmur
• Aortic stenosis
• Flow murmur

Pulmonic area
Ejection-type murmur
• Pulmonic stenosis
• Flow murmur

Left sternal border
Early diastolic murmur
• Aortic regurgitation
• Pulmonic regurgitation

Tricuspid area
Pansystolic murmur
• Tricuspid regurgitation
• Ventricular septal defect

Mid-to-late diastolic murmur
• Tricuspid stenosis
• Atrial septal defect

Mitral area
Pansystolic murmur
• Mitral regurgitation
Mid-to-late diastolic murmur
• Mitral stenosis

Figure 2.11. **Locations of maximum intensity of common murmurs.**

will become easier as you learn more about the pathophysiology of these conditions and as your experience in physical diagnosis grows. For now, just remember that the information is here, and refer to it as needed. Tables 2.2 and 2.3 and Figure 2.11 summarize features of the heart sounds and murmurs described in this chapter.

Acknowledgments

Contributors to the previous editions of this chapter were Nicole Martin, MD; Oscar Benavidez, MD; Bradley S. Marino, MD; Allan Goldblatt, MD; and Leonard S. Lilly, MD.

Additional Reading

Bickley LS. *Bates' Guide to Physical Examination and History Taking*. 10th ed. Philadelphia, PA: Lippincott Williams & Wilkins; 2008.

Constant J. *Essentials of Bedside Cardiology*. 2nd ed. Totowa, NJ: Humana Press; 2003.

LeBlond RF, DeGowin RL, Brown DD. *DeGowin's Diagnostic Examination*. 9th ed. New York, NY: McGraw-Hill; 2008.

Orient JM, Sapira JD. *Sapira's Art and Science of Bedside Diagnosis*. 3rd ed. Philadelphia, PA: Lippincott Williams & Wilkins; 2005.

Simel DL, Rennie D. *The Rational Clinical Examination: Evidence-Based Clinical Diagnosis*. New York, NY: McGraw-Hill; 2009.

Cardiac Imaging and Catheterization

Henry Jung
Ken Young Lin
Patricia Challender Come

Imaging plays a central role in the assessment of cardiac function and pathology. Traditional modalities such as chest radiography, echocardiography (echo), cardiac catheterization with angiography, and nuclear imaging are fundamental in the diagnosis and management of cardiovascular diseases. These procedures are being increasingly supplemented by newer techniques, including computed tomography (CT) and magnetic resonance imaging (MRI).

This chapter presents an overview of imaging studies as they are used to assess the cardiovascular disorders described later in this book. On first reading, it would be beneficial to familiarize yourself with the information, but not to memorize the details. This chapter is meant as a reference for diagnosis of conditions that will be explained in more detail in subsequent chapters.

CARDIAC RADIOGRAPHY

The extent of penetration of x-rays through the body is inversely proportional to tissue density. Air-filled tissues, such as the lung, absorb few x-rays and expose the underlying film (or electronic recording sensor), causing it to appear black. In contrast, dense materials, such as bone, absorb more radiation and appear white, or radiopaque. For a boundary to show between two structures, they must differ

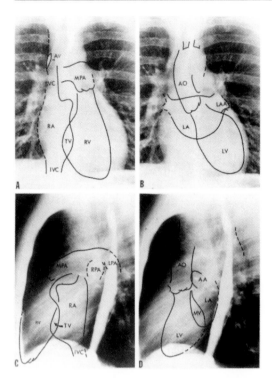

Figure 3.1. Posteroanterior (A and B) and lateral (C and D) chest radiographs of a person without cardiopulmonary disease, illustrating cardiac chambers and valves. AO, aorta; AV, azygos vein; IVC, inferior vena cava; LA, left atrium; LAA, left atrial appendage; LPA, left pulmonary artery; LV, left ventricle; MPA, main pulmonary artery; MV, mitral valve; RA, right atrium; RPA, right pulmonary artery; RV, right ventricle; SVC, superior vena cava; TV, tricuspid valve. (Reprinted with permission from Come PC, ed. *Diagnostic Cardiology: Noninvasive Imaging Techniques*. Philadelphia, PA: J.B. Lippincott; 1985.)

in density. Myocardium, valves, and other intracardiac structures have densities similar to that of adjacent blood; consequently, radiography cannot delineate these structures unless they happen to be calcified. Conversely, heart borders adjacent to a lung are depicted clearly because the heart and an air-filled lung have different densities.

Frontal and lateral radiographs are routinely used to assess the heart and lungs (Fig. 3.1). The *frontal* view is usually a posterior–anterior image in which the x-rays are transmitted from behind (i.e., posterior to) the patient, pass through the body, and are then captured by the film (or electronic sensor) placed against the anterior chest. This positioning places the heart close to the x-ray recording film plate so that its image is only minimally distorted,

allowing for an accurate assessment of size. In the standard *lateral* view, the patient's left side is placed against the film plate and the x-rays pass through the body from right to left. The frontal radiograph is particularly useful for assessing the size of the left ventricle, left atrial appendage, pulmonary artery, aorta, and superior vena cava; the lateral view evaluates right ventricular size, posterior borders of the left atrium and ventricle, and the anteroposterior diameter of the thorax.

Cardiac Silhouette

Chest radiographs are useful to evaluate the size of heart chambers and the pulmonary consequences of cardiac disease. Alterations in chamber size are reflected by changes in the cardiac silhouette. In the frontal view of adults, an enlarged heart is identified by a **cardiothoracic ratio** (the maximum width of the heart divided by the maximum internal diameter of the thoracic cage) of greater than 50%.

In certain situations, the cardiac silhouette inaccurately reflects heart size. For example, an elevated diaphragm, or narrow chest anteroposterior diameter, may cause the silhouette to expand transversely such that the heart appears larger than its actual dimensions. Therefore, the chest anteroposterior diameter should be assessed on the lateral view before concluding the heart is truly enlarged. The presence of a pericardial effusion around the heart can also widen the cardiac silhouette because fluid and myocardial tissue affect x-ray penetration similarly.

Radiographs can depict dilatation of individual cardiac chambers. Ventricular hypertrophy alone (i.e., without dilatation) may not result in radiographic abnormalities, because it generally occurs at the expense of the cavity's internal volume and produces little or no change in overall cardiac size. Major causes of chamber and great vessel dilatation include heart failure, valvular lesions, abnormal intracardiac and extracardiac communications (shunts), and certain pulmonary disorders. Because dilatation takes time to develop, recent lesions, such as *acute* mitral valve insufficiency, may present without apparent cardiac enlargement.

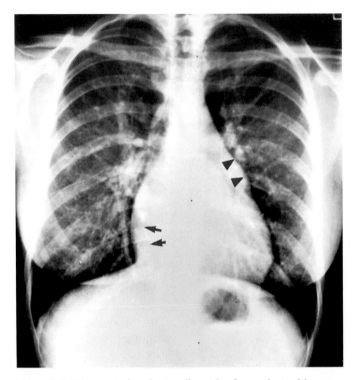

Figure 3.2. Posteroanterior chest radiograph of a patient with severe mitral stenosis and secondary pulmonary vascular congestion. The radiograph shows a prominent left atrial appendage *(arrowheads)* with consequent straightening of the left-heart border and suggestion of a double-density right cardiac border *(arrows)* produced by the enlarged left atrium. The aortic silhouette is small, which suggests chronic low cardiac output. Radiographic signs of pulmonary vascular congestion include increased caliber of upper-zone pulmonary vessel markings and decreased caliber of lower-zone vessels.

The pattern of chamber enlargement may suggest specific disease entities. For example, dilatation of the left atrium and right ventricle, accompanied by signs of pulmonary hypertension, suggests mitral stenosis (Fig. 3.2). In contrast, dilatation of the pulmonary artery and right heart chambers, but without enlargement of the left-sided heart dimensions, suggests pulmonary vascular obstruction or increased pulmonary artery blood flow (e.g., due to an atrial septal defect; Fig. 3.3).

Chest radiographs can also detect dilatation of the aorta and pulmonary artery. Causes of aortic enlargement include aneurysm, dissection, and aortic valve disease (Fig. 3.4). Normal aging and atherosclerosis may also cause the aorta to become dilated and tortuous. The pulmonary artery may be enlarged in patients with left-to-right shunts, which cause increased pulmonary blood flow, and in those with pulmonary hypertension of diverse causes (see Fig. 3.3). Isolated enlargement of the proximal left pulmonary artery is seen in some patients with pulmonic stenosis.

Pulmonary Manifestations of Heart Disease

The appearance of the pulmonary vasculature reflects abnormalities of pulmonary arterial and venous pressures and pulmonary blood flow. Increased pulmonary venous pressure, as occurs in left-heart failure, causes increased vascular markings, redistribution of blood flow from the bases to the apices of the lungs (termed *cephalization* of vessels), pulmonary edema, and pleural effusions (Fig. 3.5). Blood flow redistribution appears as an increase in the number or width of vascular markings at the

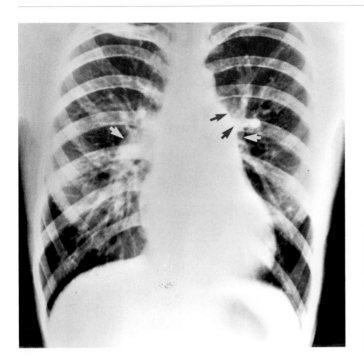

Figure 3.3. Posteroanterior chest radiograph of a patient with pulmonary hypertension secondary to an atrial septal defect. Radiographic signs of pulmonary hypertension include pulmonary artery dilatation *(black arrows;* compare with the appearance of left atrial appendage dilatation in Fig. 3.2) and large central pulmonary arteries *(white arrows)* associated with small peripheral vessels (a pattern known as peripheral pruning).

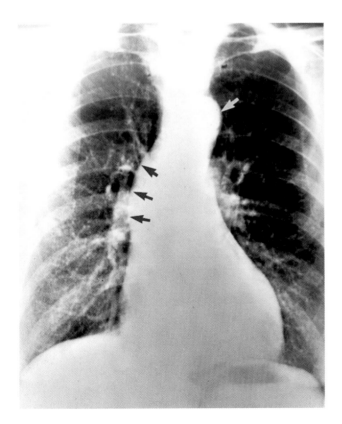

Figure 3.4. Posteroanterior chest radiograph of a patient with aortic stenosis and insufficiency secondary to a bicuspid aortic valve. In addition to dilatation of the ascending aorta *(black arrows)*, the transverse aorta *(white arrow)* is prominent.

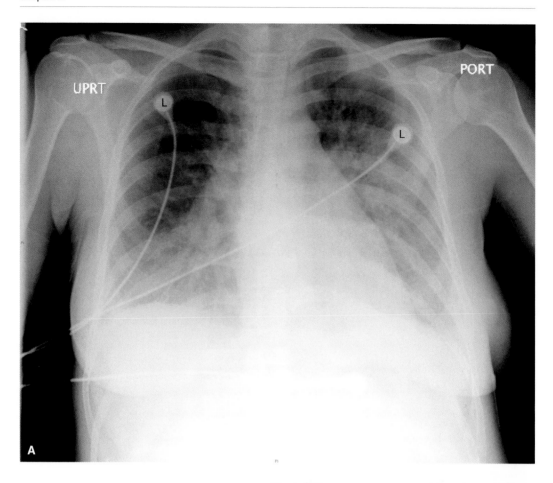

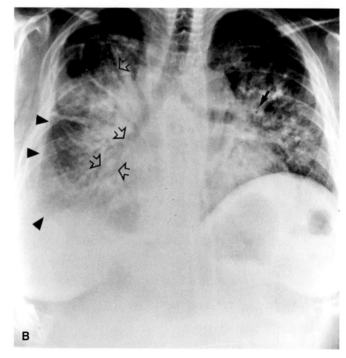

Figure 3.5. **Radiographs of patients with congestive heart failure.** These are anteroposterior views (which may exaggerate the size of the heart because it is further from the x-ray film), taken with portable x-ray machines at the bedside. **A.** Mild congestive heart failure. Pulmonary congestion is indicated by vascular redistribution from the bases to the apices of the lungs. The white spots labeled "L" are electrocardiographic leads on the patient's chest. **B:** Severe congestive heart failure. Increased pulmonary vascular markings are present throughout the lung fields, along with peribronchiolar cuffing *(black arrow)* and pleural effusion, which is indicated by blunting of the costodiaphragmatic angle and tracking up the right lateral hemithorax *(black arrowheads)*. The presence of interstitial and alveolar edema produces perihilar haziness and air bronchograms *(open arrows)*, which occur when the radiolucent bronchial tree is contrasted with opaque edematous lung tissue.

Table 3.1. Chest Radiography of Common Cardiac Disorders

Disorder	Findings
Congestive heart failure	• Vascular redistribution from bases to apices of the lungs • Interstitial and alveolar edema • Air bronchograms • Pleural effusions
Pulmonic valve stenosis	• Poststenotic dilatation of pulmonary artery
Aortic valve stenosis	• Poststenotic dilatation of ascending aorta
Aortic regurgitation	• Left ventricular enlargement • Dilated aorta
Mitral stenosis	• Enlarged left atrium • Signs of pulmonary venous congestion
Mitral regurgitation	• Left atrial dilatation • Left ventricular dilatation

apex. Interstitial and alveolar forms of pulmonary edema produce opacity radiating from the hilar region bilaterally (known as a "butterfly" pattern) and air bronchograms, respectively (Fig. 3.5B). **Kerley B lines** (short horizontal parallel lines at the periphery of the lungs adjacent to the pleura, most often at the lung bases) depict fluid in interlobular spaces that results from interstitial edema. Pleural effusions cause blunting of the costodiaphragmatic angles.

Changes in pulmonary blood flow may also alter the appearance of the pulmonary vessels. For example, focal oligemia (reduction in the size of blood vessels due to decreased blood flow) is occasionally observed distal to a pulmonary embolism (termed the *Westermark sign*). The finding of enlarged central pulmonary arteries, but small peripheral vessels (termed *peripheral pruning*), suggests pulmonary hypertension (see Fig. 3.3).

Table 3.1 summarizes the major radiographic findings in common forms of cardiac disease.

ECHOCARDIOGRAPHY

Echocardiography plays an essential role in the diagnosis and serial evaluation of many cardiac disorders. It is safe, noninvasive, and relatively inexpensive. High-frequency (ultrasonic) waves generated by a piezoelectric element travel through the body and are reflected at interfaces where there are differences in the acoustic impedance of adjacent tissues. The reflected waves return to the transducer and are recorded. The machine measures the time elapsed between the initiation and reception of the sound waves, allowing it to calculate the distance between the transducer and each anatomic reflecting surface. Images are then constructed from these calculations.

Three types of imaging are routinely performed during an echocardiographic examination: M-mode, two-dimensional (2D), and Doppler. Each type of imaging can be performed from various body locations. Most commonly, *transthoracic* studies are performed, in which images are obtained by placing the transducer on the surface of the chest. When greater structural detail is required, *transesophageal* imaging is performed.

M-mode echocardiography, the oldest form of cardiac ultrasonography, provides data from only one ultrasonic beam and is now rarely used by itself. It supplements the other modalities to provide accurate measurements of wall thicknesses and timing of valve movements.

In **2D echocardiography**, multiple ultrasonic beams are transmitted from the transducer through a wide arc. The returning signals are integrated to produce 2D images of the heart on a video monitor. As a result, this technique depicts anatomic relationships and defines the movement of cardiac structures relative to one another. Wall and valve motion abnormalities, and many types of intracardiac masses (e.g., vegetations, thrombi, tumors), can be depicted.

Each 2D plane (Fig. 3.6) delineates only part of a given cardiac structure. Optimal evaluation of the entire heart is achieved by using combinations of views. In transthoracic echocardiography (TTE), in which the transducer is placed against the patient's skin, these include the parasternal long axis, parasternal short axis, apical four-chamber, apical two-chamber, apical

three-chamber (also known as apical long axis), and subcostal views. The *parasternal long axis* view is recorded with the transducer in the third or fourth intercostal space to the left of the sternum. This view is particularly useful for evaluation of the left atrium, mitral valve, left ventricle, and left ventricular outflow tract (LVOT), which includes the aortic valve and adjacent interventricular septum. To obtain *parasternal short axis* views, the transducer is rotated 90° from its position for the long axis view. The short axis images depict transverse planes of the heart. Several different levels are imaged to assess the aortic valve, mitral valve, and left ventricular wall motion.

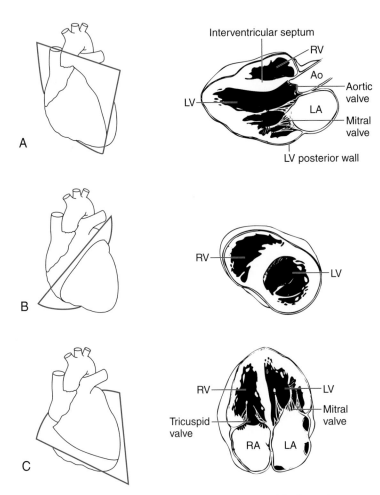

Figure 3.6. Transthoracic two-dimensional echocardiographic views. A. Parasternal long axis view. **B.** Parasternal short axis view. Notice that the left ventricle appears circular in this view, while the right ventricle is crescent shaped. **C.** Apical four-chamber view. Ao, aorta; LA, left atrium; LV, left ventricle; RA, right atrium; RV, right ventricle. (Modified from Sahn DJ, Anderson F. *Two-Dimensional Anatomy of the Heart.* New York, NY: John Wiley & Sons; 1982.)

Apical TTE views are produced when the transducer is placed at the point of maximal apical impulse. The *apical four-chamber* view evaluates the mitral and tricuspid valves as well as the atrial and ventricular chambers, including the motion of the lateral, septal, and apical left ventricular walls. The *apical two-chamber* view shows only the left side of the heart, and it depicts movement of the anterior, inferior, and apical walls.

In some patients, such as those with obstructive airways disease, the parasternal and apical views do not adequately show cardiac structures because the excessive underlying air attenuates the acoustic signal. In such patients, the *subcostal* view, in which the transducer is placed inferior to the rib cage, may provide a better ultrasonic window.

Doppler imaging depicts blood flow direction and velocity, and identifies regions of vascular turbulence. Additionally, it permits estimation of pressure gradients within the heart and great vessels. Doppler studies are based on the physical principle that waves reflected from a moving object undergo a frequency shift according to the moving object's velocity relative to the source of the waves. Color flow mapping converts the Doppler signals to a scale of colors that represent direction, velocity, and turbulence of blood flow in a semiquantitative way. The colors are superimposed on 2D images and show the location of stenotic and regurgitant valvular lesions and of abnormal communications within the heart and great vessels. For example, Doppler echocardiography in a patient with mitral regurgitation shows a jet of retrograde flow into the left atrium during systole (Fig. 3.7).

Sound frequency shifts are converted by the echo machine into blood flow velocity measurements by the following relationship:

$$v = \frac{fs \cdot c}{2f_o(\cos \theta)}$$

where v equals the blood flow velocity (m/sec); fs, the Doppler frequency shift (kHz); c, the velocity of sound in body tissue (m/sec); f_o, the frequency of the sound pulse emitted from the transducer (MHz); and θ, the angle between the transmitted sound pulse and the mean axis of blood flow.

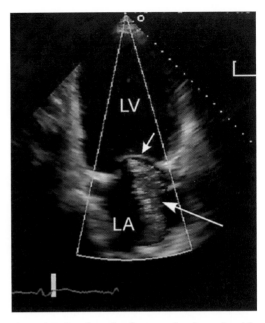

Figure 3.7. Doppler color flow mapping (reproduced in gray tones) of mitral regurgitation (MR). The Doppler image, recorded in systole, is superimposed on an apical view of the left ventricle (LV), left atrium (LA), and mitral valve *(short arrow)*. The retrograde flow of MR into the LA is indicated by the *long arrow*.

Transesophageal echocardiography (TEE) uses a miniaturized transducer mounted at the end of a modified endoscope to transmit and receive ultrasound waves from within the esophagus, thus producing very clear images of the neighboring cardiac structures (Fig. 3.8) and much of the thoracic aorta. Modern probes permit multiplanar imaging and Doppler interrogation. TEE is particularly helpful in the assessment of aortic and atrial abnormalities, conditions that are less well visualized by conventional transthoracic echo imaging. For example, TEE is more sensitive than transthoracic echo for the detection of thrombus within the left atrial appendage (Fig. 3.9). The proximity of the esophagus to the heart makes TEE imaging particularly advantageous in patients for whom transthoracic echo images are unsatisfactory (e.g., those with chronic obstructive lung disease).

TEE is also advantageous in the evaluation of patients with prosthetic heart valves. During standard transthoracic imaging, artificial mechanical valves reflect a large portion of ultrasound waves, thus interfering with

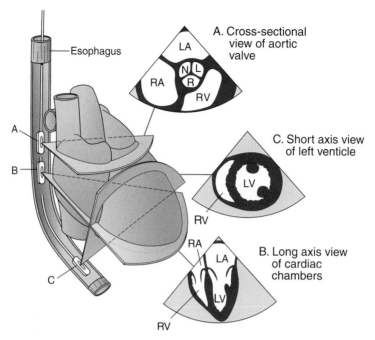

Figure 3.8. **Transesophageal echocardiographic views.** LA, left atrium; LV, left ventricle; RA, right atrium; RV, right ventricle; N, noncoronary cusp of aortic valve; L, left coronary cusp of aortic valve; R, right coronary cusp of aortic valve.

visualization of more posterior structures (termed *acoustic shadowing*). TEE aids visualization in such patients and is therefore the most sensitive noninvasive technique for evaluating perivalvular leaks.

TEE is commonly used to evaluate patients with cerebral ischemic events (i.e., strokes) of unexplained etiology, because it can identify cardiovascular sources of embolism with high sensitivity. These etiologies include intracardiac thrombi or tumors, atherosclerotic debris within the aorta, and valvular vegetations. TEE is also highly sensitive and specific for the detection of aortic dissection.

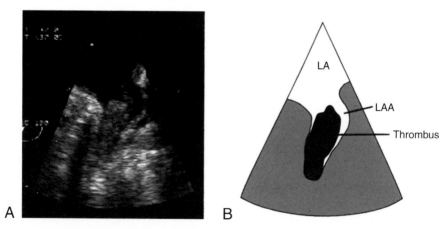

Figure 3.9. **Echocardiographic imaging of an intracardiac thrombus. A.** Transesophageal echocardiographic image demonstrates thrombus within the left atrial appendage. (Courtesy of Scott Streckenbach, MD, Massachusetts General Hospital, Boston, MA.) **B.** Schematic drawing of same image. LA, left atrium; LAA, left atrial appendage.

In the operating room, TEE permits immediate evaluation after surgical repair of cardiac lesions. In addition, imaging of ventricular wall motion can identify periods of myocardial ischemia during surgery.

The newest ultrasound imaging modality in development, and entering clinical usage, is **3D echocardiography**. The spatial reconstructions afforded by this technique are of particular promise in the assessment of valvular defects, intracardiac masses, and congenital malformations.

Contrast echocardiography is sometimes used to supplement standard imaging to evaluate for abnormal intracardiac shunts. In this technique, often called a "bubble study," an echocardiographic contrast agent (e.g., agitated saline) is rapidly injected into a peripheral vein. Using standard imaging, the contrast can be visualized passing through the cardiac chambers. Normally, there is rapid opacification of the right-sided chambers, but because the contrast is filtered out (harmlessly) in the lungs, it does not reach the left-sided chambers. Conversely, in the presence of an intracardiac shunt with abnormal right-to-left heart blood flow, or in the presence of an intrapulmonary shunt, bubbles

of contrast will appear in the left-sided chambers as well. Newer perfluorocarbon-based contrast agents have been developed with sufficiently small particle size to intentionally pass *through* the pulmonary circulation. These agents are used to opacify the left ventricular cavity and, via the coronary arteries, the myocardium, enabling superior assessment of LV contraction and myocardial perfusion.

Echocardiographic techniques can identify valvular lesions, complications of coronary artery disease (CAD), septal defects, intracardiac masses, cardiomyopathy, ventricular hypertrophy, pericardial disease, aortic disease, and congenital heart disease. Typical evaluation includes assessment of cardiac chamber sizes, wall thicknesses, wall motion, valvular function, blood flow, and intracardiac hemodynamics. A few of these topics are highlighted here.

Ventricular Assessment

Echocardiography allows measurement of ventricular wall thickness and mass (Fig. 3.10), and calculation of the **ejection fraction**, a measure of contractile function (see Chapter 9). Furthermore,

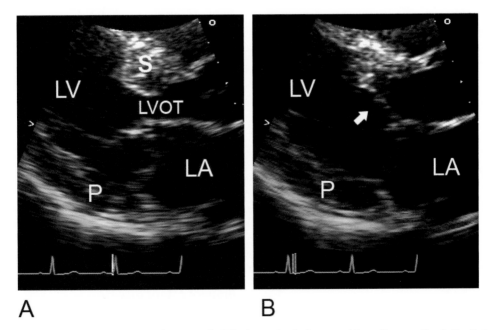

A.

B.

Figure 3.10. Left ventricular outflow tract (LVOT) obstruction in hypertrophic cardiomyopathy. Notice that the interventricular septum (S) is thicker and more echogenic than the posterior wall (P). **A.** Before ventricular contraction, the LVOT is only slightly narrowed. **B.** During contraction, the rapidly flowing blood through the LVOT incites a Venturi effect and abnormally draws the mitral valve apparatus anteriorly toward the hypertrophied septum *(arrow)*, creating a functional obstruction. LA, left atrium; LV, left ventricle.

2D echocardiography depicts regional ventricular wall motion abnormalities, a sign of CAD, and displays right ventricular function qualitatively.

Diastolic dysfunction (e.g., caused by ischemic disease, ventricular hypertrophy, or restrictive cardiomyopathy; see Chapter 9) can be evaluated by Doppler techniques. For example, **Doppler tissue imaging** is a modality that can readily record the maximum velocity of mitral annular movement in early diastole, an indicator of the left ventricle's ability to relax normally. Doppler measurement of flow velocity across the mitral valve in early, compared with late, diastole also provides information about diastolic function.

Valvular Lesions

Echocardiography can determine underlying causes of valvular abnormalities, and Doppler imaging quantitates the degree of valvular stenosis and regurgitation. The pressure gradient across a stenotic valve can be calculated from the maximum blood flow velocity (v) measured distal to the valve, using the simplified *Bernoulli equation*:

$$\text{Pressure gradient} = 4 \times v^2$$

As an example, if the peak velocity recorded distal to a stenotic aortic valve is 5 m/sec, then the calculated peak pressure gradient across the valve = $4 \times 5^2 = 100$ mm Hg.

Other calculations permit noninvasive determination of the cross-sectional area of stenotic valves. The *continuity equation* is often used to calculate aortic valve area. This equation assumes that blood flow (F, expressed in cc/sec) is the same at the aortic valve orifice (AV) as at a neighboring position along the flow stream (e.g., in the LVOT):

$$F_{\text{LVOT}} = F_{\text{AV}}$$

As shown in Figure 3.11, blood flow at any position along a flow stream can also be expressed as the product of the Doppler velocity (V, in cm/sec) and cross-sectional area (A, in cm²) at that level. If location 1 in Figure 3.11 represents a position in the LVOT and location 2 represents the aortic valve, then

$$A_{\text{LVOT}} \times V_{\text{LVOT}} = A_{\text{AV}} \times V_{\text{AV}}$$

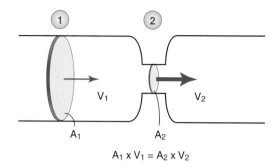

$$A_1 \times V_1 = A_2 \times V_2$$

Figure 3.11. The continuity equation. Within a closed flow stream, the volume rate of flow at any point (calculated as the cross-sectional area at that site multiplied by the maximum flow velocity at the same location) is equal to the volume rate of flow at sequential points. Thus, cross-sectional area and velocity at any location are inversely proportional to one another. Here, location 2 is narrower than location 1. Therefore, the velocity at location 2 must be greater for the same volume to pass per unit time.

The cross-sectional area of the LVOT (A_{LVOT}) is calculated simply as $\pi(d/2)^2$, where d represents the LVOT diameter, measured from the parasternal long axis view. The velocities (V_{LVOT} and V_{AV}) are measured by Doppler interrogation, from the apical four-chamber view. The equation can then be solved for the aortic valve area (A_{AV}):

$$A_{\text{AV}} = \frac{A_{\text{LVOT}} \times V_{\text{LVOT}}}{V_{\text{AV}}}$$

Color Doppler analysis provides a qualitative assessment of the severity of regurgitant valve lesions. In mitral regurgitation (see Fig. 3.7), for example, the ratio of the regurgitant jet color Doppler area to the entire left atrial area has traditionally been used to classify the regurgitation as mild, moderate, or severe. More quantitative evaluation of mitral regurgitation can now be performed by what is known as the proximal isovelocity surface area (PISA) method. This technique uses advanced color Doppler techniques to calculate the regurgitant volume and effective regurgitant orifice area, two values that predict clinical outcomes in patients with chronic mitral regurgitation.

Coronary Artery Disease

Echocardiography demonstrates ventricular wall motion abnormalities associated with infarcted or ischemic myocardium. The location and degree of abnormal systolic contraction and decreased systolic wall thickening indicate the extent of an infarction and implicate the responsible coronary artery. Echocardiography also detects complications of infarction including thrombus formation, papillary muscle rupture, ventricular septal rupture, and aneurysm.

Although echocardiography can depict those *consequences* of CAD, transthoracic echo resolution in adults is insufficient to satisfactorily image the coronary arteries themselves. However, **stress echocardiography** is a technique that aids in the diagnosis of CAD. This technique produces transient left ventricular regional wall motion abnormalities after exercise or with the infusion of specific pharmacologic agents (e.g., dobutamine), as a sign of inducible myocardial ischemia (see Chapter 6).

Cardiomyopathy

Cardiomyopathies are heart muscle disorders that occur in three forms: dilated, hypertrophic,

and restrictive (see Chapter 10). Echocardiography can distinguish these and permits assessment of the severity of systolic and diastolic dysfunction. For example, Figure 3.10 depicts the asymmetrically thickened ventricular walls of hypertrophic cardiomyopathy.

Pericardial Disease

2D echocardiography can identify abnormalities in the pericardial cavity (e.g., excessive pericardial fluid and tumor). Tamponade and constrictive pericarditis, the main consequences of pericardial disease (see Chapter 14), are associated with particular echocardiographic abnormalities. In tamponade, the increased intrapericardial pressure compresses the cardiac chambers and results in diastolic "collapse" of the right atrium and right ventricle (Fig. 3.12). Constrictive pericarditis is associated with increased thickness of the

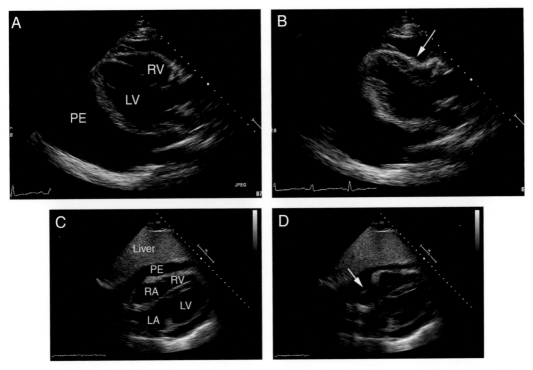

Figure 3.12. Echocardiogram of a patient with a pericardial effusion causing cardiac tamponade. A. Parasternal long axis image showing a large pericardial effusion (PE) surrounding the heart. This frame was obtained in systole and shows normal appearance of the left (LV) and right (RV) ventricles during that phase. **B.** Same image as **A**, but this frame was obtained in early diastole and shows collapse of the RV free wall *(arrow)* due to compression by the effusion. **C.** Subcostal view, obtained in systole, demonstrating the PE surrounding the right atrium (RA), RV, left atrium (LA), and LV. **D.** Same image as **C**, obtained during diastole, showing inward collapse of the RA *(arrow)*.

Table 3.2. Echocardiography in Common Cardiac Disorders

Disorder	Findings
Valvular lesions	
Mitral stenosis	• Enlarged left atrium • Thickened mitral valve leaflets • Decreased movement and separation of mitral valve leaflets • Decreased mitral valve orifice
Mitral regurgitation	• Enlarged left atrium (if chronic) • Enlarged left ventricle (if chronic) • Systolic flow from left ventricle into left atrium by Doppler
Aortic stenosis	• Thickened aortic valve cusps • Decreased valve orifice • Increased left ventricular wall thickness
Aortic regurgitation	• Enlarged left ventricle • Abnormalities of aortic valve or aortic root
Left ventricular function	
Myocardial infarction and complications	• Abnormal regional ventricular wall motion • Thrombus within left ventricle • Aneurysm of ventricular wall • Septal rupture (abnormal Doppler flow) • Papillary muscle rupture
Cardiomyopathies Dilated	• Enlarged ventricular chamber sizes • Decreased systolic contraction
Hypertrophic	• Normal or decreased ventricular chamber sizes • Increased ventricular wall thickness • Diastolic dysfunction (assessed by Doppler)
Restrictive	• Normal or decreased ventricular chamber sizes • Increased ventricular wall thickness • Ventricular contractile function often normal • Diastolic dysfunction (assessed by Doppler) • Enlarged atria

pericardial echo, abnormal patterns of diastolic left ventricular wall motion, alterations in pulmonary and hepatic venous flow patterns, and exaggerated changes in mitral and tricuspid valve inflow velocities during respiration.

Table 3.2 summarizes the echocardiographic features of common cardiac diseases.

CARDIAC CATHETERIZATION

To diagnose many cardiovascular abnormalities, intravascular catheters are inserted to measure pressures in the heart chambers, to determine cardiac output and vascular resistances, and to inject radiopaque material to examine heart structures and blood flow. In

1929, Werner Forssmann performed the first cardiac catheterization, *on himself*, thus ushering in the era of invasive cardiology. Much of what is known about the pathophysiology of valvular heart disease and congestive heart failure comes from decades of subsequent hemodynamic research in the cardiac catheterization laboratory.

Measurement of Pressure

Before catheterization of an artery or vein, the patient is mildly sedated, and a local anesthetic is used to numb the skin site of catheter entry. The catheter, attached to a pressure transducer outside the body, is then introduced into the appropriate blood vessel. To measure pressures in the right atrium, right ventricle, and pulmonary artery, a catheter is inserted into a femoral, brachial, or jugular *vein*. Pressures in the aorta and left ventricle are measured via catheters inserted into a brachial or femoral *artery*. Once

in the blood vessel, the catheter is guided by fluoroscopy (continuous x-ray images) to the area of study, where pressure measurements are made. Figure 3.13 depicts normal intracardiac and intravascular pressures.

The measurement of right-heart pressures is performed with a specialized balloon-tipped catheter (a common version of which is known as the Swan–Ganz catheter) that is advanced through the right side of the heart with the aid of normal blood flow, and into the pulmonary artery. As it travels through the right side of the heart, recorded pressure measurements identify the catheter tip's position (see Box 3.1).

Right Atrial Pressure

Right atrial pressure is equal to the central venous pressure (estimated by the jugular venous pressure on physical examination) because no obstructing valves impede blood return from the veins into the right atrium. Similarly, right

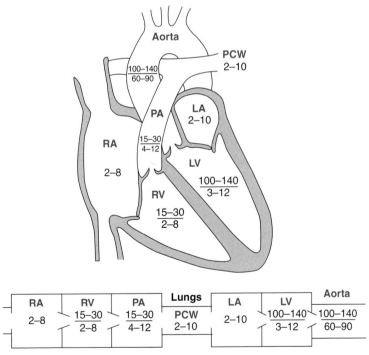

Figure 3.13. Diagrams indicating normal pressures in the cardiac chambers and great vessels. The top figure shows the normal anatomic relationship of the cardiac chambers and great vessels, whereas the figure on the bottom shows a simplified schematic to clarify the pressure relationships. Numbers indicate pressures in mm Hg. LA, left atrial mean pressure; LV, left ventricular pressure; PA, pulmonary artery pressure; PCW, pulmonary capillary wedge mean pressure; RA, right atrial mean pressure; RV, right ventricular pressure.

BOX *3.1* Intracardiac Pressure Tracings

When a catheter is inserted into a systemic vein and advanced into the right side of the heart, each cardiac chamber produces a characteristic pressure curve. It is important to distinguish these recordings from one another to localize the position of the catheter tip and to derive appropriate physiologic information.

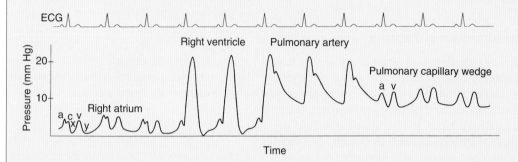

The normal *right atrial (RA)* pressure demonstrates three positive deflections (see the figure in Box 2.1 for an enlarged view): the *a* wave reflects RA contraction at the end of diastole, the *c* wave results from bulging of the tricuspid valve toward the right atrium as it closes in early systole, and the *v* wave represents passive filling of the right atrium from the systemic veins during systole, when the tricuspid valve is closed. The downward deflection that follows the *c* wave is known as the *x* descent, and the downward deflection after the *v* wave is called the *y* descent. Often the *a* and *c* waves merge so that only two major positive deflections are seen. In patients with atrial fibrillation, the *a* wave is absent because there is no organized left atrial contraction.

As the catheter is advanced into the *right ventricle (RV)*, a dramatic increase in systolic pressure is seen. The RV systolic waveform is characterized by a rapid upstroke and downstroke. In diastole, there is a gradual continuous increase in RV pressure as the chamber fills with blood.

As the catheter is moved forward into the *pulmonary artery (PA)*, the systolic pressure remains the same as that in the RV (as long as there is no obstruction to RV outflow, such as pulmonic valve stenosis). However, three characteristics of the recording indicate entry into the pulmonary artery: (1) the PA diastolic pressure is higher than that of the RV; (2) the descending systolic portion of the PA tracing inscribes a dicrotic wave, a small transient pressure increase that occurs after the systolic peak and is related to pulmonic valve closure; and (3) the diastolic portion of the PA tracing is downsloping compared with the upsloping RV diastolic pressure.

Further advancement of the catheter into a branch of the pulmonary artery results in the *pulmonary capillary wedge (PCW)* tracing, which reflects the left atrial pressure (see Fig. 3.14). Its characteristic shape is similar to the RA tracing, but the pressure values are usually higher and the tracing is often less clear (with the *c* wave not observed) because of damped transmission through the capillary vessels.

atrial pressure normally equals right ventricular pressure during diastole because the right heart functions as a "common chamber" when the tricuspid valve is open. The mean right atrial pressure is *reduced* when there is intravascular volume depletion. It is *elevated* in right ventricular failure, right-sided valvular disease, and cardiac tamponade (in which the cardiac chambers are surrounded by high-pressure pericardial fluid; see Chapter 14).

Certain abnormalities cause characteristic changes in individual components of the right atrial (and therefore jugular venous) pressure (Table 3.3). For example, a prominent *a* wave is seen in tricuspid stenosis and right ventricular hypertrophy. In these conditions, the

Table 3.3. Causes of Increased Intracardiac Pressures	
Chamber and Measurement	*Causes*
Right atrial pressure	• Right ventricular failure • Cardiac tamponade
a wave	• Tricuspid stenosis • Right ventricular hypertrophy • Atrioventricular dissociation
v wave	• Tricuspid regurgitation
Right ventricular pressure	
Systolic	• Pulmonic stenosis • Right ventricular failure • Pulmonary hypertension
Diastolic	• Right ventricular failure • Cardiac tamponade • Right ventricular hypertrophy
Pulmonary artery pressure	

Systolic and diastolic	• Pulmonary hypertension
	  • Left-sided heart failure
	  • Chronic lung disease
	  • Pulmonary vascular disease

Systolic only	• Increased flow (left-to-right shunt)
Pulmonary artery wedge pressure	• Left-sided heart failure • Mitral stenosis or regurgitation • Cardiac tamponade
a wave	• Left ventricular hypertrophy
v wave	• Mitral regurgitation • Ventricular septal defect

right atrium contracts vigorously against the obstructing tricuspid valve or stiffened right ventricle, respectively, generating a prominent pressure wave. Similarly, amplified "cannon" *a* waves may be produced by conditions of atrioventricular dissociation (see Chapter 12), when the right atrium contracts against a closed tricuspid valve. A prominent *v* wave is observed in tricuspid regurgitation because normal right atrial filling is augmented by the regurgitated blood in systole.

Right Ventricular Pressure

Right ventricular systolic pressure is increased by pulmonic valve stenosis or pulmonary hypertension. Right ventricular diastolic pressure increases when the right ventricle is subjected to pressure or volume overload and may be a sign of right-heart failure.

Pulmonary Artery Pressure

Elevation of systolic and diastolic pulmonary artery pressures occurs in three conditions: (1) *left*-sided heart failure; (2) parenchymal lung disease (e.g., chronic bronchitis or end-stage emphysema); and (3) pulmonary vascular disease (e.g., pulmonary embolism, primary pulmonary hypertension, or acute respiratory distress syndrome). Normally, the pulmonary artery diastolic pressure is equivalent to the left atrial pressure because of the low resistance of the pulmonary vasculature that separates them. If the left atrial pressure rises because of left-sided heart failure, both systolic and diastolic pulmonary artery pressures increase in an obligatory manner to maintain forward flow through the lungs. This situation leads to "passive" pulmonary hypertension.

In certain conditions, however, pulmonary vascular resistance becomes abnormally high, causing pulmonary artery diastolic pressure to be elevated compared with left atrial pressure. For example, pulmonary vascular obstructive disease may develop as a complication of a chronic left-to-right cardiac shunt, such as an atrial or ventricular septal defect (see Chapter 16).

Pulmonary Artery Wedge Pressure

If a catheter is advanced into the right or left pulmonary artery, its tip will ultimately reach one of the small pulmonary artery branches and temporarily occlude forward blood flow beyond it. During that time, a column of stagnant blood stands between the catheter tip and the portions of the pulmonary capillary and pulmonary venous segments distal to it (Fig. 3.14). That column of blood acts as an extension of the catheter, and the pressure recorded through the catheter reflects that of the downstream chamber—namely, the left atrium. Such a pressure measurement is termed the *pulmonary artery wedge pressure* or *pulmonary capillary wedge pressure (PCW)*

and closely matches the left atrial pressure in most individuals. Furthermore, while the mitral valve is open during diastole, the pulmonary venous bed, left atrium, and left ventricle normally share the same pressures. Thus, the PCW can be used to estimate the left ventricular diastolic pressure, a measurement of ventricular preload (see Chapter 9). As a result, measurement of PCW may be useful in managing certain critically ill patients in the intensive care unit.

Elevation of the mean PCW is seen in left-sided heart failure and in mitral stenosis or regurgitation. The individual components of the PCW tracing can also become abnormally high. The *a* wave may be increased in conditions of decreased left ventricular compliance, such as left ventricular hypertrophy or acute myocardial ischemia. The *v* wave is greater than normal when there is increased left atrial filling during ventricular contraction, as in mitral regurgitation.

Measurement of Blood Flow

Cardiac output is measured by either the thermodilution method or the Fick technique. In the **thermodilution method,** saline of a known temperature is injected rapidly through a catheter side port into the right side of the heart, at a specific distance from the distal tip of the catheter. The catheter tip, positioned in the pulmonary artery, contains a thermistor that registers the change in temperature induced

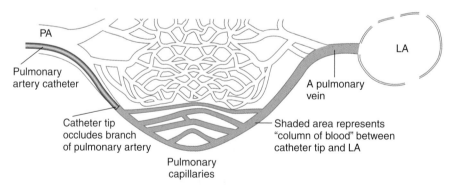

Figure 3.14. Diagram of a pulmonary artery catheter inserted into a branch of the pulmonary artery (PA). Flow is occluded in the arterial, arteriolar, and capillary vessels beyond the catheter; thus, these vessels act as a conduit that transmits the left atrial (LA) pressure to the catheter tip.

by the injected saline. The cardiac output is proportional to the rate of the temperature change and is automatically calculated by the equipment.

The **Fick method** relies on the principle that the quantity of oxygen consumed by tissues is related to the amount of O_2 content removed from blood as it flows through the tissue capillary bed:

$$O_2 \text{ consumption} = O_2 \text{ content removed} \times \text{Flow}$$
$$\left(\frac{\text{mL } O_2}{\text{min}}\right) \qquad \left(\frac{\text{mL } O_2}{\text{mL blood}}\right) \qquad \left(\frac{\text{mL blood}}{\text{min}}\right)$$

Or, in more applicable terms:

$$O_2 \text{ consumption} =$$
$$AVO_2 \text{ difference} \times \text{Cardiac output}$$

where the arteriovenous O_2 (AVO_2) difference equals the difference in oxygen content between the arterial and venous compartments. Total body oxygen consumption can be determined by analyzing expired air from the lungs, and arterial and venous O_2 content is measured in blood samples. By rearranging the terms, the cardiac output can be calculated:

$$\text{Cardiac output} = \frac{O_2 \text{ consumption}}{AVO_2 \text{ difference}}$$

For example, if the arterial blood in a normal adult contains 190 mL of O_2 per liter and the venous blood contains 150 mL of O_2 per liter, the arteriovenous difference is 40 mL of O_2 per liter. If this patient has a measured O_2 consumption of 200 mL/min, the calculated cardiac output is 5 L/min.

In many forms of heart disease, the cardiac output is lower than normal. In that situation, the total body oxygen consumption does not change significantly; however, a greater percentage of O_2 is extracted per volume of circulating blood by the metabolizing tissues. The result is a lower-than-normal venous O_2 content and therefore an increased AVO_2 difference. In our example, if the patient's venous blood O_2 content fell to 100 mL/L, the AVO_2 difference would increase to 90 mL/L and the calculated cardiac output would be reduced to 2.2 L/min.

Because the normal range of cardiac output varies with a patient's size, it is common to report the **cardiac index**, which is equal to the cardiac output divided by the patient's body surface area (normal range of cardiac index = 2.6–4.2 L/min/m²).

Calculation of Vascular Resistance

Once pressures and cardiac output have been determined, pulmonary and systemic vascular resistances can be calculated, based on the principle that the pressure difference across a vascular bed is proportional to the product of flow and resistance. The calculations are:

$$PVR = \frac{MPAP - LAP}{CO} \times 80$$

PVR, pulmonary vascular resistance (dynes-sec-cm⁻⁵)

MPAP, mean pulmonary artery pressure (mm Hg)

LAP, mean left atrial pressure (mm Hg)

CO, cardiac output (L/min)

$$SVR = \frac{MAP - RAP}{CO} \times 80$$

SVR, systemic vascular resistance (dynes-sec-cm⁻⁵)

MAP, mean arterial pressure (mm Hg)

RAP, mean right atrial pressure (mm Hg)

CO, cardiac output (L/min)

The normal PVR ranges from 20 to 130 dynes-sec-cm⁻⁵. The normal SVR is 700 to 1,600 dynes-sec-cm⁻⁵.

Contrast Angiography

This technique uses radiopaque contrast to visualize regions of the cardiovascular system. A catheter is introduced into an appropriate vessel and guided under fluoroscopy to the site of injection. Following administration of the contrast agent, x-rays are transmitted through the area of interest. A continuous series of x-ray exposures is recorded to produce a motion picture cineangiogram (often simply called a "cine," or "angiogram").

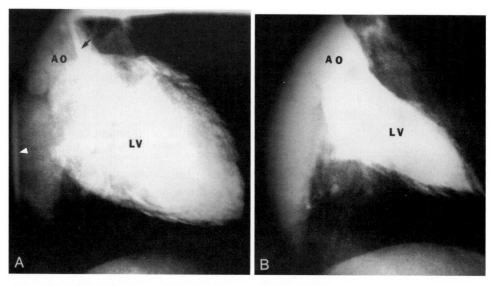

Figure 3.15. **Left ventriculogram, in diastole (A) and systole (B) in the right anterior oblique projection, from a patient with normal ventricular contractility.** A catheter *(arrow)* is used to inject contrast into the left ventricle (LV). The catheter can also be seen in the descending aorta *(arrowhead)*. AO, aortic root.

Digital subtraction angiography (DSA) is commonly used in vascular imaging. Electronic processing of digitalized x-ray images subtracts the background of soft tissue and bone, thus enhancing the blood vessel or chamber into which contrast was injected. DSA has advantages over conventional angiography: smaller catheters may be used, the amount of contrast agent required may be lower, and better image quality is usually achieved.

Selective injection of contrast into specific heart chambers can be used to identify valvular insufficiency, intracardiac shunts, thrombi within the heart, and congenital malformations, and is also used to measure ventricular contractile function (Fig. 3.15).

A widespread application of contrast injection is **coronary artery angiography**, to examine the location and severity of coronary atherosclerotic lesions. To maximize the test's sensitivity and reproducibility, each patient is imaged in several standard views. When necessary, angioplasty and stent placement can be performed (Figs. 3.16 and 3.17; see Chapter 6).

A small risk is associated with catheterization and contrast angiography. Complications are uncommon but include myocardial perforation by the catheter, precipitation of arrhythmias

and conduction blocks, damage to vessel walls, hemorrhage, dislodgement of atherosclerotic plaques, pericardial tamponade (see Chapter 14), and infection. The contrast medium itself can cause anaphylaxis and renal toxicity.

Table 3.4 summarizes the catheterization findings in common cardiac abnormalities. Therapeutic interventional catheterization techniques are described in Chapter 6.

NUCLEAR IMAGING

Heart function can be evaluated using injected, radioactively labeled tracers and γ-camera detectors. The resulting images reflect the distribution of the tracers within the cardiovascular system. Nuclear techniques are used to assess myocardial perfusion, to image blood passing through the heart and great vessels, to localize and quantify myocardial ischemia and infarction, and to assess myocardial metabolism.

Assessment of Myocardial Perfusion

Ischemia and infarction resulting from CAD can be detected by myocardial perfusion imaging using various radioisotopes, including compounds labeled with thallium-201 (^{201}Tl)

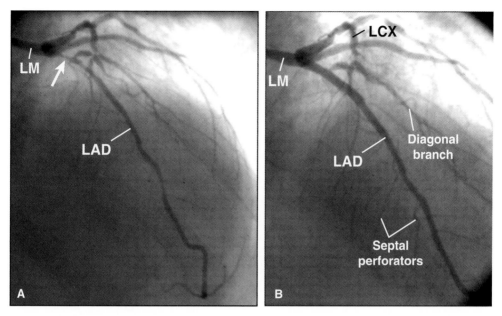

Figure 3.16. Cardiac catheterization and stenting of a proximal left anterior descending artery (LAD) stenosis, shown in an anteroposterior cranial projection. A. When contrast agent is injected into the left main coronary artery (LM), the left circumflex artery (LCX) fills normally but the LAD is almost completely occluded at its origin *(white arrow)*. **B.** After the stenosis is successfully stented, the LAD and its branches fill robustly.

and technetium-99m (^{99m}Tc). Of the latter, currently ^{99m}Tc-sestamibi and ^{99m}Tc-tetrofosmin are widely used. Both ^{201}Tl- and ^{99m}Tc-labeled compounds are sensitive for the detection of ischemic or scarred myocardium, but each has distinct advantages. For example, the

^{99m}Tc-labeled agents provide better image quality and are superior for detailed single photon emission computed tomography (SPECT, as in Fig. 3.18). Conversely, enhanced detection of myocardial cellular viability is possible with ^{201}Tl imaging.

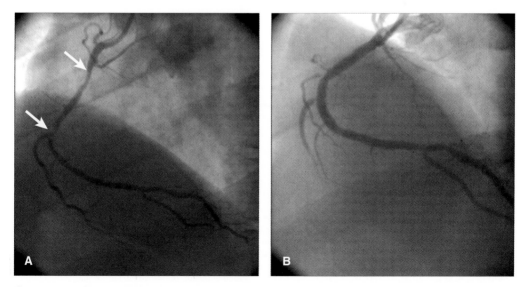

Figure 3.17. Cardiac catheterization and stenting of right coronary artery (RCA) stenoses. Both images are obtained in the left anterior oblique (LAO) projection. **A.** The stenotic segment is located between the *white arrows*. **B.** After stenting, the caliber of the vessel and flow have improved.

Table 3.4. Cardiac Catheterization and Angiography in Cardiac Disorders

Disorder	Finding
Coronary artery disease	• Identification of atherosclerotic lesions
Mitral regurgitation	• Large systolic *v* wave in left atrial pressure tracing
Mitral stenosis	• Abnormally high pressure gradient between left atrium and left ventricle in diastole
Tricuspid insufficiency	• Large systolic *v* wave in the right atrial pressure tracing
Aortic stenosis	• Systolic pressure gradient between left ventricle and aorta
Congestive heart failure	• Reduced ejection fraction (see Chapter 9) if systolic dysfunction • Elevated diastolic pressure with normal ejection fraction if diastolic dysfunction

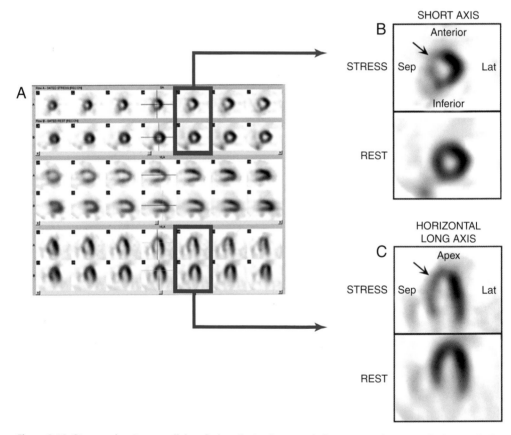

Figure 3.18. Stress and rest myocardial perfusion single photon emission computed tomography images (using 99mTc-tetrofosmin) of a patient with a high-grade stenosis within the proximal left anterior descending coronary artery. A. Miniaturized reproduction of the complete scan showing tomographic images in each of the three views. The first, third, and fifth rows demonstrate images during stress, and the second, fourth, and sixth rows are matching images acquired at rest. **B,C.** Enlarged selected panels from **A** showing stress and rest images in the short axis and horizontal long axis views. The arrows indicate regions of decreased perfusion during stress but normal perfusion on the matching resting scans, consistent with inducible ischemia. Lat, lateral wall of the LV; Sep, septal wall. (Courtesy of Marcelo Di Carli, MD, Brigham and Women's Hospital, Boston, MA.)

In the case of ^{201}Tl imaging, the radio-isotope is injected intravenously while the patient is exercising on a treadmill or stationary bicycle. Because thallium is a potassium analogue, it enters normal myocytes, a process thought to be partially governed by the sodium–potassium ATPase pump. The intracellular concentration of thallium, estimated by the density of the image, depends on vascular supply (perfusion) and membrane function (tissue viability). In the normal heart, the radionuclide scan shows a homogenous distribution of thallium in the myocardial tissue. Conversely, myocardial regions that are scarred (by previous infarction) or have reduced perfusion during exercise (i.e., transient myocardial ischemia) do not accumulate as much thallium as normal heart muscle. Consequently, these areas will appear on the thallium scan as light or "cold" spots.

When evaluating for myocardial ischemia, an initial set of images is taken right after exercise and ^{201}Tl injection. Well-perfused myocardium will take up more tracer than ischemic or infarcted myocardium at this time. Delayed images are acquired several hours later, because ^{201}Tl accumulation does not remain fixed in myocytes. Rather, continuous redistribution of the isotope occurs across the cell membrane. After 3 to 4 hours of redistribution, when additional images are obtained, all viable myocytes will have equal concentrations of ^{201}Tl. Consequently, any uptake abnormalities on the initial exercise scan that were caused by myocardial *ischemia* will have resolved (i.e., filled in) on the delayed scan (and are therefore termed "reversible" defects), and those representing *infarcted* or scarred myocardium will persist as cold spots ("fixed" defects).

Of note, some myocardial segments that demonstrate persistent ^{201}Tl defects on both stress and redistribution imaging are falsely characterized as nonviable, scarred tissue. Sometimes these areas represent ischemic, noncontractile, but metabolically active areas that have the potential to regain function if an adequate blood supply is restored. For example, such areas may represent **hibernating myocardium,** segments that demonstrate diminished contractile function owing to chronic reduction of coronary blood flow (see Chapter 6). This viable state (in which the affected cells can be predicted to regain function following coronary revascularization) can often be differentiated from irreversibly scarred myocardium by repeat imaging at rest after the injection of additional ^{201}Tl to enhance uptake by viable cells.

^{99m}Tc-sestamibi (commonly referred to as MIBI) is the most widely used ^{99m}Tc-labeled compound. This agent is a large lipophilic molecule that, like thallium, is taken up in the myocardium in proportion to blood flow. The uptake mechanism differs in that the compound crosses the myocyte membrane passively, driven by the negative membrane potential. Once inside the cell, it further accumulates in mitochondria, driven by that organelle's even more negative membrane potential. The myocardial distribution of MIBI reflects perfusion at the moment of injection, and in contrast to thallium, it remains fixed intracellularly, that is, it *does not redistribute over time.* Consequently, performing a MIBI procedure is more flexible, as images can be obtained up to 4 to 6 hours after injection and repeated as necessary. A MIBI study is usually performed as a 1-day protocol in which an initial injection of a small tracer dose and imaging are performed at rest. Later, a larger tracer dose is given after exercise, and imaging is repeated.

Stress nuclear imaging studies with either ^{201}Tl- or ^{99m}Tc-labeled compounds have greater sensitivity and specificity than standard exercise electrocardiography for the detection of ischemia but are more expensive and should be ordered judiciously. Nuclear imaging is particularly appropriate for patients with certain baseline electrocardiogram (ECG) abnormalities of the ST segment that preclude accurate interpretation of a standard exercise test. Examples include patients with electronic pacemaker rhythms, those with left bundle branch block, those with ST abnormalities due to left ventricular hypertrophy, and those who take certain medications that alter the ST segment, such as digoxin. Nuclear scans also provide more accurate anatomic localization of the ischemic segment(s) and quantification of the extent of ischemia compared with standard exercise testing. In addition, electronic synchronizing (gating) of nuclear images to the ECG cycle permits wall motion analysis.

Patients with orthopedic or neurologic conditions, as well as those with severe physical deconditioning or chronic lung disease, may be unable to perform an adequate exercise test on a treadmill or bicycle. In such patients, stress images can be obtained instead by administering pharmacologic agents, such as adenosine or dipyridamole. These agents induce diffuse coronary vasodilation, augmenting blood flow to myocardium perfused by healthy coronary arteries. Since ischemic regions are already maximally dilated (because of local metabolite accumulation), the drug-induced vasodilation causes a "steal" phenomenon, *reducing* isotope uptake in regions distal to significant coronary stenoses (see Chapter 6). Alternatively, dobutamine (see Chapter 17) can be infused intravenously to increase myocardial oxygen demand as a means to assess for ischemia.

Radionuclide Ventriculography

Radionuclide ventriculography (RVG, also known as blood pool imaging) is used to analyze right and left ventricular function. A radioisotope (usually ^{99m}Tc) is bound to red blood cells or to human serum albumin and then injected as a bolus. Nuclear images are obtained at fixed time intervals as the labeled material passes through the heart and great vessels. Multiple images are displayed sequentially to produce a dynamic picture of blood flow. Calculations, such as determination of the ejection fraction, are based on the difference between radioactive counts present in the ventricle at end diastole and at end systole. Therefore, measurements are largely independent of any assumptions of ventricular geometry and are highly reproducible. Studies suggest that RVG and echocardiography provide similar left ventricular ejection fraction values, but unlike echocardiography, RVG can also calculate an accurate right ventricular ejection fraction.

RVG is commonly used to assess baseline cardiac function in patients scheduled to undergo potentially cardiotoxic chemotherapy (e.g., doxorubicin) and to follow cardiac function over time in such patients. In addition, first-pass imaging permits recognition and quantification of cardiac and vascular shunts (described in Chapter 16).

Assessment of Myocardial Metabolism

Positron emission tomography (PET) is a specialized nuclear imaging technique used to assess myocardial perfusion and viability. PET imaging employs positron-emitting isotopes (e.g., rubidium-82, nitrogen-13, and fluorine-18) attached to metabolic or flow tracers. Sensitive detectors measure positron emission from the tracer molecules.

Myocardial perfusion is commonly assessed using nitrogen-13–labeled ammonia or rubidium-82. Both are taken up by myocytes in proportion to blood flow. *Myocardial viability* can be determined by PET by studying glucose utilization in myocardial tissue. In normal myocardium under fasting conditions, glucose is used for approximately 20% of energy production, with free fatty acids providing the remaining 80%. In ischemic conditions, however, metabolism shifts toward glucose use, and the more ischemic the myocardial tissue, the stronger the reliance on glucose. Fluoro-18 deoxyglucose (^{18}FDG), created by substituting fluorine-18 for hydrogen in 2-deoxyglucose, is used to study glucose uptake. This substance competes with glucose both for transport into myocytes and for subsequent phosphorylation. Unlike glucose, however, ^{18}FDG is not metabolized and becomes trapped within the myocyte.

Combined evaluation of perfusion and ^{18}FDG metabolism allows assessment of both regional blood flow and glucose uptake, respectively. PET scanning thus helps determine whether areas of ventricular contractile dysfunction with decreased flow represent irreversibly damaged scar tissue, or whether the region is still viable (e.g., hibernating myocardium). In scar tissue, both blood flow to the affected area and ^{18}FDG uptake are decreased. Because the myocytes in this region are permanently damaged, such tissue is not likely

Table 3.5. Nuclear Imaging in Cardiac Disorders	
Disorder	*Findings*
Myocardial ischemia	
Stress-delayed reinjection ^{201}Tl	• Low uptake during stress with complete or partial fill-in with delayed or reinjection images
Rest–stress ^{99m}Tc-labeled compounds	• Normal uptake at rest with decreased uptake during stress
PET (N-13 ammonia/^{18}FDG)	• Decreased flow with normal or increased ^{18}FDG uptake during stress
Myocardial infarction	
Stress-delayed reinjection ^{201}Tl	• Low uptake during stress and low uptake after reinjection
Rest–stress ^{99m}Tc-labeled compounds	• Low uptake in rest and stress images
PET (N-13 ammonia/^{18}FDG)	• Decreased flow and decreased ^{18}FDG uptake at rest
Hibernating myocardium	
Rest-delayed ^{201}Tl	• Complete or partial fill-in of defects after reinjection
PET (N-13 ammonia/^{18}FDG)	• Decreased flow and normal or increased ^{18}FDG uptake at rest
Assessment of ventricular function	
^{99m}Tc RBC-gated radionuclide ventriculography	• Assessment of global left and right ventricular function

^{18}FDG, fluoro-18 deoxyglucose; N-13, nitrogen-13; PET, positron emission tomography; RBC, red blood cell; ^{99m}Tc, technetium-99m; ^{201}Tl, thallium-201.

to benefit from revascularization. Hibernating myocardium, in contrast, shows decreased blood flow but normal or elevated ^{18}FDG uptake. Such tissue may benefit from revascularization procedures (see Chapter 6).

Table 3.5 summarizes the radionuclide-imaging abnormalities associated with common cardiac conditions.

COMPUTED TOMOGRAPHY

CT uses thin x-ray beams to obtain a large series of axial plane images. An x-ray tube is programmed to rotate around the body, and the generated beams are partially absorbed by body tissues. The remaining beams emerge and are captured by electronic detectors, which relay information to a computer for image composition. CT scanning typically requires administration of an intravenous contrast agent to distinguish intravascular contents (i.e., blood)

from neighboring soft tissue structures (e.g., myocardium).

Applications of CT in cardiac imaging include assessment of the great vessels, pericardium, myocardium, and coronary arteries. CT is used to diagnose aortic dissections and aneurysms (Fig. 3.19). It can identify abnormal pericardial fluid, thickening, and calcification. Myocardial abnormalities, such as regional hypertrophy or ventricular aneurysms, and intracardiac thrombus formation can be distinctly visualized by CT. A limitation of conventional CT techniques is the artifact generated by patient motion (i.e., breathing) during image acquisition. Modern **spiral CT** imaging allows more rapid image acquisition, often during a single breath-hold, at relatively lower radiation doses than conventional CT. Spiral CT is particularly important in the diagnosis of pulmonary embolism. When an intravenous iodine-based contrast agent is administered, emboli create the appearance of

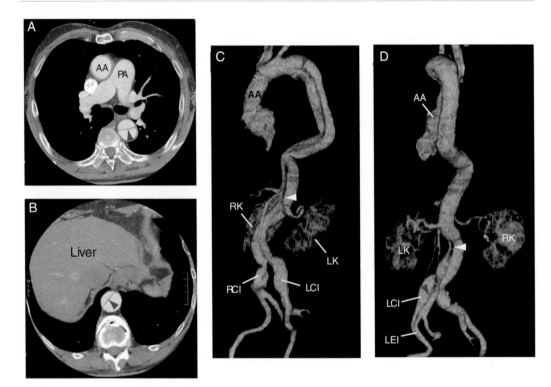

Figure 3.19. Computed tomography (CT) imaging of aortic dissection. A,B. Axial images demonstrate an intimal flap *(colored arrowheads)* separating the true and false lumens of the descending thoracic and abdominal aorta. C. CT angiography (CTA) with three-dimensional reconstructions. In this left anterior oblique view, the origin of the dissection *(colored arrowhead)* is apparent in the distal portion of the aortic arch. The dissection continues to the level of the renal arteries *(white arrowhead)* and beyond. D. In this CTA left posterior oblique view, the dissection extends to the infrarenal aorta *(white arrowhead)* and involves the left common and external iliac arteries *(colored arrowhead)*. AA, ascending aorta; LCI, left common iliac artery; LEI, left external iliac artery; LK, left kidney; PA, main pulmonary artery; RCI, right common iliac artery; RK, right kidney. (Courtesy of Suhny Abbara, MD, Massachusetts General Hospital, Boston, MA.)

"filling defects" in otherwise contrast-enhanced pulmonary vessels (Fig. 3.20).

Electron beam computed tomography (EBCT) uses a direct electron beam to acquire images in a matter of milliseconds. Rapid succession of images depicts cardiac structures at multiple times during a single cardiac cycle. Displaying these images in a cine format can provide estimates of left ventricular volumes and ejection fraction. Capable of detecting coronary artery calcification, EBCT has been used primarily to screen for CAD. Because calcified coronary artery plaques have a radiodensity similar to that of bone, they appear attenuated (white) on CT. The *Agatson score*, a measure of total coronary artery calcium, correlates well with atherosclerotic plaque burden, and predicts the risk of coronary events, independently of other cardiac risk factors.

Newer CT technology can characterize atherosclerotic stenoses in great detail. Current **multidetector row CT** scanners acquire as many as 320 anatomic sections with each rotation, providing excellent spatial resolution. Administration of intravenous contrast and computer reformatting allows visualization of the arterial lumen and regions of coronary narrowings (Fig. 3.21). Because image acquisition is timed with the cardiac cycle, a relatively low heart rate is desirable, such that a β-blocker is often administered prior to scanning.

CT is not as sensitive as conventional angiography for the detection of coronary lesions, and it cannot adequately evaluate stenosis within coronary artery stents. In addition, this technique results in significant radiation exposure. However, CT is rapid,

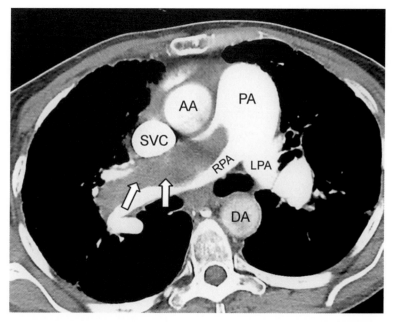

Figure 3.20. Spiral computed tomography image demonstrating a massive pulmonary embolism. The white arrows point to a large thrombus within the right pulmonary artery. It appears as a filling defect within the otherwise contrast-enhanced pulmonary vasculature. AA, ascending aorta; DA, descending aorta; LPA, left pulmonary artery; PA, main pulmonary artery; RPA, right pulmonary artery; SVC, superior vena cava.

relatively inexpensive, and significantly less invasive than conventional angiography. Its role in assessing patients with symptoms suggestive of CAD and for following the progression of known coronary disease is under active evaluation.

MAGNETIC RESONANCE IMAGING

MRI uses a powerful magnetic field to obtain detailed images of internal structures. This technique is based on the magnetic polarity of hydrogen nuclei, which align themselves with an applied magnetic field. Radio frequency excitation causes the nuclei to move out of alignment momentarily. As they return to their resting states, the nuclei emit signals that are translated into computer-generated images. Therefore, MRI requires no ionized radiation. Among all the imaging modalities, MRI is best at differentiating tissue contrasts (blood, fluid, fat, and myocardium) and can often do so even without the use of contrast agents. The addition of gadolinium-

based contrast allows further characterization of cardiac structures and tissues.

The detail of soft tissue structures is often exquisitely demonstrated in magnetic resonance images (Fig. 3.22). Cardiac MRI has an established role in evaluating congenital anomalies, such as shunts, and diseases of the aorta, including aneurysm and dissection. It is also used to assess left and right ventricular mass and volume, intravascular thrombus, cardiomyopathies, and neoplastic disease (Fig. 3.23). ECG-gated and cine MRI techniques capture images at discrete times in the cardiac cycle, and permit evaluation of valvular and ventricular function.

Two applications of cardiac MRI deserve special mention. **Coronary magnetic resonance angiography (coronary MRA)** is a noninvasive, contrast-free angiographic imaging modality. Laminar blood flow appears as bright signal intensity, whereas turbulent blood flow, at the site of stenosis, results in less bright or absent signal intensity. This technique has shown high sensitivity and accuracy for the detection

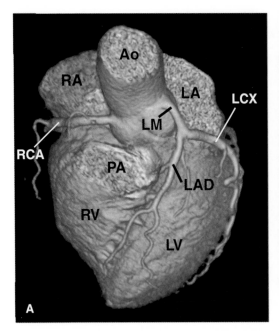

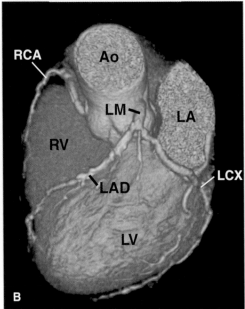

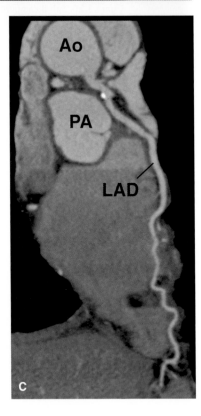

Figure 3.21. **Computed tomography (CT) coronary angiography.** After a patient is imaged in a high-resolution axial CT scanner, three-dimensional reconstructions (termed *volume renderings*) are generated by a computer. **A.** Volume rendering of a normal CT angiogram. **B.** Volume rendering of a CT angiogram that demonstrates diffuse coronary artery disease. Notice that the caliber of each vessel is irregular along its length. **C.** This curved reformat of the left anterior descending artery (LAD) depicts the entire course of the vessel in a single, flat image, making it easier to detect stenoses. None are present here. Ao, aorta; LA, left atrium; LCX, left circumflex artery; LM, left main coronary artery; LV, left ventricle; PA, pulmonary artery; RA, right atrium; RCA, right coronary artery; RV, right ventricle. (Courtesy of Suhny Abbara, MD, Massachusetts General Hospital, Boston, MA.)

of important CAD in the left main coronary artery and in the proximal and midportions of the three major coronary vessels. Coronary MRA is also useful in delineating coronary artery congenital anomalies.

In **contrast-enhanced MRI**, a gadolinium-based agent is administered intravenously to identify infarcted (irreversibly damaged) myocardium and to differentiate it from impaired (but viable) muscle segments. This technique

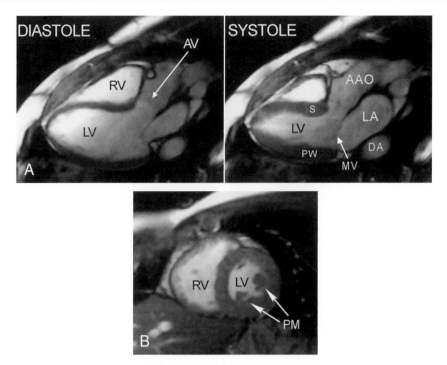

Figure 3.22. **Cardiac magnetic resonance images of a normal person. A.** Three-chamber long axis view of the heart in diastole and systole showing the left ventricle (LV), right ventricle (RV), and left atrium (LA). The mitral valve (MV), aortic valve (AV), ascending aorta (AAO), and descending aorta (DA) are also imaged. **B.** Midventricular short axis view demonstrating the LV, RV, and left ventricular papillary muscles (PMs). PW, posterior wall; S, septum. (Courtesy of Raymond Y. Kwong, MD, Brigham and Women's Hospital, Boston, MA.)

is based on the fact that gadolinium is excluded from viable cells with intact cell membranes but can permeate and concentrate in infarcted zones, producing "hyperenhancement" on the image (Fig. 3.24). In addition, the transmural extent of myocardial scar can be depicted, and infarcting tissue can also be differentiated from acute myocarditis, a condition that may present with similar clinical features (see Chapter 10).

SUMMARY

This chapter has presented an overview of imaging and catheterization techniques available to assess cardiac structure and function. Many of these tools are expensive and yield similar information. For example, estimates of ventricular contractile function can be made by echocardiography, nuclear imaging, contrast angiography, gated CT, or MRI. Myocardial viability can be assessed using nuclear imaging

studies, gadolinium MRI, or dobutamine echocardiography.

Determining the single best test for any given patient depends on a number of factors. One is the ease by which images may be obtained. In a critically ill patient, bedside echocardiography provides a readily acquired measure of left ventricular systolic function. Conversely, obtaining similar information from a nuclear or magnetic resonance study would require a trip to the respective scanner. Another factor to consider is the degree of invasiveness of a given imaging technique. Expense, available equipment, and institutional expertise also play roles in selecting an imaging approach. When used appropriately, each of these tools can provide important information to guide the diagnosis and management of cardiovascular disorders.

Table 3.6 summarizes common uses of the imaging techniques. The listed clinical conditions are described in greater detail in subsequent chapters.

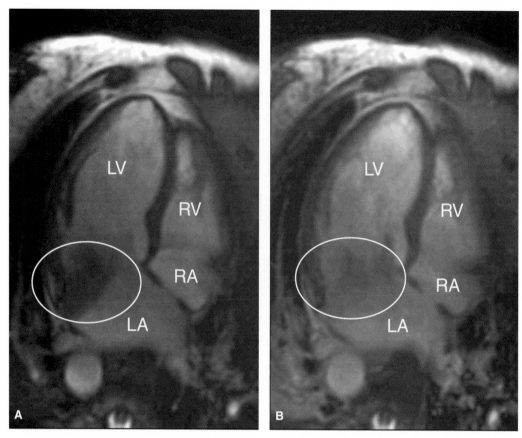

Figure 3.23. Magnetic resonance imaging of an intracardiac mass. Both images are apical four-chamber views. **A.** Before a gadolinium-based contrast agent is administered, an abnormal left atrial mass (indicated by the oval) demonstrates diminished signal relative to the surrounding tissue. In this respect, it resembles a nonvascular thrombus. **B.** After contrast injection, the mass enhances similar to the surrounding tissue, indicating that it is vascularized. Biopsy revealed a spindle-cell carcinoma. LA, left atrium; LV, left ventricle; RA, right atrium; RV, right ventricle. (Courtesy of Raymond Y. Kwong, MD, Brigham and Women's Hospital, Boston, MA.)

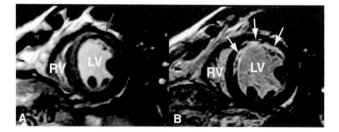

Figure 3.24. Gadolinium-enhanced magnetic resonance images demonstrating a region of nonviable myocardium. Both images are short axis views. **A.** Imaging before administration of gadolinium demonstrates thinning of the anterior and anteroseptal myocardium *(colored arrow)* suggestive of infarcted tissue. **B.** After contrast injection, the anterior and anteroseptal segments of the left ventricle selectively enhance *(white arrows)*, indicating that scar tissue is present. Because more than half the thickness of the ventricular wall is scarred, coronary revascularization would have a low likelihood of improving contractile function of these myocardial segments. LV, left ventricle; RV, right ventricle. (Courtesy of Raymond Y. Kwong, MD, Brigham and Women's Hospital, Boston, MA.)

Table 3.6. Summary of Cardiac Imaging Techniques

Imaging Technique	Findings	Examples of Clinical Uses
Chest radiography	• Cardiac and mediastinal contours • Pulmonary vascular markings	• Detect chamber dilatation • Identify consequences of stenotic and regurgitant valve lesions and intracardiac shunts • Visualize pulmonary signs of heart failure
Transthoracic echocardiography (TTE)	• Wall thickness, chamber dimensions • Anatomic relationships and motion of cardiac structures • Flow direction, turbulence, and velocity measurements • Echo contrast studies • Stress echocardiography	• Assess global and segmental ventricular contraction • Identify valvular abnormalities and vegetations • Diagnose consequences of myocardial infarction (e.g., ventricular aneurysm, papillary muscle rupture, intraventricular thrombus) • Identify myocardial, pericardial, and congenital abnormalities
Transesophageal echocardiography (TEE)	• Similar to TTE but higher resolution	• Visualize intracardiac thrombus • Evaluate prosthetic valves and perivalvular leaks • Identify valvular vegetations and myocardial abscess in endocarditis • Diagnose aortic dissection
Cardiac catheterization	• Pressure measurement • Contrast angiography	• Evaluate intracardiac pressures (e.g., in valvular disease, heart failure, pericardial disease) • Visualize ventricular contractile function, regurgitant valve lesions • Identify coronary anatomy and severity of stenoses
Nuclear SPECT imaging (using ^{99m}Tc-labeled compounds or ^{201}Tl)	• Regional myocardial perfusion • Myocardial viability	• Detect, quantify, and localize myocardial ischemia • Perform stress testing in patients with baseline ECG abnormalities • Distinguish viable myocardium from scar tissue
Radionuclide ventriculography	• Ventricular contractile function	• Calculate ventricular ejection fraction and quantitate intracardiac shunts
Positron emission tomography (PET)	• Myocardial perfusion and metabolism	• Evaluate contractile function • Distinguish viable myocardium from scar tissue
Computed tomography (CT)	• Anatomy and structural relationships	• Diagnose disease of the great vessels (aortic dissection, pulmonary embolism) • Assess pericardial disease and myocardial abnormalities • Detect coronary artery calcification and stenoses
Magnetic resonance imaging (MRI)	• Detailed soft tissue anatomy	• Assess myocardial structure and function (e.g., ventricular mass and volume, neoplastic disease, intracardiac thrombus, cardiomyopathies) • Diagnose aortic and pericardial disease

ECG, electrocardiogram; SPECT, single photon emission computed tomography; ^{99m}Tc, technetium-99m; ^{201}Tl, thallium-201.

Acknowledgments

The authors are grateful to Suhny Abbara, MD; Sharmila Dorbala, MD; Raymond Y. Kwong, MD; and Jeffrey Popma, MD, for their helpful suggestions. Contributors to the previous editions of this chapter were Nicole Martin, MD; Deborah Bucino, MD; Sharon Horesh, MD; Shona Pendse, MD; Albert S. Tu, MD; Patrick Yachimski, MD, and Patricia C. Come, MD.

Additional Reading

Baim D, Grossman W. *Grossman's Cardiac Catheterization, Angiography and Intervention*. 7th ed. Philadelphia, PA: Lippincott Williams & Wilkins; 2005.

Bengel FM, Higuchi T, Javadi MS, et al. Cardiac positron emission tomography. *J Am Coll Cardiol*. 2009;54:1–15.

Dewey M. *Coronary CT Angiography*. Berlin: Springer; 2009.

Di Carli MF. Hybrid imaging: integration of nuclear imaging and cardiac CT. *Cardiol Clin*. 2009;27: 257–263.

Douglas PS, Khandheria B, Stainback RF, et al. ACCF/ASE/ACEP/ASNC/SCAI/SCCT/SCMR 2007 appropriateness criteria for transthoracic and transesophageal echocardiography. *J Am Coll Cardiol*. 2007;50:187–204.

Douglas PS, Khandheria B, Stainback RF, et al. ACCF/ASE/ACEP/AHA/ASNC/SCAI/SCCT/SCMR 2008 appropriateness criteria for stress echocardiography. *Circulation*. 2008;117:1478–1497.

Fazel R, Krumholz HM, Wang Y, et al. Exposure to low-dose ionizing radiation from medical imaging procedures. *N Engl J Med*. 2009;361:849–857.

Hendel RC, Berman DS, Di Carli MF, et al. ACCF/ASNC/ACR/AHA/ASE/SCCT/SCMR/SNM 2009 appropriate use criteria for cardiac radionuclide imaging. *Circulation*. 2009;119:561–587.

Kern MJ, Samady H. Current concepts of integrated coronary physiology in the catheterization laboratory. *J Am Coll Cardiol*. 2010;55:173–185.

Kim HW, Farzaneh-Far A, Kim RJ. Cardiovascular magnetic resonance in patients with myocardial infarction. *J Am Coll Cardiol*. 2010;55:1–16.

Kurt M, Shaikh KA, Peterson L, et al. Impact of contrast echocardiography on evaluation of ventricular function and clinical management in a large prospective cohort. *J Am Coll Cardiol*. 2009;53:802–810.

Min JK, Shaw LJ, Berman DS. The present state of coronary computed tomographic angiography. *J Am Coll Cardiol*. 2010;55:957–965.

Otto CM. *Textbook of Clinical Echocardiography*. 4th ed. Philadelphia, PA: Elsevier Saunders; 2009.

Pennell DJ. Cardiovascular magnetic resonance. *Circulation*. 2010;121:692–705.

Perrino AC, Reeves ST. *A Practical Approach to Transesophageal Echocardiography*. 2nd ed. Philadelphia, PA: Lippincott Williams & Wilkins; 2008.

Schuijf JD, van Werkhoven JM, Pundziute G, et al. Invasive versus noninvasive evaluation of coronary artery disease. *JACC Cardiovasc Imaging*. 2008;1:190–199.

The Electrocardiogram

Stephen R. Pomedli
Leonard S. Lilly

Cardiac contraction relies on the organized flow of electrical impulses through the heart. The electrocardiogram (ECG) is an easily obtained recording of that activity and provides a wealth of information about cardiac structure and function. This chapter presents the electrical basis of the ECG in health and disease and leads the reader through the basics of interpretation. To become fully adept at this technique and to practice the principles described here, you may wish to consult one of the complete electrocardiographic textbooks listed at the end of this chapter.

ELECTRICAL MEASUREMENT—SINGLE-CELL MODEL

This section begins by observing the propagation of an electrical impulse along a single cardiac muscle cell, illustrated in Figure 4.1. On the right side of the diagram, a voltmeter records the electrical potential at the cell's surface on graph paper. In the resting state, the cell is polarized; that is, the entire outside of the cell is electrically positive with respect to the inside, because of the ionic distribution across the cell membrane, as described in Chapter 1. In this resting state, the voltmeter electrodes, which are placed on opposite outside surfaces of the cell, do not record any electrical activity, because there is no electrical potential difference between them (the myocyte surface is homogeneously charged).

This equilibrium is disturbed, however, when the cell is stimulated (see Fig. 4.1B). During the action potential, cations rush across the sarcolemma into the cell and the polarity at the stimulated region transiently reverses such that the outside becomes negatively charged with respect to the inside; that is, the region **depolarizes**. At that moment, an electrical potential is created on the cell surface between the depolarized area (negatively charged surface) and the still-polarized (positively charged surface) portions of the cell. As a result, an electrical current begins to flow between these two regions.

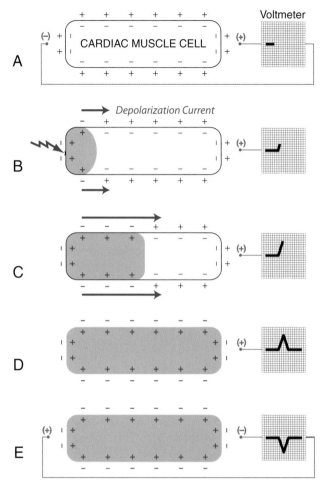

Figure 4.1. Depolarization of a single cardiac muscle cell. A. In the resting state, the surface of the cell is positively charged relative to the inside. Because the surface is homogeneously charged, the voltmeter electrodes outside the cell do not record any electrical potential difference ("flat line" recording). **B.** Stimulation of the cell initiates depolarization (shaded area); the outside of the depolarized region becomes negatively charged relative to the inside. Because the current of depolarization is directed toward the (+) electrode of the voltmeter, an upward deflection is recorded. **C.** Depolarization spreads, creating a greater upward deflection by the recording electrode. **D.** The cell has become fully depolarized. The surface of the cell is now completely negatively charged compared with the inside. Because the surface is again homogeneously charged, a flat line is recorded by the voltmeter. **E.** Notice that if the position of the voltmeter electrodes had been reversed, the electrical current would have been directed away from the (+) electrode, causing the deflection to be downward.

By convention, the direction of an electrical current is said to flow from areas that are negatively charged to those that are positively charged. When a depolarization current is directed toward the (+) electrode of the voltmeter, an *upward* deflection is recorded. Conversely, if it is directed away from the (+) electrode, a *downward* deflection is recorded.

Because the depolarization current in this example proceeds from left to right—that is, toward the (+) electrode—an upward deflection is recorded by the voltmeter. As the wave of depolarization propagates rightward along the cell, additional electrical forces directed toward the (+) electrode record an even greater upward deflection (see Fig. 4.1C). Once the cell has become fully depolarized (see Fig. 4.1D), its outside is completely negatively charged with respect to the inside, the opposite of the initial resting condition. However, because the surface charge is homogeneous once again, the external electrodes measure a potential difference of zero and the voltmeter records a neutral "flat line" at this time.

Note that in Figure 4.1E, if the voltmeter electrode positions had been reversed, such that the (+) pole was placed to the *left* of the cell, then as the wave of depolarization proceeds toward the right, the current would be directed *away* from the (+) electrode and the recorded deflection would be *downward*. This relationship should be kept in mind when the polarity of ECG leads is described below.

Depolarization initiates myocyte contraction and is then followed by **repolarization**, the process by which the cellular charges return to the resting state. In Figure 4.2, as

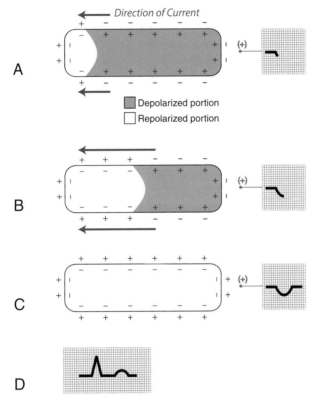

Figure 4.2. Sequence of repolarization of a single cardiac muscle cell. A. As repolarization commences, positive charges reemerge on the surface of the cell, and a current flows from the still negatively charged surface areas to the repolarized region (blue arrows). Because the current is directed away from the (+) electrode of the voltmeter, a downward deflection is recorded. **B.** Repolarization progresses. **C.** Repolarization has completed, and the outside surface of the cell is once again homogeneously charged, so that no further electrical potential is detected (flat line once again). **D.** Sequence of cardiac depolarization and repolarization as measured by an ECG machine at the skin surface. As described in the text, repolarization actually proceeds in the direction *opposite* to that of depolarization in the intact heart, such that the deflections of repolarization are inverted compared to the schematics presented in parts **A–C** of this figure. Therefore, *the deflections of depolarization and repolarization of the normal heart are oriented in the same direction.* Note that the wave of repolarization is more prolonged and of lower amplitude than that of depolarization.

the left side of the cardiac muscle cell in our example begins to repolarize, its surface charge becomes positive once again. An electrical potential is therefore generated and current flows from the still negatively charged surface toward the positively charged region. Since this current is directed away from the voltmeter's (+) electrode, a downward deflection is recorded, opposite to that which was observed during the process of depolarization.

Repolarization is a slower process than depolarization, so the inscribed deflection of repolarization is usually wider and of lower magnitude. Once the cell has returned to the resting state, the surface charges are once again homogeneous and no further electrical potential is detected, resulting in a neutral flat line on the voltmeter recording (see Fig. 4.2C).

The depolarization and repolarization of a single cardiac muscle cell have been considered here. As a wave of depolarization spreads through the entire heart, each cell generates electrical forces, and it is the sum of these forces, measured at the skin's surface, that is recorded by the ECG machine.

It is important to note that in the intact heart the sequence by which regions repolarize is actually *opposite* to that of their depolarization. This occurs because myocardial action potential durations are more prolonged in cells near the inner endocardium (the first cells stimulated by Purkinje fibers) than in myocytes near the outer epicardium (the last

cells to depolarize). Thus, the cells close to the endocardium are the first to depolarize but are the last to repolarize. As a result, the direction of repolarization recorded by the ECG machine is usually the *inverse* of what was presented in the single cell example in Figure 4.2. That is, unlike the single cell model, the electrical deflections of depolarization and repolarization in the intact heart are usually oriented in the *same* direction on the ECG tracing (see Fig. 4.2D).

The direction and magnitude of the deflections on an ECG recording depend on how the generated electrical forces are aligned to a set of specific reference axes, known as ECG leads, as described in the next section.

ELECTROCARDIOGRAPHIC LEAD REFERENCE SYSTEM

When the first device to produce an ECG was invented over a century ago, the recording was made by dunking the patient's arms and legs into large buckets of electrolyte solution that were wired to the machine. That process was likely fairly messy and fortunately is no longer necessary. Instead, wire electrodes are placed directly on the skin, held in place by adhesive tabs, on each of the four limbs and on the chest in the standard arrangement shown in Figure 4.3. The right-leg electrode is not used for the measurement but serves as an electrical ground. Table 4.1 lists the standard locations of the chest electrodes.

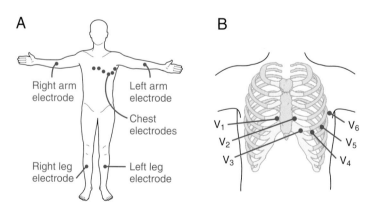

A

Right arm electrode

Left arm electrode

Chest electrodes

Right leg electrode

Left leg electrode

B

V_1

V_2

V_3

V_6

V_5

V_4

Figure 4.3. Placement of electrocardiogram (ECG) electrodes. A. Standard positions. **B.** Close-up view of chest electrode placement, at the standard positions listed in Table 4.1.

Table 4.1. Positions of ECG Chest Electrodes

V_1	4th ICS, 2 cm to the right of sternum
V_2	4th ICS, 2 cm to the left of sternum
V_3	Midway between V_2 and V_4
V_4	5th ICS, left midclavicular line
V_5	5th ICS, left anterior axillary line
V_6	5th ICS, left midaxillary line

ICS, intercostal space.

A complete ECG (termed a "12-lead ECG") is produced by recording electrical activity between the electrodes in specific patterns. This results in six reference axes in the body's frontal plane (termed *limb leads*) plus six in the transverse plane (termed *chest leads*). Figure 4.4 demonstrates the orientation of the six limb leads, which are electronically constructed as described in the following paragraphs.

The ECG machine records lead **aVR** by selecting the right-arm electrode as the (+) pole with respect to the other electrodes. This is known as a **unipolar** lead, because there is no single (−) pole; rather, the other limb electrodes are averaged to create a composite (−) reference. When the instantaneous electrical activity of the heart points in the direction of the right arm, an upward deflection is recorded in lead aVR. Conversely, when electrical forces are directed away from the right arm, the ECG inscribes a downward deflection in aVR.

Similarly, lead **aVF** is recorded by setting the left leg as the (+) pole, such that a positive deflection is recorded when forces are directed toward the feet. Lead **aVL** is selected when the left-arm electrode is made the (+) pole and it records an upward deflection when electrical activity is aimed in that direction.

In addition to these three unipolar leads, three **bipolar** limb leads are part of the standard ECG recording (see Fig. 4.4). Bipolar indicates that one limb electrode is the (+) pole and another single electrode provides

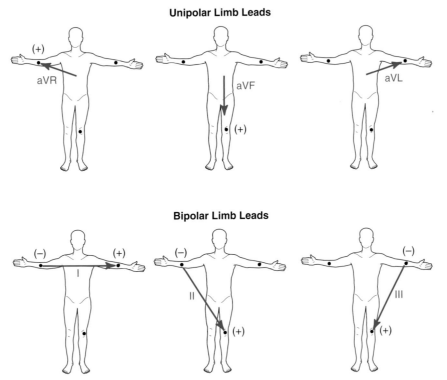

Unipolar Limb Leads

Bipolar Limb Leads

Figure 4.4. The six limb leads are derived from the electrodes placed on the arms and left leg. **Top,** Each unipolar lead has a single (+) designated electrode; the (−) pole is an average of the other electrodes. **Bottom,** Each bipolar lead has specific (−) and (+) designated electrodes.

Table 4.2. Limb Leads		
Lead	*(+) Electrode*	*(−) Electrode*
Bipolar leads		
I	LA	RA
II	LL	RA
III	LL	LA
Unipolar leads		
aVR	RA	a
aVL	LA	a
aVF	LL	a

a(−) Electrode constructed by combining other limb electrodes.
LA, left arm; LL, left leg; RA, right arm.

the (−) reference. In this case, the ECG machine inscribes an upward deflection if electrical forces are heading toward the (+) electrode and records a downward deflection if the forces are heading toward the (−) electrode. A simple mnemonic to remember the orientation of the bipolar leads is that the lead name indicates the number of *l*'s in the placement sites. For example, lead I connects the *l*eft arm to the right arm, lead II connects the right arm to the *l*eft *l*eg, and lead III connects the *l*eft arm to the *l*eft *l*eg. Table 4.2 summarizes how the six limb leads are derived.

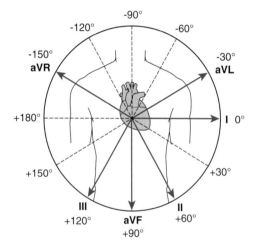

Figure 4.5. The axial reference system is created by combining the six limb leads shown in Figure 4.4. Each lead has a (+) region indicated by the arrowhead and a (−) region indicated by the dashed line.

By overlaying these six limb leads, an axial reference system is established (Fig. 4.5). In the figure, each lead is presented with its (+) pole designated by an arrowhead and the (−) aspect by dashed lines. Note that each 30° sector of the circle falls along the (+) or (−) pole of one of the standard six ECG limb leads. Also note that the (+) pole of lead I points to 0° and that, by convention, measurement of the angles proceeds clockwise from 0° as +30°, +60°, and so forth. The complete ECG recording provides a simultaneous "snapshot" of the heart's electrical activity, taken from the perspective of each of these lead reference axes.

Figure 4.6 demonstrates how the magnitude and direction of electrical activity are represented by the ECG recording in each lead. This figure should be studied until the following four points are clear:

1. An electrical force directed toward the (+) pole of a lead results in an upward deflection on the ECG recording of that lead.
2. Forces that head away from the (+) electrode result in a downward deflection in that lead.
3. The magnitude of the deflection, either upward or downward, reflects how parallel the electrical force is to the axis of the lead being examined. The more parallel the electrical force is to the lead, the greater the magnitude of the deflection.
4. An electrical force directed perpendicular to an electrocardiographic lead does not register any activity by that lead (a flat line on the recording).

The six standard limb leads examine the electrical forces in the frontal plane of the body. However, because electrical activity travels in three dimensions, recordings from a perpendicular plane are also essential (Fig. 4.7A). This is accomplished by the use of the six electrodes placed on the anterior and left lateral aspect of the chest (see Fig. 4.3B), creating the chest (also termed "precordial") leads. The orientation of these leads around the heart in the cross-sectional plane is shown in Figure 4.7B. These are unipolar leads and, as with the unipolar

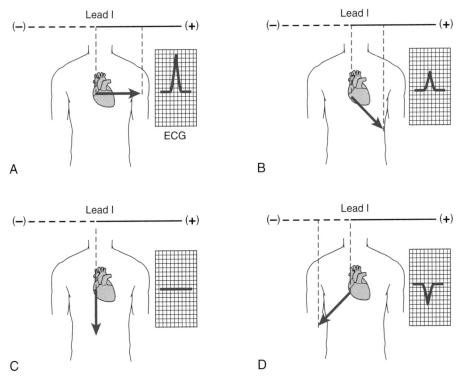

Figure 4.6. Relationship of the magnitude and direction of electrical activity to the ECG lead. A. The electrical vector is oriented parallel to lead I and directed toward the (+) electrode; therefore, a tall upward deflection is recorded by the lead. **B.** The vector is still oriented toward the (+) electrode of lead I but not parallel to the lead, so that only a component of the force is recorded. Thus, the recorded deflection is still upward but of lower amplitude compared with that shown in **A. C.** The electrical vector is perpendicular to lead I so that no deflection is generated. **D.** The vector is directed toward the (−) region of lead I, causing the ECG to record a downward deflection.

limb leads, electrical forces directed *toward* these individual (+) electrodes result in an upward deflection on the recording of that lead, and forces heading *away* record a downward deflection.

A complete ECG prints samples from each of the six limb leads and each of the six chest leads in a standard order, examples of which are presented later in this chapter (see Figs. 4.28–4.36).

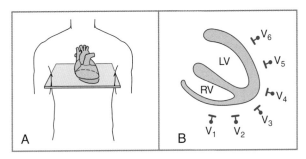

Figure 4.7. The chest (precordial) leads. A. The cross-sectional plane of the chest. **B.** Arrangement of the six chest electrodes shown in the cross-sectional plane. Note that the right ventricle is anterior to the left ventricle.

SEQUENCE OF NORMAL CARDIAC ACTIVATION

Conduction of electrical impulses through the heart is an orderly process. The normal beat begins at the sinoatrial node, located at the junction of the right atrium and the superior vena cava (Fig. 4.8). The wave of depolarization spreads rapidly through the right and left atria and then reaches the atrioventricular (AV) node, where it encounters an expected delay. The impulse then travels rapidly through the bundle of His and into the right and left bundle branches. These divide into the Purkinje fibers, which radiate toward the myocardial fibers, stimulating them to depolarize and contract.

Each heartbeat is represented on the ECG by three major deflections that record the sequence of electrical propagation (see Fig. 4.8B). The **P wave** represents depolarization of the atria.

Following the P wave, the tracing returns to its baseline as a result of the conduction delay at the AV node. The second deflection of the ECG, the **QRS complex**, represents depolarization of the ventricular muscle cells. After the QRS complex, the tracing returns to baseline once again, and after a brief delay, repolarization of the ventricular cells is signaled by the **T wave**. Occasionally, an additional small deflection follows the T wave (the **U wave**), which is believed to represent late phases of ventricular repolarization.

The QRS complex may take one of several shapes but can always be subdivided into individual components (Fig. 4.9). If the first deflection of the QRS complex is *downward*, it is known as a Q wave. However, if the initial deflection is upward, then that particular complex *does not have a Q wave.* The R wave is defined as the first *upward* deflection, whether or not a Q wave is present. Any downward

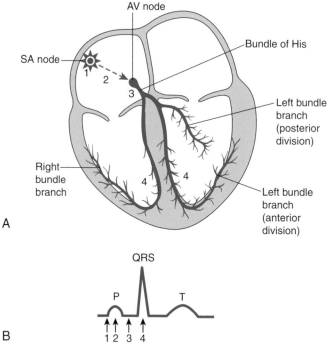

Figure 4.8. Cardiac conduction pathway. A. The electrical impulse begins at the sinoatrial (SA) node (1) then traverses the atria (2). After a delay at the AV node (3), conduction continues through the bundle of His and into the right and left bundle branches (4). The latter divide into Purkinje fibers, which stimulate contraction of the myocardial cells. **B.** Corresponding waveforms on the ECG recording: (1) the SA node discharges (too small to generate any deflection on ECG), (2) P wave inscribed by depolarization of the atria, (3) delay at the AV node, and (4) depolarization of the ventricles (QRS complex). The T wave represents ventricular repolarization.

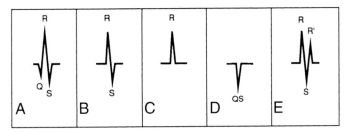

Figure 4.9. **Examples of QRS complexes. A.** The first deflection is downward (Q wave), followed by an upward deflection (R wave), and then another downward wave (S wave). **B.** Because the first deflection is upward, this complex does *not* have a Q wave; rather, the downward deflection *after* the R wave is an S wave. **C.** A QRS complex without downward deflections lacks Q and S waves. **D.** QRS composed of only a downward deflection; this is a Q wave but is often referred to as a QS complex. **E.** A second upward deflection (seen in bundle branch blocks) is referred to as R′.

deflection *following* the R wave is known as an S wave. Figure 4.9 demonstrates several common variations of the QRS complex. In certain pathologic states, such as bundle branch blocks, additional deflections may be inscribed, as shown in the figure. Please study Figure 4.9 until you can confidently differentiate a Q from an S wave.

Figure 4.10 illustrates the course of normal ventricular depolarization as it is recorded by two of the ECG leads: aVF and aVL. The recording in aVF represents electrical activity from the perspective of the inferior (i.e., underside) aspect of the heart, and aVL records from the perspective of the left lateral side. Recall that in the resting state, the surfaces of myocardial cells are homogeneously charged such that no electrical activity is detected by the external ECG leads and zero voltage is recorded by the machine.

The initial portion of ventricular myocardium that is stimulated to depolarize with each cardiac cycle is the midportion of the interventricular septum, on the left side. Because depolarization reverses the cellular charge, the surface of that region becomes negative with respect to the inside, and an electrical potential is generated (see Fig. 4.10B, arrow). The initial current is directed toward the right ventricle and inferiorly. Because the force is directed *away* from the (+) pole region of lead aVL, an initial *downward* deflection is recorded in that lead. At the same time, the electrical force is directed *toward* the (+) pole region of lead aVF, causing an initial *upward*

deflection to be recorded there. As the wave of depolarization spreads through the ventricular myocardium, the progression of net electrical vectors is depicted by the series of arrows in Figure 4.10.

As the lateral walls of the ventricles are depolarized, the forces of the thicker left side outweigh those of the right. Therefore, the arrow's orientation is increasingly directed toward the left ventricle (leftward and posteriorly). At the completion of depolarization, the myocytes are again homogeneously charged, no further net electrical force is generated, and the ECG voltage recording returns to baseline in both leads. Thus, in this example of depolarization in a normal heart, lead aVL inscribes an initial small Q wave followed by a tall R wave. Conversely, in lead aVF, there is an initial upward deflection (R wave) followed by a downward S wave.

The sequence of ventricular depolarization in the horizontal plane of the body is evident on examining the six chest leads (Fig. 4.11). Once again, recall that the first region to depolarize is the midportion of the interventricular septum on the left side. Depolarization proceeds from there toward the right ventricle (which is anterior to the left ventricle), then toward the cardiac apex, and finally around the lateral walls of both ventricles. Because the initial forces are directed anteriorly—that is, toward the (+) pole of V_1—the initial deflection recorded by lead V_1 is upward. These same initial forces are directed away from V_6 (which overlies the lateral wall of the left ventricle),

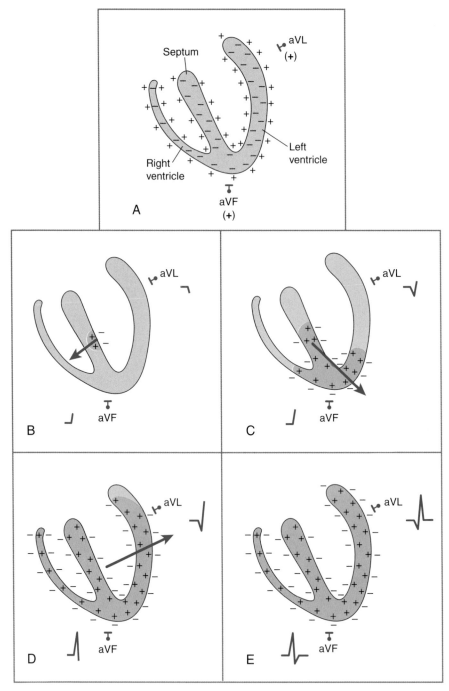

Figure 4.10. Normal ventricular depolarization as recorded by leads aVL and aVF. A. In the resting state, the surface is homogeneously charged so that the leads do not record any electrical potential. **B.** The first area to depolarize is the left side of the ventricular septum. This results in forces heading away from aVL (downward deflection on aVL recording) but toward the (+) region of aVF, such that an upward deflection is recorded by that lead. **C** and **D.** Depolarization continues; the forces from the thicker-walled left ventricle outweigh those of the right, such that the electrical vector swings leftward and posteriorly toward aVL (upward deflection) and away from aVF. **E.** At the completion of depolarization, the surface is again homogeneously charged, and no further electrical forces are recorded.

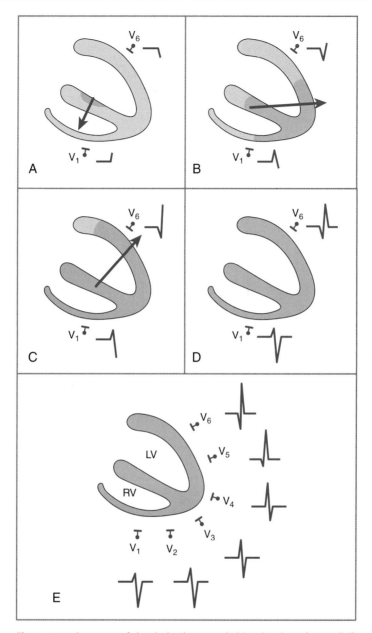

Figure 4.11. Sequence of depolarization recorded by the chest (precordial) leads. A–D. Depolarization begins at the left side of the septum. The electrical vector then progresses posteriorly toward the thick-walled left ventricle. Thus, V_1, which is an anterior lead, records an initial upward deflection followed by a downward wave, whereas V_6, a posterior lead, inscribes the opposite. **E.** In the normal pattern of the QRS from V_1 to V_6, the R wave becomes progressively taller and the S wave less deep.

so an initial downward deflection is recorded there. As the wave of depolarization spreads, the forces of the left ventricle outweigh those of the right, and the vector swings posteriorly toward the bulk of the left ventricular muscle. As the forces swing away from lead V_1, the

deflection there becomes *downward*, whereas it becomes more *upright* in lead V_6. Leads V_2 through V_5 record intermediate steps in this process, such that the R wave becomes progressively taller from lead V_1 through lead V_6 (see Fig. 4.11E), a pattern known as "R wave progression." Typically, the height of the R wave becomes greater than the depth of the S wave in lead V_3 or V_4; the lead in which this occurs is termed the "transition" lead.

INTERPRETATION OF THE ELECTROCARDIOGRAM

From a technical standpoint, the ECG is recorded on a special grid divided into lines spaced 1 mm apart in both the horizontal and the vertical directions. Each fifth line is made heavier to facilitate measurement. On the vertical axis, voltage is measured in millivolts (mV), and in the standard case, each 1-mm line separation represents 0.1 mV. The horizontal axis represents time. Because the standard recording speed is 25 mm/sec, each 1 mm division represents 0.04 sec and each heavy line (5 mm) represents 0.2 sec (Fig. 4.12).

Many cardiac disorders alter the ECG recording in a diagnostically useful way, and it is important to interpret each tracing in a standard fashion to avoid missing subtle abnormalities. Here is a commonly followed sequence of analysis, followed by a description of each:

1. Check voltage calibration
2. Heart rhythm
3. Heart rate
4. Intervals (PR, QRS, QT)
5. Mean QRS axis
6. Abnormalities of the P wave
7. Abnormalities of the QRS (hypertrophy, bundle branch block, infarction)
8. Abnormalities of the ST segment and T wave

Calibration

ECG machines routinely inscribe a 1.0-mV vertical signal at the beginning or end of each 12-lead tracing to document the voltage calibration of the machine. In the normal case, each 1-mm vertical box on the ECG paper represents 0.1 mV, so that the calibration signal records a 10-mm deflection (e.g., as shown later in Fig. 4.28). However, in patients with markedly

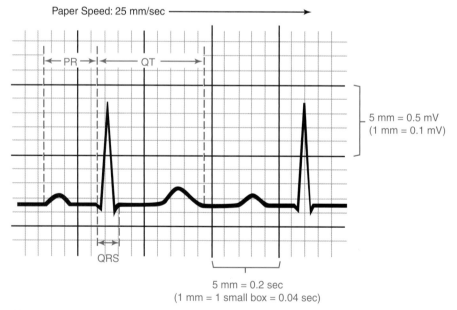

Figure 4.12. **Enlarged view of an ECG strip.** The paper travels through the machine at 25 mm/sec, so that each 1 mm on the horizontal axis represents 0.04 sec. Each 1 mm on the vertical axis represents 0.1 mV. Measurements in this example are as follows: PR interval (from the beginning of the P wave to the beginning of the QRS) = 4 small boxes = 0.16 sec; QRS duration (from the beginning to the end of the QRS complex) = 1.75 small boxes = 0.07 sec; and QT interval (from the beginning of the QRS to the end of the T wave) = 8 small boxes = 0.32 sec. The corrected QT interval = $\frac{QT}{\sqrt{R-R}}$. Because the R–R interval = 15 small boxes (0.6 sec), the corrected QT interval = $\frac{0.32}{\sqrt{0.6}}$ = 0.41 sec.

increased voltage of the QRS complex (e.g., some patients with left ventricular hypertrophy or bundle branch blocks), the very large deflections do not fit on the standard tracing. To facilitate interpretation in such a case, the recording is often purposely made at half the standard voltage (i.e., each 1-mm box = 0.2 mV), and this is indicated on the ECG tracing by a change in the height of the 1.0-mV calibration signal (at half the standard voltage, the signal would be 5 mm tall). It is important to check the height of the calibration signal on each ECG to ensure that the voltage criteria used to define specific abnormalities are applicable.

Heart Rhythm

The normal cardiac rhythm, initiated by depolarization of the sinus node, is known as **sinus rhythm** and is present if (1) every P wave is followed by a QRS; (2) every QRS is preceded by a P wave; (3) the P wave is upright in leads I, II, and III; and (4) the PR interval is greater than 0.12 sec (3 small boxes). If the heart rate in sinus rhythm is between 60 and 100 bpm, then **normal sinus rhythm** is present. If less than 60 bpm, the rhythm is **sinus bradycardia;** if greater than 100 bpm, the rhythm is **sinus tachycardia**. Other abnormal rhythms (termed *arrhythmias* or *dysrhythmias*) are described in Chapters 11 and 12.

Heart Rate

The standard ECG paper speed is 25 mm/sec. Therefore,

$$\text{Heart rate (bpm)} = \frac{25 \text{ mm/sec} \times 60 \text{ sec/min}}{\text{Number of mm between beats}}$$

or more simply, as shown in Figure 4.13:

$$\text{Heart rate (bpm)} = \frac{1,500}{\text{Number of small boxes between two consecutive beats}}$$

It is rarely necessary, however, to determine the *exact* heart rate, and a more rapid determination can be made with just a bit of memorization. Simply "count off" the number of large boxes between two consecutive QRS complexes, using the sequence

300—150—100—75—60—50

which corresponds to the heart rate in beats per minute, as illustrated in Figure 4.13 (Method 2).

When the rhythm is *irregular*, the heart rate may be approximated by counting the number of complexes during 6 sec of the recording and multiplying that number by 10. ECG paper often has time markers, spaced 3 sec apart, printed at the top or bottom of the tracing that facilitates this measurement (see Fig. 4.13, Method 3).

Intervals (PR, QRS, QT)

The PR interval, QRS interval, and QT interval are measured as demonstrated in Figure 4.12. For each of these, it is appropriate to take the measurement in the lead in which the interval is the longest in duration (the intervals can vary a bit in each lead). The **PR interval** is measured from the onset of the P wave to the onset of the QRS. The **QRS interval** is measured from the beginning to the end of the QRS complex. The **QT interval** is measured from the beginning of the QRS to the end of the T wave. The normal ranges of the intervals are listed in Table 4.3, along with conditions associated with abnormal values.

Because the QT interval varies with heart rate (the faster the heart rate, the shorter the QT), the **corrected QT interval** is determined by dividing the measured QT by the square root of the R−R interval (see Fig. 4.12). When the heart rate is in the normal range (60 to 100 bpm), a rapid visual rule can be applied: if the QT interval is less than half the interval between two consecutive QRS complexes, then the QT interval is within the normal range.

Mean QRS Axis

The mean QRS axis represents the average of the instantaneous electrical forces generated during the sequence of ventricular depolarization as measured in the frontal plane. The normal value is between −30° and +90° (Fig. 4.14). A mean axis that is more negative than −30° implies **left axis deviation**, whereas an axis greater than +90° represents **right axis deviation**. The mean axis can be determined precisely by plotting the QRS complexes of

| Method 1 | First, count the number of small boxes (1 mm each) between two adjacent QRS complexes (i.e., between 2 "beats"). Then, since the standard paper speed is 25 mm/sec:

$$\text{Heart Rate (beats/min)} = \frac{(25 \text{ mm/sec} \times 60 \text{ sec/min})}{\text{Number of mm between beats}} = \frac{1{,}500}{\text{number of mm between beats}}$$

In this example, there are 23 mm between the first 2 beats.

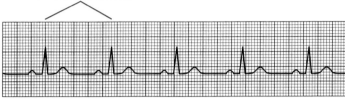

23 mm between beats

Therefore, the heart rate $= \dfrac{1{,}500}{23} = 65$ bpm

Method 1 is particularly helpful for measuring fast heart rates (>100 bpm)

| Method 2 | The "count-off" method requires memorizing the sequence:

300—150—100—75—60—50

Then use this sequence to count the number of large boxes between two consecutive beats:

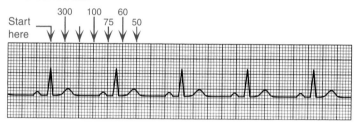

The second QRS falls between 75 and 60 bpm; therefore, the heart rate is approximately midway between them ~67 bpm. Knowing that the heart rate is approximately 60–70 bpm is certainly close enough.

| Method 3 | ECG recording paper often indicates 3-sec time markers at the top or bottom of the tracing:

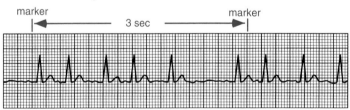

To calculate the heart rate, count the number of QRS complexes between the 3-sec markers (= 6 beats in this example) and multiply by 20. Thus, the heart rate here is approximately 120 bpm.

It's even easier (and more accurate) to count the number of complexes between the first and third markers on the strip (representing 6 sec of the recording) and then multiply by 10 to determine the heart rate.

Method 3 is particularly helpful for measuring irregular heart rates.

Figure 4.13. **Methods to calculate heart rate.**

Table 4.3. Electrocardiographic Intervals

Interval	Normal	Decreased Interval	Increased Interval
PR	0.12–0.20 sec (3–5 small boxes)	• Preexcitation syndrome • Junctional rhythm	• First-degree AV block
QRS	≤0.10 sec (≤2.5 small boxes)		• Bundle branch blocks • Ventricular ectopic beat • Toxic drug effect (e.g., certain antiarrhythmic drugs—see Chapter 17) • Severe hyperkalemia
QT	Corrected QT[a] ≤0.44 sec	• Hypercalcemia • Tachycardia	• Hypocalcemia • Hypokalemia (↑ QU interval owing to ↑ U wave) • Hypomagnesemia • Myocardial ischemia • Congenital prolongation of QT • Toxic drug effect (e.g., certain antiarrhythmic drugs—see Chapter 17)

[a]Corrected QT $= \dfrac{QT}{\sqrt{R-R}}$.

different leads on the axial reference diagram for the limb leads (see Fig. 4.5), but this is tedious and is rarely necessary. The following rapid approach to axis determination generally provides sufficient accuracy.

First, recall from Figure 4.5 that each ECG lead has a (+) region and a (−) region. Electrical activity directed toward the (+) half results in an upward deflection, whereas activity toward the (−) half results in a downward

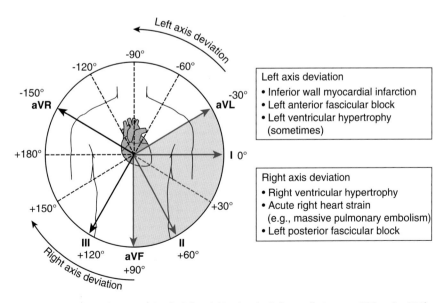

Figure 4.14. A normal mean QRS axis falls within the shaded area (between −30° and +90°). A mean axis more negative than −30° is termed *left axis deviation*, whereas an axis more positive than +90° is *right axis deviation*. The figure shows common conditions that result in axis deviation.

deflection on the ECG recording of that lead. To determine whether the axis is normal or abnormal, examine the QRS complexes in limb leads I and II. As illustrated in Figure 4.15, if the QRS is primarily positive in both of these leads (i.e., the upward deflection is greater than the downward deflection in each of them), then the mean vector falls within the normal range and no further calculation is necessary. However, if the QRS in *either* lead I or II is not primarily upward, then the axis is *abnormal*, and the approximate axis should then be determined by the more precise method described in the following paragraphs. Please be aware that some other books recommend examining leads I and aVF, rather than leads I and II, to determine whether the mean axis falls in the normal range. However, using leads I and aVF for this purpose would erroneously classify a mean axis between 0° and −30° as being abnormal.

In order to determine the mean axis with greater precision when necessary, first consider the special example in Figure 4.16. The sequence of a ventricular depolarization is represented in this figure by vectors *a* through *e*, along with the corresponding deflections on the ECG recording of lead I.

If the QRS complex is mainly upward in limb lead I, then the mean axis falls within the "+" region of that lead, shown as the shaded half of the circle below.

Similarly, if the QRS is predominantly upward in limb lead II, then the mean axis falls within the "+" half of lead II, shown as the shaded half here:

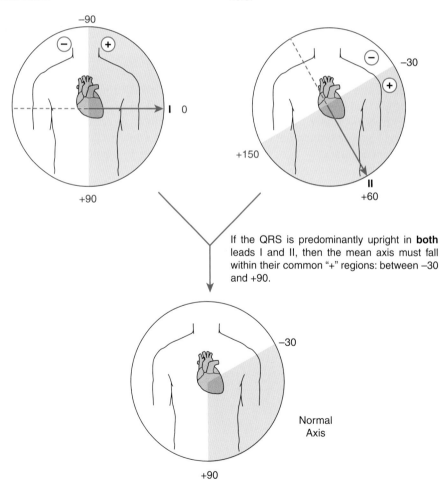

If the QRS is predominantly upright in **both** leads I and II, then the mean axis must fall within their common "+" regions: between −30 and +90.

Figure 4.15. **The mean axis is within the normal range if the QRS complex is predominantly upright in limb leads I and II.**

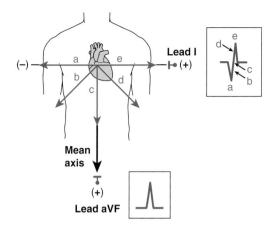

Figure 4.16. Sequence of ventricular depolarization when the mean axis is +90°. Because the mean axis is perpendicular to limb lead I, an isoelectric QRS complex (height of upward deflection = height of downward deflection) is recorded by that lead (see text for details).

The initial deflection (representing left septal depolarization) points to the patient's right side. Because it is directed completely away from the (+) pole of lead I, a strong downward deflection is recorded by the lead. As depolarization continues, the arrow swings downward and to the left, resulting in less negative deflections in lead I. After arrow c, the electrical vector swings into the positive region of lead I, so that upward deflections are recorded.

In this special example, in which electrical forces begin exactly opposite lead I's (+) electrode and terminate when pointed directly at that electrode, note that the mean electrical vector points straight downward (in the direction of arrow c), *perpendicular* to the lead I axis. Also note the configuration of the inscribed QRS complex in lead I. There is a downward deflection, followed by an upward deflection of equal magnitude (when the upward and downward deflections of a QRS are of equal magnitude, it is termed an **isoelectric complex**). Thus, *when an ECG limb lead inscribes an isoelectric QRS complex, it indicates that the mean electrical axis of the ventricles is perpendicular to that particular lead.*

Therefore, an easy way to determine the mean QRS axis is to glance at the six limb lead recordings and observe which one has the most isoelectric-appearing complex: the mean axis is simply perpendicular to it. One step remains. When the mean axis is perpendicular to a lead, it could be perpendicular in either a clockwise *or* a counterclockwise direction. In the example of Figure 4.16, the isoelectric complex appears in lead I, such that the mean vector could be at +90° *or* it could be at −90°, because both are perpendicular. To determine which of these is correct requires inspecting the recording of the ECG lead that is perpendicular to the one inscribing the isoelectric complex (and is therefore parallel to the mean axis). If the QRS is predominantly upright in that perpendicular lead, then the mean vector points toward the (+) pole of that lead. If it is predominantly negative, then it points away from the lead's (+) pole. In the example, the isoelectric complex appears in lead I; therefore, the next step is to inspect the perpendicular lead, which is aVF (see Fig. 4.5 if this relationship is not clear). Because the QRS complex in aVF is primarily upward, the mean axis points toward its (+) pole, which is in fact located at +90°.

To summarize, the mean QRS axis is calculated as follows:

1. Inspect limb leads I and II. If the QRS is primarily upward in both, then the axis is normal and you are done. If not, then proceed to the next step.

2. Inspect the six limb leads and determine which one contains the QRS that is most isoelectric. The mean axis is perpendicular to that lead.

3. Inspect the lead that is perpendicular to the lead containing the isoelectric complex. If the QRS in that perpendicular lead is primarily upward, then the mean axis points to the (+) pole of that lead. If primarily negative, then the mean QRS points to the (−) pole of that lead.

Conditions that result in left or right axis deviation are listed in Figure 4.14. In addition, the vertical position of the heart in many normal children and adolescents may result in a mean axis that is slightly rightward (>+90°).

In some patients, isoelectric complexes are inscribed in *all* the limb leads. That situation arises when the heart is tilted, so that the mean

QRS points straight forward or back from the frontal plane, as it may be in patients with chronic obstructive lung disease; in such a case, the mean axis is said to be *indeterminate*.

Abnormalities of the P Wave

The P wave represents depolarization of the right atrium followed quickly by the depolarization of the left atrium; the two components are nearly superimposed on one another (Fig. 4.17). The P wave is usually best visualized in lead II, the lead that is most parallel to the flow of electrical current through the atria from the sinoatrial to the AV node. When the *right* atrium is enlarged, the initial component of the P wave is larger than normal (the P is taller than 2.5 mm in lead II).

Left atrial enlargement is best observed in lead V_1. Normally, V_1 inscribes a P wave with an initial positive deflection reflecting right atrial depolarization (directed anteriorly), followed by a negative deflection, owing to the left atrial forces oriented posteriorly (see Fig. 1.2 for anatomic relationships). Left atrial enlargement is therefore manifested by a greater-than-normal negative deflection (at least 1 mm wide and 1 mm deep) in lead V_1 (see Fig. 4.17).

Abnormalities of the QRS Complex

Ventricular Hypertrophy

Hypertrophy of the left or right ventricle causes the affected chamber to generate greater-than-normal electrical activity. Ordinarily, the thicker-walled left ventricle produces forces that are more prominent than those of the right. However, in **right ventricular hypertrophy**, the augmented right-sided forces may outweigh those of the left. Therefore, chest leads V_1 and V_2, which overlie the right ventricle, record greater-than-normal upward deflections: the R wave becomes taller than the S wave in those leads, the opposite of the normal situation (Fig. 4.18). In addition, the increased right ventricular mass shifts the mean axis of the heart, resulting in right axis deviation (mean axis $>+90°$).

In **left ventricular hypertrophy**, greater-than-normal forces are generated by that chamber, which simply exaggerates the normal situation. Leads that directly overlie the left ventricle (chest leads V_5 and V_6 and limb leads I and aVL) show taller-than-normal R waves. Leads on the other side of the heart (V_1 and V_2) demonstrate the opposite: deeper-than-normal

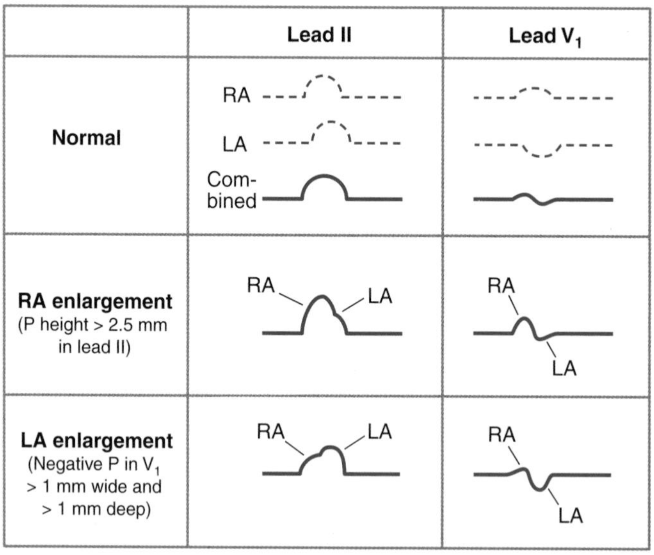

	Lead II	Lead V$_1$
Normal	RA LA Combined	
RA enlargement (P height > 2.5 mm in lead II)	RA LA	RA LA
LA enlargement (Negative P in V$_1$ > 1 mm wide and > 1 mm deep)	RA LA	RA LA

Figure 4.17. The P wave represents superimposition of right atrial (RA) and left atrial (LA) depolarization. RA depolarization occurs slightly earlier than LA depolarization. In RA enlargement, the initial component of the P wave is prominent (>2.5 mm tall) in lead II. In LA enlargement, there is a large terminal downward deflection in lead V_1 (>1 mm wide and >1 mm deep).

A

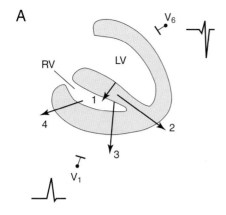

RIGHT VENTRICULAR HYPERTROPHY

• R > S in lead V₁
• Right axis deviation

B

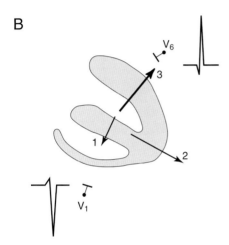

LEFT VENTRICULAR HYPERTROPHY

• S in V₁ *plus*
  R in V₅ or V₆ ≥ 35 mm *or*
• R in aVL > 11 mm *or*
• R in lead I > 15 mm

Figure 4.18. **Ventricular hypertrophy.** The arrows indicate the sequence of average electrical forces during ventricular depolarization. **A.** Right ventricular (RV) hypertrophy. The RV forces outweigh those of the left, resulting in tall R waves in leads V_1 and V_2 and a deep S wave in lead V_6. **B.** Left ventricular (LV) hypertrophy exaggerates the normal pattern of depolarization, with greater-than-normal forces directed toward the LV, resulting in a tall R wave in V_6 and a deep S wave in lead V_1.

S waves. Many criteria have been proposed for the diagnosis of left ventricular hypertrophy by ECG. Three of the most helpful criteria are listed in Figure 4.18.

Bundle Branch Blocks

Interruption of conduction through the right or left bundle branches may develop from ischemic or degenerative damage. As a result, the affected ventricle does not depolarize in the normal sequence. Rather than rapid uniform stimulation by the Purkinje fibers, the cells of that ventricle must rely on relatively slow myocyte-to-myocyte spread of electrical activity traveling from the unaffected ventricle. This delayed pro-

cess prolongs depolarization and widens the QRS complex. A normal QRS duration is ≤0.10 sec (≤2.5 small boxes). When a bundle branch block widens the QRS duration to 0.10–0.12 sec (2.5–3.0 small boxes), an *incomplete* bundle branch block is present. If the QRS duration is greater than 0.12 sec (3.0 small boxes), *complete* bundle branch block is identified.

In **right bundle branch block** (RBBB) (Fig. 4.19; see also Fig. 4.29), normal depolarization of the right ventricle is interrupted. In this case, initial depolarization of the ventricular septum (which is stimulated by a branch of the left bundle) is unaffected so that the normal small R wave in lead V_1 and small Q wave in lead V_6 are recorded. As the wave of depolarization

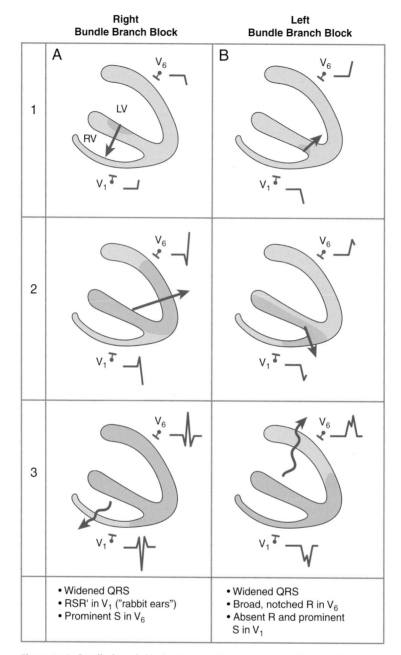

Figure 4.19. Bundle branch blocks. Interruption of conduction through the right or left bundles results in delayed, slowed activation of the respective ventricle and widening of the QRS complex. In **right bundle branch block**, normal initial activation of the septum (1) is followed by depolarization of the left ventricle (2). Slow cell-to-cell spread activates the right ventricle (RV) *after* the left ventricle (LV) has nearly fully depolarized, so that the late forces generated by the RV are unopposed. Therefore, V_1 records an abnormal terminal upward deflection (R'), and V_6 records an abnormal, terminal deep S wave (3). In **left bundle branch block**, the initial septal depolarization is blocked, such that initial forces are oriented from right to left. Thus, the normal initial R wave in V_1 and Q wave in V_6 are absent (1). After the RV depolarizes (2), late, slow activation of the LV results in a terminal upward deflection in V_6 and downward deflection in V_1 (3).

spreads down the septum and into the left ventricular free wall, the sequence of depolarization is indistinguishable from normal, because left ventricular forces *normally* outweigh those of the right. However, by the time the left ventricle has almost fully depolarized, slow cell-to-cell spread has finally reached the "blocked" right ventricle and depolarization of that chamber begins, unopposed by left ventricular activity (because that chamber has nearly fully depolarized). This prolonged depolarization process widens the QRS complex and produces a late depolarization current in the direction of the anteriorly situated right ventricle. Since the terminal portion of the QRS complex in RBBB represents these right ventricular forces acting alone, the ECG records an abnormal terminal *upward* deflection (known as R' wave) over the right ventricle in lead V_1 and a downward deflection (S wave) in V_6 on the opposite side of the heart. The appearance of the QRS complex in lead V_1 in RBBB (upward R, downward S, then upward R') is often described as having the appearance of "rabbit ears."

Left bundle branch block (LBBB) produces even more prominent QRS abnormalities. In this situation, normal initial depolarization of the left septum does *not* occur; rather, the right side of the ventricular septum is first to depolarize, through branches of the right bundle. Thus, the initial forces of depolarization are directed toward the left ventricle instead of the right (see Fig. 4.19; see also Fig. 4.30). Therefore, an initial *downward* deflection is recorded in V_1 and the normal small Q wave in V_6 is absent. Only after depolarization of the right ventricle does slow cell-to-cell spread reach the left ventricular myocytes. These slowly conducted forces inscribe a widened QRS complex with abnormal terminally upward deflections in the leads overlying the left ventricle (e.g., V_5 and V_6), as shown in Figure 4.19.

Fascicular Blocks

Recall from Chapter 1 that the left bundle branch subdivides into two main divisions, termed fascicles: the left anterior fascicle and left posterior fascicle. Although LBBB implies that conduction is blocked in the entire left bundle branch, impairment can also occur in just one of the two fascicles, resulting in left anterior or left posterior fascicular blocks (also termed *hemiblocks*). The main significance of fascicular blocks in ECG interpretation is that they can markedly alter the mean ECG axis.

Anatomically, the anterior fascicle of the left bundle runs along the front of the left ventricle toward the anterior papillary muscle (which is located in the anterior and superior portion of the chamber), whereas the posterior fascicle travels to the posterior papillary muscle (which is located in the posterior, inferior, and medial aspect of the left ventricle). Under normal conditions, conduction via the left anterior and left posterior fascicles proceeds simultaneously, such that electrical activation of the left ventricle is uniform, spreading outward from the bases of the two papillary muscles. However, if conduction is blocked in one of the two divisions, then initial LV depolarization arises exclusively from the unaffected fascicle (Fig. 4.20).

In the case of **left anterior fascicular block (LAFB),** left ventricular activation begins via the left posterior fascicle alone, at the posterior papillary muscle, and then spreads to the rest of the ventricle. Because the left posterior fascicle first activates the posterior, inferior, medial region of the left ventricle, the initial impulses are directed downward (i.e., toward the feet) and toward the patient's right side (see Fig. 4.20). This results in a positive deflection (initial small R wave) in the inferior leads (leads II, III, and aVF) and a negative deflection (small Q wave) in the left lateral leads, I and aVL. As depolarization then spreads upward and to the left, toward the "blocked" anterior, superior, and lateral regions of the left ventricle, a positive deflection (R wave) is inscribed in leads I and aVL, while a negative deflection (S wave) develops in the inferior leads. The predominance of these leftward forces, resulting from the abnormal activation of the anterior superior left ventricular wall, results in *left axis deviation* (generally more negative than −45°). A complete 12-lead ECG demonstrating the pattern of LAFB is shown later (see Fig. 4.34).

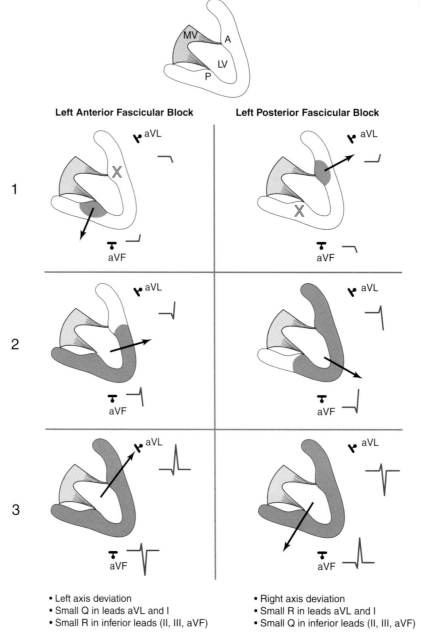

Left Anterior Fascicular Block **Left Posterior Fascicular Block**

- Left axis deviation
- Small Q in leads aVL and I
- Small R in inferior leads (II, III, aVF)

- Right axis deviation
- Small R in leads aVL and I
- Small Q in inferior leads (II, III, aVF)

Figure 4.20. Left anterior and left posterior fascicular blocks and their patterns in the ECG limb leads. The schematic at the top of the figure shows the left ventricle (LV) in the frontal plane. The mitral valve (MV) chordae tendineae insert into the anterior (A) and posterior (P) papillary muscles, which are important landmarks: the anterior fascicle of the left bundle branch courses toward the anterior papillary muscle, whereas the posterior fascicle travels to the posterior papillary muscle (the fascicles are not shown). Notice that the anterior papillary muscle is *superior* to the posterior papillary muscle. **Left side of figure:** In left anterior fascicular block, activation begins solely in the region of the posterior papillary muscle (1) because initial conduction to the anterior papillary muscle is blocked (denoted by the *X*). As a result, the initial forces of depolarization are directed downward toward the feet, producing an initial positive deflection (R wave) in lead aVF and a negative deflection (Q wave) in lead aVL. As the wave of depolarization spreads toward the left side and superiorly, aVF begins to register a negative deflection and aVL starts to record a positive deflection (2). Panel 3 shows the complete QRS complexes at the end of depolarization. **Right side of figure:** In left posterior fascicular block (denoted by the *X*), LV activation begins solely in the region of the anterior papillary muscle (1). Thus, the initial forces are directed upward and toward the patient's left side, producing an initial R wave in aVL and a Q wave in aVF. Panels 2 and 3 show how the spread of depolarization travels in the direction opposite that of LAFB.

Left posterior fascicular block (LPFB) is less common than LAFB. In LPFB, ventricular activation begins via the left anterior fascicle at the base of the anterior papillary muscle (see Fig. 4.20). As that anterosuperior left ventricular region depolarizes, the initial forces are directed upward and to the patient's left (creating a positive R wave in leads I and aVL and a negative Q wave in the inferior leads). As the impulse then spreads downward and to the right toward the initially blocked region, an S wave is inscribed in leads I and aVL, while an R wave is recorded in leads II, III, and aVF. Because the bulk of these delayed forces head toward the patient's right side, *right axis deviation* of the QRS mean axis occurs (see Fig. 4.36).

In contrast to RBBBs and LBBBs, LAFB and LPFB do not result in significant widening of the QRS because rapidly conducting Purkinje fibers bridge the territories served by the anterior and posterior fascicles. Therefore, although the sequence of conduction is altered, the total time required for depolarization is usually only slightly prolonged. Also note that although LBBBs and RBBBs are most easily recognized by analyzing the patterns of depolarization in the precordial (chest) leads, in the case of LAFB and LPFB, it is the recordings in the limb leads (as in Fig. 4.20) that are most helpful.

Pathologic Q waves in Myocardial Infarction

As you will learn in Chapter 7, sudden occlusion of a coronary artery typically results in a syndrome known as *acute ST segment elevation myocardial infarction*. When this occurs, a sequence of abnormalities of the ST segment and T wave evolves over a period of hours, as

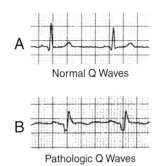

Figure 4.21. Normal versus pathologic Q waves. Compared with the small Q waves generated during normal depolarization (**A**), pathologic Q waves are more prominent with a width ≥1 mm (1 small box) and depth >25% of the height of the QRS complex (**B**).

described in the next section. Unless reperfusion of the occluded artery is quickly achieved, irreversible necrosis of the heart muscle served by that vessel ensues and is marked by the formation of **pathologic Q waves** on the electrocardiographic QRS complex.

Recall that it is normal for small initial Q waves to appear in some ECG leads. For example, initial septal depolarization routinely inscribes small Q waves in leads V_6 and aVL. Such physiologic Q waves are of short duration (≤0.04 sec, or 1 small box) and of low magnitude (<25% of the QRS total height). In distinction, pathologic Q waves are more prominent (Fig. 4.21), having a width ≥1 small box in duration and a depth >25% of the total height of the QRS. The ECG lead groupings in which pathologic Q waves appear reflect the anatomic site of the infarction (Table 4.4; also see Fig. 4.23).

Pathologic Q waves develop in the leads overlying infarcted tissue because necrotic muscle does not generate electrical forces. Rather, the ECG electrode over that region detects

Table 4.4. Localization of Myocardial Infarction

Anatomic Site	Leads with Abnormal ECG Complexes[a]	Coronary Artery Most Often Responsible
Inferior	II, III, aV_F	RCA
Anteroseptal	V_1–V_2	LAD
Anteroapical	V_3–V_4	LAD (distal)
Anterolateral	V_5–V_6, I, aV_L	CFX
Posterior	V_1–V_2 (tall R wave, not Q wave)	RCA

[a]Pathologic Q waves in all of leads V_1–V_6 implies an "extensive anterior MI" usually associated with a proximal left coronary artery occlusion.
CFX, left circumflex coronary artery; LAD, left anterior descending coronary artery; RCA, right coronary artery.

electrical currents from the healthy tissue on *opposite* regions of the ventricle, which are directed *away* from the infarct and the recording electrode, thus inscribing the downward deflection (Fig. 4.22). Q waves are permanent evidence of an ST-elevation type of myocardial infarction; only rarely do they disappear over time.

Notice in Table 4.4 that in the case of a posterior wall myocardial infarction (see Fig. 4.23A), it is not pathologic Q waves that are evident on the ECG. Because standard electrodes are not typically placed on the patient's back overlying the posterior wall, other leads must be relied on to indirectly identify the presence of such an infarction. Chest leads V_1 and V_2, which are directly opposite the posterior wall, record the *inverse* of what leads placed on the back would demonstrate. Therefore, *taller-than-normal R waves in leads V_1 and V_2* are the equivalent of pathologic Q waves in the diagnosis of a posterior wall MI. It may be recalled that right ventricular hypertrophy (RVH) also produces tall R waves in leads V_1 and V_2. These conditions can be distinguished, however, as RVH causes right axis deviation, which is not a feature of posterior wall MI.

It is important to note that if a Q wave appears in only a single ECG lead, it is not diagnostic of an infarction. True pathologic Q waves should appear in the groupings listed in Table 4.4 and Figure 4.23. For example, if a pathologic Q wave is present in lead III but not in II or aVF, it likely does not indicate an infarction. Also, Q waves are *disregarded* in lead aVR because electrical forces are *normally* directed away from the right arm. Finally, in the presence of LBBB, Q waves are usually not helpful in the diagnosis of MI because of the markedly abnormal pattern of depolarization in that condition.

ST Segment and T Wave Abnormalities

Transient Myocardial Ischemia

Among the most important abnormalities of the ST segments and T waves are those related to coronary artery disease. Because ventricular repolarization is very sensitive to myocardial perfusion, reversible deviations

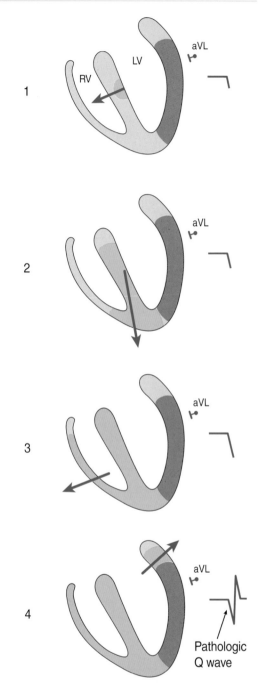

Figure 4.22. Sequence of depolarization recorded by lead aVL, overlying a lateral wall infarction (dark gray region). A pathologic Q wave is recorded because the necrotic muscle does not generate electrical forces; rather, at the time when the lateral wall *should* be depolarizing (**panel 3**), the activation of the healthy muscle on the *opposite* side of the heart is unopposed, such that net forces are directed away from aVL. The terminal R wave recorded by aVL reflects depolarization of the remaining viable myocardium beyond the infarct.

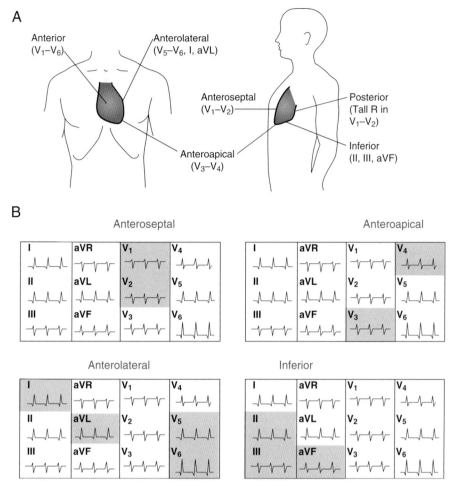

Figure 4.23. Relationship between ECG leads and cardiac anatomic regions. A. The lead groupings listed in parentheses represent each region. **B.** Miniaturized 12-lead ECG schematic drawings showing the standard orientation of printed samples from each lead. The major anatomic groupings are shaded and labeled in each drawing. While the presence of pathologic Q waves in leads V_1 and V_2 are indicative of anteroseptal infarction, be aware that *tall initial R waves* in those leads can indicate a posterior wall infarction, as described in the text.

of the ST segments and T waves (usually depression of the ST segment and/or inversion of the T wave) are common during transient episodes of myocardial ischemia, as will be explained in Chapter 6.

Acute ST Segment Elevation MI

As described in the previous section, pathologic Q waves are associated with one type of myocardial infarction (ST segment elevation myocardial infarction [STEMI]) but do not differentiate between an acute event and an MI that occurred weeks or years earlier. However, an *acute* STEMI

results in a temporal sequence of ST and T wave abnormalities that permits this distinction (Fig. 4.24). The initial abnormality is elevation of the ST segment, often with a peaked appearance of the T wave. At this early stage, myocardial cells are still viable and Q waves have not yet developed. In patients who achieve successful acute coronary reperfusion (by fibrinolytic therapy or percutaneous coronary intervention, as described in Chapter 7), the ST segments return to baseline and the sequence of changes described in the next paragraph do not occur.

In patients who *do not* achieve successful acute reperfusion, within several hours myocyte

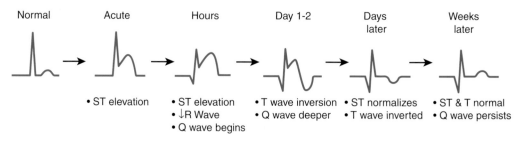

Normal	Acute	Hours	Day 1-2	Days later	Weeks later

| | • ST elevation | • ST elevation
• ↓R Wave
• Q wave begins | • T wave inversion
• Q wave deeper | • ST normalizes
• T wave inverted | • ST & T normal
• Q wave persists |

Figure 4.24. ECG evolution during acute ST elevation myocardial infarction (also termed "acute Q wave myocardial infarction"). However, as described in Chapter 7, if successful early reperfusion of the coronary occlusion is achieved, the elevated ST segments return to baseline without subsequent T wave inversion or Q wave development.

death leads to loss of the amplitude of the R wave and pathologic Q waves begin to be inscribed by the ECG leads positioned over the infarction territory. During the first 1 to 2 days following infarction, the ST segments remain elevated, the T wave inverts, and the Q wave deepens. Several days later, the ST segment elevation returns to baseline, but the T waves remain inverted. Weeks or months following the infarct, the ST segment and T waves have usually returned to normal, but the pathologic Q waves persist, a permanent marker of the MI. If the ST segment *remains* elevated several weeks later, it is likely that a bulging fibrotic scar (ventricular aneurysm) has developed at the site of infarction.

These evolutionary changes of the QRS, ST, and T waves are recorded by the leads overlying the zone of infarction (see Table 4.4 and Fig. 4.23). Typically, *reciprocal* changes are observed in leads opposite that site. For example, in acute anteroseptal MI, ST segment elevation is expected in chest leads V_1 and V_2; simultaneously, however, reciprocal changes (ST *depression*) may be inscribed by the leads overlying the opposite (inferior) region, namely in leads II, III, and aVF. An example of reciprocal ST changes is shown later in Figure 4.32.

The mechanism by which ST segment deviations develop during acute MI has not been established with certainty. It is believed, however, that the abnormality results from injured myocardial cells immediately adjacent to the infarct zone producing abnormal diastolic or systolic currents. One explanation, the *diastolic current theory*, contends that these damaged cells are capable of depolarization but are abnormally "leaky," allowing ionic flow that prevents the cells from fully repolarizing (Fig. 4.25). Because

the surface of such partially depolarized cells in the resting state would be relatively negatively charged compared with normal fully repolarized zones, an electrical current is generated between the two regions. This current is directed away from the more negatively charged ischemic area, causing the baseline of the ECG leads overlying that region to *shift downward*. Because the ECG machine records only *relative* position, rather than absolute voltages, the downward deviation of the baseline is not apparent. Following ventricular depolarization (indicated by the QRS complex), after *all* the myocardial cells have fully depolarized (including those of the injured zone), the net electrical potential surrounding the heart is *true zero*. However, compared with the abnormally displaced downward baseline, the ST segment *appears* elevated (see Fig. 4.25). As the myocytes then repolarize, the injured cells return to the abnormal state of diastolic ion leak, and the ECG again inscribes the abnormally depressed baseline. Thus, ST elevation in acute STEMI may in part simply reflect an abnormal shift of the recording baseline.

The *systolic current theory* of ST segment shifts contends that in addition to altering the resting membrane potential, ischemic injury shortens the action potential duration of affected cells. As a result, the ischemic cells repolarize faster than neighboring normal myocytes. Since the positive surface charge of the damaged myocytes is restored earlier that that of the normal cells, a voltage gradient develops between the two zones, creating an electrical current directed *toward* the ischemic area. This gradient occurs during the ST interval of the ECG, resulting in ST elevation in the leads overlying the ischemic region (Fig. 4.26).

ST Segment Elevation MI

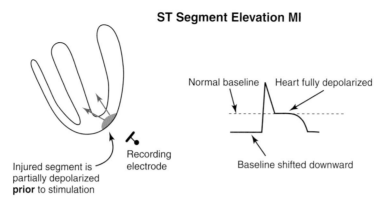

Normal baseline

Heart fully depolarized

Recording electrode

Injured segment is partially depolarized **prior** to stimulation

Baseline shifted downward

Non-ST Segment Elevation MI

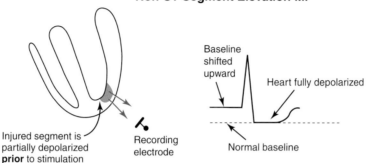

Baseline shifted upward

Heart fully depolarized

Injured segment is partially depolarized **prior** to stimulation

Recording electrode

Normal baseline

Figure 4.25. ST deviations in acute MI: diastolic injury current. Top, Ionic leak results in partial depolarization of injured myocardium in diastole, prior to electrical stimulation, which produces forces heading away from that site and shifts the ECG baseline downward. This is not noticeable on the ECG because only relative, not absolute, voltages are recorded. Following stimulation, when the entire myocardium has fully depolarized, the voltage is true zero but gives the appearance of ST elevation compared with the abnormally depressed baseline. **Bottom,** In non-ST segment elevation MI, the process is similar, but the ionic leak typically arises from the subendocardial tissue. As a result, the partial depolarization before stimulation results in electrical forces directed *toward* the recording electrode; hence, the baseline is shifted *upward*. When fully depolarized, the voltage is true zero, but the ST segment *appears* depressed compared with the shifted baseline.

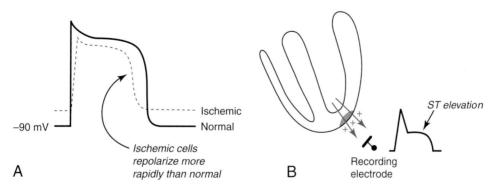

−90 mV

Ischemic

Normal

Ischemic cells repolarize more rapidly than normal

A

ST elevation

Recording electrode

B

Figure 4.26. ST deviation in acute ST segment elevation MI: systolic injury current. A. Compared with normal myocytes (solid line), ischemic myocytes (dashed line) display a reduced resting membrane potential and repolarize more rapidly. **B.** More rapid repolarization causes the surface of the ischemic zone to be relatively positively charged at the time the ST segment is inscribed. The associated electrical current (arrows) is directed *toward* the recording electrode overlying that site, so that the ST segment is abnormally elevated.

Acute Non-ST Segment Elevation MI

As described in Chapter 7, not all acute myocardial infarctions result in ST segment elevation and potential Q wave development. A more limited type of infarction, known as acute *non-ST elevation MI*, typically results from an acute *partially* occlusive coronary thrombus. In such infarctions, it is ST segment depression and/or T wave inversion, rather than ST elevation, that appears in the leads overlying the infarcting myocardium.

The extent of myocardial damage with this form of infarction is less than in STEMI, often involving only the subendocardial layers of the myocardium. As a result, pathologic Q waves do not develop, because the remaining viable cells are able to generate some electrical activity.

In non-ST elevation MI, the diastolic current theory maintains that diastolic ionic leak of injured cells adjacent to the subendocardial infarct zone generates electrical forces directed from the inner endocardium to the outer epicardium and therefore toward the overlying ECG electrode. Thus, the baseline of the ECG is shifted *upward* (see Fig. 4.25, bottom). Following full cardiac depolarization, the electrical potential of the heart returns to true zero but, relative to the abnormal baseline, gives the appearance of ST segment *depression*.

In addition to myocardial ischemia and infarction, there are several other causes of ST segment and T wave abnormalities that result from alterations in myocyte repolarization. The most commonly encountered of these are illustrated in Figure 4.27.

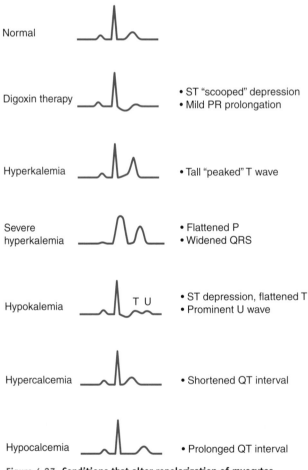

Normal

Digoxin therapy
• ST "scooped" depression
• Mild PR prolongation

Hyperkalemia
• Tall "peaked" T wave

Severe hyperkalemia
• Flattened P
• Widened QRS

Hypokalemia
• ST depression, flattened T
• Prominent U wave

Hypercalcemia
• Shortened QT interval

Hypocalcemia
• Prolonged QT interval

Figure 4.27. Conditions that alter repolarization of myocytes and therefore result in ST segment and T wave abnormalities.

SUMMARY

The ECG provides a wealth of information about the structure and integrity of the heart and is one of the most important diagnostic tools in cardiology. With the knowledge of this chapter in hand, the reader should be well prepared to practice analyzing ECGs in any of the complete ECG texts listed under "Additional Reading." Table 4.5 summarizes the suggested sequence of ECG interpretation. Sample normal and abnormal ECGs, with their interpretations, are presented in Figures 4.28 through 4.36. Disturbances of the cardiac rhythm can be identified by electrocardiography and are described in Chapters 11 and 12.

Table 4.5. Summary of Sequence of ECG Interpretation

1. Calibration
- Check 1.0 mV vertical box inscription (normal standard = 10 mm)

2. Rhythm
- Sinus rhythm is present if
  - Each P wave is followed by a QRS complex
  - Each QRS is preceded by a P wave
  - P wave is upright in leads I, II, and III
  - PR interval is >0.12 sec (3 small boxes)
- If these criteria are not met, determine type of arrhythmia (see Chapter 12)

3. Heart rate
- Use one of three methods:
  - 1,500/(number of mm between beats)
  - Count-off method: 300—150—100—75—60—50
  - Number of beats in 6 sec × 10
- Normal rate = 60–100 bpm (bradycardia <60, tachycardia >100)

4. Intervals
- Normal PR = 0.12–0.20 sec (3–5 small boxes)
- Normal QRS ≤ 0.10 sec (≤2.5 small boxes)
- Normal QT ≤ half the R–R interval, if heart rate normal

5. Mean QRS axis
- Normal if QRS is primarily upright in leads I and II (+90° to −30°)
- Otherwise, determine axis by isoelectric/perpendicular method

6. P wave abnormalities
- Inspect P in leads II and V_1 for left and right atrial enlargement

7. QRS wave abnormalities
- Inspect for left and right ventricular hypertrophy
- Inspect for bundle branch blocks
- Inspect for pathologic Q waves: What anatomic distribution?

8. ST segment or T wave abnormalities
- Inspect for ST elevations:
  - ST segment elevation MI
  - Pericarditis (see Chapter 14)
- Inspect for ST depressions or T wave inversions:
  - Myocardial ischemia or non-ST elevation MI
  - Usually accompany ventricular hypertrophy or bundle branch blocks
  - Metabolic or chemical abnormalities (see Fig. 4.27)

9. Compare with patient's previous ECGs

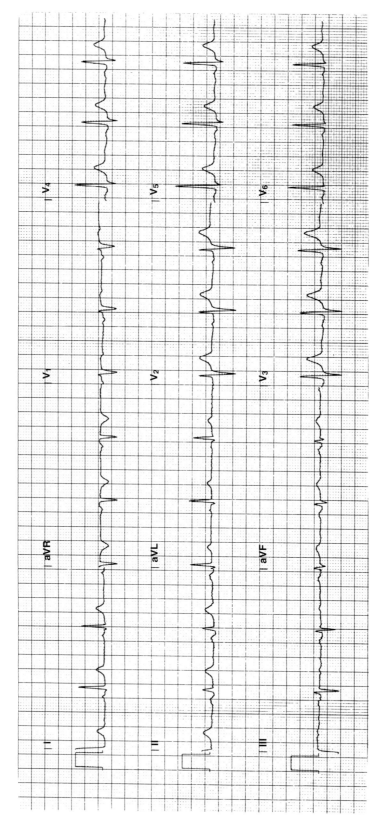

Figure 4.28. **12-lead ECG (normal).** The rectangular upward deflection at the beginning of each line is the voltage calibration signal (1 mV). *Rhythm:* normal sinus. *Rate:* 70 bpm. *Intervals:* PR, 0.17; QRS, 0.06; QT, 0.40 sec. *Axis:* 0° (QRS is isoelectric in lead aVF). The P wave, QRS complex, ST segment, and T waves are normal. Notice the gradual increase in R wave height between leads V_1 through V_6.

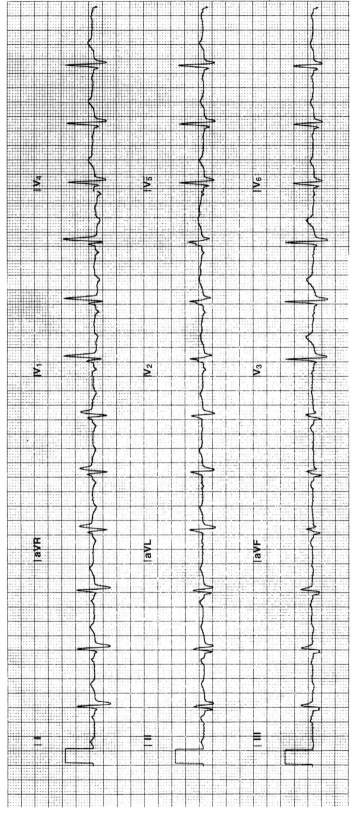

Figure 4.29. **12-lead ECG (abnormal).** *Rhythm:* normal sinus. *Rate:* 75 bpm. *Intervals:* PR, 0.16; QRS, 0.15; QT, 0.42 sec. *Axis:* indeterminate (isoelectric in all limb leads). *P wave:* left atrial enlargement (1 mm wide and 1 mm deep in lead V_1). *QRS:* widened with RSR' in lead V_1 consistent with right bundle branch block (RBBB). Also, pathologic Q waves are in leads II, III, and aVF, consistent with inferior wall myocardial infarction (an old one, because the ST segments do not demonstrate an acute injury pattern).

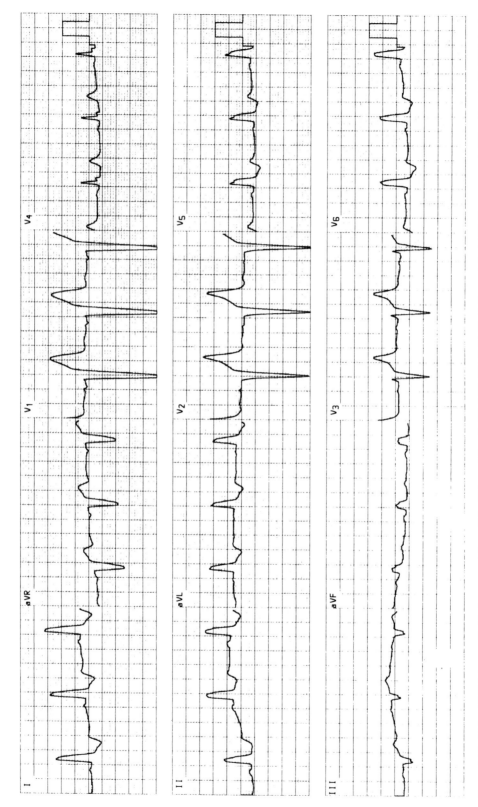

Figure 4.30. 12-lead ECG (abnormal). *Rhythm:* normal sinus. *Rate:* 68 bpm. *Intervals:* PR, 0.16; QRS, 0.16; QT, 0.40 sec. *Axis:* +15°. *P wave:* normal. *QRS:* widened with RR' in leads V₄–V₆ consistent with left bundle branch block (LBBB). The ST segment and T wave abnormalities are secondary to LBBB.

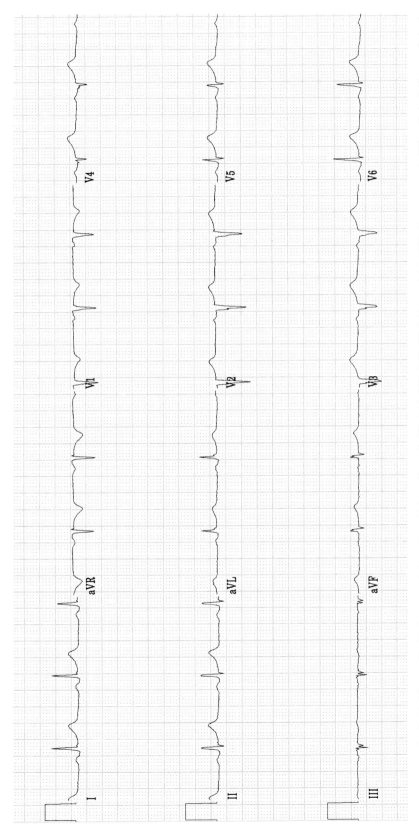

Figure 4.31. 12-lead ECG (abnormal). *Rhythm:* normal sinus. *Rate:* 66 bpm. *Intervals:* PR, 0.16; QRS, 0.08; QT, 0.40 sec. *Axis:* +10°. *P wave:* normal. *QRS:* pathologic Q waves in leads V₁–V₄, consistent with anteroseptal and anteroapical myocardial infarction (MI). The *ST segment and T waves* do not demonstrate an acute injury pattern; thus, the MI is old.

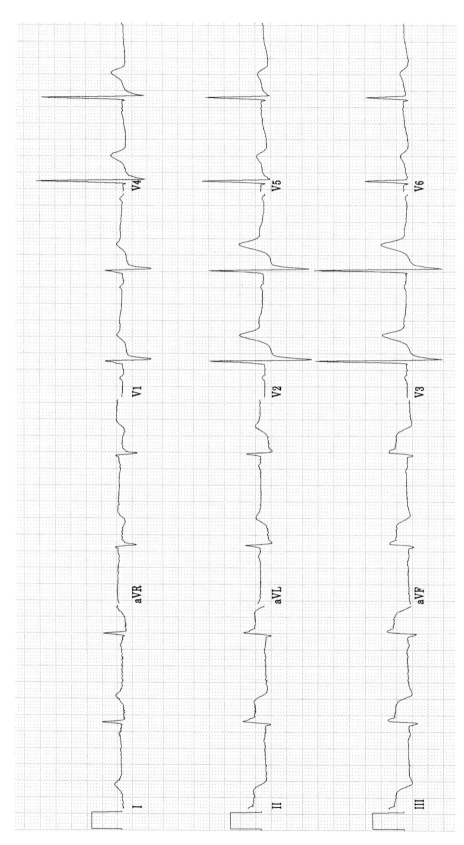

Figure 4.32. 12-lead ECG (abnormal). *Rhythm:* sinus bradycardia. *Rate:* 55 bpm. *Intervals:* PR, 0.20 (in aVF); QRS, 0.10; QT, 0.44 sec. *Axis:* normal (QRS is predominantly upright in leads I and II). *P wave:* normal. *QRS:* voltage in chest leads is prominent but does not meet criteria for ventricular hypertrophy; pathologic Q waves are present in II, III, and aVF, indicating inferior wall MI, and the tall R wave in V$_2$ is suggestive of posterior MI involvement as well. Marked *ST segment elevation* is apparent in II, III, and aVF, indicating that this is an *acute MI.* Note the reciprocal ST segment depression in leads I and aVL.

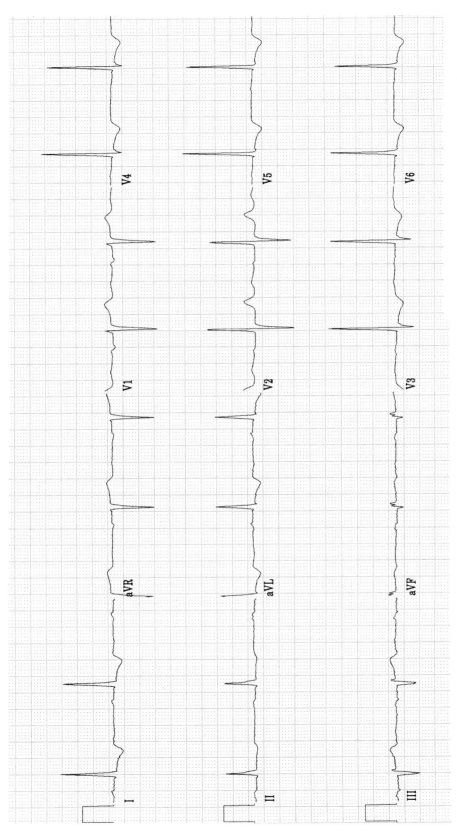

Figure 4.33. **12-lead ECG (abnormal).** *Rhythm:* sinus bradycardia. *Rate:* 55 bpm. *Intervals:* PR, 0.24 (first-degree AV block; see Chapter 12); QRS, 0.09; QT, 0.44 sec. *Axis:* 0°. *P wave:* normal. *QRS:* left ventricular hypertrophy (LVH): S in V_1 (14 mm) + R in V_5 (22 mm) > 35 mm. Pathologic Q waves in leads III and aVF raise the possibility of an old inferior MI. The *ST segment depression and T wave inversion* are secondary to the abnormal repolarization resulting from LVH.

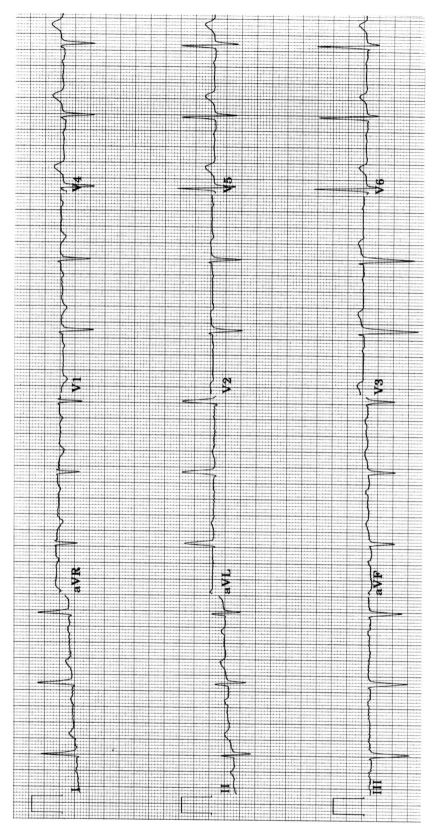

Figure 4.34. 12-lead ECG (abnormal). *Rhythm:* normal sinus. *Rate:* 68 bpm. *Intervals:* PR, 0.24 (first-degree AV block; see Chapter 12); QRS, 0.10; QT, 0.36 sec. *Axis:* −45° (left axis deviation). *P wave:* left atrial enlargement (terminal deflection of P wave in V_1 is 1 mm wide and 1 mm deep—just barely). *QRS:* pattern of left anterior fascicular block (LAFB; see Fig. 4.20). The abnormally small R waves in leads V_2–V_4 are associated with LAFB resulting from the reduction of initial anterior forces. The *ST segment and T waves* are unremarkable.

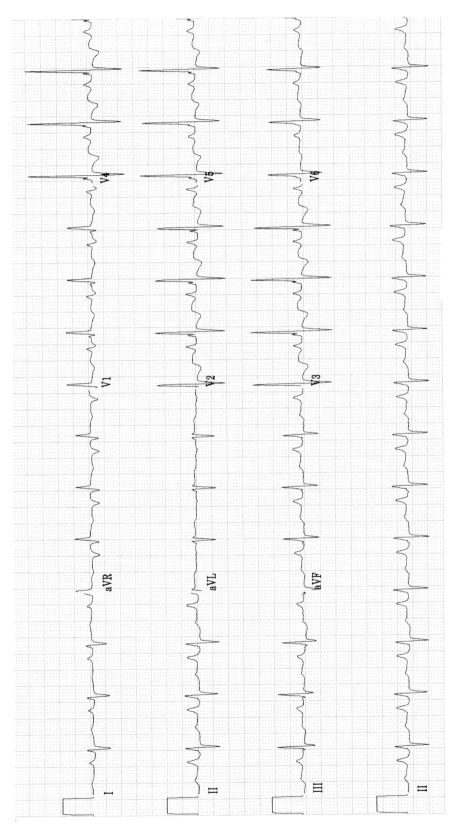

Figure 4.35. 12-lead ECG (abnormal). *Rhythm:* normal sinus. *Rate:* 95 bpm. *Intervals:* PR, 0.20; QRS, 0.10; QT, 0.34 sec. *Axis:* +160° (right axis deviation [RAD]). *P wave:* right atrial enlargement (P wave in lead II is >2.5 mm tall). *QRS:* right ventricular hypertrophy (RVH): R > S in V₁ with RAD. The T waves are inverted in the anterior leads, at least in part reflecting abnormal repolarization owing to RVH.

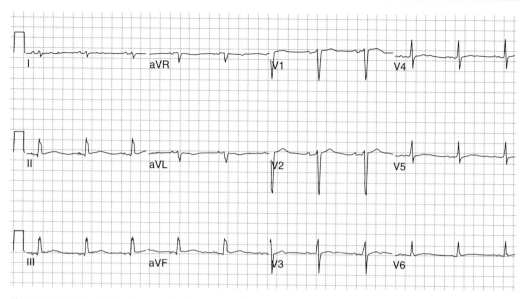

Figure 4.36. 12-lead ECG (abnormal). *Rhythm:* normal sinus. *Rate:* 62 bpm. *Intervals:* PR, 0.14; QRS, 0.10; QT, 0.52 (corrected QT, 0.53, which is prolonged). *Axis:* +95° (right axis deviation [RAD]). *QRS:* pattern of left posterior fascicular block (LPFB), with small R wave in leads I and aVL, small Q wave in leads II, III, and aVF, and RAD (see Fig. 4.20 for further description of LPFB). The prolonged QT interval in this patient is the result of antiarrhythmic medication.

Acknowledgments

Contributors to the previous editions of this chapter were Lilit Garibyan, MD; Kyle Low, MD; Price Kerfoot, MD; and Leonard S. Lilly, MD.

Additional Reading

Dubin D. *Rapid Interpretation of EKGs*. 6th ed. Tampa, FL: Cover Publishing; 2000.

Goldberger AL, Goldberger E. *Clinical Electrocardiography: A Simplified Approach*. 7th ed. St. Louis, MO: Mosby; 2006.

O'Keefe JH Jr, Hammill SC, Freed MS, et al. *The Complete Guide to ECGs*. 3rd ed. Sudbury, MA: Jones and Bartlett Publishers; 2008.

Surawicz B, Knilans TK. *Chou's Electrocardiography in Clinical Practice*. 6th ed. Philadelphia, PA: Saunders; 2008.

Surawicz B, Childers R, Deal BJ, et al. AHA/ACC/HRS recommendations for the standardization and interpretation of the electrocardiogram (Parts I–VI). *J Am Coll Cardiol.* 2007;49:1109–1135 and 2009; 53:976–1011.

Wagner GS. *Marriott's Practical Electrocardiography*. 11th ed. Baltimore, MD: Lippincott Williams & Wilkins; 2007.

Atherosclerosis

Jordan B. Strom
Peter Libby

Atherosclerosis is the leading cause of mortality and morbidity in the developed world. Through its major manifestations of cardiovascular disease and stroke, it likely will become the leading global killer by the year 2020. Commonly known as "hardening of the arteries," atherosclerosis derives its name from the Greek roots *athere-*, meaning "gruel," and *-skleros*, meaning "hardness."

Recent evidence has demonstrated that atherosclerosis is a chronic inflammatory condition and that its pathogenesis involves lipids, thrombosis, elements of the vascular wall, and immune cells. The process of atherogenesis can smolder throughout adulthood, punctuated by acute cardiovascular events.

This chapter consists of two sections. The first part describes the normal arterial wall, the pathogenesis of atherosclerotic plaque formation, and pathologic complications that lead to clinical symptoms. The second section relates findings from population studies to attributes that lead to this condition, thereby offering opportunities for prevention and treatment.

VASCULAR BIOLOGY OF ATHEROSCLEROSIS

Normal Arterial Wall

The arterial wall consists of three layers (Fig. 5.1): the **intima**, closest to the arterial lumen and therefore most "intimate" with the blood; the **media**, which is the middle layer; and the outer layer, the **adventitia**. The intimal surface consists of a single layer of endothelial cells that acts as a metabolically active barrier between circulating blood and the vessel wall. The media is the thickest layer of the normal artery. Boundaries of elastin, known as the internal and external elastic laminae, separate this middle layer from the intima and adventitia, respectively. The media consists of smooth muscle cells and extracellular matrix, and subserves the contractile and elastic functions of the vessel. The elastic component, more prominent in large arteries (e.g., the aorta and its primary branches), stretches during the high pressure of systole and then recoils during diastole, propelling blood forward. The muscular component, more prominent in smaller arteries such as arterioles, constricts or relaxes to alter vessel resistance and therefore luminal blood flow (flow = pressure/resistance; see Chapter 6). The adventitia contains the nerves, lymphatics, and blood vessels (vasa vasorum) that nourish the cells of the arterial wall.

Far from an inert conduit, the living arterial wall is a scene of dynamic interchange between its cellular components—most importantly, endothelial cells, vascular smooth muscle cells, and their surrounding extracellular

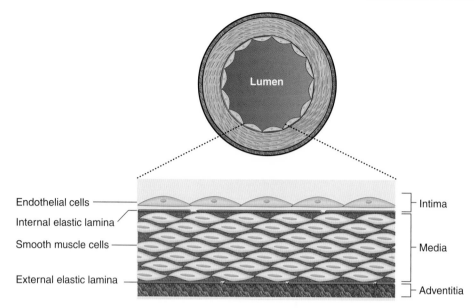

Figure 5.1. Schematic diagram of the arterial wall. The intima, the innermost layer, overlies the muscular media demarcated by the internal elastic lamina. The external elastic lamina separates the media from the outer layer, the adventitia.

matrix. An understanding of the dysfunction that leads to atherosclerosis requires knowledge of the normal function of these components.

Endothelial Cells

In a healthy artery, the endothelium performs structural, metabolic, and signaling functions that maintain homeostasis of the vessel wall. The tightly adjoined endothelial cells form a barrier that contains blood within the lumen of the vessel and limits the passage of large molecules from the circulation into the subendothelial space.

As blood traverses the vascular tree, it encounters antithrombotic molecules produced by the normal endothelium that prevent it from clotting. Some of these molecules reside on the endothelial surface (e.g., heparan sulfate, thrombomodulin, and plasminogen activators; see Chapter 7), while other antithrombotic products of the endothelium enter the circulation (e.g., prostacyclin and nitric oxide [NO]; see Chapter 6). Although a net anticoagulant state normally prevails, the endothelium can also produce prothrombotic molecules when subjected to various stressors.

Endothelial cells also secrete substances that modulate contraction of smooth muscle cells in the underlying medial layer. These substances include vasodilators (e.g., NO and prostacyclin) and vasoconstrictors (e.g., endothelin) that alter the resistance of the vessel and therefore luminal blood flow. In a normal artery, the predominance of vasodilator substances results in net smooth muscle relaxation. Several of the aforementioned endothelial products also function within the vessel wall to inhibit proliferation of smooth muscle cells into the intima, thus enforcing their normal residence within the media.

Endothelial cells can also modulate the immune response. In the absence of pathologic stimulation, healthy arterial endothelial cells resist leukocyte adhesion and thereby oppose local inflammation. However, endothelial cells in postcapillary venules respond to local injury or infection by secreting chemokines—chemicals that attract white blood cells to the area. Such stimulation also causes endothelial cells to produce cell surface adhesion molecules, which anchor mononuclear cells to the endothelium and facilitate their migration to the site of injury. These effects may be mediated in part via

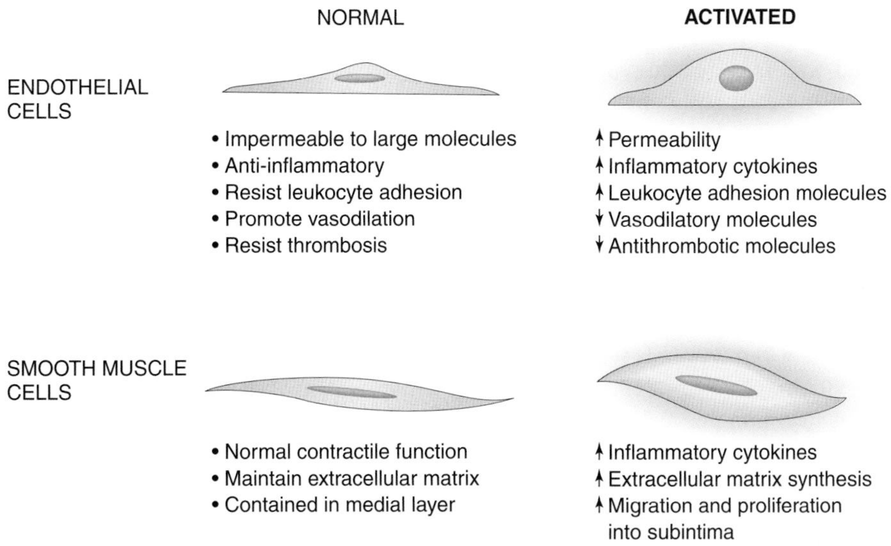

NORMAL   **ACTIVATED**

ENDOTHELIAL
CELLS

- Impermeable to large molecules
- Anti-inflammatory
- Resist leukocyte adhesion
- Promote vasodilation
- Resist thrombosis

↟ Permeability
↟ Inflammatory cytokines
↟ Leukocyte adhesion molecules
↡ Vasodilatory molecules
↡ Antithrombotic molecules

SMOOTH MUSCLE
CELLS

- Normal contractile function
- Maintain extracellular matrix
- Contained in medial layer

↟ Inflammatory cytokines
↟ Extracellular matrix synthesis
↟ Migration and proliferation
  into subintima

Figure 5.2. Endothelial and smooth muscle cell activation by inflammation. Normal endothelial and smooth muscle cells maintain the integrity and elasticity of the normal arterial wall while limiting immune cell infiltration. Inflammatory activation of these vascular cells corrupts their normal functions and favors proatherogenic mechanisms that drive plaque development.

Kruppel-like factor 2 (KLF2), a gene regulator in endothelial cells. As described later, under the adverse influences present during atherogenesis, endothelial cells similarly recruit leukocytes to the vessel wall.

Thus, the normal endothelium provides a protective, nonthrombogenic surface with homeostatic vasodilatory and anti-inflammatory properties (Fig. 5.2).

Vascular Smooth Muscle Cells

Smooth muscle cells within the vessel wall have both contractile and synthetic capabilities. Various vasoactive substances modulate the contractile function, resulting in vasoconstriction or vasodilation. Such agonists include circulating molecules (e.g., angiotensin II), those released from local nerve terminals (e.g., acetylcholine), and others originating from the overlying endothelium (e.g., endothelin and NO).

Normal biosynthetic functions of smooth muscle cells include production of the collagen, elastin, and proteoglycans that form the vascular extracellular matrix (see Fig. 5.2). Smooth muscle cells can also synthesize vasoactive and inflammatory mediators, including interleukin-6 (IL-6) and tumor necrosis factor-α (TNF-α), which promote leukocyte proliferation and induce endothelial expression of leukocyte adhesion molecules (LAM). These synthetic functions become more prominent at sites of atherosclerotic plaque and may contribute to their pathogenesis.

Extracellular Matrix

In healthy arteries, fibrillar collagen, proteoglycans, and elastin make up most of the extracellular matrix in the medial layer. Interstitial collagen fibrils, constructed from intertwining helical proteins, possess great biomechanical strength, while elastin provides flexibility. Together these components maintain the structural integrity of the vessel, despite the high pressure within the lumen. The extracellular matrix also regulates the growth of its resident cells. Native fibrillar collagen, in particular, can inhibit smooth muscle cell proliferation in vitro. Furthermore, the matrix influences cellular responses to stimuli—matrix-bound cells respond in a specific manner to growth factors and are less likely to undergo apoptosis (programmed cell death).

Atherosclerotic Arterial Wall

The arterial wall is a dynamic and regulated system, but noxious elements can disturb normal homeostasis and pave the way for atherogenesis. For example, as described later, vascular endothelial and smooth muscle cells react readily to inflammatory mediators such as IL-1 and TNF-α. These inflammatory agents can also activate vascular cells to *produce* IL-1 and TNF-α—contrary to past dogma stating that only cells of the immune system synthesize such cytokines.

Realizing that immune cells were not the only source of proinflammatory agents, investigations into the role of "activated" endothelial and smooth muscle cells in atherogenesis burgeoned. This fundamental research has identified several key components that contribute to the atherosclerotic inflammatory process, including endothelial dysfunction, accumulation of lipids within the intima, recruitment of leukocytes and smooth muscle cells to the vessel wall, formation of foam cells, and deposition of extracellular matrix (Fig. 5.3), as described in the following sections. Rather than follow a sequential path,

the cells of atherosclerotic lesions continuously interact and compete with each other, shaping the plaque over decades into one of many possible profiles. This section categorizes these mechanisms into three pathologic stages: the fatty streak, plaque progression, and plaque disruption (Fig. 5.4).

Fatty Streak

Fatty streaks represent the earliest visible lesions of atherosclerosis. On gross inspection, they appear as areas of yellow discoloration on the artery's inner surface, but they neither protrude substantially into the arterial lumen nor impede blood flow. Surprisingly, fatty streaks exist in the aorta and coronary arteries of most people by age 20. They do not cause symptoms, and in some locations in the vasculature, they may regress over time. Although the precise initiation of fatty streak development is not known, observations in animals suggest that various stressors cause early endothelial dysfunction, as described in the next section. Such dysfunction allows entry and modification of lipids within the subendothelial space, where they serve as

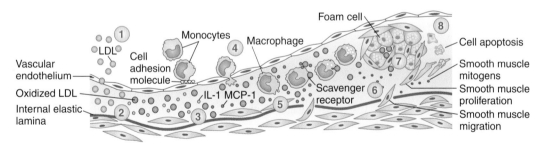

Figure 5.3. Schematic diagram of the evolution of atherosclerotic plaque. (1) Accumulation of lipoprotein particles in the intima. The darker color depicts modification of the lipoproteins (e.g., by oxidation or glycation). (2) Oxidative stress, including constituents of mLDL, induces local cytokine elaboration. (3) These cytokines promote increased expression of adhesion molecules that bind leukocytes and of chemoattractant molecules (e.g., monocyte chemoattractant protein 1 [MCP-1]) that direct leukocyte migration into the intima. (4) After entering the artery wall in response to chemoattractants, blood monocytes encounter stimuli such as macrophage colony–stimulating factor (M-CSF) that augment their expression of scavenger receptors. (5) Scavenger receptors mediate the uptake of modified lipoprotein particles and promote the development of foam cells. Macrophage foam cells are a source of additional cytokines and effector molecules such as superoxide anion (O_2^-) and matrix metalloproteinases. (6) Smooth muscle cells migrate into the intima from the media. Note the increasing intimal thickness. (7) Intimal smooth muscle cells divide and elaborate extracellular matrix, promoting matrix accumulation in the growing atherosclerotic plaque. In this manner, the fatty streak evolves into a fibrofatty lesion. (8) In later stages, calcification can occur (not depicted) and fibrosis continues, sometimes accompanied by smooth muscle cell death (including programmed cell death, or apoptosis), yielding a relatively acellular fibrous capsule surrounding a lipid-rich core that may also contain dying or dead cells. IL-1, interleukin 1; LDL, low-density lipoprotein. (Modified from Zipes D, Libby P, Bonow RO, et al., eds. *Braunwald's Heart Disease: A Textbook of Cardiovascular Medicine.* 7th ed. Philadelphia, PA: Elsevier Saunders; 2005:925.)

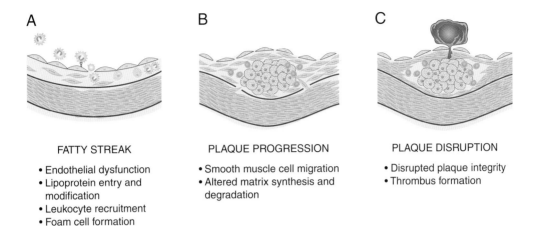

A

FATTY STREAK

- Endothelial dysfunction
- Lipoprotein entry and modification
- Leukocyte recruitment
- Foam cell formation

B

PLAQUE PROGRESSION

- Smooth muscle cell migration
- Altered matrix synthesis and degradation

C

PLAQUE DISRUPTION

- Disrupted plaque integrity
- Thrombus formation

Figure 5.4. **Stages of plaque development. A.** The fatty streak develops as a result of endothelial dysfunction, lipoprotein entry and modification, leukocyte recruitment, and foam cell formation. **B.** Plaque progression is characterized by migration of smooth muscle cells into the intima, where they divide and elaborate extracellular matrix. The fibrous cap contains a lipid core. **C.** Hemodynamic stresses and degradation of extracellular matrix increase the susceptibility of the fibrous cap to rupture, allowing superimposed thrombus formation. (Modified from Libby P, Ridker PM, Maseri A. Inflammation and atherosclerosis. *Circulation.* 2002;105:1136.)

proinflammatory mediators that initiate leukocyte recruitment and foam cell formation—the pathologic hallmarks of the fatty streak (Fig. 5.5).

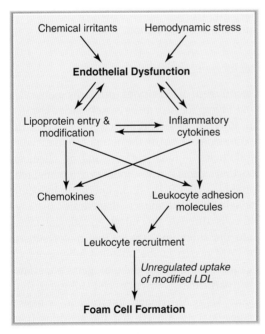

Figure 5.5. **Endothelial dysfunction is the primary event in plaque initiation.** Physical and chemical stressors alter the normal endothelium, allowing lipid entry into the subintima and promoting inflammatory cytokine release. This cytokine- and lipid-rich environment promotes recruitment of leukocytes to the subintima, where they may become foam cells—a prominent inflammatory participant.

Endothelial Dysfunction

Injury to the arterial endothelium represents a primary event in atherogenesis. Such injury can result from exposure to diverse agents, including physical forces and chemical irritants.

The predisposition of certain regions of arteries (e.g., branch points) to develop atheromata supports the role of hydrodynamic stress. In straight sections of arteries, the normal laminar (i.e., smooth) shear forces favor the endothelial production of NO, which is an endogenous vasodilator, an inhibitor of platelet aggregation, and an anti-inflammatory substance (see Chapter 6). Moreover, laminar flow not only activates KLF-2 as described above, but also accentuates expression of the antioxidant enzyme superoxide dismutase, which protects against reactive oxygen species produced by chemical irritants or transient ischemia. Conversely, disturbed flow occurs at arterial branch points, which impairs these locally atheroprotective endothelial functions. Accordingly, arteries with few branches (e.g., the internal mammary artery) show relative resistance to atherosclerosis, whereas bifurcated vessels (e.g., the common carotid and left coronary arteries) are common sites for atheroma formation.

Endothelial dysfunction may also result from exposure to a "toxic" chemical environment. For example, tobacco smoking, abnormal circulating lipid levels, and diabetes—all known risk factors for atherosclerosis—can promote endothelial dysfunction. Each of these states increases endothelial production of reactive oxygen species—notably, superoxide anion—which interact with other intracellular molecules to influence the metabolic and synthetic functions of the endothelium. In such an environment, the cells promote local inflammation.

When physical and chemical stressors interrupt normal endothelial homeostasis, an activated state ensues, manifested by impairment of the endothelium's role as a permeability barrier, release of inflammatory cytokines, increased production of cell surface adhesion molecules that recruit leukocytes, altered release of vasoactive substances (e.g., prostacyclin and NO), and interference with normal antithrombotic properties. These undesired effects of endothelial dysfunction lay the groundwork for subsequent events in the development of atherosclerosis (see Fig. 5.2).

Lipoprotein Entry and Modification

The activated endothelium no longer serves as an effective barrier to the passage of circulating lipoproteins into the arterial wall (see Box 5.1 for a summary of the major lipoprotein pathways). Increased endothelial permeability allows the entry of low-density lipoprotein (LDL) into the intima, a process facilitated by an elevated circulating LDL concentration. In addition to high LDL concentrations from excessive dietary intake, several monogenic causes of elevated LDL exist, including mutations in the LDL receptor, apolipoprotein B, and PCSK9, a protease involved in regulation of the LDL receptor. Once within the intima, LDL accumulates in the subendothelial space by binding to components of the extracellular matrix known as proteoglycans. This "trapping" increases the residence time of LDL within the vessel wall, where the lipoprotein may undergo chemical modifications that appear critical to the development of atherosclerotic lesions.

Hypertension, a major risk factor for atherosclerosis, may promote retention of lipoproteins in the intima by accentuating the production of LDL-binding proteoglycans by smooth muscle cells.

Oxidation is one type of modification that befalls LDL trapped in the subendothelial space. It can result from the local action of reactive oxygen species and pro-oxidant enzymes derived from activated endothelial or smooth muscle cells, or from macrophages that penetrate the vessel wall. In addition, the microenvironment of the subendothelial space can sequester oxidized LDL from antioxidants in the plasma. In diabetic patients with sustained hyperglycemia, *glycation* of LDL can occur—a modification that may ultimately render LDL antigenic and proinflammatory. These biochemical modifications of LDL act early and contribute to the inflammatory mechanisms initiated by endothelial dysfunction, and they may continue to promote inflammation throughout the lifespan of the plaque. In the fatty streak, and likely throughout plaque development, modified LDL (mLDL) promotes leukocyte recruitment and foam cell formation.

Leukocyte Recruitment

Recruitment of leukocytes (primarily monocytes and T lymphocytes) to the vessel wall is a key step in atherogenesis. The process depends on the expression of LAM on the normally nonadherent endothelial luminal surface, and on chemoattractant signals (e.g., monocyte chemotactic protein 1 [MCP-1], IL-8, interferon-inducible protein-10) that direct diapedesis (passage of cells through the intact endothelial layer) into the subintimal space. Two major subsets of LAM persist in the inflamed atherosclerotic plaque: the immunoglobulin gene superfamily (particularly, vascular cell adhesion molecule 1 [VCAM-1] and intercellular adhesion molecule 1 [ICAM-1]) and the selectins (particularly, E- and P-selectin). Despite the central role of T lymphocytes in the immune system, plaque LAM and chemoattractant signals direct mainly monocytes to the forming lesion. Recent research shows that hypercholesterolemia favors accumulation in blood of a particularly proinflammatory subset of monocytes, characterized by expression of high levels of proinflammatory cytokines (e.g., IL-1 and TNF-1), distinguished in mice by expression of the cell surface marker Ly6c. Although outnumbered by macrophages, T lymphocytes localize within plaques at all stages, where they likely furnish an important additional source of cytokines.

mLDL and proinflammatory cytokines can induce LAM and chemoattractant cytokine (chemokine) expression independently, but mLDL also potently stimulates endothelial and smooth muscle cells to *produce* proinflammatory cytokines, thereby reinforcing the direct action. This dual ability of mLDL to promote leukocyte recruitment and inflammation directly and indirectly persists throughout atherogenesis.

Foam Cell Formation

After monocytes adhere to and penetrate the intima, they differentiate into phagocytic macrophages and imbibe lipoproteins to form foam cells. It is important to note that foam cells do not arise from uptake of LDL by the classic cell–surface LDL-receptor mechanism described in Box 5.1, because the high cholesterol content within these cells actually suppresses expression of the receptor. Furthermore, the classic LDL receptor does not recognize chemically mLDL. Rather, macrophages rely on a family of "scavenger" receptors that preferentially bind and internalize mLDL. Unlike uptake via the classic LDL receptor, mLDL ingestion by scavenger receptors evades negative feedback inhibition and permits engorgement of the macrophages with cholesterol and cholesteryl ester, resulting in the typical appearance of foam cells. Although such uptake initially may be beneficial (by sequestering proinflammatory mLDL particles), the impaired efflux of these cells, as compared to the amount of influx, leads to local accumulation in the plaque, mitigating their protective role and fueling foam cell apoptosis and release of proinflammatory cytokines that promote atherosclerotic plaque progression. The lipid-rich center of a plaque, formed by necrotic foam cells, is often called the *necrotic core*.

Plaque Progression

Whereas endothelial cells play a central role in formation of the fatty streak, smooth muscle cell migration into the intima dominates early plaque progression. During decades of development, the typical atherosclerotic plaque acquires a distinct thrombogenic lipid core that underlies a protective fibrous cap. Not all fatty streaks progress into fibrofatty lesions, and it is unknown why some evolve and others do not.

Early plaque growth shows a compensatory outward remodeling of the arterial wall that preserves the diameter of the lumen and permits plaque accumulation without limitation of blood flow, hence producing no ischemic symptoms. This stage can even evade detection by angiography. Later plaque growth, however, can outstrip the compensatory arterial enlargement, restrict the vessel lumen, and impede perfusion. Such flow-limiting plaques can result in tissue ischemia, causing symptoms such as angina pectoris (see Chapter 6) or intermittent claudication of the extremities (see Chapter 15).

Most acute coronary syndromes (acute myocardial infarction and unstable angina pectoris) result when the fibrous cap of an atherosclerotic plaque ruptures, exposing prothrombotic molecules within the lipid core and precipitating an acute thrombus that suddenly occludes the arterial lumen. As described in this section, the extracellular matrix plays a pivotal role in fortifying the fibrous cap, isolating the thrombogenic plaque interior from coagulation substrates in the circulation.

Smooth Muscle Cell Migration

The transition from fatty streak to fibrous atheromatous plaque involves the migration of smooth muscle cells from the arterial media into the intima, proliferation of the smooth muscle cells within the intima, and secretion of extracellular matrix macromolecules by the smooth muscle cells. Foam cells, activated platelets entering through microfissures in the plaque surface, and endothelial cells all elaborate substances that

BOX *5.1*   The Lipoprotein Transport System

Lipoproteins ferry water-insoluble fats through the bloodstream. These particles consist of a lipid core surrounded by more hydrophilic phospholipid, free cholesterol, and apolipoproteins (also called *apoproteins*). The apoproteins present on various classes of lipoprotein molecules serve as the "conductors" of the system, directing the lipoproteins to specific tissue receptors and mediating enzymatic reactions. Five major classes of lipoproteins exist, distinguished by their densities, lipid constituents, and associated apoproteins. In order of increasing density, they are **chylomicrons, very low density lipoproteins (VLDL), intermediate-density lipoproteins (IDL), low-density lipoproteins (LDL), and high-density lipoproteins (HDL)**. The major steps in the lipoprotein pathways are labeled in the accompanying figure and described as follows. The key apoproteins (apo) at each stage are indicated in the figure in parentheses.

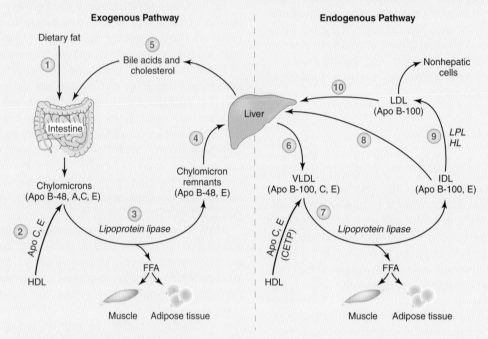

Exogenous (Intestinal) Pathway

1. Dietary fats are absorbed by the small intestine and repackaged as chylomicrons, accompanied by apo B-48. Chylomicrons are large particles, particularly rich in triglycerides, that enter the circulation via the lymphatic system.

2. Apo E and subtypes of apo C are transferred to chylomicrons from HDL particles in the bloodstream.

3. Apo C (subtype CII) enhances interactions of chylomicrons with *lipoprotein lipase (LPL)* on the endothelial surface of adipose and muscle tissue. This reaction hydrolyzes the triglycerides within chylomicrons into free fatty acids (FFA), which are stored by adipose tissue or used for energy in cardiac and skeletal muscle.

4. Chylomicron remnants are removed from the circulation by the liver, mediated by apo E.

5. One fate of cholesterol in the liver is incorporation into bile acids, which are exported to the intestine, completing the exogenous pathway cycle.

Endogenous (Hepatic) Pathway

Because dietary fat availability is not constant, the endogenous pathway provides a reliable supply of triglycerides for tissue energy needs:

6. The liver packages cholesterol and triglycerides into VLDL particles, accompanied by apo B-100 and phospholipid. The triglyceride content of VLDL is much higher than that of cholesterol, but this is the main means by which the liver releases cholesterol into the circulation.

7. VLDL is catabolized by LPL (similar to chylomicrons, as described in step 3), releasing fatty acids to muscle and adipose tissue. During this process, VLDL also interacts with HDL, exchanging some of its triglyceride for apo C subtypes, apo E, and cholesteryl ester from HDL. The latter exchange (important in reverse cholesterol transport, as described in the next section) is mediated by cholesteryl ester transfer protein (CETP).

8. Approximately 50% of the VLDL remnants (termed intermediate-density lipoproteins [IDL]) are then cleared in the liver by hepatic receptors that recognize apo E.

9. The remaining IDL is catabolized further by LPL and hepatic lipase (HL), which remove additional triglyceride, apo E, and apo C, forming LDL particles.

10. Plasma clearance of LDL occurs primarily via LDL receptor–mediated endocytosis in the liver and peripheral cells, directed by LDL's apo B-100 and apo E.

Cholesterol Homeostasis and Reverse Cholesterol Transport

Intracellular cholesterol content is tightly maintained by de novo synthesis, cellular uptake, storage, and efflux from the cell. The enzyme *HMG-CoA reductase* is the rate-limiting element of cholesterol biosynthesis, and cellular uptake of cholesterol is controlled by receptor-mediated endocytosis of circulating LDL (see step 10). When intracellular cholesterol levels are low, the transcription factor *sterol regulatory element binding protein (SREBP)* is released from the endoplasmic reticulum. The active fragment of SREBP enters the nucleus to increase transcription of HMG-CoA reductase and the LDL receptor—which, through their subsequent actions, tend to normalize the intracellular cholesterol content.

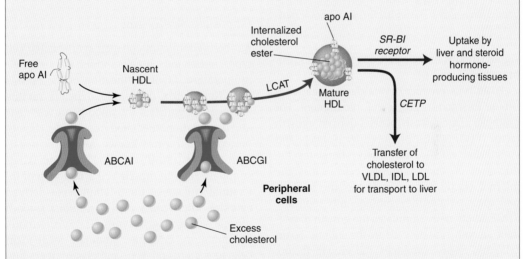

Under conditions of intracellular cholesterol excess (Figure above), peripheral cells increase the transcription of the ATP-binding cassette A1 and G1 genes (ABCA1 and ABCG1, respectively). The ABCA1 gene codes for a transmembrane protein transporter that initiates efflux of cholesterol from the cell to lipid-poor circulating apo AI (which is synthesized by the liver and intestine), thus forming nascent (immature) HDL particles. ABCG1 facilitates further efflux of cholesterol to form more mature HDL particles. As free cholesterol is acquired by circulating HDL, it is esterified by *lecithin cholesterol acyltransferase (LCAT)*, an enzyme activated by apo AI. The hydrophobic cholesterol esters move into the particle's core. Most cholesterol esters in HDL can then be exchanged in the circulation (via the enzyme CETP) with any of the apo B–containing lipoproteins (i.e., VLDL, IDL, LDL), which deliver the cholesterol back to the liver. HDL can also transport cholesterol to the liver and steroid hormone–producing tissues via the SR-B1 scavenger receptor.

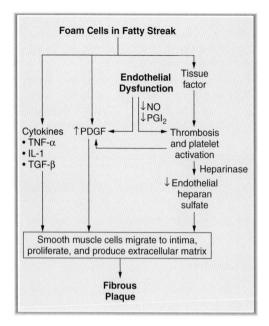

Figure 5.6. Progression from the fatty streak involves the migration and proliferation of smooth muscle cells. Substances released from foam cells, dysfunctional endothelial cells, and platelets contribute to this process. IL-1, interleukin-1; NO, nitric oxide; PDGF, platelet-derived growth factor; PGI$_2$, prostacyclin; TGF-β, transforming growth factor-β; TNF-α, tumor necrosis factor-α.

signal smooth muscle cell migration and proliferation (Fig. 5.6).

Foam cells produce several factors that contribute to smooth muscle cell recruitment. For example, they release platelet-derived growth factor (PDGF)—also produced by platelets and endothelial cells—which likely stimulates the migration of smooth muscle cells across the internal elastic lamina and into the subintimal space, where they subsequently replicate. PDGF additionally stimulates the growth of resident smooth muscle cells in the intima. Foam cells also release cytokines and growth factors (e.g., TNF-α, IL-1, fibroblast growth factor, and transforming growth factor-β [TGF-β]) that further incite smooth muscle cell proliferation and synthesis of extracellular matrix proteins. Furthermore, these stimulatory cytokines induce smooth muscle cell and leukocyte activation, promoting further cytokine release, thus reinforcing and maintaining inflammation in the lesion.

According to the traditional concept, plaques grow gradually and continuously, but

current evidence suggests that this progression may be punctuated by subclinical events with bursts of smooth muscle replication. For example, morphologic evidence of resolved intraplaque hemorrhages indicates that small breaches in plaque integrity can occur without clinical symptoms or signs. At the cellular level, such breaches expose tissue factor from foam cells, which activates coagulation and microthrombus formation. Activated platelets within such microthrombi release additional potent factors—including PDGF and heparinase—that can spur a local wave of smooth muscle cell migration and proliferation. Heparinase degrades heparan sulfate, a polysaccharide in the extracellular matrix that normally inhibits smooth muscle cell migration and proliferation. Moreover, other forms of lymphocytes—such as Treg and Th2 lymphocytes—may produce factors, including TGF-β and IL-10, respectively, which can inhibit smooth muscle cell proliferation and thus regulate plaque growth.

Extracellular Matrix Metabolism

As the predominant collagen-synthesizing cell type, smooth muscle cells should, through their proliferation, favor fortification of the fibrous cap. Net matrix deposition depends on the balance of synthesis by smooth muscle cells and degradation, mediated in part by a class of proteolytic enzymes known as matrix metalloproteinases (MMP). While PDGF and TGF-β stimulate smooth muscle cell production of interstitial collagens, the T-lymphocyte–derived cytokine interferon-γ (IFN-γ) *inhibits* smooth muscle cell collagen synthesis. Furthermore, inflammatory cytokines stimulate local foam cells to secrete collagen- and elastin-degrading MMP, thereby weakening the fibrous cap and predisposing it to rupture (Fig. 5.7).

Plaque Disruption

Plaque Integrity

The tug of war between matrix synthesis and degradation continues over decades, but not without consequences. Death of smooth muscle and foam cells, either owing to excess

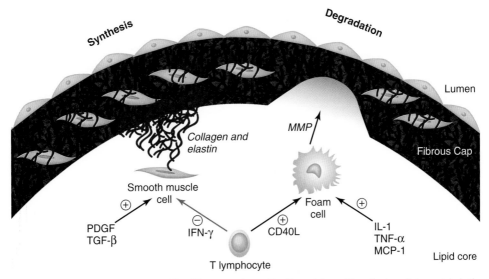

Figure 5.7. Matrix metabolism underlies fibrous cap integrity. The net deposition of extracellular matrix is the result of competing synthesis and degradation reactions. Smooth muscle cells synthesize the bulk of the fibrous cap constituents, such as collagen and elastin. Foam cells elaborate destructive proteolytic enzymes, such as the collagen-degrading matrix metalloproteinases and the elastolytic cathepsins. T-lymphocyte–derived factors favor destruction of the fibrous cap. All plaque residents, however, contribute to the cytokine milieu of the plaque, providing multiple activating and inhibitory stimuli as shown. IFN-γ, interferon-γ; IL-1, interleukin-1; MCP-1, monocyte chemoattractant protein 1; PDGF, platelet-derived growth factor; TGF-β, transforming growth factor-β; TNF-α, tumor necrosis factor-α. (Modified from Libby P. The molecular bases of acute coronary syndromes. *Circulation*. 1995;91:2844–2850; Young JL, Libby P, Schönbeck U. Cytokines in the pathogenesis of atherosclerosis. *Thromb Haemost*. 2002;88:554–567.)

inflammatory stimulation or by contact activation of apoptosis pathways, liberates cellular contents, contributing imbibed lipids and cellular debris to the growing lipid core. The size of the lipid core has biomechanical implications for the stability of the plaque. With increasing size and protrusion into the arterial lumen, mechanical stress focuses on the plaque border abutting normal tissue, the so-called shoulder region. In addition to bearing increased stress, local accumulation of foam cells and T lymphocytes at this site accelerates degradation of extracellular matrix, making this region the most common site of plaque rupture.

The net deposition and distribution of the fibrous cap is an important determinant of overall plaque integrity. Whereas lesions with thick fibrous caps may cause pronounced arterial narrowing, they have less propensity to rupture. Conversely, plaques that have thinner caps (and often appear less obstructive by angiography) tend to be fragile, and more likely to rupture and incite thrombosis. Current clinical terminology describes the extreme spectrums of integrity as "stable plaques" (marked by a thick fibrous cap and small lipid core) or "vulnerable plaques" (marked by a thin fibrous cap, rich lipid core, extensive macrophage infiltrate, and a paucity of smooth muscle cells; Fig. 5.8). Despite the common use of these terms, it is important to recognize that this distinction oversimplifies the heterogeneity of plaques and may overestimate the ability to foresee a plaque's "clinical future" based on structural information.

Thrombogenic Potential

Rupture of atherosclerotic plaque does not inevitably cause major clinical events such as myocardial infarction and stroke. As described in the previous section, small non-occlusive thrombi may reabsorb into the plaque, stimulating further smooth muscle growth and fibrous deposition (see Fig. 5.8). It is in large part the balance between the thrombogenic and fibrinolytic potential of the plaque, and the fluid phase of blood,

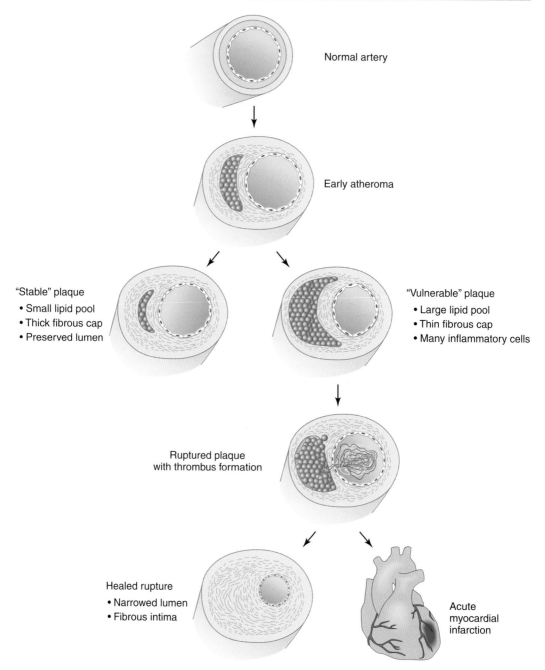

Figure 5.8. Stable versus vulnerable plaques. Stable plaque is characterized by a small lipid core and a thick fibrous cap, whereas vulnerable plaque tends to have a large lipid core and a relatively thin fibrous cap. The latter is subject to rupture, resulting in thrombosis. A resulting occlusive clot can cause an acute cardiac event, such as myocardial infarction. A lesser thrombus may resorb, but the wound-healing response stimulates smooth muscle cell proliferation and collagen production, thereby thickening the fibrous cap and narrowing the vessel lumen further. (Modified from Libby P. Inflammation in atherosclerosis. *Nature*. 2002;420:868–874.)

that determines whether disruption of the fibrous cap leads to a transient, nonobstructive mural thrombus or to a completely occlusive clot.

The probability of a major thrombotic event reflects the balance between the competing processes of coagulation and fibrinolysis. Inflammatory stimuli common in

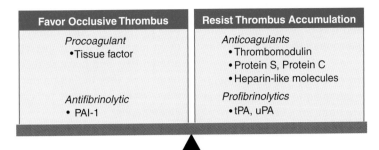

Favor Occlusive Thrombus	Resist Thrombus Accumulation
Procoagulant • Tissue factor	*Anticoagulants* • Thrombomodulin • Protein S, Protein C • Heparin-like molecules
Antifibrinolytic • PAI-1	*Profibrinolytics* • tPA, uPA

Figure 5.9. Competing factors in thrombosis. The clinical manifestations of plaque disruption rely not only on the stability of the fibrous cap, but also on the thrombogenic potential of the plaque core. The balance of physiologic mediators dictates the prominence of the thrombus, resulting in either luminal occlusion or resorption into the plaque. PAI-1, plasminogen activator inhibitor 1; tPA, tissue plasminogen activator; uPA, urokinase-type plasminogen activator.

the plaque microenvironment (e.g., CD40L) elicit tissue factor, the initiator of the extrinsic coagulation pathway, from many plaque components, including smooth muscle cells, endothelial cells, and macrophage-derived foam cells. Beyond enhancing expression of the potent procoagulant tissue factor, inflammatory stimuli further support thrombosis by favoring the expression of antifibrinolytics (e.g., plasminogen activator inhibitor-1) over the expression of anticoagulants (e.g., thrombomodulin, heparin-like molecules, protein S) and profibrinolytic mediators (e.g., tissue plasminogen activator and urokinase-type plasminogen activator; Fig. 5.9). Moreover, as described earlier, the activated endothelium also promotes thrombin formation, coagulation, and fibrin deposition at the vascular wall.

A person's propensity toward coagulation may be enhanced by genetics (e.g., the presence of a procoagulant prothrombin gene mutation), comorbid conditions (e.g., diabetes), and/or lifestyle factors (e.g., smoking, visceral obesity). Consequently, the concept of the "vulnerable plaque" has expanded to that of the "vulnerable patient," to acknowledge other contributors to a person's vascular risk.

Complications of Atherosclerosis

Atherosclerotic plaques do not distribute homogeneously throughout the vasculature. They usually develop first in the dorsal aspect of the abdominal aorta and proximal coronary arteries, followed by the popliteal arteries, descending thoracic aorta, internal carotid arteries, and renal arteries. Therefore, the regions perfused by these vessels most commonly suffer the consequences of atherosclerosis.

Complications of atherosclerotic plaques—including calcification, rupture, hemorrhage, and embolization—can have dire clinical consequences due to acute restriction of blood flow or alterations in vessel wall integrity. These complications, which are discussed in greater detail in later chapters, include the following:

• Calcification of atherosclerotic plaque, which imparts a pipe-like rigidity to the vessel wall and increases its fragility.

• Rupture or ulceration of atherosclerotic plaque, which exposes procoagulants within the plaque to circulating blood, causing a thrombus to form at that site. Such thrombosis can occlude the vessel and result in infarction of the involved organ. Alternatively, the thrombus material can incorporate into the lesion and add to the bulk of the plaque.

• Hemorrhage into the plaque owing to rupture of the fibrous cap or of the microvessels that form within the lesion. The resulting intramural hematoma may further narrow the vessel lumen.

• Embolization of fragments of disrupted atheroma to distal vascular sites.

• Weakening of the vessel wall: the fibrous plaque subjects the neighboring medial layer to increased pressure, which may provoke atrophy and loss of elastic tissue with subsequent expansion of the artery, forming an aneurysm.

- Microvessel growth within plaques, providing a source for intraplaque hemorrhage and further leukocyte trafficking.

The complications of atherosclerotic plaque may result in specific clinical consequences in different organ systems (Fig. 5.10). In the case of coronary plaque, lesions with gradually progressive expansion and a thick fibrous cap tend to narrow the vessel lumen and cause intermittent chest discomfort on exertion (angina pectoris). In contrast, plaque that does not compromise the vessel lumen but has characteristics of vulnerability (a thin fibrous cap and large lipid core) can rupture, leading to acute thrombosis and myocardial infarction (see Chapter 7). Such nonstenotic plaques are often numerous and dispersed throughout the arterial tree, and because they do not limit arterial flow, they do not produce symptoms and often evade detection by exercise testing or angiography.

The description presented here of atherogenesis and its complications can explain the limitations of widely employed treatments. For example, percutaneous intervention (angioplasty and stent placement) of symptomatic coronary stenoses effectively relieves angina pectoris, but does not necessarily prevent future myocardial infarction or prolong life. This disparity likely reflects the multiplicity of nonocclusive plaques at risk of precipitating thrombotic events. It follows that lifestyle modifications and drug therapies

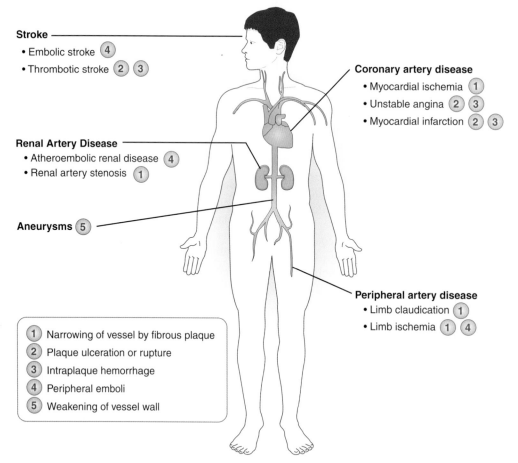

Figure 5.10. Clinical sequelae of atherosclerosis. Complications of atherosclerosis arise from the mechanisms listed in the figure.

that curb the risk factors for plaque formation, and lessen features associated with "vulnerability," furnish a critical foundation for preventing progression and complications of atherosclerosis.

ATHEROSCLEROSIS RISK FACTORS

In the early 20th century, it was widely believed that atherosclerosis was an inevitable process of aging. But in 1948, the landmark Framingham Heart Study began to examine the relationship between specific attributes and cardiovascular disease, establishing the concept of atherosclerotic risk factors. Among later studies, the Multiple Risk Factor Intervention Trial (MRFIT) screened more than 325,000 men to correlate risk factors with subsequent cardiovascular disease and mortality. These studies and others have established the importance of modifiable risk factors for atherosclerosis, including aberrant levels of circulating lipids (dyslipidemia), tobacco smoking, hypertension, diabetes mellitus, and lack of physical activity and obesity (Table 5.1). Major nonmodifiable risk factors include advanced age, male sex, and heredity—that is, a history of coronary heart disease among first-degree relatives at a young age (before age 55 for a male relative or before age 65 for a female relative).

In addition to these standard predictors, certain biologic markers associated with the development of cardiovascular events have been undergoing rigorous evaluation as "novel" risk markers. These include elevated circulating levels of the amino acid metabolite homocysteine, the special lipoprotein particle

Lp(a), and certain markers of inflammation, including the acute-phase reactant C-reactive protein (CRP). Furthermore, recent genome-wide association studies (GWAS) have sought to identify variants in genetic loci associated with increased cardiovascular risk.

The following sections address these risk factors and biologic markers.

Traditional Risk Factors

Dyslipidemia

A large and consistent body of evidence establishes abnormal circulating lipid levels as a major risk factor for atherosclerosis. Observational studies have shown that in the United States and other societies where there is high consumption of saturated fat and prevalent hypercholesterolemia, there is greater mortality from coronary disease than in countries with traditionally low saturated fat intake and low serum cholesterol levels (e.g., rural Japan and certain Mediterranean nations). Similarly, data from the Framingham Heart Study and other cohorts have shown that the risk of ischemic heart disease increases with higher total serum cholesterol levels. The coronary risk is approximately twice as high for a person with a total cholesterol level of 240 mg/dL compared with a person whose cholesterol level is 200 mg/dL.

In particular, elevated levels of circulating LDL correlate with an increased incidence of atherosclerosis and coronary artery disease. When present in excess, LDL can accumulate in the subendothelial space and undergo the chemical modifications that further damage the intima, as described earlier, initiating and perpetuating the development of atherosclerotic lesions. Thus, LDL is commonly known as "bad cholesterol." Conversely, elevated high-density lipoprotein (HDL) particles appear to protect against atherosclerosis, likely because of HDL's ability to transport cholesterol away from the peripheral tissues back to the liver for disposal (termed "reverse cholesterol transport"; see Box 5.1) and because of its putative antioxidative and anti-inflammatory properties. Thus, HDL has earned the moniker "good cholesterol."

Table 5.1. Common Cardiovascular Risk Factors

Modifiable risk factors
Dyslipidemia (elevated LDL, decreased HDL)
Tobacco smoking
Hypertension
Diabetes mellitus, metabolic syndrome
Lack of physical activity

Nonmodifiable risk factors
Advanced age
Male gender
Heredity

Elevated serum LDL may persist for many reasons, including a high-fat diet or abnormalities in the LDL-receptor clearance mechanism. Patients with genetic defects in the LDL receptor, which leads to a condition known as *familial hypercholesterolemia*, cannot remove LDL from the circulation efficiently. Heterozygotes with this condition have one normal and one defective gene coding for the receptor. They display high plasma LDL levels and develop premature atherosclerosis. Homozygotes who *completely* lack functional LDL receptors may experience vascular events, such as acute myocardial infarction, as early as the first decade of life.

Increasing evidence also implicates triglyceride-rich lipoproteins, such as very low density lipoprotein (VLDL) and intermediate-density lipoprotein (IDL), in the development of atherosclerosis. However, it remains undetermined whether these particles participate directly in atherogenesis or simply keep company with low levels of HDL cholesterol. Of note, poorly controlled type 2 diabetes mellitus commonly associates with the combination of hypertriglyceridemia and low HDL levels.

Lipid-Altering Therapy

Strategies that improve abnormal lipid levels can limit the consequences of atherosclerosis. Many large studies of patients with coronary disease show that dietary or pharmacologic reduction of serum cholesterol can slow the progression of atherosclerotic plaque. These trials form the basis of the screening guidelines devised by the National Cholesterol Education Program panel, which recommend a fasting lipid profile every five years for all adults. The guidelines specify an "optimal" LDL cholesterol level as <100 mg/dL. Patients with established atherosclerosis, or those who have equivalent risk (e.g., diabetes), should receive treatment to attain this goal. An even lower goal of <70 mg/dL is recommended for patients with atherosclerotic disease at the highest risk of future vascular events—those who have recently sustained an acute coronary syndrome (see Chapter 7) and those with multiple risk factors, especially diabetes, the metabolic syndrome (described later in this chapter), or tobacco smoking.

Diet and exercise comprise two important components of the risk-reduction arsenal. For example, the Lyon Diet Heart Study demonstrated that patients with coronary disease who were randomized to a Mediterranean-style diet decreased their risk of recurrent cardiac events. The diet implemented in this study included replacement of saturated fats with polyunsaturated fats (particularly α-linolenic acid, an omega-3 fatty acid). In vitro evidence indicates that polyunsaturated fats may activate a transcription factor (peroxisome proliferator-activated receptor-α [PPAR-α], or its obligate partner, retinoid X receptor), which increases expression of the major HDL apoprotein (apo AI) and the enzyme lipoprotein lipase, and inhibits cytokine-induced expression of LAM on endothelial cells. These actions may oppose atherogenesis. Physical activity and loss of excess weight can also improve the lipid profile, notably by lowering triglycerides and raising HDL.

When lifestyle modifications fail to achieve target values, pharmacologic agents can improve abnormal lipid levels. The major groups of lipid-altering agents (see Chapter 17) include HMG-CoA reductase inhibitors (also known as statins), niacin, fibric acid derivatives, cholesterol intestinal absorption inhibitors, and bile acid–binding agents. The statins have emerged as the most effective LDL-lowering drugs. They inhibit the rate-limiting enzyme responsible for cholesterol biosynthesis. The resulting reduction in intracellular cholesterol concentration promotes increased LDL-receptor expression and thus augmented clearance of LDL particles from the bloodstream. Statins also lower the rate of VLDL synthesis by the liver (thus lowering circulating triglyceride levels), and raise HDL by an unknown mechanism.

Major clinical trials evaluating statin therapy have demonstrated reductions in ischemic cardiac events, the occurrence of strokes, and (in many cases) mortality rates (Fig. 5.11). The benefits documented in these studies have extended to people with wide ranges of LDL, with or without known preexisting atherosclerotic disease. Furthermore, the effect

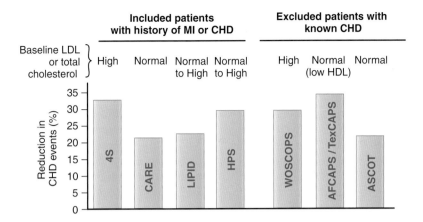

4S: Scandinavian Simvastatin Survival Study. *Lancet.* 1994;344:1383–1389.

AFCAPS/TexCAPS: The Air Force/Texas Coronary Atherosclerosis Prevention Study. *JAMA.* 1998;279:1615–1622.

ASCOT: Anglo-Scandinavian Cardiac Outcomes Trial—Lipid Lowering Arm. *Lancet.* 2003;361:1149–1158.

CARE: Cholesterol And Recurrent Events. *N Engl J Med.* 1996;335:1001–1009.

HPS: Heart Protection Study. *Lancet.* 2004;363:757–767.

LIPID: The Long-term Intervention with Pravastatin in Ischaemic Disease. *N Engl J Med.* 1998;339:1349–1357.

WOSCOPS: West of Scotland Coronary Primary Prevention Study. *N Engl J Med.* 1995;333:1301–1307.

Figure 5.11. Statins reduce cardiovascular risk. Several major clinical studies have supported the beneficial role of statin-induced lipid lowering in reducing coronary heart disease (CHD) events. Regardless of baseline serum cholesterol levels, the benefits of statins extend to patients with an established history of coronary disease and to patients with significant risk factors who do not have such a history. HDL, high-density lipoprotein; LDL, low-density lipoprotein.

may depend on the degree of LDL lowering achieved, as demonstrated by the PROVE IT-TIMI 22 and TNT studies, which showed that *intensive* statin therapy (yielding lower LDL levels) improves cardiovascular outcomes in acute and chronic coronary heart disease more than moderate-dose statins.

The clinical benefits of statins likely derive from several mechanisms. The combination of lowering LDL and raising HDL may reduce the lipid content of atherosclerotic plaques and thus favorably affect their biologic activity. Other potentially beneficial actions (so-called "pleiotropic effects") include increased NO synthesis, enhanced fibrinolytic activity, inhibition of smooth muscle proliferation and monocyte recruitment, and reduction in macrophage production of matrix-degrading enzymes. In vitro studies suggest that statins may also reduce inflammation by inhibiting the macrophage cytokines TNF-α, IL-1, and IL-6, thereby reducing endothelial expression of LAM and macrophage tissue factor production. Some of these pleiotropic effects may result from activation of the transcription factor KLF2 and interference with prenylation of small G proteins implicated in the regulation of inflammatory functions of vascular cells and leukocytes. Clinical trials have supported an anti-inflammatory action of statins because they reduce plasma levels of CRP, a serum marker of inflammation described later. It should be noted, however, that it is experimentally difficult to separate the LDL-lowering effect of statins from their anti-inflammatory mechanisms because of the prominent role of oxidized LDL in initiating inflammatory cascades. Nonetheless, accumulating clinical and experimental data suggest that at least part of the benefit of statins derives from mechanisms other than LDL lowering.

Tobacco Smoking

Numerous studies have shown that tobacco smoking increases the risk of atherosclerosis and ischemic heart disease. Even minimal smoking increases the risk, and the heaviest smokers have the greatest risk of cardiovascular events.

Tobacco smoking could lead to atherosclerotic disease in several ways, including enhanced oxidative modification of LDL, decreased circulating HDL levels, endothelial dysfunction owing to tissue hypoxia and increased oxidant stress, increased platelet adhesiveness, increased expression of soluble LAM, inappropriate stimulation of the sympathetic nervous system by nicotine, and displacement of oxygen by carbon monoxide from hemoglobin. Extrapolation from animal experiments suggests that smoking not only accelerates atherogenesis, but also increases the propensity for thrombosis—both components of the "vulnerable patient."

Fortunately, smoking cessation can reverse some of the adverse outcomes. People who stop smoking greatly reduce their likelihood of coronary heart disease, compared with those who continue to smoke. In one study, after three years of cessation, the risk of coronary artery disease for former smokers became similar to subjects who never smoked.

Hypertension

Elevated blood pressure (either systolic or diastolic) augments the risk of developing atherosclerosis, coronary heart disease, and stroke (see Chapter 13). The association of elevated blood pressure with cardiovascular disease does not appear to have a specific threshold. Rather, risk increases continuously with progressively higher pressure values. Systolic pressure predicts adverse outcomes more reliably than does diastolic pressure, particularly in older persons.

Hypertension may accelerate atherosclerosis in several ways. Animal studies have shown that elevated blood pressure injures vascular endothelium and may increase the permeability of the vessel wall to lipoproteins. In addition to causing direct endothelial damage, increased hemodynamic stress can augment the number of scavenger receptors on macrophages, thus enhancing the development of foam cells. Cyclic circumferential strain, increased in hypertensive arteries, can enhance smooth muscle cell production of proteoglycans that bind and retain LDL particles, promoting their accumulation in the intima and facilitating their oxidative modification. Angiotensin II, a mediator of hypertension, acts not only as a vasoconstrictor, but also as a stimulator of oxidative stress (through activation of NADPH oxidases, a source of superoxide anion, O_2) and as a proinflammatory cytokine. Thus, hypertension may also promote atherogenesis by contributing to a pro-oxidant and inflammatory state.

Antihypertensive Therapy

Like dyslipidemias, treatment of hypertension should start with lifestyle modifications, but often requires pharmacologic intervention. The Dietary Approaches to Stop Hypertension (DASH) studies demonstrate that a diet high in fruits and vegetables, with dairy products low in fat and an overall reduced sodium content, significantly improves systolic and diastolic blood pressures. Regular exercise can also reduce resting blood pressure levels. Many medications effectively lower blood pressure, as described in Chapters 13 and 17.

Diabetes Mellitus and the Metabolic Syndrome

The global incidence of diabetes mellitus is estimated at 170 million people and projected to grow 40% worldwide by 2030. In the United States alone, 18.2 million people are diabetic, and projections suggest that one in every three children born in 2000 will eventually develop the condition. With a three- to fivefold increased risk of acute coronary events, 80% of diabetic patients succumb to atherosclerosis-related conditions, including coronary heart disease, stroke, and peripheral artery disease. Accordingly, some consider diabetes an atherosclerotic risk equivalent, elevating it to the same risk category as that of people with a history of myocardial infarction.

The predisposition of diabetic patients to atherosclerosis may relate in part to the non-enzymatic glycation of lipoproteins (which enhances uptake of cholesterol by scavenger macrophages, as described earlier), or to a pro-thrombotic tendency and antifibrinolytic state that is often present. Diabetics frequently have impaired endothelial function, gauged by the reduced bioavailability of NO and increased leukocyte adhesion. Tight control of serum glucose levels in diabetic patients reduces the risk of *microvascular* complications, such as retinopathy and nephropathy. At least one study has also demonstrated a reduction in *macrovascular* outcomes, such as myocardial infarction and stroke, in patients with type 1 diabetes who followed an intense antidiabetic regimen. In addition, control of hypertension and dyslipidemia in diabetic patients convincingly reduces the risk of cardiac and cerebrovascular complications.

The **metabolic syndrome** (previously known as the "insulin resistance syndrome" or "syndrome X") is a descriptor for a clustering of risk factors, including hypertension, hyper-triglyceridemia, reduced HDL, cellular insulin resistance (often leading to glucose intolerance), and visceral obesity (excessive adipose tissue in the abdomen). This constellation associates with a high risk for atherosclerosis in both diabetic and nondiabetic patients, and the National Health and Nutrition Examination Survey estimates that an astounding 44% of Americans have the metabolic syndrome based on current guidelines. The presence of insulin resistance in this syndrome appears to promote atherogenesis long before affected persons develop overt diabetes.

Lack of Physical Activity

Exercise may mitigate atherogenesis in several ways. In addition to its beneficial effects on the lipid profile and blood pressure, exercise enhances insulin sensitivity and endothelial production of NO. Long-term prospective studies of both men and women indicate that even modest activities, such as brisk walking, for as little as 30 minutes per day can protect against cardiovascular mortality.

Estrogen Status

Cardiovascular disease dominates over other causes of mortality in women, including breast and other cancers. Before menopause, women have a lower incidence of coronary events than men. After menopause, however, men and women have similar rates. This observation suggests that estrogen (the levels of which decline after menopause) may have atheroprotective properties. Physiologic estrogen levels in premenopausal women raise HDL and lower LDL. Experimentally, estrogen also exhibits potentially beneficial antioxidant and antiplatelet actions and improves endothelium-dependent vasodilation.

Early observational studies suggested that hormone therapy reduced the risk of coronary artery disease in postmenopausal women, prompting many physicians to prescribe such medications for cardiovascular prevention purposes. However, the Heart and Estrogen/Progestin Replacement Study demonstrated an association between such hormone use and an early *increased* risk of vascular events in women with preexisting coronary disease. Subsequent randomized primary prevention studies from the Women's Health Initiative were terminated prematurely because estrogen-plus-progestin treatment increased cardiovascular risk by 24% overall, with a striking 81% higher risk during the first year of therapy. Of note, these troubling outcomes did not appear in the cohort of patients randomized to the estrogen-only arm of the study. Further analyses will help determine if safe hormone therapies are possible. Meanwhile, because currently available clinical trial data do not show that gonadal hormone therapy is cardioprotective and that it may actually be harmful, such therapy should not be commenced for the sole goal of reducing cardiovascular risk.

Biomarkers of Cardiovascular Risk

Despite identification of the well-established risk factors just described, one out of five cardiovascular events occurs in patients lacking these attributes. In conjunction with growing knowledge about the pathogenesis of atherosclerosis, several novel markers of risk have emerged. These biomarkers serve three primary roles: (1) as a means to help stratify the risk of atherosclerotic disease and thus guide the choice of therapies, (2) as clinical measures to assess treatment success, and (3) as potential targets of new therapeutic regimens.

Homocysteine

Some studies have shown a significant relationship between elevated circulating levels of the amino acid homocysteine and the incidence of coronary, cerebral, and peripheral artery disease. The mechanism by which homocysteine might increase atherosclerotic risk remains undetermined, but current evidence suggests that abnormally high levels may promote oxidative stress, vascular inflammation, and platelet adhesiveness. Although folic acid and other vitamin B supplements reduce high serum homocysteine levels, clinical trials have not shown that such therapy reduces atherosclerotic disease or its complications.

Lipoprotein (a)

Lipoprotein (a), referred to as Lp(a) and pronounced "L-P-little-a," has been identified as an independent risk factor for coronary artery disease in some studies. Lp(a) is a variant of LDL whose major apolipoprotein (apo B-100) links by a disulfide bridge to another protein, apo(a). Apo(a) structurally resembles plasminogen, a plasma protein important in the endogenous lysis of fibrin clots (see Chapter 7). Thus, the detrimental effect attributed to Lp(a) may relate to competition with normal plasminogen activity. Lp(a) is able to enter the arterial intima, and in vitro studies have shown that it encourages inflammation and thrombosis.

Lp(a) levels in the population are skewed and not normally distributed, showing a trailing prevalence of the higher levels. As with homocysteine, not all population studies support a link between Lp(a) and cardiovascular events, though people with the highest Lp(a) levels do appear to be at increased risk. Recent GWAS and Mendelian randomization analyses also support a causal link between Lp(a) and cardiovascular events.

Diet and exercise have little impact on Lp(a) levels. Of current lipid-lowering agents, niacin has the greatest effect on Lp(a), lowering its concentration by as much as 20%. However, thus far, there is no evidence that reduction of Lp(a) by drug therapy improves cardiovascular outcomes.

C-Reactive Protein and Other Markers of Inflammation

Because the pathogenesis of atherosclerosis involves inflammation at every stage, markers of inflammation have undergone evaluation as predictors of cardiac risk. Recall that the process of lipoprotein entry and modification in the vessel wall triggers the release of cytokines, followed by leukocyte infiltration, more cytokine release, and smooth muscle migration into—and proliferation within—the intima. Involved cytokines (e.g., IL-6) mobilize to the liver and incite increased production of acute-phase reactants, including CRP, fibrinogen, and serum amyloid A.

Of these molecules, CRP has shown the greatest promise as a marker of low-grade systemic inflammation associated with atherosclerotic disease. Large studies of apparently healthy men and women indicate that those with higher basal CRP levels have a greatly increased risk of adverse cardiovascular outcomes, independent of serum cholesterol levels. Recent prospective studies affirm high-sensitivity CRP as an independent predictor of myocardial infarction, stroke, peripheral artery disease, and sudden cardiac death. Although it serves as a marker of risk not captured by traditional algorithms, there is no convincing evidence that CRP itself is actually a mediator of atherogenesis.

Recent data support the use of CRP levels to guide therapy. The JUPITER trial, a study of 17,800 healthy individuals with above-median levels of CRP but without elevated LDL, demonstrated a reduced incidence of major cardiovascular events among patients who were treated with a statin.

Genetics

Genetic predisposition, as reflected by family history, represents a major nonmodifiable risk factor for atherosclerosis. While directly causative genes remain elusive, recent GWAS have identified a number of loci associated with atherosclerotic disease. The strongest connection with CAD and myocardial infarction localizes to chromosome 9p21.3. This region contains genes that code for two cyclin-dependent kinase inhibitors that are involved in regulation of the cell cycle and may participate in TGF-β inhibitory pathways. Other associations with CAD include loci on chromosome 6q25.1, which maps to a gene that encodes a mitochondrial C1-tetrahydrofolate synthase involved in methionine synthesis, and chromosome 2q36.3, a region devoid of known functional genes. It is too early to know whether such findings will ultimately result in enhanced identification, prevention, and treatment of atherosclerotic disease.

Infectious Agents in Atherogenesis

Several studies have identified infectious agents (e.g., herpes viruses, *Chlamydia pneumoniae*) within some atherosclerotic lesions, raising the question of their potential role in atherogenesis. These studies have generated substantial controversy, and proof of a causal role is lacking. Although it is unclear if infections truly play a role in atherogenesis, viral and microbial products could plausibly drive aspects of atherogenesis. To date, a number of well-powered trials have not shown that antibiotic treatment directed against infectious agents reduces the risk of future cardiac events in survivors of acute coronary syndromes.

Outlook

Despite accumulating knowledge of the pathogenesis of atherosclerosis and its clinical sequelae, this disease remains a major cause of death in the modern world. Although improvements in cardiovascular care have reduced age-adjusted mortality from this condition, it will continue to be a menace as the population ages and as developing countries embrace the adverse dietary and activity habits of a Western lifestyle. Ongoing research of the biology of atherosclerosis, as well as advances in therapeutic procedures and medications, will undoubtedly continue to further our abilities to combat this condition. Yet we have not fully capitalized on what we already know—that much cardiovascular risk is modifiable. Effective control of the risk factors described earlier remains a critical component to tame this global scourge. It is here that the patient–physician relationship and the role of medical professionals as community leaders advocating healthy lifestyles remain of cardinal importance.

SUMMARY

1. Early in atherogenesis, injurious and inflammatory stimuli activate endothelial and smooth muscle cells. The resulting cascade of events recruits immune cells to the vessel wall, fueling a persistent inflammatory state believed to underlie progression of the disease (see Fig. 5.2).

2. Mechanisms that contribute to atherosclerosis shape the forming plaque over decades (see Figs. 5.3 through 5.7). Plaques can display features associated with clinical stability or propensity to provoke thrombotic events (so-called "vulnerable" plaques; see Fig. 5.8).

3. Clinical expression of atherosclerosis commonly results from narrowing of the vessel lumen, from calcification or weakening of the arterial wall, or from plaque disruption with superimposed thrombus formation. Common manifestations include angina pectoris, myocardial infarction, stroke, and peripheral arterial disease (see Fig. 5.10).

4. Modifiable risk factors for atherosclerosis include dyslipidemia, smoking, hypertension, and diabetes. Nonmodifiable risk factors include advanced age, male gender, and a family history of premature coronary disease. Novel biomarkers, such as CRP, may prove useful in further defining risk.

Acknowledgments

Contributors to the previous editions of this chapter were James L. Young, MD; Rushika Fernandopulle, MD; Gopa Bhattacharyya, MD; Mary Beth Gordon, MD; and Joseph Loscalzo, MD, PhD.

Additional Reading

Ding K, Kullo IJ. Genome-wide association studies for atherosclerotic vascular disease and its risk factors. *Circ Cardiovasc Genet*. 2009;2:63–72.

Emerging Risk Factors Collaboration. Lipoprotein(a) concentration and the risk of coronary heart disease, stroke, and nonvascular mortality. *JAMA*. 2009;302:412–423.

Epstein SE, Zhu J, Najafi AH, et al. Insights into the role of infection in atherogenesis and in plaque rupture. *Circulation*. 2009;119:3133–3141.

Iqbal R, Anand S, Ounpuu S, et al. Dietary patterns and the risk of acute myocardial infarction in 52 countries: results of the INTERHEART study. *Circulation*. 2008;118:1929–1937.

Kuklina EV, Yoon PW, Keenan NL. Trends in high levels of low-density lipoprotein cholesterol in the United States, 1999–2006. *JAMA*. 2009;302:2104–2110.

Libby P, Nahrendorf M, Pitter MJ, et al. Diversity of denizens of the atherosclerotic plaque: not all monocytes are created equal. *Circulation*. 2008;117:3168–3170.

Libby P, Ridker PM, Hansson GK. Inflammation in atherosclerosis: from pathophysiology to practice. *J Am Coll Cardiol*. 2009;54:2129–2138.

Melander O, Newton-Cheh C, Almgren P, et al. Novel and conventional biomarkers for prediction of incident cardiovascular events in the community. *JAMA*. 2009;302:49–57.

Miller DT, Ridker PM, Libby P, et al. Atherosclerosis: the path from genomics to therapeutics. *J Am Coll Cardiol*. 2007;49:1589–1599.

O'Keefe JH, Carter MD, Lavie CJ. Primary and secondary prevention of cardiovascular diseases: a practical evidence-based approach. *Mayo Clin Proc*. 2009;84:741–757.

Ridker PM. C-reactive protein: eighty years from discovery to emergence as a major risk marker for cardiovascular disease. *Clin Chem*. 2009;5:209–215.

Ridker PM, Danielson E, Fonseca FA, et al. Rosuvastatin to prevent vascular events in men and women with elevated C-reactive protein. *N Engl J Med*. 2008;359:2195–2207.

Samani NJ, Erdmann J, Hall AS, et al. Genomewide association analysis of coronary artery disease. *N Engl J Med*. 2007;357:443–453.

Schunkert H, Götz A, Braund P, et al. Repeated replication and a prospective meta-analysis of the association between chromosome 9p21.3 and coronary artery disease. *Circulation*. 2008;117:1675–1684.

Ischemic Heart Disease

June-Wha Rhee
Marc S. Sabatine
Leonard S. Lilly

In 1772, the British physician William Heberden reported a disorder in which patients developed an uncomfortable sensation in the chest when walking. Labeling it *angina pectoris*, Heberden noted that this discomfort would disappear soon after the patient stood still but would recur with similar activities. Although he did not know the cause, it is likely that he was the first to describe the symptoms of ischemic heart disease, a condition of imbalance between myocardial oxygen supply and demand most often caused by atherosclerosis of the coronary arteries. Ischemic heart disease now afflicts millions of Americans and is the leading cause of death in industrialized nations.

The clinical presentation of ischemic heart disease can be highly variable and forms a spectrum of syndromes (Table 6.1). For example, ischemia may be accompanied by the same exertional symptoms described by Heberden. In other cases, it may occur without any clinical manifestations at all, a condition termed *silent ischemia*. This chapter describes the causes and consequences of chronic ischemic heart disease syndromes and provides a framework for the diagnosis and treatment of affected patients.

Angina pectoris remains the most common manifestation of ischemic heart disease and literally means "strangling in the chest." Although other conditions may lead to similar discomfort, *angina* refers specifically to the uncomfortable sensation in the chest and neighboring structures that arises from an

Table 6.1. Clinical Definitions

Syndrome	Description
Ischemic heart disease	Condition in which imbalance between myocardial oxygen supply and demand results in myocardial hypoxia and accumulation of waste metabolites, most often caused by atherosclerotic disease of the coronary arteries (often termed *coronary artery disease*)
Angina pectoris	Uncomfortable sensation in the chest and neighboring anatomic structures produced by myocardial ischemia
Stable angina	Chronic pattern of transient angina pectoris, precipitated by physical activity or emotional upset, relieved by rest within a few minutes; episodes often associated with temporary depression of the ST segment, but permanent myocardial damage does not result
Variant angina	Typical anginal discomfort, usually *at rest*, which develops because of coronary artery spasm rather than an increase of myocardial oxygen demand; episodes often associated with transient shifts of the ST segment, usually ST elevation (also termed *Prinzmetal angina*)
Silent ischemia	Asymptomatic episodes of myocardial ischemia; can be detected by electrocardiogram and other laboratory techniques
Unstable angina	Pattern of increased frequency and duration of angina episodes produced by less exertion or at rest; high frequency of progression to myocardial infarction if untreated
Myocardial infarction	Region of myocardial necrosis usually caused by prolonged cessation of blood supply; most often results from acute thrombus at site of coronary atherosclerotic stenosis; may be first clinical manifestation of ischemic heart disease, or there may be a history of angina pectoris

imbalance between myocardial oxygen supply and demand.

DETERMINANTS OF MYOCARDIAL OXYGEN SUPPLY AND DEMAND

In the normal heart, the oxygen requirements of the myocardium are continuously matched by the coronary arterial supply. Even during vigorous exercise, when the metabolic needs of the heart increase, so does the delivery of oxygen to the myocardial cells so that the balance is maintained. The following sections describe the key determinants of myocardial oxygen supply and demand in a normal person (Fig. 6.1) and how they are altered by the presence of atherosclerotic coronary artery disease (CAD).

Myocardial Oxygen Supply

The supply of oxygen to the myocardium depends on the **oxygen content** of the blood and the rate of **coronary blood flow**. The oxygen content is determined by the hemoglobin concentration and the degree of systemic oxygenation. In the absence of anemia or lung disease, oxygen content remains fairly constant. In contrast, coronary blood flow is much more dynamic, and regulation of that flow is responsible for matching the oxygen supply with metabolic requirements.

As in all blood vessels, coronary artery flow (Q) is directly proportional to the vessel's perfusion pressure (P) and is inversely proportional to coronary vascular resistance (R). That is,

$$Q \propto \frac{P}{R}$$

However, unlike other arterial systems in which the greatest blood flow occurs during systole, *the predominance of coronary perfusion takes place during diastole*. The reason for this is that systolic flow is impaired by the

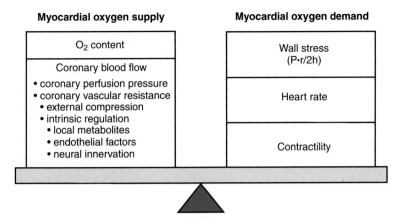

Myocardial oxygen supply

| O$_2$ content |
| Coronary blood flow |
| • coronary perfusion pressure
• coronary vascular resistance
• external compression
• intrinsic regulation
• local metabolites
• endothelial factors
• neural innervation |

Myocardial oxygen demand

| Wall stress
(P·r/2h) |
| Heart rate |
| Contractility |

Figure 6.1. Major determinants of myocardial oxygen supply and demand. *P*, ventricular pressure; *r*, ventricular radius; *h*, ventricular wall thickness.

compression of the small coronary branches as they course through the contracting myocardium. Coronary flow is unimpaired in diastole because the relaxed myocardium does not compress the coronary vasculature. Thus, in the case of the coronaries, **perfusion pressure** can be approximated by the aortic diastolic pressure. Conditions that decrease aortic diastolic pressure (such as hypotension or aortic valve regurgitation) decrease coronary artery perfusion pressure and may lessen myocardial oxygen supply.

Coronary vascular resistance is the other major determinant of coronary blood flow. In the normal artery, this resistance is dynamically modulated by (1) forces that externally compress the coronary arteries and (2) factors that alter intrinsic coronary tone.

External Compression

External compression is exerted on the coronary vessels during the cardiac cycle by contraction of the surrounding myocardium. The degree of compression is directly related to intramyocardial pressure and is therefore greatest during systole, as described in the previous section. Moreover, when the myocardium contracts, the subendocardium, adjacent to the high intraventricular pressure, is subjected to greater force than are the outer muscle layers. This is one reason that the subendocardium is the region most vulnerable to ischemic damage.

Intrinsic Control of Coronary Arterial Tone

Unlike most tissues, the heart cannot increase oxygen extraction on demand because in its basal state it removes nearly as much oxygen as possible from its blood supply. Thus, *any additional oxygen requirement must be met by an increase in blood flow*, and autoregulation of coronary vascular resistance is the most important mediator of this process. Factors that participate in the regulation of coronary vascular resistance include the accumulation of local metabolites, endothelium-derived substances, and neural innervation.

Metabolic Factors

The accumulation of local metabolites significantly affects coronary vascular tone and acts to modulate myocardial oxygen supply to meet changing metabolic demands. During states of hypoxemia, aerobic metabolism and oxidative phosphorylation in the mitochondria are inhibited. High-energy phosphates, including adenosine triphosphate (ATP), cannot be regenerated. Consequently, adenosine diphosphate (ADP) and adenosine monophosphate (AMP) accumulate and are subsequently degraded to adenosine. Adenosine is a potent vasodilator and is thought to be the prime metabolic mediator of vascular tone. By binding to receptors on vascular smooth muscle, adenosine decreases calcium entry into cells, which leads to relaxation, vasodilatation, and

BOX *6.1*   Endothelium-Derived Relaxing Factor, Nitric Oxide, and the Nobel Prize

Normal arterial endothelial cells synthesize potent vasodilator substances that contribute to the modulation of vascular tone. Among the first of these to be identified were prostacyclin (an arachidonic acid metabolite) and a substance termed endothelium-derived relaxing factor (EDRF).

EDRF was first studied in the 1970s. In experimental preparations, it was shown that acetylcholine (ACh) has two opposite actions on blood vessels. Its direct effect on vascular smooth muscle cells is to cause vasoconstriction, but when an intact endothelial lining overlies the smooth muscle cells, vasodilation occurs instead. Subsequent experiments showed that ACh causes the endothelial cells to release a chemical mediator (that was termed EDRF), which quickly diffuses to the adjacent smooth muscle cells and results in their relaxation with subsequent vasodilation of the vessel.

Subsequent research demonstrated that the mysterious EDRF is actually the nitric oxide (NO) radical. Binding of ACh (or another endothelial-dependent vasodilator such as serotonin or histamine) to endothelial cells catalyzes the formation of NO from the amino acid L-arginine (see figure). NO then diffuses to the adjacent vascular smooth muscle, where it activates guanylyl cyclase (G-cyclase). G-cyclase in turn forms cyclic guanosine monophosphate (cGMP), which results in smooth muscle cell relaxation through mechanisms that involve a reduction in cytosolic Ca^{++}.

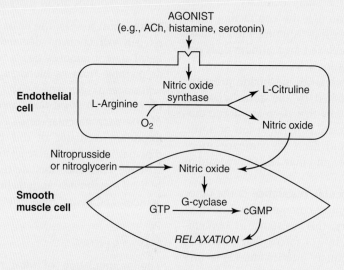

In contrast to the endothelial-dependent vasodilators, some agents cause smooth muscle relaxation *independent* of the presence of endothelial cells. For example, the drugs sodium nitroprusside and nitroglycerin result in vasodilation by providing an exogenous source of NO to vascular smooth muscle cells, thereby activating G-cyclase and forming cGMP without endothelial cell participation.

In the cardiac catheterization laboratory, the intracoronary administration of ACh in a normal person causes vasodilation of the vessel, presumably through the release of NO. However, in conditions of endothelial dysfunction, such as atherosclerosis, intracoronary ACh administration results in paradoxical *vasoconstriction* instead. This likely reflects reduced production of NO by the dysfunctional endothelial cells, resulting in unopposed direct vasoconstriction of the smooth muscle by ACh. Of particular interest is that the loss of vasodilatory response to infused ACh is evident in persons with certain cardiac risk factors (e.g., elevated LDL cholesterol, hypertension, cigarette smoking) even before the physical appearance of atheromatous plaque. Thus, the impaired release of NO may be an early and sensitive predictor for the later development of atherosclerotic lesions.

The significance of these discoveries was highlighted in 1998, when the Nobel Prize in medicine was awarded to the scientists who discovered the critical role of NO as a cardiovascular signaling molecule.

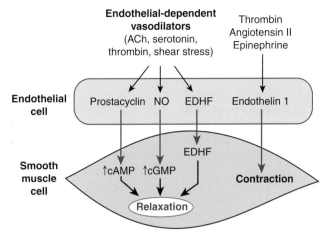

Figure 6.2. Endothelium-derived vasoactive substances and their regulators. Endothelium-derived vasodilators are shown on the left and include nitric oxide (NO), prostacyclin, and endothelium-derived hyperpolarizing factor (EDHF). Endothelin 1 is an endothelium-derived vasoconstrictor. In the normal state, the vasodilator influence predominates over that of vasoconstriction. ACh, acetylcholine.

increased coronary blood flow. Other metabolites that act locally as vasodilators include lactate, acetate, hydrogen ions, and carbon dioxide.

Endothelial Factors

Endothelial cells of the arterial wall produce numerous vasoactive substances that contribute to the regulation of vascular tone. *Vasodilators* produced by the endothelium include nitric oxide (NO), prostacyclin, and endothelium-derived hyperpolarizing factor (EDHF). Endothelin 1 is an example of an endothelium-derived *vasoconstrictor.*

The discovery and significance of **endothelium-derived NO** are highlighted in Box 6.1. In brief, NO regulates the vascular tone by diffusing into and then relaxing neighboring arterial smooth muscle by a cyclic guanosine monophosphate (cGMP)–dependent mechanism. The production of NO by normal endothelium occurs in the basal state and is additionally stimulated by many substances and conditions. For example, its release is augmented when the endothelium is exposed to acetylcholine (ACh), thrombin, products of aggregating platelets (e.g., serotonin and ADP), or even the shear stress of blood flow. Although the *direct* effect of many of these

substances on vascular smooth muscle is to cause *vasoconstriction*, the induced release of NO from the normal endothelium results in *vasodilatation* instead (Fig. 6.2).

Prostacyclin, an arachidonic acid metabolite, has vasodilator properties similar to those of NO (see Fig. 6.2). It is released from endothelial cells in response to many stimuli, including hypoxia, shear stress, ACh, and platelet products (e.g., serotonin). It causes relaxation of vascular smooth muscle by a cyclic AMP-dependent mechanism.

EDHF also appears to have important vasodilatory properties. Like endothelial-derived NO, it is a diffusible substance released by the endothelium that hyperpolarizes (and therefore relaxes) neighboring vascular smooth muscle cells. EDHF is released by many of the same factors that stimulate NO, including ACh and normal pulsatile blood flow. In the coronary circulation, EDHF appears to be more important in modulating relaxation in small arterioles than in the large conduit arteries.

Endothelin 1 is a potent vasoconstrictor produced by endothelial cells that partially counteracts the actions of the endothelial vasodilators. Its expression is stimulated by several factors, including thrombin, angiotensin II, epinephrine, and the shear stress of blood flow.

Under normal circumstances, the healthy endothelium promotes vascular smooth muscle *relaxation* (vasodilatation) through elaboration of substances such as NO and prostacyclin, the influences of which predominate over the endothelial vasoconstrictors (see Fig. 6.2). However, as described later in the chapter, dysfunctional endothelium (e.g., in atherosclerotic vessels) secretes reduced amounts of vasodilators, causing the balance to shift toward vasoconstriction instead.

Neural Factors

The neural control of vascular resistance has both sympathetic and parasympathetic components. Under normal circumstances, the contribution of the parasympathetic nervous system appears minor, but *sympathetic receptors* play an important role. Coronary vessels contain both α-adrenergic and β_2-adrenergic receptors. Stimulation of α-adrenergic receptors results in vasoconstriction, whereas β_2-receptors promote vasodilatation.

It is the interplay among the metabolic, endothelial, and neural regulating factors that determines the net impact on coronary vascular tone. For example, catecholamine stimulation of the heart may initially cause coronary *vasoconstriction* via the α-adrenergic receptor neural effect. However, catecholamine stimulation also increases myocardial oxygen consumption through increased heart rate and contractility (β_1-adrenergic effect), and the resulting increased production of local metabolites induces net coronary *dilatation* instead.

Myocardial Oxygen Demand

The three major determinants of myocardial oxygen demand are (1) ventricular wall stress, (2) heart rate, and (3) contractility (which is also termed the *inotropic state*). Additionally, very small amounts of oxygen are consumed in providing energy for basal cardiac metabolism and electrical depolarization.

Ventricular **wall stress** (σ) is the tangential force acting on the myocardial fibers, tending to pull them apart, and energy is expended in opposing that force. Wall stress is related to intraventricular pressure (P), the radius of the ventricle (r), and ventricular wall thickness (h) and is approximated by Laplace's relationship:

$$\sigma = \frac{P \times r}{2h}$$

Thus, wall stress is directly proportional to systolic ventricular pressure. Circumstances that increase pressure development in the left ventricle, such as aortic stenosis or hypertension, increase wall stress and myocardial oxygen consumption. Conditions that decrease ventricular pressure, such as antihypertensive therapy, reduce myocardial oxygen consumption.

Because wall stress is also directly proportional to the radius of the left ventricle, conditions that augment left ventricular (LV) filling (e.g., mitral or aortic regurgitation) raise wall stress and oxygen consumption. Conversely, any physiologic or pharmacologic maneuver that decreases LV filling and size (e.g., nitrate therapy) reduces wall stress and myocardial oxygen consumption.

Finally, wall stress is *inversely* proportional to ventricular wall thickness because the force is spread over a greater muscle mass. A hypertrophied heart has lower wall stress and oxygen consumption per gram of tissue than a thinned-wall heart. Thus, when hypertrophy develops in conditions of chronic pressure overload, such as aortic stenosis, it serves a compensatory role in reducing oxygen consumption.

The second major determinant of myocardial oxygen demand is **heart rate**. If the heart rate accelerates—during physical exertion, for example—the number of contractions and the amount of ATP consumed per minute increases and oxygen requirements rise. Conversely, slowing the heart rate (e.g., with a β-blocker drug) decreases ATP utilization and oxygen consumption.

The third major determinant of oxygen demand is myocardial **contractility**, a measure of the force of contraction (see Chapter 9). Circulating catecholamines, or the administration of positive inotropic drugs, directly increase the force of contraction, which augments oxygen utilization. Conversely, negative inotropic effectors, such as β-adrenergic-blocking drugs, decrease myocardial oxygen consumption.

In the normal state, autoregulatory mechanisms adjust coronary tone to match myocardial oxygen supply with oxygen requirements. In the absence of obstructive coronary disease, these mechanisms maintain a fairly constant rate of coronary flow, as long as the aortic perfusion pressure is approximately 60 mm Hg or greater. In the setting of advanced coronary atherosclerosis, however, the fall in perfusion pressure distal to the arterial stenosis, along with dysfunction of the endothelium of the involved segment, sets the stage for a mismatch between the available blood supply and myocardial metabolic demands.

PATHOPHYSIOLOGY OF ISCHEMIA

The traditional view has been that myocardial ischemia in CAD results from fixed atherosclerotic plaques that narrow the vessel's lumen and limit myocardial blood supply. However, recent research has demonstrated that the reduction of blood flow in this condition results from the *combination* of fixed vessel narrowing *and* abnormal vascular tone, contributed to by atherosclerosis-induced endothelial cell dysfunction.

Fixed Vessel Narrowing

The hemodynamic significance of fixed atherosclerotic coronary artery stenoses relates to both the fluid mechanics and the anatomy of the vascular supply.

Fluid Mechanics

Poiseuille's law states that for flow through a vessel,

$$Q = \frac{\Delta P \pi r^4}{8 \eta L}$$

in which Q is flow, ΔP is the pressure difference between the points being measured, r is the vessel radius, η is the fluid viscosity, and L is the vessel length. By analogy to Ohm's law, flow is also equal to the pressure difference divided by the resistance (R) to flow:

$$Q = \frac{\Delta P}{R}$$

By combining these two formulas and rearranging, resistance to blood flow in a vessel can be expressed as:

$$R = \frac{8 \eta L}{\pi r^4}$$

Thus, vascular resistance is governed, in part, by the geometric component L/r^4. That is, the hemodynamic significance of a stenotic lesion depends on its length and, far more importantly, on the degree of vessel narrowing (i.e., the reduction of r) that it causes.

Anatomy

The coronary arteries consist of large, proximal epicardial segments and smaller, distal resistance vessels (arterioles). The proximal vessels are subject to overt atherosclerosis that results in stenotic plaques. The distal vessels are usually free of flow-limiting plaques and can adjust their vasomotor tone in response to metabolic needs. These resistance vessels serve as a reserve, increasing their diameter with exertion to meet increasing oxygen demand and dilating, even at rest, if a proximal stenosis is sufficiently severe.

The hemodynamic significance of a coronary artery narrowing depends on both the degree of stenosis of the epicardial portion of the vessel and the amount of *compensatory vasodilatation* the distal resistance vessels are able to achieve (Fig. 6.3). If a stenosis narrows the lumen diameter by less than 60%, the maximal potential blood flow through the artery is not significantly altered and, in response to exertion, the resistance vessels can dilate to provide adequate blood flow. When a stenosis narrows the diameter by more than approximately 70%, resting blood flow is normal, but maximal blood flow is reduced even with full dilatation of the resistance vessels. In this situation, when oxygen demand increases (e.g., from the elevated heart rate and force of contraction during physical exertion), coronary flow reserve is inadequate, oxygen demand exceeds supply, and myocardial ischemia results. If the stenosis compromises the vessel lumen by more than approximately 90%, then even with maximal dilatation of the resistance vessels, blood flow

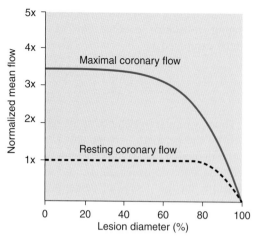

Figure 6.3. Resting and maximal coronary blood flows are affected by the magnitude of proximal arterial stenosis (percent lesion diameter). The dotted line indicates resting blood flow, and the solid line represents maximal blood flow (i.e., when there is full dilatation of the distal resistance vessels). Compromise of maximal blood flow is evident when the proximal stenosis reduces the coronary lumen diameter by more than ~70%. Resting flow may be compromised if the stenosis exceeds ~90%. (Modified from Gould KL, Lipscomb K. Effects of coronary stenoses on coronary flow reserve and resistance. *Am J Cardiol.* 1974;34:50.)

may be inadequate to meet basal requirements and ischemia can develop *at rest.*

Although collateral connections (see Chapter 1) may become apparent between unobstructed coronaries and sites distal to atherosclerotic stenoses, and such flow can buffer the fall in myocardial oxygen supply, it is often not sufficient to prevent ischemia during exertion in critically narrowed vessels.

Endothelial Cell Dysfunction

In addition to fixed vessel narrowing, the other major contributor to reduced myocardial oxygen supply in chronic CAD is endothelial dysfunction. Abnormal endothelial cell function can contribute to the pathophysiology of ischemia in two ways: (1) by inappropriate vasoconstriction of coronary arteries and (2) through loss of normal antithrombotic properties.

Inappropriate Vasoconstriction

In normal persons, physical activity or mental stress results in measurable coronary artery *vasodilatation.* This effect is thought to be

regulated by activation of the sympathetic nervous system, with increased blood flow and shear stress stimulating the release of endothelial-derived vasodilators, such as NO. It is postulated that in typical people, the relaxation effect of NO outweighs the direct α-adrenergic constrictor effect of catecholamines on arterial smooth muscle, such that vasodilatation results. However, in patients with dysfunctional endothelium (e.g., atherosclerosis), an *impaired release of endothelial vasodilators* leaves the direct catecholamine effect unopposed, such that relative vasoconstriction occurs instead. The resultant decrease in coronary blood flow contributes to ischemia. Even the vasodilatory effect of local metabolites (such as adenosine) is attenuated in patients with dysfunctional endothelium, further uncoupling the regulation of vascular tone from metabolic demands.

In patients with risk factors for CAD, such as hypercholesterolemia, diabetes mellitus, hypertension, and cigarette smoking, impaired endothelial-dependent vasodilation is noted even *before* visible atherosclerotic lesions have developed. This suggests that endothelial dysfunction occurs very early in the atherosclerotic process.

Inappropriate vasoconstriction also appears to be important in acute coronary syndromes, such as unstable angina and myocardial infarction (MI). As described in Chapter 7, the usual cause of acute coronary syndromes is disruption of atherosclerotic plaque, with superimposed platelet aggregation and thrombus formation. Normally, the products of platelet aggregation in a developing clot (e.g., serotonin and ADP) result in vasodilatation because they stimulate the endothelial release of NO. However, with dysfunctional endothelium, the direct *vasoconstricting* actions of platelet products predominate (Fig. 6.4), further compromising flow through the arterial lumen.

Loss of Normal Antithrombotic Properties

In addition to their vasodilatory actions, factors released from endothelial cells (including NO and prostacyclin) also exert antithrombotic properties by interfering with platelet aggregation (see Fig. 6.4). However, in states of endothelial

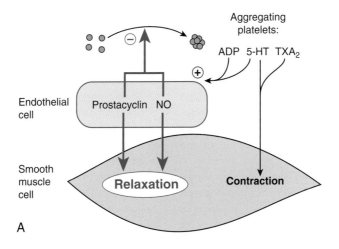

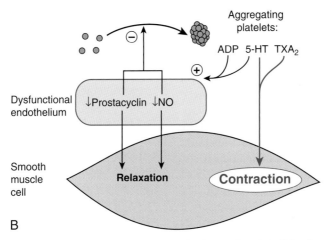

Figure 6.4. **The interaction between platelets and endothelial cells.**
A. Normal endothelium. Aggregating platelets release thromboxane (TXA$_2$)
and serotonin (5-HT), the direct vascular effects of which cause contraction
of vascular smooth muscle and vasoconstriction. However, platelet products
(e.g., ADP and 5-HT) also stimulate the endothelial release of the potent
vasodilators nitric oxide (NO) and prostacyclin, such that the net effect is
smooth muscle relaxation instead. Endothelial production of NO and prostacyclin also serves antithrombotic roles, which limit further platelet aggregation.
B. Dysfunctional endothelium demonstrates impaired release of the vasodilator substances, such that net smooth muscle *contraction* and *vasoconstriction*
supervene. The reduced endothelial release of NO and prostacyclin diminishes
their antiplatelet effect, such that thrombosis proceeds unchecked.

cell dysfunction, release of these substances is
reduced; therefore, the antithrombotic effect is
attenuated. Thus, in syndromes characterized by
thrombosis (i.e., the acute coronary syndromes
described in Chapter 7), the impaired release of
NO and prostacyclin allows platelets to aggregate
and to secrete their potentially harmful procoagulants and vasoconstrictors.

Other Causes of Myocardial Ischemia

In addition to atherosclerotic CAD, other conditions may result in an imbalance between myocardial oxygen supply and demand and result
in ischemia. Other common causes of decreased
myocardial oxygen supply include (1) decreased
perfusion pressure due to hypotension (e.g., in

a patient with hypovolemia or septic shock) and (2) a severely decreased blood oxygen content (e.g., marked anemia, or impaired oxygenation of blood by the lungs). For example, a patient with massive bleeding from the gastrointestinal tract may develop myocardial ischemia and angina pectoris, even in the absence of atherosclerotic coronary disease, because of reduced oxygen supply (i.e., the loss of hemoglobin and hypotension).

On the other side of the balance, a profound increase in myocardial oxygen demand can cause ischemia even in the absence of coronary atherosclerosis. This can occur, for example, with rapid tachycardias, acute hypertension, or severe aortic stenosis.

CONSEQUENCES OF ISCHEMIA

The consequences of ischemia reflect the inadequate myocardial oxygenation and local accumulation of metabolic waste products. For example, during ischemia, myocytes convert from aerobic to anaerobic metabolic pathways. The reduced generation of ATP impairs the interaction of the contractile proteins and results in a transient reduction of both ventricular systolic contraction and diastolic relaxation (both of which are energy-dependent processes). The consequent elevation of LV diastolic pressure is transmitted (via the left atrium and pulmonary veins) to the pulmonary capillaries and can precipitate pulmonary congestion and the symptom of shortness of breath (dyspnea). In addition, metabolic products such as lactate, serotonin, and adenosine accumulate locally. It is suspected that one or more of these compounds activate peripheral pain receptors in the C7 through T4 distribution and may be the mechanism by which the discomfort of angina is produced. The accumulation of local metabolites and transient abnormalities of myocyte ion transport may also precipitate arrhythmias (see Chapter 11).

The ultimate fate of myocardium subjected to ischemia depends on the severity and duration of the imbalance between oxygen supply and demand. It was previously thought that ischemic cardiac injury results in either irreversible myocardial necrosis (i.e., MI) or rapid and full recovery of myocyte function (e.g., after a brief episode of typical angina).

It is now known that in addition to those outcomes, ischemic insults can sometimes result in a period of prolonged contractile dysfunction *without* myocyte necrosis, and recovery of normal function may ultimately follow.

For example, **stunned myocardium** refers to tissue that, after suffering an episode of severe acute, transient ischemia (but not necrosis), demonstrates prolonged systolic dysfunction even after the return of normal myocardial blood flow. In this setting, the functional, biochemical, and ultrastructural abnormalities following ischemia are reversible and contractile function gradually recovers. The mechanism responsible for this delayed recovery of function involves myocyte calcium overload and the accumulation of oxygen-derived free radicals during ischemia. In general, the magnitude of stunning is proportional to the degree of the preceding ischemia, and this state is likely the pathophysiologic response to an ischemic insult that just falls short of causing irreversible necrosis.

In contrast, **hibernating myocardium** refers to tissue that manifests *chronic* ventricular contractile dysfunction due to a persistently reduced blood supply, usually because of multivessel CAD. In this situation, irreversible damage has not occurred and ventricular function can promptly improve if appropriate blood flow is restored (e.g., by coronary angioplasty or bypass surgery). The clinical importance of stunned or hibernating myocardium is summarized in Box 6.2.

Ischemic Syndromes

Depending on the underlying pathophysiologic process and the timing and severity of a myocardial ischemic insult, a spectrum of distinct clinical syndromes may result, as illustrated in Figure 6.5.

Stable Angina

Chronic *stable angina* is manifested as a pattern of predictable, transient chest discomfort during exertion or emotional stress. It is generally caused by fixed, obstructive atheromatous plaque in one or more coronary arteries (see Fig. 6.5B). The pattern of symptoms is

BOX 6.2   Clinical Relevance of Stunned and Hibernating Myocardium

The concepts of stunned and hibernating myocardium are very important in the clinical setting. Such regions of myocardium contract poorly when imaged (e.g., by echocardiography or contrast angiography) and can appear indistinguishable from irreversibly infarcted heart muscle. However, they can be differentiated from necrotic regions by special imaging studies (e.g., dobutamine echocardiography, thallium-201 viability study, or positron emission tomography; see Chapter 3). That distinction influences the decision of whether to undertake mechanical reperfusion procedures (percutaneous or surgical), because stunned or hibernating myocardium would be expected to improve with mechanical revascularization, whereas truly infarcted myocardium would not.

usually related to the degree of stenosis. As described in the earlier section on pathophysiology, when atherosclerotic stenoses narrow a coronary artery lumen diameter by more than approximately 70%, the reduced flow capacity may be sufficient to serve the low cardiac oxygen needs at rest but is insufficient to compensate for any significant increase in oxygen demand (see Fig. 6.3). During physical exertion, for example, activation of the sympathetic

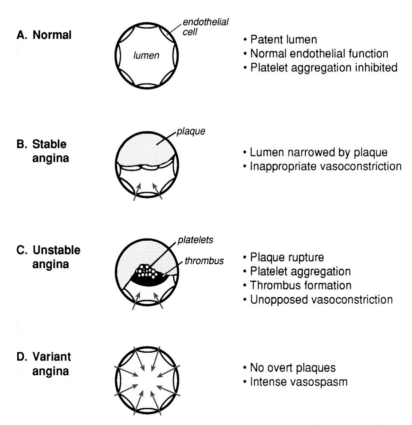

A. Normal
- endothelial cell
- lumen
  - • Patent lumen
  - • Normal endothelial function
  - • Platelet aggregation inhibited

B. Stable angina
- plaque
  - • Lumen narrowed by plaque
  - • Inappropriate vasoconstriction

C. Unstable angina
- platelets
- thrombus
  - • Plaque rupture
  - • Platelet aggregation
  - • Thrombus formation
  - • Unopposed vasoconstriction

D. Variant angina
  - • No overt plaques
  - • Intense vasospasm

Figure 6.5. **Pathophysiologic findings in anginal syndromes. A.** Normal coronary arteries are widely patent, and the endothelium functions normally. **B.** In stable angina, atherosclerotic plaque and inappropriate vasoconstriction (caused by dysfunctional endothelium) reduce the vessel lumen's size and coronary blood flow. **C.** In unstable angina, disruption of the plaque triggers platelet aggregation, thrombus formation, and vasoconstriction, all of which contribute to reduced coronary blood supply. **D.** In variant angina, atherosclerotic plaques are absent; rather, ischemia is due to intense vasospasm that reduces myocardial oxygen supply.

nervous system results in increased heart rate, blood pressure, and contractility, all of which augment myocardial oxygen consumption. During the period that oxygen demand exceeds available supply, myocardial ischemia results, often accompanied by the chest discomfort of angina pectoris. The ischemia and symptoms persist until the increased demand is alleviated and oxygen balance is restored.

Potentially contributing to the inadequate oxygen supply in stable angina is inappropriate coronary vasoconstriction caused, at least in part, by atherosclerosis-associated endothelial dysfunction. Recall that normally, the high myocardial oxygen demand during exertion is balanced by an increased supply of blood as the accumulation of local metabolites induces vasodilatation. With endothelial cell dysfunction, however, vasodilatation is impaired and the vessels may paradoxically vasoconstrict instead, in response to exercise-induced catecholamine stimulation of α-adrenergic receptors on the coronary artery smooth muscle cells.

As a result, the extent of coronary artery narrowing in patients with atherosclerosis is not necessarily constant. Rather, it can vary from moment to moment because of changes in the superimposed coronary vascular tone. For some patients with stable angina, alterations in tone play a minimal role in the decreased myocardial oxygen supply, and the level of physical activity required to precipitate angina is fairly constant. These patients have *fixed-threshold angina*. In other cases, the degree of dynamic obstruction caused by vasoconstriction or vasospasm plays a more prominent role, and such patients may have *variable-threshold angina*. For example, on a given day, a patient with variable-threshold angina can exert herself or himself without chest discomfort, but on another day, the same degree of myocardial oxygen demand *does* produce symptoms. The difference reflects alterations in vascular tone over the sites of fixed stenosis. Other clinical features of chronic stable angina are described in greater detail later in the chapter.

Unstable Angina

A patient with chronic stable angina may experience a sudden increase in the tempo and duration of ischemic episodes, occurring with lesser degrees of exertion and even at rest. This acceleration of symptoms is known as *unstable angina*, which can be a precursor to an acute MI. Unstable angina and acute MI are also known as *acute coronary syndromes* and result from specific pathophysiologic mechanisms, most commonly rupture of an unstable atherosclerotic plaque with subsequent platelet aggregation and thrombosis (see Fig. 6.5C). These syndromes are described in detail in Chapter 7.

Variant Angina

A small minority of patients manifest episodes of focal *coronary artery spasm* in the absence of overt atherosclerotic lesions, and this syndrome is known as *variant angina* or *Prinzmetal angina*. In this case, intense vasospasm alone reduces coronary oxygen supply and results in angina (see Fig. 6.5D). The mechanism by which such profound spasm develops is not completely understood but may involve increased sympathetic activity in combination with endothelial dysfunction. It is thought that many patients with variant angina may actually have early atherosclerosis manifested only by a dysfunctional endothelium, because the response to endothelium-dependent vasodilators (e.g., ACh and serotonin) is often abnormal.

Variant angina often occurs at rest because ischemia in this case results from transient reduction of the coronary oxygen supply rather than an increase in myocardial oxygen demand.

Silent Ischemia

Episodes of cardiac ischemia sometimes occur in the absence of perceptible discomfort or pain, and such instances are referred to as *silent ischemia*. These asymptomatic episodes can occur in patients who on other occasions experience typical *symptomatic* angina. Conversely, in some patients, silent ischemia may be the *only* manifestation of CAD. It may be difficult to diagnose silent ischemia on clinical grounds, but its presence can be detected by laboratory techniques such as continuous ambulatory electrocardiography or it can be elicited by exercise stress testing, as described later in the chapter. One study estimated that silent ischemic episodes occur in 40% of patients with stable symptomatic angina and in 2.5% to 10% of asymptomatic middle-aged men. When considering the importance of anginal discomfort as a physiologic warning signal, the asymptomatic nature of silent ischemia becomes all the more concerning.

The reason why some episodes of ischemia are silent whereas others are symptomatic has not been elucidated. The degree of ischemia cannot fully explain the disparity, because even MI may present without symptoms in some patients. Silent ischemia has been reported to be more common among diabetic patients (possibly due to impaired pain sensation from peripheral neuropathy), the elderly, and in women.

Syndrome X

The term *syndrome X* refers to patients with typical symptoms of angina pectoris who have no evidence of significant atherosclerotic coronary stenoses on coronary angiograms. Some of these patients may show definite laboratory signs of ischemia during exercise testing. The pathogenesis of ischemia in this situation may be related to inadequate vasodilator reserve of the coronary resistance vessels. It is thought that the resistance vessels (which are too small to be visualized by coronary angiography) may not dilate appropriately during periods of increased myocardial oxygen demand. Microvascular dysfunction, vasospasm, and hypersensitive pain perception may each contribute to this syndrome. Patients with syndrome X have a better prognosis than those with overt atherosclerotic disease.

CLINICAL FEATURES OF CHRONIC STABLE ANGINA

History

The most important part of the clinical evaluation of ischemic heart disease is the history described by the patient. Because chest pain is such a common complaint, it is important to focus on the characteristics that help distinguish myocardial ischemia from other causes of discomfort. From a diagnostic standpoint, it would be ideal to interview and examine a patient during an actual episode of angina, but most people are asymptomatic during routine clinic examinations. Therefore, a careful history probing several features of the discomfort should be elicited.

Quality

Angina is most often described as a "pressure," "discomfort," "tightness," "burning," or "heaviness" in the chest. It is rare that the sensation is actually described as a "pain," and often a patient will correct the physician who refers to the anginal symptom as such. Sometimes, a patient likens the sensation to "an elephant sitting on my chest." Anginal discomfort is neither sharp nor stabbing, and it does not vary significantly with inspiration or movement of the chest wall. It is a steady discomfort that lasts a few minutes, yet rarely more than 5 to 10 minutes. It *always* lasts more than a few seconds, and this helps to differentiate it from sharper and briefer musculoskeletal pains.

While describing angina, the patient may place a clenched fist over his or her sternum, referred to as the **Levine sign**, as if defining the constricting discomfort by that tight grip.

Location

Anginal discomfort is usually *diffuse* rather than localized to a single point. It is most often located in the retrosternal area or in the left precordium but may occur anywhere in the chest, back, arms, neck, lower face, or upper abdomen. It often radiates to the shoulders and inner aspect of the arms, especially on the left side.

Accompanying Symptoms

During the discomfort of an acute anginal attack, generalized sympathetic and parasympathetic stimulation may result in *tachycardia*, *diaphoresis*, and *nausea*. Ischemia also results in transient dysfunction of LV systolic contraction and diastolic relaxation. The resultant elevation of LV diastolic pressure is transmitted to the pulmonary vasculature and often causes *dyspnea* during the episode. Transient *fatigue* and *weakness* are also common, particularly in elderly patients. When such symptoms occur as a consequence of myocardial ischemia but are unaccompanied by typical chest discomfort, they are referred to as "anginal equivalents."

Precipitants

Angina, when not caused by pure vasospasm, is precipitated by conditions that increase myocardial oxygen demand (e.g., increased heart rate, contractility, or wall stress). These include physical exertion, anger, and other emotional excitement. Additional factors that increase myocardial oxygen demand and can precipitate anginal discomfort in patients with CAD include a large meal or cold weather. The latter induces peripheral vasoconstriction, which in turn augments myocardial wall stress as the left ventricle contracts against the increased resistance.

Angina is generally relieved within minutes after the cessation of the activity that precipitated it and even more quickly (within 3 to 5 minutes) by sublingual nitroglycerin. This response can help differentiate myocardial ischemia from many of the other conditions that produce chest discomfort.

Patients who experience angina primarily due to increased coronary artery tone or vasospasm often develop symptoms at rest, independent of activities that increase myocardial oxygen demand.

Frequency

Although the level of exertion necessary to precipitate angina may remain fairly constant, the frequency of episodes varies considerably because patients quickly learn which activities cause their discomfort and avoid them. It is thus important to inquire about reductions in activities of daily living when taking the history.

Risk Factors

In addition to the description of chest discomfort, a careful history should uncover risk factors that predispose to atherosclerosis and CAD, including cigarette smoking, dyslipidemia, hypertension, diabetes, and a family history of premature coronary disease (see Chapter 5).

Differential Diagnosis

Several conditions can give rise to symptoms that mimic the transient chest discomfort of angina pectoris, including other cardiac causes (e.g., pericarditis), gastrointestinal disorders (e.g., gastroesophageal reflux, esophageal spasm, or biliary pain), and musculoskeletal conditions (including chest wall pain, spinal osteoarthritis, and cervical radiculitis). The history remains of paramount importance in distinguishing myocardial ischemia from these disorders. In contrast to angina pectoris, gastrointestinal causes of recurrent chest pain are often precipitated by certain foods and are unrelated to exertion. Musculoskeletal causes of chest discomfort tend to be more superficial or can be localized to a discrete spot (i.e., the patient can point to the pain with one finger) and often vary with changes in position. Similarly, the presence of pleuritic pain (sharp pain aggravated by respiratory movements) argues against angina as the cause; this symptom is more likely a result of pericarditis, or an acute pulmonary condition such as pulmonary embolism or acute pneumothorax. Useful differentiating features of recurrent chest pain are listed in Table 6.2.

Physical Examination

If it is possible to examine a patient *during* an anginal attack, several transient physical signs may be detected (Fig. 6.6). An increased heart rate and blood pressure are common because of the augmented sympathetic response. Myocardial ischemia may lead to papillary muscle dysfunction and therefore mitral regurgitation. Ischemia-induced regional ventricular contractile abnormalities can sometimes be detected as an abnormal bulging impulse on palpation of the left chest. Ischemia decreases ventricular compliance, producing a stiffened ventricle and therefore an S_4 gallop on physical examination during atrial contraction (see Chapter 2). However, if the patient is free of chest discomfort during the examination, there may be *no* abnormal cardiac physical findings.

Physical examination should also assess for signs of atherosclerotic disease in more accessible vascular beds. For example, carotid bruits may indicate the presence of cerebrovascular disease, whereas femoral artery bruits or diminished

Table 6.2. Causes of Recurrent Chest Pain

Condition	Differentiating Features
Cardiac	
Myocardial ischemia	• Retrosternal tightness or pressure; typically radiates to neck, jaw, or left shoulder and arm • Lasts a few minutes (usually <10) • Brought on by exertion, relieved by rest or nitroglycerin • ECG: transient ST depressions or elevations, or flattened or inverted T waves
Pericarditis	• Sharp, pleuritic pain that varies with position; friction rub on auscultation • Can last for hours to days • ECG: diffuse ST elevations and PR depression
Gastrointestinal	
Gastroesophageal reflux	• Retrosternal burning • Precipitated by certain foods, worsened by supine position, unaffected by exertion • Relieved by antacids
Peptic ulcer disease	• Epigastric ache or burning • Occurs after meals, unaffected by exertion • Relieved by antacids, not by nitroglycerin
Esophageal spasm	• Retrosternal pain accompanied by dysphagia • Precipitated by meals, unaffected by exertion • May be relieved by nitroglycerin
Biliary colic	• Constant, deep pain in right upper quadrant; can last for hours • Brought on by fatty foods, unaffected by exertion • Not relieved by antacids or nitroglycerin
Musculoskeletal	
Costochondral syndrome	• Sternal pain worsened by chest movement • Costochondral junctions tender to palpation • Relieved by anti-inflammatory drugs, not by nitroglycerin
Cervical radiculitis	• Constant ache or shooting pains, may be in a dermatomal distribution • Worsened by neck motion

ECG, electrocardiogram.

pulses in the lower extremities can be a clue to peripheral arterial disease (see Chapter 15).

Diagnostic Studies

Once angina is suspected, several diagnostic procedures may be helpful in confirming myocardial ischemia as the cause. Because many of these tests are costly, it is important to choose the appropriate studies for each patient.

Electrocardiogram

One of the most useful tools is an electrocardiogram (ECG) obtained during an anginal episode. Although this is easy to arrange when symptoms occur in hospitalized patients, it may not be possible to "catch" episodes in people seen on an outpatient basis. During myocardial ischemia, ST segment and T wave changes commonly appear (Fig. 6.7). Acute ischemia usually results in transient horizontal or downsloping ST segment depressions and T wave flattening or inversions. Occasionally, ST segment *elevations* are seen, suggesting more severe transmural myocardial ischemia, and can also be observed during the intense vasospasm of variant angina. In contrast to the ECG of a patient with an acute MI, the

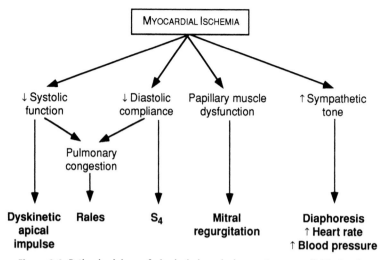

Figure 6.6. **Pathophysiology of physical signs during acute myocardial ischemia.**

ST deviations seen in patients with stable angina quickly normalize with resolution of the patient's symptoms. In fact, ECGs obtained during periods free of ischemia are completely normal in approximately half of patients with stable angina. In others, chronic "nondiagnostic" ST and T wave deviations may be present. Evidence of a previous MI (e.g., pathologic Q waves) on the ECG also points to the presence of underlying coronary disease.

Stress Testing

Because ECGs obtained during or between episodes of chest discomfort may be normal, such tracings do not rule out underlying ischemic heart disease. For this reason, provocative

exercise or **pharmacologic stress tests** are valuable diagnostic and prognostic aids.

Standard Exercise Testing

For many patients suspected of having CAD, a standard exercise test is performed. During this test, the patient exercises on a treadmill or a stationary bicycle to progressively higher workloads and is observed for the development of chest discomfort or excessive dyspnea. The heart rate and ECG are continuously monitored, and blood pressure is checked at regular intervals. The test is continued until angina develops, signs of myocardial ischemia appear on the ECG, a target heart rate is achieved (85% of the maximal predicted heart rate [MHR]; the

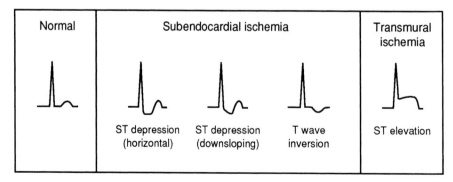

Figure 6.7. **Common transient ECG abnormalities during ischemia.** Subendocardial ischemia causes ST segment depressions and/or T wave flattening or inversions. Severe transient transmural ischemia can result in ST segment *elevations*, similar to the early changes in acute myocardial infarction. When transient ischemia resolves, so do the electrocardiographic changes.

MHR is calculated as 220 beats/min minus the patient's age), or the patient becomes too fatigued to continue.

The test is considered *positive* if the patient's typical chest discomfort is reproduced or if ECG abnormalities consistent with ischemia develop (i.e., >1 mm horizontal or downsloping ST segment depressions). Among patients who later undergo diagnostic coronary angiography, standard exercise testing has a sensitivity of approximately 65% to 70% and specificity of 75% to 80% for the detection of anatomically significant CAD.

The stress test is considered *markedly positive* if one or more of the following signs of severe ischemic heart disease occur: (1) ischemic ECG changes develop in the first 3 minutes of exercise or persist 5 minutes after exercise has stopped; (2) the magnitude of the ST segment depressions is >2 mm; (3) the systolic blood pressure abnormally falls during exercise (i.e., resulting from ischemia-induced impairment of contractile function); (4) high-grade ventricular arrhythmias develop; or (5) the patient cannot exercise for at least 2 minutes because of cardiopulmonary limitations. Patients with markedly positive tests are more likely to have severe multivessel coronary disease.

The utility of a stress test may be affected by the patient's medications. For example, β-blockers or certain calcium channel blockers (verapamil, diltiazem) may blunt the ability to achieve the target heart rate. In these situations, one must consider the purpose of the stress test. If it is to determine whether ischemic heart disease is present, then those medications are typically withheld for 24 to 48 hours before the test. On the other hand, if the patient has known ischemic heart disease and the purpose of the test is to assess the efficacy of the current medical regimen, testing should be performed while the patient takes his or her usual antianginal medications.

Nuclear Imaging Studies

Because the standard exercise test relies on ischemia-related changes on the ECG, the test is less useful in patients with baseline abnormalities of the ST segments (e.g., as seen in left bundle branch block or LV hypertrophy).

In addition, the standard exercise stress test sometimes yields equivocal results in patients for whom the clinical suspicion of ischemic heart disease is high. In these situations, radionuclide imaging can be combined with exercise testing to overcome these limitations and to increase the sensitivity and specificity of the study.

During myocardial perfusion imaging (see Chapter 3), a radionuclide (commonly either a technetium-99m-labeled compound or thallium-201) is injected intravenously at peak exercise, after which imaging is performed. The radionuclide accumulates in proportion to the degree of perfusion of viable myocardial cells. Therefore, areas of poor perfusion (i.e., regions of ischemia) during exercise do not accumulate radionuclide and appear as "cold spots" on the image. However, irreversibly infarcted areas also do not take up the radionuclide, and they too will appear as cold spots. To differentiate between transient ischemia and infarcted tissue, imaging is also performed at rest (either before, or several hours after, the exercise portion of the test). If the cold spot fills in, a region of *transient ischemia* has been identified. If the cold spot remains unchanged, a region of irreversible *infarction* is likely.

Standard radionuclide exercise tests are 80% to 90% sensitive and approximately 80% specific for the detection of clinically significant CAD. Positron emission tomography (PET; see Chapter 3), another form of nuclear stress imaging that is not as widely available, offers superior spatial and temporal resolution, with sensitivity and specificity of approximately 90%. Because these techniques are expensive, their use in screening for CAD should be reserved for (1) patients in whom baseline ECG abnormalities preclude interpretation of a standard exercise test or for (2) improvement in test sensitivity when standard stress test results are discordant with the clinical suspicion of coronary disease.

Exercise Echocardiography

Exercise testing with *echocardiographic* imaging is another technique to diagnose myocardial ischemia in patients with baseline ST or T wave abnormalities or in those with equivocal standard stress tests. In this procedure, LV contractile function is assessed by echocardiography at baseline and immediately after treadmill or bicycle exercise. The test indicates inducible myocardial ischemia if regions of ventricular contractile dysfunction develop with exertion and has a sensitivity of approximately 80% and a specificity of about 90% for the detection of clinically significant CAD.

Pharmacologic Stress Tests

For patients unable to exercise (e.g., those with hip or knee arthritis), *pharmacologic* stress testing can be performed instead using various agents, including the inotrope *dobutamine* (which increases myocardial oxygen demand by stimulating the heart rate and force of contraction) or the vasodilators *dipyridamole* or *adenosine.* Dipyridamole blocks the cellular uptake and destruction of adenosine and thereby increases adenosine's circulating concentration. When adenosine binds to its vascular receptors, coronary vasodilatation results. As ischemic regions are already maximally dilated (in compensation for the epicardial coronary stenoses), the drug-induced vasodilatation increases flow to the myocardium perfused by healthy coronary arteries and thus "steals" blood away from the diseased segments. These pharmacologic interventions are coupled (in place of exercise) with nuclear imaging or echocardiography, as described above, to reveal regions of impaired myocardial perfusion.

Coronary Angiography

The most direct means of identifying coronary artery stenoses is by coronary angiography, in which atherosclerotic lesions are visualized radiographically following the injection of radiopaque contrast material into the artery (Fig. 6.8; see Chapter 3). Although generally safe, the procedure is associated with a small risk of complications directly related to its invasive nature. Therefore, coronary angiography is typically reserved for patients whose anginal symptoms do not respond adequately to pharmacologic therapy, for those with an unstable presentation, or when the results of

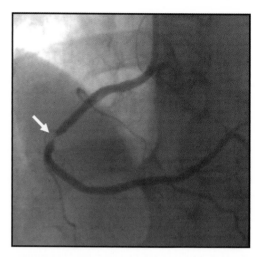

Figure 6.8. Example of coronary angiography. Injection of the right coronary artery demonstrates a stenosis in the midportion of the vessel, indicated by the arrow. (Courtesy of Pinak B. Shah, MD, Brigham and Women's Hospital, Boston, MA.)

noninvasive testing are so abnormal that severe CAD warranting revascularization is likely.

Although coronary angiography is considered the "gold standard" for the diagnosis of CAD, it should be noted that it provides only anatomic information. The clinical significance of lesions detected by angiography depends not only on the degree of narrowing but also on the pathophysiologic consequences. Therefore, treatment decisions are made not only on the finding of such stenoses but even more so on their functional effects, manifested by the patient's symptoms, the viability of the myocardium segment served by stenotic vessels, and the degree of ventricular contractile dysfunction. Furthermore, standard arteriography does not reveal the composition of coronary atherosclerotic plaque or its vulnerability to rupture (see Chapter 5).

Noninvasive Imaging of Coronary Arteries

Cardiac computed tomography (CT) can visualize cardiac anatomy in great detail (see Chapter 3). It is particularly sensitive for the detection of coronary artery calcification, which correlates well with the severity of CAD. Concurrent administration of intravenous contrast and multidetector scanning permits visualization of the coronary lumen and stenoses (see Fig. 3.21). CT is not as sensitive as conventional angiography for definition of coronary lesions, and its most helpful role at present is to exclude significant CAD in patients with chest pain and a low clinical suspicion of serious coronary disease.

Natural History

The patient with chronic angina may show no change in a stable pattern of ischemia for many years. In some patients, however, the course may be punctuated by the occurrence of unstable angina, MI, or sudden cardiac death. These complications are often related to acute thrombosis at the site of disrupted athero- sclerotic plaque (see Chapter 7). Why some patients, but not others, sustain these compli- cations remains a subject of intense clinical and basic science investigation and may relate to the vulnerability of plaque to rupture.

Before the current era of sophisticated phar- macotherapy and coronary revascularization procedures, studies showed that the annual mortality rate of patients with CAD corre- sponded to the number of vessels containing significant stenoses. For example, patients with advanced stenoses within a single coro- nary vessel could expect an annual mortality rate of <4%. Those with two involved vessels had a mortality rate of 7% to 10%, and those with advanced, three-vessel disease showed a 10% to 12% annual mortality rate. If the left main artery was significantly stenosed, the mortality rate was greatly increased (15% to 25%). These outcomes were worse in corre- sponding patients with subnormal ventricular contractile function.

More recent studies have confirmed that the location and extent of coronary stenoses are important but also that other critical predictors of mortality include (1) the extent of impaired LV contractile function, (2) poor exercise ca- pacity, and (3) the magnitude of clinical an- ginal symptoms. These predictors are taken into account when contemplating treatment decisions.

The mortality associated with CAD has declined significantly in recent decades: the age-adjusted death rate has fallen by more than 50%. This is likely related to (1) athero- sclerotic risk reduction through improved

lifestyle changes (e.g., less tobacco use, less dietary fat consumption, and more exercise); (2) improved therapeutic strategies and lon- gevity following acute coronary syndromes (see Chapter 7); and (3) advances in the pharmacologic and mechanical therapies for chronic CAD.

TREATMENT

The goals of therapy in chronic ischemic heart disease are to decrease the frequency of anginal attacks, to prevent acute coronary syndromes such as MI, and to prolong survival. A long- term crucial step is to address the risk factors that led to the development of atherosclerotic coronary disease. Data convincingly demon- strate the benefit of smoking cessation, choles- terol improvement, blood pressure control, and serum glucose control in lowering the risk of coronary disease events (see Chapter 5). Im- provements in other risk factors for CAD, in- cluding obesity and physical inactivity, are also likely to reduce the risk of adverse outcomes although the benefits of these interventions are less well documented.

The following sections describe medical and surgical strategies to (1) reduce ischemia and its symptoms by restoring the balance be- tween myocardial oxygen supply and demand and (2) prevent acute coronary syndromes and death in patients with chronic CAD.

Medical Treatment of an Acute Episode of Angina

When experiencing acute angina, the patient should cease physical activity. Sublingual nitroglycerin, an organic nitrate, is the drug of choice in this situation. Placed under the tongue, this medication produces a slight burning sensation as it is absorbed through the mucosa, and it begins to take effect in 1 to 2 minutes. Nitrates relieve ischemia primarily through vascular smooth muscle relaxation, particularly *venodilatation.* Venodilatation reduces venous return to the heart, with a subsequent decline in LV volume (a determi- nant of wall stress). The latter decreases myo- cardial oxygen consumption, thus helping to restore oxygen balance in the ischemic heart.

A second action of nitrates is to dilate the coronary vasculature, with subsequent augmentation of coronary blood flow. This effect may be of little value in patients with angina in whom maximal coronary dilatation has already resulted from the accumulation of local metabolites. However, when coronary vasospasm plays a role in the development of ischemia, nitrate-induced coronary vasodilatation may be particularly beneficial.

Medical Treatment to Prevent Recurrent Ischemic Episodes

Pharmacologic agents are also the first line of defense in the *prevention* of anginal attacks. The goal of these agents is to decrease the cardiac workload (i.e., reduce myocardial oxygen demand) and to increase myocardial perfusion. The three classes of medications most commonly used are the organic nitrates, β-adrenergic blockers, and calcium channel blockers (Table 6.3).

Organic nitrates (e.g., nitroglycerin, isosorbide dinitrate, isosorbide mononitrate), as previously mentioned, relieve ischemia primarily through venodilatation (i.e., lower wall stress results from a smaller ventricular radius) and possibly through coronary vasodilatation. The organic nitrates are the oldest of the antianginal drugs and come in several preparations (also described in Chapter 17). Sublingual nitroglycerin tablets or sprays are used in the treatment of acute attacks because of their rapid onset of action. In addition, when taken immediately before a person engages in activities known to provoke angina, these rapidly acting nitrates are useful as *prophylaxis* against anginal attacks.

Longer-acting anginal prevention can be achieved through a variety of nitrate preparations, including oral tablets of isosorbide dinitrate (or mononitrate) or a transdermal nitroglycerin patch, which is applied once a day. A limitation to chronic nitrate therapy is the development of drug tolerance (i.e., decreased

Table 6.3. Pharmacologic Agents Used in the Prevention and Treatment of Angina

Drug Class	Mechanism of Action	Adverse Effects

Organic nitrates	↓ *Myocardial O$_2$ demand*
	  ↓ Preload (venodilatation)
	↑ *O$_2$ supply*
	  ↑ Coronary perfusion
	  ↓ Coronary vasospasm
		• Headache
		• Hypotension
		• Reflex tachycardia

β-Blockers	↓ *Myocardial O$_2$ demand*
	  ↓ Contractility
	  ↓ Heart rate
		• Excessive bradycardia
		• ↓ LV contractile function
		• Bronchoconstriction
		• May worsen diabetic control
		• Fatigue

Calcium channel blockers (agent specific; see footnote)	↓ *Myocardial O$_2$ demand*
	  ↓ Preload (venodilatation)
	  ↓ Wall stress (↓BP)
	  ↓ Contractility (V, D)
	  ↓ Heart rate (V, D)
	↑ *O$_2$ supply*
	  ↑ Coronary perfusion
	  ↓ Coronary vasospasm
		• Headache, flushing
		• ↓ LV contraction (V, D)
		• Marked bradycardia (V, D)
		• Edema (especially N, D)
		• Constipation (especially V)

Ranolazine	↓ *Late phase inward sodium current*	• Dizziness, headache • Constipation, nausea

BP, blood pressure; D, diltiazem; LV, left ventricular; N, nifedipine and other dihydropyridine calcium channel antagonists; V, verapamil.

effectiveness of the drug during continued administration), which occurs to some degree in most patients. This undesired effect can be overcome by providing a nitrate-free interval for several hours each day, usually while the patient sleeps.

There is no evidence that nitrates improve survival or prevent infarctions in patients with chronic CAD, and they are used purely for symptomatic relief. Common side effects include headache, lightheadedness, and palpitations induced by vasodilatation and reflex sinus tachycardia. The latter can be prevented by combining a β-blocker with the nitrate regimen.

β-Blockers (see Chapter 17) exert their antianginal effect primarily by reducing myocardial oxygen demand. They are directed against β-receptors, of which there are two classes: β_1-adrenergic receptors are restricted to the myocardium, whereas β_2-adrenergic receptors are located throughout blood vessels and the bronchial tree. The stimulation of β_1-receptors by endogenous catecholamines and exogenous sympathomimetic drugs increases heart rate and contractility. Consequently, β-adrenergic *antagonists* decrease the force of ventricular contraction and heart rate, thereby relieving ischemia by reducing myocardial oxygen demand. In addition, slowing the heart rate may benefit myocardial oxygen supply by augmenting the time spent in diastole, the phase when coronary perfusion primarily occurs.

In addition to suppressing angina, several studies have shown that β-blockers decrease the rates of recurrent infarction and mortality following an acute MI (see Chapter 7). Moreover, they have been shown to reduce the likelihood of an initial MI in patients with hypertension. Thus, β-blockers are first-line chronic therapy in the treatment of CAD.

β-Blockers are generally well tolerated but have several potential side effects. For example, they may precipitate bronchospasm in patients with underlying asthma by antagonizing β_2-receptors in the bronchial tree. Although β_1-selective blockers are theoretically less likely to exacerbate bronchospasm in such patients, drug selectivity for the β_1-receptor is not complete, and in general, all β-blockers should be used cautiously, or avoided, in patients with significant obstructive airway disease.

β-Blockers are also generally not used in patients with acutely *decompensated* LV dysfunction because they could intensify heart failure symptoms by further reducing inotropy. (However, as described in Chapter 9, β-blockers actually *improve* outcomes in patients with stable chronic heart failure conditions.) β-Blockers are also relatively contraindicated in patients with marked bradycardia or certain types of heart block to avoid additional impairment of electrical conduction.

β-Blockers sometimes cause fatigue and sexual dysfunction. They should be used with caution in insulin-treated diabetic patients because they can mask tachycardia and other catecholamine-mediated responses that can warn of hypoglycemia. One might also expect that β-blockers would decrease myocardial blood perfusion by blocking the vasodilating β_2-adrenergic receptors on the coronary arteries. However, this effect is usually attenuated by autoregulation and vasodilation of the coronary vessels owing to the accumulation of local metabolites.

Calcium channel blockers (see Chapter 17) antagonize voltage-gated L-type calcium channels, but the actions of the individual drugs of this group vary. The dihydropyridines (e.g., nifedipine and amlodipine) are potent vasodilators. They relieve myocardial ischemia by (1) decreasing oxygen demand (*venodilation* reduces ventricular filling and size, *arterial dilation* reduces the resistance against which the left ventricle contracts, and both actions reduce wall stress) and (2) increasing myocardial oxygen supply via coronary dilatation. By the latter mechanism, they are also potent agents for the relief of coronary artery vasospasm.

Nondihydropyridine calcium channel blockers (verapamil and diltiazem) also act as vasodilators but are not as potent in this regard as the dihydropyridines. However, these agents have additional beneficial antianginal effects stemming from their more potent cardiac depressant actions: they reduce the force of ventricular contraction (contractility) and slow the heart rate. Accordingly, verapamil and diltiazem also decrease myocardial oxygen demand by these mechanisms.

Questions have been raised about the safety of *short-acting* calcium channel–blocking drugs in the treatment of ischemic heart disease. In meta-analyses of randomized trials, these drugs have been associated with an *increased* incidence of MI and mortality. The adverse effect may relate to the rapid hemodynamic effects and blood pressure swings induced by the short-acting agents. Therefore, only *long-acting* calcium channel blockers (i.e., preparations taken once a day) are recommended in the treatment of chronic angina, generally as second-line drugs if symptoms are not controlled by β-blockers and nitrates.

The three standard groups of antianginal drugs described in this section can be used alone or in combination. However, care should be taken in combining a β-blocker with a nondihydropyridine calcium channel blocker (verapamil or diltiazem) because the additive negative chronotropic effect can cause excessive bradycardia and the combined negative inotropic effect could precipitate heart failure in patients with LV contractile dysfunction.

Ranolazine, a fourth type of anti-ischemic therapy, is the most recent to become available. This medication has been shown to decrease the frequency of anginal episodes and improve exercise capacity in patients with chronic CAD but differs from other anti-ischemic drugs in that it does not affect the heart rate or blood pressure. Although its mechanism of action has not been fully elucidated, it is believed to inhibit the late phase of the action potential's inward sodium current (I_{Na}^+) in ventricular myocytes. That late phase tends to be abnormally enhanced in ischemic myocardium, and the associated increased sodium influx results in higher-than-normal intracellular Ca^{++} (mediated by the trans-sarcolemmal Na^+–Ca^{++} exchanger; see Fig. 1.10). Such calcium overload is thought to result in impaired diastolic relaxation and contractile inefficiency. Inhibition of the late I_{Na}^+ by ranolazine counters these pathologic effects. Recent studies have supported ranolazine's effectiveness in reducing angina and its long-term safety, when used alone or in combination with other antianginal agents.

Although useful in controlling symptoms of angina, none of the antianginal drug groups has been shown to slow or reverse the atherosclerotic process responsible for the arterial lesions of chronic CAD. Moreover, although β-blockers have demonstrated mortality benefits in patients after MI, none of these agents has been shown to improve longevity in patients with chronic stable angina and preserved LV function.

Medical Treatment to Prevent Acute Cardiac Events

Platelet aggregation and thrombosis are key elements in the pathophysiology of acute MI and unstable angina (see Chapter 7). **Antiplatelet therapy** reduces the risk of these acute coronary syndromes in patients with chronic angina and should be a standard part of the regimen used to treat CAD. **Aspirin** has antithrombotic actions through inhibition of platelet aggregation (and therefore reduces the release of platelet-derived procoagulants and vasoconstrictors) as well as anti-inflammatory properties that may be important in stabilizing atheromatous plaque. Unless contraindications are present (e.g., allergy or gastric bleeding), aspirin should be continued indefinitely in all patients with CAD.

Clopidogrel, a thienopyridine, is one of a group of novel antiplatelet agents that block the platelet $P2Y_{12}$ ADP receptor, thereby preventing platelet activation and aggregation (see Chapter 17). It can be used as an antiplatelet substitute in patients who are allergic to aspirin. In addition, the combination of aspirin and clopidogrel is superior to aspirin alone in reducing death and ischemic complications in patients with acute coronary syndromes and in those undergoing elective percutaneous coronary stenting. Similarly, in patients with a history of MI, long-term treatment with aspirin plus clopidogrel is associated with fewer subsequent cardiac events than aspirin alone.

Lipid-regulating therapy also reduces cardiovascular clinical events. In particular, HMG-CoA reductase inhibitors ("statins"; see Chapter 17) lower MI and death rates in patients with established coronary disease and in those at high risk of developing CAD. The benefits of statin therapy are believed to extend beyond their lipid-altering effects, because there is evidence that they decrease vascular inflammation and improve endothelial cell dysfunction and thus may help stabilize atherosclerotic plaques. All patients with CAD should have their LDL cholesterol maintained at <100 mg/dL. Moreover, trials of patients with established atherosclerotic disease have demonstrated that *intensive* lipid lowering (with high-dose statin therapy) is superior to *moderate* lipid-lowering therapy in preventing ischemic events and cardiovascular death. As a result, current national guidelines include an optional goal of LDL <70 mg/dL for patients with known CAD, especially those at highest risk (e.g., following an acute coronary syndrome or those with multiple major risk factors, especially diabetes or continued smoking).

Angiotensin-converting enzyme (ACE) inhibitors, known to be beneficial in the treatment of hypertension (see Chapter 13), heart failure (see Chapter 9), and following MI (see Chapter 7), have been studied more recently as chronic therapy for patients with stable CAD not complicated by heart failure. Some (but not all) of these trials have shown reduced rates of death, MI, and stroke. Thus, many cardiologists recommend that an ACE inhibitor be included in the medical regimen of patients with chronic CAD.

Revascularization

Patients with angina that becomes asymptomatic during pharmacologic therapy are usually followed along by their physicians with continued emphasis on cardiac risk factor reduction. However, coronary revascularization is pursued if (1) the patient's symptoms of angina do not respond adequately to antianginal drug therapy, (2) unacceptable side effects of medications occur, or (3) the patient is found to have high-risk coronary disease for which revascularization is known to improve survival (as described in the next section). The two techniques used to accomplish mechanical revascularization are percutaneous coronary intervention (PCI) and coronary artery bypass graft (CABG) surgery.

PCIs include **percutaneous transluminal coronary angioplasty (PTCA)**, a procedure performed under fluoroscopy in which a balloon-tipped catheter is inserted through a peripheral artery (usually, femoral, brachial, or radial) and maneuvered into the stenotic segment of a coronary vessel. The balloon at the end of the catheter is then inflated under high pressure to dilate the stenosis, after which the balloon is deflated

and the catheter is removed from the body. The improvement in the size of the coronary lumen increases coronary perfusion and myocardial oxygen supply. Effective dilatation of the stenosis results from compression of the atherosclerotic plaque and often by creating a fracture within the lesion and stretching the underlying media. The risk of MI during the procedure is less than 1.5%, and mortality is less than 1%. Unfortunately, approximately one third of patients who undergo balloon angioplasty develop recurrent symptoms within 6 months owing to restenosis of the dilated artery and require additional coronary interventions.

For this reason **coronary stents** were developed, for implantation at the time of PCI, and have been shown to significantly reduce the rate of restenosis. Such stents are slender, cage-like metal support devices that in their collapsed configuration can be threaded into the region of stenosis by a catheter. Once in position, the stent is expanded into its open position by inflating a high-pressure balloon in its interior (Fig. 6.9). The balloon and attached

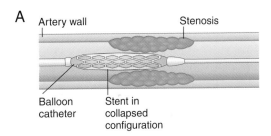

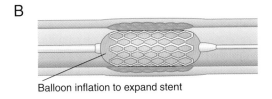

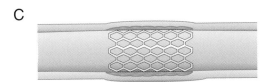

Figure 6.9. Placement of a coronary artery stent. A. A stent, in its original collapsed state, is advanced into the coronary stenosis on a balloon catheter. **B.** The balloon is inflated to expand the stent. **C.** The balloon is deflated and the catheter is removed from the body, leaving the stent permanently in place.

catheter are then removed, but the stent is left permanently in place to serve as a scaffold to maintain arterial patency. Because stents are thrombogenic, a combination of oral antiplatelet agents (commonly, aspirin plus clopidogrel) is crucial after stent implantation.

Compared with conventional balloon angioplasty, stent implantation decreases restenosis rates and reduces the need for repeat PCIs. Although restenosis resulting from vessel elastic recoil is greatly diminished by standard metal stent placement, neointimal proliferation (i.e., migration of smooth muscle cells and production of extracellular matrix) remains an important cause of in-stent restenosis and recurrent anginal symptoms.

To address the problem of in-stent restenosis after PCI, **drug-eluting stents** were devised. These special stents are fabricated with a polymer coat that incorporates an antiproliferative medication such as *sirolimus* (an immunosuppressive agent that inhibits T-cell activation), *everolimus* (an immunosuppressive similar to sirolimus), or *paclitaxel* (which interferes with cellular microtubule function). The medication is released from the stent over a period of 2 to 4 weeks, and this approach has shown great effect at preventing neointimal proliferation and reducing the need for repeat revascularization by more than half. However, just as neointimal proliferation is slowed, so too is protective endothelialization of the stent. The delay in endothelial cell coverage of the metal struts leaves patients at risk for thrombus formation within the stent should antiplatelet agents be discontinued prematurely. Therefore, prolonged courses of combination antiplatelet therapy (e.g., aspirin plus clopidogrel for at least 12 months) followed by aspirin indefinitely are necessary for patients who receive drug-eluting stents.

Although percutaneous revascularization techniques are generally superior to standard medical therapy for relief of angina, it is important to note that in the setting of stable coronary disease (i.e., not an acute coronary syndrome), they have not been shown to reduce the risk of MI or death.

CABG surgery entails grafting portions of a patient's native blood vessels to bypass obstructed coronary arteries. Two types of surgical grafts

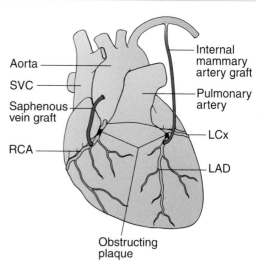

Figure 6.10. Coronary artery bypass surgery. Two types of bypasses are illustrated: 1) The left internal mammary artery originates from the left subclavian artery, and in this schematic, it is anastomosed to the left anterior descending (LAD) coronary artery distal to obstructing plaque; 2) One end of a saphenous vein graft is sutured to the proximal aorta and the other end to the right coronary artery (RCA) distal to a stenotic segment.

are used (Fig. 6.10). The first employs native veins—typically, a section of the saphenous vein (a "superfluous" vessel removed from the leg) that is sutured from the base of the aorta to a coronary segment downstream from the region of stenosis. The second method uses arterial grafts—most commonly, an internal mammary artery (IMA, a "superfluous" branch of each subclavian artery)—that can be directly anastomosed distal to a stenotic coronary site. Vein grafts have a patency rate of up to 80% at 12 months but are vulnerable to accelerated atherosclerosis; 10 years after surgery, more than 50% have occluded. In contrast, IMA grafts are more resistant to atherosclerosis with a patency rate of 90% at 10 years. Therefore, IMA grafts are often used to perfuse sites of critical flow such as the left anterior descending artery. Clinical trial evidence supports the use of aggressive lipid-lowering drug therapy after CABG to improve the long-term patency rates of bypass grafts.

In recent years, less invasive surgical alternatives to conventional CABG have been explored. These include "minimally invasive" operations with smaller incisions, the use of transcutaneous ports with videoscopic robotic assistance,

Table 6.4. Relative Advantages of Coronary Revascularization Procedures

Percutaneous Coronary Interventions (PCI)	Coronary Artery Bypass Graft Surgery (CABG)
Less invasive than CABG	More effective for long-term relief of angina than PCI or pharmacologic therapy
Shorter hospital stay and easier recuperation than CABG	Most complete revascularization
Superior to pharmacologic therapy for relief of angina	Improved survival in patients with • >50% left main stenosis • 3-vessel CAD, especially if LV contractile function is impaired • 2-vessel disease with tight (>75%) LAD stenosis, especially if LV contractile function is impaired • Diabetes and multivessel disease

CAD, coronary artery disease; LV, left ventricle; LAD, left anterior descending coronary artery; MI, myocardial infarction.

and "off-pump" procedures, which avoid the use of cardiopulmonary bypass (heart-lung) machines. Current studies are examining the advantages and limitations of these techniques in comparison with standard CABG.

Medical Versus Revascularization Therapy

Many patients with chronic, stable angina can be successfully managed with pharmacologic therapy alone. However, if anginal symptoms prove refractory to optimal medical therapy, or if intolerable drug side effects develop, coronary angiography is usually recommended for further therapeutic planning. For patients whose angina *is* controlled by medications, it is standard to perform non-invasive testing (e.g., exercise testing, echocardiography) to identify those with high-risk disease, because the long-term prognosis for such patients can be improved by coronary revascularization.

Once the coronary anatomy is defined, the decision to proceed with percutaneous intervention or bypass graft surgery depends on several considerations, including those listed in Table 6.4. In general, patients with persistent episodes of angina and significant stenoses in one to two coronary arteries are good candidates for PCI, as are certain lower-risk patients with three-vessel disease. Conversely, patients who fare better over the long term with CABG include those with significant (>50%) stenosis

of the left main coronary artery and patients with multivessel disease who also have reduced LV contractile function.

Each of the previously described approaches for the treatment of coronary disease is benefiting from rapidly developing research advancements. New surgical techniques (increased use of various arterial grafts, less invasive operations), new drug-eluting stents (e.g., incorporation of bioabsorbable/biodegradable polymers to decrease late stent thrombosis), novel adjuncts to stenting (potent antithrombotic drugs), and progress in pharmacologic management (e.g., aggressive use of statins and antithrombotic drugs) will likely further improve outcomes and better define the best therapeutic approaches for specific subsets of patients with chronic CAD.

SUMMARY

1. Cardiac ischemia results from an imbalance between myocardial oxygen supply and demand. Myocardial oxygen supply is determined by the oxygen content of the blood and coronary blood flow. The latter is dependent on the coronary perfusion pressure and coronary vascular resistance. Key regulators of myocardial oxygen demand include myocardial wall stress, heart rate, and contractility.

2. In the presence of atherosclerotic disease, myocardial oxygen supply is compromised.

Atherosclerotic plaques cause vascular lumen narrowing and reduce coronary blood flow. In addition, atherosclerosis-associated endothelial cell dysfunction causes inappropriate vasoconstriction of the coronary resistance vessels.

3. Angina pectoris is the most frequent symptom of intermittent ischemia, and its diagnosis relies heavily on the patient's description of the discomfort. Angina may be accompanied by signs and symptoms of adrenergic stimulation, pulmonary congestion, and transient LV systolic and diastolic dysfunction.

4. The diagnosis of angina can be aided by laboratory studies, including the ECG (ST segment and T wave abnormalities), exercise (or pharmacologic) stress testing, and conventional or CT angiography.

5. Standard pharmacologic therapy for chronic angina includes agents to prevent ischemia and relieve symptoms (mainly organic nitrates, β-blockers, calcium channel antagonists, alone or in combination) as well as agents that reduce the risk of acute coronary syndromes and death (e.g., aspirin, antilipidemic therapy, and consideration of ACE inhibitors). Modifiable risk factors for atherosclerosis should be corrected.

6. Revascularization with PCI or CABG surgery may provide relief from ischemia in patients with chronic angina who are refractory to, or unable to tolerate, medical therapy. CABG confers improved survival rates to certain high-risk groups.

Acknowledgments

Contributors to the previous editions of this chapter were Haley Naik, MD, Christopher P. Chiodo, MD, Carey Farquhar, MD, Anurag Gupta, MD, Rainu Kaushal, MD, William Carlson, MD, Michael E. Mendelsohn, MD, Patrick T. O'Gara, MD, Marc S. Sabatine, MD, and Leonard S. Lilly, MD.

Additional Reading

Abrams J. Chronic stable angina. *N Eng J Med.* 2005; 352:2524–2533.

The BARI 2D Study Group. A randomized trial of therapies for type 2 diabetes and coronary artery disease. *N Engl J Med.* 2009;360:2503–2515.

Fraker TD Jr, Fihn SD, Gibbons RJ, et al. 2007 chronic angina focused update of the ACC/AHA 2002 guidelines for the management of patients with chronic stable angina: a report of the American College of Cardiology/American Heart Association Task Force on Practice Guidelines Writing Group to develop the focused update of the 2002 guidelines. *Circulation.* 2007;116:2762–2772.

Hannan EL, Wu C, Walford G, et al. Drug-eluting stents vs. coronary-artery bypass grafting in multivessel coronary disease. *N Engl J Med.* 2008;358:331–341.

King SB III, Smith SC Jr, Hirshfeld JW Jr, et al. 2007 Focused Update of the ACC/AHA/SCAI. 2005 Guideline Update for Percutaneous Coronary Intervention: a report of the American College of Cardiology/American Heart Association Task Force on Practice Guidelines. *Circulation.* 2008;117:261–295.

Nash DT, Nash SD. Ranolazine for chronic stable angina. *Lancet.* 2008;372:1335–1341.

Patel MR, Dehmer GJ, Hirshfeld JW, et al. ACCF/SCAI/STS/AATS/AHA/ASNC 2009 appropriateness criteria for coronary revascularization: a report of the American College of Cardiology Foundation Appropriateness Criteria Task Force, Society for Cardiovascular Angiography and Interventions, Society of Thoracic Surgeons, American Association for Thoracic Surgery, American Heart Association, and the American Society of Nuclear Cardiology. *Circulation.* 2009;119:1330–1352.

Serruys PW, Kutryk MJB, Ong ATL. Coronary-artery stents. *N Engl J Med.* 2006;354:483–495.

Serruys PW, Morice MC, Kappetein AP, et al. SYNTAX Investigators. Percutaneous coronary intervention versus coronary-artery bypass grafting for severe coronary artery disease. *N Engl J Med.* 2009;360:961–972.

Tonino PA, De Bruyne B, Pijls NH, et al. FAME Study Investigators. Fractional flow reserve versus angiography for guiding percutaneous coronary intervention. *N Engl J Med.* 2009;360:213–224.

Acute Coronary Syndromes

June-Wha Rhee
Marc S. Sabatine
Leonard S. Lilly

Acute coronary syndromes (ACS) are life-threatening conditions that can punctuate the course of patients with coronary artery disease at any time. These syndromes form a continuum that ranges from an unstable pattern of angina pectoris to the development of a large acute myocardial infarction (MI), a condition of irreversible necrosis of heart muscle (Fig. 7.1). All ACS share a common initiating pathophysiologic mechanism, as this chapter will examine.

The frequency of ACS is staggering: more than 1.4 million people are admitted to hospitals in the United States each year with these conditions. Approximately 38% of patients who experience an ACS will die as a result. Despite these daunting statistics, mortality associated with ACS has actually substantially and continuously declined in recent decades as a result of major therapeutic and preventive advances. This chapter considers the

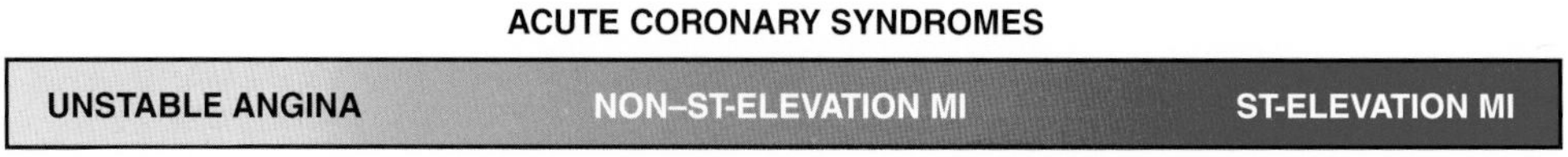

ACUTE CORONARY SYNDROMES

UNSTABLE ANGINA	NON–ST-ELEVATION MI	ST-ELEVATION MI

Figure 7.1. The continuum of acute coronary syndromes ranges from unstable angina, through non–ST-elevation myocardial infarction (MI), to ST-elevation MI.

events that lead to ACS, the pathologic and functional changes that follow, and therapeutic approaches that ameliorate the aberrant pathophysiology.

PATHOGENESIS OF ACUTE CORONARY SYNDROMES

More than 90% of ACS result from disruption of an atherosclerotic plaque with subsequent platelet aggregation and formation of an intracoronary thrombus. The thrombus transforms a region of plaque narrowing to one of severe or complete occlusion, and the impaired blood flow causes a marked imbalance between myocardial oxygen supply and demand. The form of ACS that results depends on the degree of coronary obstruction and associated ischemia (see Fig. 7.1). A *partially* occlusive thrombus is the typical cause of the closely related syndromes **unstable angina (UA)** and **non–ST-elevation myocardial infarction (NSTEMI,** historically referred to as *non–Q-wave MI*), with the latter being distinguished from the former by the presence of myocardial necrosis. At the other end of the spectrum, if the thrombus *completely* obstructs the coronary artery, the results are more severe ischemia and a larger amount of necrosis, manifesting as an **ST-elevation myocardial infarction (STEMI,** historically referred to as *Q-wave MI*).

The responsible thrombus in ACS is generated by interactions among the atherosclerotic plaque, the coronary endothelium, circulating platelets, and the dynamic vasomotor tone of the vessel wall, which overwhelm the natural antithrombotic mechanisms described in the next section.

Normal Hemostasis

When a normal blood vessel is injured, the endothelial surface becomes disrupted and thrombogenic connective tissue is exposed. *Primary hemostasis* is the first line of defense

against bleeding. This process begins within seconds of vessel injury and is mediated by circulating platelets, which adhere to collagen in the vascular subendothelium and aggregate to form a "platelet plug." While the primary hemostatic plug forms, the exposure of subendothelial tissue factor triggers the plasma coagulation cascade, initiating the process of *secondary hemostasis*. The plasma coagulation proteins involved in secondary hemostasis are sequentially activated at the site of injury and ultimately form a fibrin clot by the action of thrombin. The resulting clot stabilizes and strengthens the platelet plug.

The normal hemostatic system minimizes blood loss from injured vessels, but there is little difference between this physiologic response and the pathologic process of coronary thrombosis triggered by disruption of atherosclerotic plaques.

Endogenous Antithrombotic Mechanisms

Normal blood vessels, including the coronary arteries, are replete with safeguards that prevent spontaneous thrombosis and occlusion, some examples of which are shown in Figure 7.2.

Inactivation of Clotting Factors

Several natural inhibitors tightly regulate the coagulation process to oppose clot formation and maintain blood fluidity. The most important of these are antithrombin, proteins C and S, and tissue factor pathway inhibitor (TFPI).

Antithrombin is a plasma protein that irreversibly binds to thrombin and other clotting factors, inactivating them and facilitating their clearance from the circulation (see mechanism 1 in Fig. 7.2). The effectiveness of antithrombin is increased 1,000-fold by binding to heparan sulfate, a heparin-like molecule normally present on the luminal surface of endothelial cells.

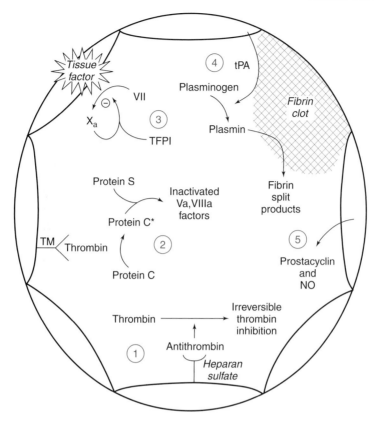

Figure 7.2. Endogenous protective mechanisms against thrombosis and vessel occlusion. (1) Inactivation of thrombin by antithrombin (AT), the effectiveness of which is enhanced by binding of AT to heparan sulfate. (2) Inactivation of clotting factors Va and VIIIa by activated protein C (protein C*), an action that is enhanced by protein S. Protein C is activated by the thrombomodulin (TM)–thrombin complex. (3) Inactivation of factor VII/tissue factor complex by tissue factor pathway inhibitor (TFPI). (4) Lysis of fibrin clots by tissue plasminogen activator (tPA). (5) Inhibition of platelet activation by prostacyclin and NO.

Protein C/protein S/thrombomodulin form a natural anticoagulant system that inactivates the "acceleration" factors of the coagulation pathway (i.e., factors Va and VIIIa). Protein C is synthesized in the liver and circulates in an inactive form. Thrombomodulin is a thrombin-binding receptor normally present on endothelial cells. Thrombin bound to thrombomodulin cannot convert fibrinogen to fibrin (the final reaction in clot formation). Instead, the thrombin–thrombomodulin complex activates protein C. Activated protein C degrades factors Va and VIIIa (see mechanism 2 in Fig. 7.2), thereby inhibiting coagulation. The presence of protein S in the circulation enhances the inhibitory function of protein C.

TFPI is a plasma serine protease inhibitor that is activated by coagulation factor Xa. The combined factor Xa–TFPI binds to and inactivates the complex of tissue factor with factor VIIa that normally triggers the extrinsic coagulation pathway (see mechanism 3 in Fig. 7.2). Thus, TFPI serves as a negative feedback inhibitor that interferes with coagulation.

Lysis of Fibrin Clots

Tissue plasminogen activator (tPA) is a protein secreted by endothelial cells in response to many triggers of clot formation. It cleaves the protein plasminogen to form active plasmin, which in turn enzymatically degrades fibrin clots (see mechanism 4 in Fig. 7.2). When tPA binds to fibrin in a forming clot, its ability to convert plasminogen to plasmin is greatly enhanced.

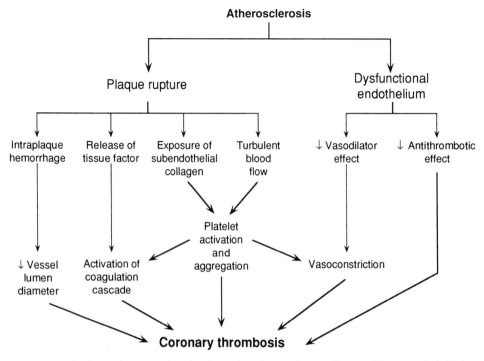

Figure 7.3. Mechanisms of coronary thrombus formation. Factors that contribute to this process include plaque disruption (e.g., rupture) and inappropriate vasoconstriction and loss of normal antithrombotic defenses because of dysfunctional endothelium.

Endogenous Platelet Inhibition and Vasodilatation

Prostacyclin is synthesized and secreted by endothelial cells (see mechanism 5 in Fig. 7.2), as described in Chapter 6. Prostacyclin increases platelet levels of cyclic AMP and thereby strongly inhibits platelet activation and aggregation. It also *indirectly* inhibits coagulation via its potent vasodilating properties. Vasodilatation helps guard against thrombosis by augmenting blood flow (which minimizes contact between procoagulant factors) and by reducing shear stress (an inducer of platelet activation).

Nitric oxide (NO) is similarly secreted by endothelial cells, as described in Chapter 6. It acts locally to inhibit platelet activation, and it too serves as a potent vasodilator.

Pathogenesis of Coronary Thrombosis

Normally, the mechanisms shown in Figure 7.2 serve to prevent spontaneous intravascular thrombus formation. However, abnormalities associated with atherosclerotic lesions may overwhelm these defenses and result in coronary thrombosis and vessel occlusion (Fig. 7.3). Atherosclerosis contributes to thrombus formation by (1) plaque rupture, which exposes the circulating blood elements to thrombogenic substances, and (2) endothelial dysfunction with the loss of normal protective antithrombotic and vasodilatory properties.

Atherosclerotic **plaque rupture** is considered the major trigger of coronary thrombosis. The underlying causes of plaque disruption are (1) chemical factors that destabilize atherosclerotic lesions and (2) physical stresses to which the lesions are subjected. As described in Chapter 5, atherosclerotic plaques consist of a lipid-laden core surrounded by a fibrous external cap. Substances released from inflammatory cells within the plaque can compromise the integrity of the fibrous cap. For example, T lymphocytes elaborate γ-interferon, which inhibits collagen synthesis by smooth muscle cells and thereby interferes with the usual strength of the cap. Additionally, cells within atherosclerotic lesions produce enzymes (e.g., metalloproteinases) that degrade the interstitial matrix, further compromising plaque stability. A weakened or thin-capped plaque is subject to rupture, particularly in its "shoulder" region (the border with the normal arterial wall that is subjected to high circumferential stress) either spontaneously or by physical forces, such as intraluminal blood pressure and torsion from the beating myocardium.

ACS sometimes occur in the setting of certain triggers, such as strenuous physical activity or emotional upset. The activation of the sympathetic nervous system in these situations increases the blood pressure, heart rate, and force of ventricular contraction—actions that may stress the atherosclerotic lesion, thereby causing the plaque to fissure or rupture. In addition, MI is most likely to occur in the early morning hours. This observation may relate to the tendency of key physiologic stressors (such as systolic blood pressure, blood viscosity, and plasma epinephrine levels) to be most elevated at that time of day, and these factors subject vulnerable plaques to rupture.

Following plaque rupture, thrombus formation is provoked via the mechanisms shown in Figure 7.3. The exposure of tissue factor from the atheromatous core triggers the coagulation pathway, while the exposure of subendothelial collagen activates platelets. Activated platelets release the contents of their granules, which include facilitators of platelet aggregation (e.g., adenosine diphosphate [ADP] and fibrinogen), activators of the coagulation cascade (e.g., factor Va), and vasoconstrictors (e.g., thromboxane and serotonin). The developing intracoronary thrombus, intraplaque hemorrhage, and vasoconstriction all contribute to narrowing the vessel lumen, creating turbulent blood flow that contributes to shear stress and further platelet activation.

Dysfunctional endothelium, which is apparent even in mild atherosclerotic coronary disease, also increases the likelihood of thrombus formation. In the setting of endothelial dysfunction, reduced amounts of vasodilators (e.g., NO and prostacyclin) are released and inhibition of platelet aggregation by these factors is impaired, resulting in the loss of a key defense against thrombosis.

Not only is dysfunctional endothelium less equipped to prevent platelet aggregation, but also is less able to counteract the vasoconstricting products of platelets. During thrombus formation, vasoconstriction is promoted both by platelet products (thromboxane and serotonin) and by thrombin within the developing clot. The *normal* platelet-associated vascular response is vasodilatation, because platelet products stimulate endothelial NO and prostacyclin release, the influences of which predominate over direct platelet-derived vasoconstrictors (see Fig. 6.4). However, reduced secretion of endothelial vasodilators in atherosclerosis allows vasoconstriction to proceed unchecked. Similarly, thrombin in a forming clot is a potent vascular smooth muscle constrictor in the setting of dysfunctional endothelium. Vasoconstriction causes torsional stresses that can contribute to plaque rupture or can transiently occlude the stenotic vessel through heightened arterial tone. The reduction in coronary blood flow caused by vasoconstriction also reduces the washout of coagulation proteins, thereby enhancing thrombogenicity.

Significance of Coronary Thrombosis

The formation of an intracoronary thrombus results in one of the several potential outcomes (Fig. 7.4). For example, plaque rupture is sometimes superficial, minor, and self-limited, such that only a small, nonocclusive thrombus forms. In this case, the thrombus may simply become incorporated into the growing atheromatous lesion through fibrotic organization, or it may be lysed by natural fibrinolytic mechanisms. Recurrent asymptomatic plaque ruptures of this type may cause gradual progressive enlargement of the coronary stenosis.

However, deeper plaque rupture may result in greater exposure of subendothelial collagen and tissue factor, with formation of a larger thrombus that more substantially occludes the vessel's lumen. Such obstruction may cause prolonged severe ischemia and the development of an ACS. If the intraluminal thrombus at the site of plaque disruption *totally* occludes the vessel, blood flow beyond the obstruction will cease, prolonged ischemia will occur, and an MI (usually an ST-elevation MI) will result.

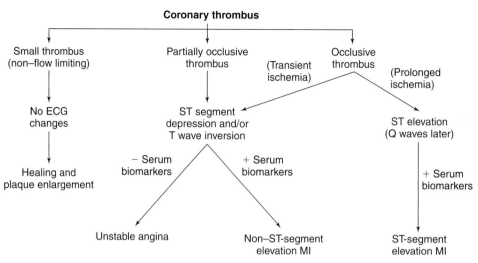

Figure 7.4. Consequences of coronary thrombosis. A small thrombus formed on superficial plaque rupture may not result in symptoms or electrocardiogram (ECG) abnormalities, but healing and fibrous organization may incorporate the thrombus into the plaque, causing the atherosclerotic lesion to enlarge. A partially occlusive thrombus (with or without superimposed vasospasm) narrows the arterial lumen, restricts blood flow, and can cause unstable angina or a non–ST-elevation MI, either of which may result in ST segment depression and/or T wave inversion on the ECG. A totally occlusive thrombus with prolonged ischemia is the most common cause of ST-elevation MI, in which the ECG initially shows ST segment elevation, followed by Q wave development. An occlusive thrombus that recanalizes, or one that develops in a region served by adequate collateral blood flow, may result in less prolonged ischemia and a non–ST-elevation MI instead. Markers of myocardial necrosis include cardiac-specific troponins and creatine kinase MB isoenzyme.

Conversely, if the thrombus *partially* occludes the vessel (or if it totally occludes the vessel but only transiently because of spontaneous recanalization or by relief of superimposed vasospasm), the severity and duration of ischemia will be less, and a smaller NSTEMI or UA is the more likely outcome. The distinction between NSTEMI and UA is based on the degree of the ischemia and whether the event is severe enough to cause necrosis, indicated by the presence of certain serum biomarkers (see Fig. 7.4). Nonetheless, NSTEMI and UA act quite alike, and the management of these entities is similar.

Occasionally, a non–ST-elevation infarct may result from total coronary occlusion. In this case, it is likely that a substantial collateral blood supply (see Chapter 1) limits the extent of necrosis, such that a larger ST-elevation MI is prevented.

Nonatherosclerotic Causes of Acute Coronary Syndromes

Infrequently, mechanisms other than acute thrombus formation can precipitate an ACS

(Table 7.1). These should be suspected when an ACS occurs in a young patient or a person with no coronary risk factors. For example, coronary emboli from mechanical or infected cardiac valves may lodge in the coronary circulation, inflammation from acute vasculitis can initiate coronary occlusion, or patients with connective tissue disorders, or peripartum women, can rarely experience a spontaneous coronary artery dissection (a tear in the vessel wall, described in Chapter 15). Occasionally, intense transient coronary spasm can sufficiently reduce myocardial blood supply to result in UA or infarction.

Another cause of ACS is cocaine abuse. Cocaine increases sympathetic tone by blocking the presynaptic reuptake of norepinephrine and by enhancing the release of adrenal catecholamines, which can lead to vasospasm and therefore decreased myocardial oxygen supply. An ACS may ensue because of increased myocardial oxygen demand resulting from cocaine-induced sympathetic myocardial stimulation (increased heart rate and blood pressure) in the face of the decreased oxygen supply.

Table 7.1. Causes of Acute Coronary Syndromes

- Atherosclerotic plaque rupture with superimposed thrombus
- Vasculitic syndromes (see Chapter 15)
- Coronary embolism (e.g., from endocarditis, artificial heart valves)
- Congenital anomalies of the coronary arteries
- Coronary trauma or aneurysm
- Severe coronary artery spasm (primary or cocaine-induced)
- Increased blood viscosity (e.g., polycythemia vera, thrombocytosis)
- Spontaneous coronary artery dissection
- Markedly increased myocardial oxygen demand (e.g., severe aortic stenosis)

PATHOLOGY AND PATHOPHYSIOLOGY

MI (either STEMI or NSTEMI) results when myocardial ischemia is sufficiently severe to cause myocyte necrosis. Although by definition UA does not result in necrosis, MI may subsequently ensue if the underlying pathophysiology of the unstable pattern of angina is not promptly corrected.

In addition to their clinical classifications, infarctions can be described pathologically by the extent of necrosis they produce within the myocardial wall. **Transmural infarcts** span the entire thickness of the myocardium and result from total, prolonged occlusion of an epicardial coronary artery. Conversely, **subendocardial infarcts** exclusively involve the innermost layers of the myocardium. The subendocardium is particularly susceptible to ischemia because it is the zone subjected to the highest pressure from the ventricular chamber, has few collateral connections that supply it, and is perfused by vessels that must pass through layers of contracting myocardium.

Infarction represents the culmination of a disastrous cascade of events, initiated by ischemia, that progresses from a potentially reversible phase to irreversible cell death. Myocardium that is supplied directly by an occluded vessel may die quickly. The adjacent tissue may not necrose immediately because it may be sufficiently perfused by nearby patent vessels. However, the neighboring cells may become increasingly ischemic over time, as demand for oxygen continues in the face of decreased oxygen supply. Thus, the region of infarction may subsequently extend outward. The amount of tissue that ultimately succumbs to infarction therefore relates to (1) the mass of myocardium perfused by the occluded vessel, (2) the magnitude and duration of impaired coronary blood flow, (3) the oxygen demand of the affected region, (4) the adequacy of collateral vessels that provide blood flow from neighboring nonoccluded coronary arteries, and (5) the degree of tissue response that modifies the ischemic process.

The pathophysiologic alterations that transpire during MI occur in two stages: early changes at the time of acute infarction and late changes during myocardial healing and remodeling.

Early Changes in Infarction

Early changes include the histologic evolution of the infarct and the functional impact of oxygen deprivation on myocardial contractility. These changes culminate in coagulative necrosis of the myocardium in 2 to 4 days.

Cellular Changes

As oxygen levels fall in the myocardium supplied by an abruptly occluded coronary vessel, there is a rapid shift from aerobic to anaerobic metabolism (Fig. 7.5). Because mitochondria can no longer oxidize fats or products of glycolysis, high-energy phosphate production drops dramatically and anaerobic glycolysis leads to the accumulation of lactic acid. This results in a lowered pH.

Furthermore, the paucity of high-energy phosphates such as adenosine triphosphate (ATP) interferes with the transmembrane Na^+-K^+-ATPase, with resultant elevation in the concentrations of intracellular Na^+ and extracellular K^+. Rising intracellular Na^+ contributes to cellular edema. Membrane leak and rising

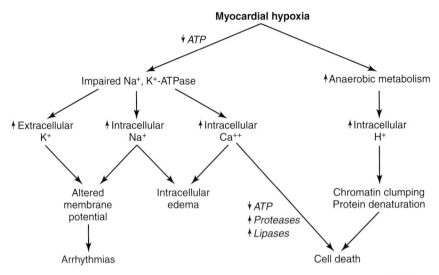

Figure 7.5. Mechanisms of cell death in myocardial infarction. Acute ischemia rapidly depletes the intracellular supply of adenosine triphosphate (ATP) as aerobic metabolism fails. Subsequent intracellular acidosis and impairment of ATP-dependent processes culminate in intracellular calcium accumulation, edema, and cell death.

extracellular K^+ concentration contributes to alterations in the transmembrane electrical potential, predisposing the myocardium to lethal arrhythmias. Intracellular calcium accumulates in the damaged myocytes and is thought to contribute to the final common pathway of cell destruction through the activation of degradative lipases and proteases.

Collectively, these metabolic changes decrease myocardial function as early as 2 minutes following occlusive thrombosis. Without intervention, *irreversible* cell injury ensues in 20 minutes and is marked by the development of membrane defects. Proteolytic enzymes leak across the myocyte's altered membrane, damaging adjacent myocardium, and the release of certain macromolecules into the circulation serves as a clinical marker of acute infarction.

Edema of the myocardium develops within 4 to 12 hours, as vascular permeability increases and interstitial oncotic pressure rises (because of the leak of intracellular proteins). The earliest histologic changes of irreversible injury are **wavy myofibers,** which appear as intercellular edema separates the myocardial cells that are tugged about by the surrounding, functional myocardium (Fig. 7.6). **Contraction bands** can often be seen near the borders of the infarct: sarcomeres are contracted and consolidated and appear as bright eosinophilic belts.

An acute inflammatory response, with infiltration of neutrophils, begins after approximately 4 hours and incites further tissue damage. Within 18 to 24 hours, **coagulation necrosis** is evident with pyknotic nuclei and bland eosinophilic cytoplasm, seen by light microscopy. These early changes are demonstrated in Figure 7.6 and summarized in Table 7.2.

Gross Changes

Gross morphologic changes do not appear until 18 to 24 hours after coronary occlusion, although certain staining techniques (e.g., tetrazolium) permit the pathologist to identify regions of infarction earlier. Most often, ischemia and infarction begin in the subendocardium and then extend laterally and outward toward the epicardium.

Late Changes in Infarction

Late pathologic changes in the course of acute MI (see Table 7.2) include (1) the clearing of necrotic myocardium and (2) the deposition of collagen to form scar tissue.

Irreversibly injured myocytes do not regenerate; rather, the cells are removed and replaced by fibrous tissue. Macrophages invade the inflamed myocardium shortly after neutrophil infiltration and remove necrotic tissue.

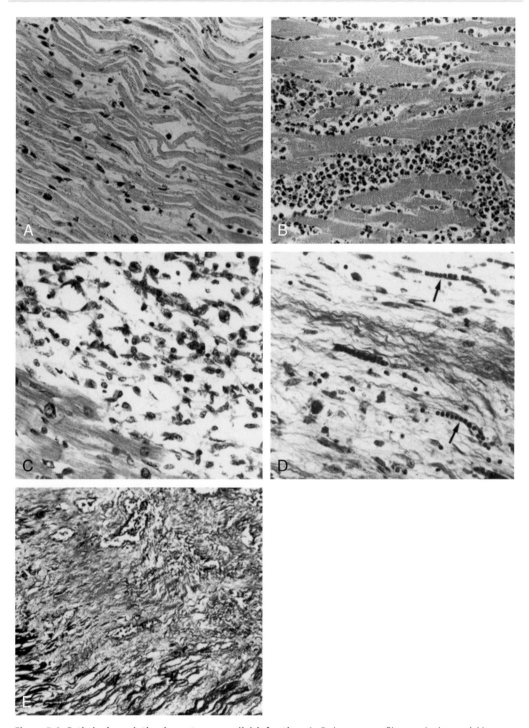

Figure 7.6. Pathologic evolution in acute myocardial infarction. A. Early wavy myofibers and edema; viable myocardium is at lower left. **B.** Coagulation necrosis and dense infiltration of neutrophils. **C.** Necrotic myocytes largely removed by phagocytes (7 to 10 days); viable myocardium at lower left. **D.** Granulation tissue with early collagen deposition; new capillaries have formed (arrows). **E.** Late fibrotic scarring. (Reprinted with permission from Schoen FJ. *Interventional and Surgical Cardiovascular Pathology—Clinical Correlations and Basic Principles*. Philadelphia, PA: Saunders; 1989:67.)

Table 7.2. Pathologic Time Line in Transmural Infarction	
Time	*Event*
Early changes	
1–2 min	ATP levels fall; cessation of contractility
10 min	50% depletion of ATP; cellular edema, decreased membrane potential and susceptibility to arrhythmias
20–24 min	Irreversible cell injury
1–3 hr	Wavy myofibers
4–12 hr	Hemorrhage, edema, PMN infiltration begins
18–24 hr	Coagulation necrosis (pyknotic nuclei with eosinophilic cytoplasm), edema
2–4 days	Total coagulation necrosis (no nuclei or striations, rimmed by hyperemic tissue); monocytes appear; PMN infiltration peaks
Late changes	
5–7 days	Yellow softening from resorption of dead tissue by macrophages
7+ days	Ventricular remodeling
7 weeks	Fibrosis and scarring complete

ATP, adenosine triphosphate; PMN, polymorphonuclear leukocyte.

This period of tissue resorption is termed **yellow softening** because connective tissue elements are destroyed and removed along with dead myocardial cells. The phagocytic clearing, combined with thinning and dilatation of the infarcted zone, results in structural weakness of the ventricular wall and the possibility of myocardial wall rupture at this stage. **Fibrosis** subsequently ensues, and scarring is complete by 7 weeks after infarction (see Fig. 7.6).

Functional Alterations

Impaired Contractility and Compliance

The destruction of functional myocardial cells in infarction quickly leads to impaired ventricular contraction **(systolic dysfunction)**. Cardiac output is further compromised because *synchronous* contraction of myocytes is lost. Specific terms are used to describe the types of wall motion abnormalities that can result. A localized region of reduced contraction is termed *hypokinetic*, a segment that does not contract at all is called *akinetic*, and a *dyskinetic* region is one that bulges *outward* during contraction of the remaining functional portions of the ventricle.

During ACS, the left ventricle is also adversely compromised by **diastolic dysfunction**. Ischemia and/or infarction impair diastolic relaxation (an energy-dependent process; see Chapter 1), which reduces ventricular compliance and contributes to elevated ventricular filling pressures.

Stunned Myocardium

Sometimes transient myocardial ischemia can result in a very prolonged, but gradually reversible, period of contractile dysfunction. For example, as described in Chapter 6, **stunned myocardium** is tissue that demonstrates prolonged systolic dysfunction after a discrete episode of severe ischemia, despite restoration of adequate blood flow, and *gradually* regains contractile force days to weeks later. Stunning may play an important role in patients with UA or in myocardium adjacent to the region of an acute infarction. In both instances, prolonged contractile dysfunction of affected ventricular segments may be evident after the event, simulating infarcted tissue. However, if the tissue is simply stunned rather than necrotic, its function will recover over time.

Ischemic Preconditioning

Brief ischemic insults to a region of myocardium may render that tissue more resistant to subsequent episodes, a phenomenon termed **ischemic preconditioning**. The clinical relevance is that patients who sustain an MI in the context of recent angina experience less morbidity and mortality than those without preceding ischemic episodes. The mechanism of this phenomenon is unknown but appears to involve multiple signaling pathways. Substances released during ischemia, including adenosine and bradykinin, are believed to be key triggers of these pathways.

Ventricular Remodeling

Following an MI, changes occur in the geometry of both the infarcted and the noninfarcted ventricular muscle. Such alterations in chamber size and wall thickness affect long-term cardiac function and prognosis.

In the early post-MI period, infarct *expansion* may occur, in which the affected ventricular segment enlarges without additional myocyte necrosis. Infarct expansion represents thinning and dilatation of the necrotic zone of tissue, likely because of "slippage" between the muscle fibers, resulting in a decreased volume of myocytes in the region. Infarct expansion can be detrimental because it increases ventricular size, which (1) augments wall stress, (2) impairs systolic contractile function, and (3) increases the likelihood of aneurysm formation.

In addition to early expansion of the infarcted territory, remodeling of the ventricle may also involve dilatation of the overworked *noninfarcted* segments, which are subjected to increased wall stress. This dilatation begins in the early postinfarct period and continues over the ensuing weeks and months. Initially, chamber dilatation serves a compensatory role because it increases cardiac output via the Frank–Starling mechanism (see Chapter 9), but progressive enlargement may ultimately lead to heart failure and predisposes to ventricular arrhythmias.

Adverse ventricular remodeling can be beneficially modified by certain interventions. At the time of infarction, for example, reperfusion therapies limit infarct size and therefore decrease the likelihood of infarct expansion. In addition, drugs that interfere with the renin–angiotensin system have been shown to attenuate progressive remodeling and to reduce short- and long-term mortality after infarction (as discussed later in the chapter).

CLINICAL FEATURES OF ACUTE CORONARY SYNDROMES

Because ACS represent disorders along a continuum, their clinical features overlap. In general, the severity of symptoms and associated laboratory findings progress from UA on one side of the continuum, through NSTEMI, to STEMI on the other end of the continuum (see Fig. 7.1). Distinguishing among these syndromes is based on the clinical presentation, electrocardiographic findings, and serum biomarkers of myocardial damage. To institute appropriate immediate therapy, the most important distinction to make is between ACS that cause ST segment elevation on the electrocardiogram (STEMI) and those acute syndromes that do not (UA and NSTEMI).

Historically, MIs have been classified as Q-wave or non–Q-wave infarctions. Dogma held that transmural infarcts produce Q waves (after an initial period of ST elevation) on the electrocardiogram (ECG), whereas subendocardial infarcts generate ST depressions without Q wave development. However, it is now known that these ECG findings do not reliably correlate with the pathologic findings and that much overlap exists among the types of infarction. Moreover, the use of Q waves to classify ACS is now less clinically important, because Q waves, unlike ST changes, may take hours or longer to develop and cannot be used to make early therapeutic decisions. Thus, in this book (and in clinical settings), the terms STEMI and NSTEMI are used instead of Q-wave and non–Q-wave MI, respectively.

Clinical Presentation

Unstable Angina

UA presents as an acceleration of ischemic symptoms in one of the following three ways: (1) a crescendo pattern in which a patient with chronic stable angina experiences a sudden increase in the frequency, duration, and/or intensity of ischemic episodes; (2) episodes of angina that occur at rest, without provocation;

or (3) the new onset of anginal episodes, described as severe, in a patient without previous symptoms of coronary artery disease. These presentations are different from the pattern of chronic stable angina, in which instances of chest discomfort are predictable, brief, and nonprogressive, occurring only during physical exertion or emotional stress. Patients with UA may progress further along the continuum of ACS and develop evidence of necrosis (i.e., acute NSTEMI or STEMI) unless the condition is recognized and promptly treated.

Acute Myocardial Infarction

The symptoms and physical findings of acute MI (both STEMI and NSTEMI) can be predicted from the pathophysiology described earlier in this chapter and are summarized in Table 7.3. The discomfort experienced during an MI resembles angina pectoris qualitatively but is usually more severe, lasts longer, and may radiate more widely. Like angina, the sensation may result from the release of mediators such as adenosine and lactate from ischemic myocardial cells onto local nerve endings. Because ischemia in acute MI persists and proceeds to necrosis, these provocative substances continue to accumulate and activate afferent nerves for longer periods. The discomfort is often referred to other regions of the C7 through T4 dermatomes, including the neck, shoulders, and arms. Initial

symptoms are usually rapid in onset and briskly crescendo to leave the victim with a profound "feeling of doom." Unlike a transient attack of angina, the pain does not wane with rest, and there may be little response to the administration of sublingual nitroglycerin.

The chest discomfort associated with an acute MI is often severe, but not always. In fact, up to 25% of patients who sustain an MI are *asymptomatic* during the acute event, and the diagnosis is made only in retrospect. This is particularly common among diabetic patients who may not adequately sense pain because of associated peripheral neuropathy.

The combination of intense discomfort and baroreceptor unloading (if hypotension is present) may trigger a dramatic sympathetic nervous system response. Systemic signs of subsequent catecholamine release include diaphoresis (sweating), tachycardia, and cool and clammy skin caused by vasoconstriction.

If the ischemia affects a sufficiently large amount of myocardium, left ventricular (LV) contractility can be reduced (systolic dysfunction), thereby decreasing the stroke volume and causing the diastolic volume and pressure within the LV to rise. The increase in LV pressure, compounded by the ischemia-induced stiffness of the chamber (diastolic dysfunction), is conveyed to the left atrium and pulmonary veins. The resultant pulmonary congestion decreases lung compliance and stimulates

Table 7.3. Signs and Symptoms of Myocardial Infarction	
1. Characteristic pain	• Severe, persistent, typically substernal
2. Sympathetic effect	• Diaphoresis • Cool and clammy skin
3. Parasympathetic (vagal effect)	• Nausea, vomiting • Weakness
4. Inflammatory response	• Mild fever
5. Cardiac findings	• S_4 (and S_3 if systolic dysfunction present) gallop • Dyskinetic bulge (in anterior wall MI) • Systolic murmur (if mitral regurgitation or VSD)
6. Other	• Pulmonary rales (if heart failure present) • Jugular venous distention (if heart failure or right ventricular MI)

MI, myocardial infarction; S_3, third heart sound; S_4, fourth heart sound; VSD, ventricular septal defect.

juxtacapillary receptors. These *J receptors* effect a reflex that results in rapid, shallow breathing and evokes the subjective feeling of dyspnea. Transudation of fluid into the alveoli exacerbates this symptom.

Physical findings during an acute MI depend on the location and extent of the infarct. The S_4 sound, indicative of atrial contraction into a noncompliant left ventricle, is frequently present (see Chapter 2). An S_3 sound, indicative of volume overload in the presence of failing LV systolic function, may also be heard. A systolic murmur may appear if ischemia-induced papillary muscle dysfunction causes mitral valvular insufficiency, or if the infarct ruptures through the interventricular septum to create a ventricular septal defect (as discussed later in the chapter).

Myocardial necrosis also activates systemic responses to inflammation. Cytokines such as interleukin 1 (IL-1) and tumor necrosis factor (TNF) are released from macrophages and vascular endothelium in response to tissue injury. These mediators evoke an array of clinical responses, including low-grade fever.

Not all patients with severe chest pain are in the midst of MI or UA. Table 7.4 lists other common causes of acute chest discomfort and clinical, laboratory, and radiographic features to differentiate them from an ACS.

Table 7.4. Conditions That May Be Confused with Acute Coronary Syndromes

Condition	Differentiating Features
Cardiac	
Acute coronary syndrome	• Retrosternal pressure, radiating to neck, jaw, or left shoulder and arm; more severe and lasts longer than previous anginal attacks • ECG: localized ST elevations or depressions
Pericarditis	• Sharp pleuritic pain (worsens with inspiration) • Pain varies with position (relieved by sitting forward) • Friction rub auscultated over precordium • ECG: diffuse ST elevations (see Chapter 14)
Aortic dissection	• Tearing, ripping pain that migrates over time (chest and back) • Asymmetry of arm blood pressures • Widened mediastinum on chest radiograph
Pulmonary	
Pulmonary embolism	• Localized pleuritic pain, accompanied by dyspnea • Pleural friction rub may be present • Predisposing conditions for venous thrombosis
Pneumonia	• Pleuritic chest pain • Cough and sputum production • Abnormal lung auscultation and percussion (i.e., consolidation) • Infiltrate on chest radiograph
Pneumothorax	• Sudden sharp, pleuritic unilateral chest pain • Decreased breath sounds and hyperresonance of affected side • Chest radiograph: increased lucency and absence of pulmonary markings
Gastrointestinal	
Esophageal spasm	• Retrosternal pain, worsened by swallowing • History of dysphagia
Acute cholecystitis	• Right upper quadrant abdominal tenderness • Often accompanied by nausea • History of fatty food intolerance

Table 7.5. Distinguishing Features of Acute Coronary Syndromes

| Feature | Unstable Angina | Myocardial Infarction | |
		NSTEMI	STEMI
Typical symptoms	Crescendo, rest, or new-onset severe angina	Prolonged "crushing" chest pain, more severe and wider radiation than usual angina	
Serum biomarkers	No	Yes	Yes
Electrocardiogram initial findings	ST depression and/or T wave inversion	ST depression and/or T wave inversion	ST elevation (and Q waves later)

NSTEMI, non–ST-elevation myocardial infarction; STEMI, ST-elevation myocardial infarction.

Diagnosis of Acute Coronary Syndromes

The diagnosis of, and distinctions among, the ACS is made on the basis of (1) the patient's presenting symptoms, (2) acute ECG abnormalities, and (3) detection of specific serum markers of myocardial necrosis (see Fig. 7.4 and Table 7.5). Specifically, UA is a clinical diagnosis supported by the patient's symptoms, transient ST abnormalities on the ECG (usually ST depression and/or T wave inversion), and the absence of serum biomarkers of myocardial necrosis. Non–ST segment elevation MI is distinguished from UA by the detection of serum markers of necrosis and often more persistent ST or T wave abnormalities. The hallmark of ST-elevation MI is an appropriate clinical history coupled with ST elevations on the ECG plus detection of serum markers of myocardial necrosis.

ECG Abnormalities

ECG abnormalities, which reflect abnormal electrical currents during ACS, are usually manifest in characteristic ways. In UA or NSTEMI, ST segment depression and/or T wave inversions are most common (Fig. 7.7). These abnormalities may be transient, occurring just during chest pain episodes in UA, or they may persist in patients with NSTEMI. In contrast, as described in Chapter 4, STEMI presents with a temporal sequence of abnormalities: initial ST segment elevation, followed over the course of several hours by inversion of the T wave and

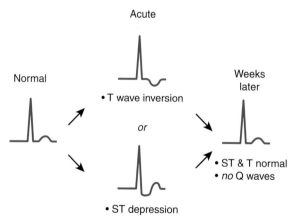

Figure 7.7. ECG abnormalities in unstable angina and non–ST-elevation myocardial infarction.

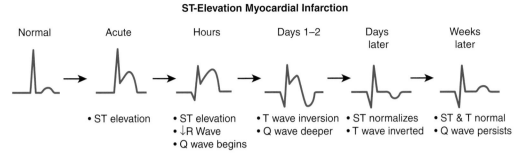

ST-Elevation Myocardial Infarction

Normal	Acute	Hours	Days 1–2	Days later	Weeks later

- ST elevation

- ST elevation
- ↓R Wave
- Q wave begins

- T wave inversion
- Q wave deeper

- ST normalizes
- T wave inverted

- ST & T normal
- Q wave persists

Figure 7.8. **ECG evolution during ST-elevation myocardial infarction.**

Q wave development (Fig. 7.8). Note that these characteristic patterns of ECG abnormalities in ACS can be minimized or aborted by early therapeutic interventions.

Serum Markers of Infarction

Necrosis of myocardial tissue causes disruption of the sarcolemma, so that intracellular macromolecules leak into the cardiac interstitium and ultimately into the bloodstream (Fig. 7.9). Detection of such molecules in the serum, particularly cardiac-specific troponins and creatine kinase MB isoenzyme, serves important diagnostic and prognostic roles. In patients with STEMI or NSTEMI, these markers rise above a threshold level in a defined temporal sequence.

Cardiac-specific Troponins

Troponin is a regulatory protein in muscle cells that controls interactions between myosin and actin (see Chapter 1). It consists of three subunits: TnC, TnI, and TnT. Although these subunits are found in both skeletal and cardiac muscles, the cardiac forms of troponin I (cTnI) and troponin T (cTnT) are structurally unique, and highly specific assays for their detection in the serum have been developed. Because their serum levels are virtually absent in healthy persons, the presence of even minor elevations of cTnI or cTnT serves as a sensitive and powerful marker of myocyte damage. The advent of increasingly sensitive troponin assays has shifted classification of some ACS presentations that would have previously been termed UA to NSTEMI instead. It should also be noted

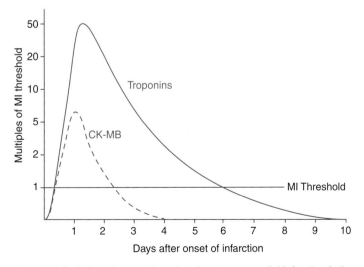

Figure 7.9. **Evolution of serum biomarkers in acute myocardial infarction (MI).**

175

that cardiac troponins can be detected in small quantities in the serum in other conditions that cause acute cardiac strain or inflammation (e.g., a heart failure exacerbation, myocarditis, hypertensive crisis, or pulmonary embolism [which can cause right ventricular strain]).

In the case of MI, cardiac troponin serum levels begin to rise 3 to 4 hours after the onset of discomfort, peak between 18 and 36 hours, and then decline slowly, allowing for detection for up to 10 to 14 days after a large MI. Thus, their measurement may be helpful for detection of MI for nearly 2 weeks after the event occurs. Given their high sensitivity and specificity, cardiac troponins are the preferred serum biomarkers to detect myocardial necrosis.

Creatine Kinase

The enzyme creatine kinase (CK) reversibly transfers a phosphate group from creatine phosphate, the endogenous storage form of high-energy phosphate bonds, to ADP, producing ATP. Because creatine kinase is found in the heart, skeletal muscle, brain, and many other organs, serum concentrations of the enzyme may become elevated following injury to any of these tissues.

There are, however, three *isoenzymes* of CK that improve diagnostic specificity of its origin: CK-MM (found mainly in skeletal muscle), CK-BB (located predominantly in the brain), and **CK-MB** (localized mainly in the heart). It should be noted that small amounts of CK-MB are found in tissues outside the heart, including the uterus, prostate, gut, diaphragm, and tongue. CK-MB also makes up 1% to 3% of the creatine kinase in skeletal muscle. In the absence of trauma to these other organs and tissues, elevation of CK-MB is highly suggestive of myocardial injury. To facilitate the diagnosis of MI using this marker, it is common to calculate the ratio of CK-MB to total CK. The ratio is usually >2.5% in the setting of myocardial injury and less than that when CK-MB elevation is from another source.

The serum level of CK-MB starts to rise 3 to 8 hours following infarction, peaks at 24 hours, and returns to normal within 48 to 72 hours (see Fig. 7.9). This temporal sequence is important because other sources of CK-MB

(e.g., skeletal muscle injury) or other non-MI cardiac conditions that raise serum levels of the isoenzyme (e.g., myocarditis) do not usually show this delayed peaking pattern. It should also be reinforced that CK-MB is not as sensitive or specific for detection of myocardial injury as is measurement of cardiac troponins.

Because troponin and CK-MB levels do not become elevated in the serum until at least a few hours after the onset of MI symptoms, a single normal value drawn early in the course of evaluation (e.g., in the hospital emergency department) does not rule out an acute MI; thus, the diagnostic utility of these biomarkers is limited in that critical period. As a result, early decision making in patients with ACS often relies most heavily on the patient's history and ECG findings.

Imaging

Sometimes the early diagnosis of MI can remain uncertain even after careful evaluation of the patient's history, ECG, and serum biomarkers. In such a situation, an additional diagnostic study that may be useful is *echocardiography*, which typically reveals abnormalities of ventricular contraction in the region of ischemia or infarction.

TREATMENT OF ACUTE CORONARY SYNDROMES

Successful management of ACS requires rapid initiation of therapy to limit myocardial damage and minimize complications. Therapy must address the intracoronary thrombus that incited the syndrome and provide anti-ischemic measures to restore the balance between myocardial oxygen supply and demand. Although certain therapeutic aspects are common to all ACS, there is a critical difference in the approach to patients who present with ST segment elevation (STEMI) compared with those without ST segment elevation (UA and NSTEMI). Patients with STEMI typically have total occlusion of a coronary artery and benefit from immediate reperfusion therapies (pharmacologic or mechanical), while patients without ST elevation do not (Fig. 7.10 and as discussed later in the chapter).

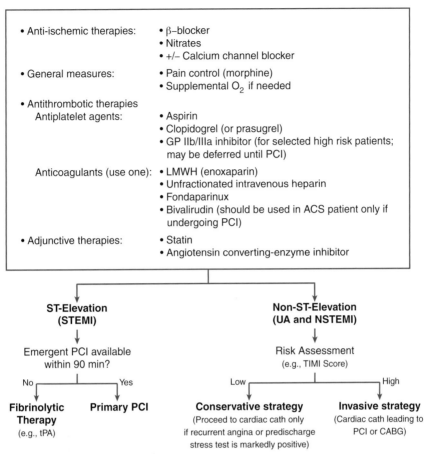

- Anti-ischemic therapies:
  - β–blocker
  - Nitrates
  - +/– Calcium channel blocker
- General measures:
  - Pain control (morphine)
  - Supplemental O$_2$ if needed
- Antithrombotic therapies
  Antiplatelet agents:
  - Aspirin
  - Clopidogrel (or prasugrel)
  - GP IIb/IIIa inhibitor (for selected high risk patients; may be deferred until PCI)
  Anticoagulants (use one):
  - LMWH (enoxaparin)
  - Unfractionated intravenous heparin
  - Fondaparinux
  - Bivalirudin (should be used in ACS patient only if undergoing PCI)
- Adjunctive therapies:
  - Statin
  - Angiotensin converting-enzyme inhibitor

ST-Elevation (STEMI)

Emergent PCI available within 90 min?

No — **Fibrinolytic Therapy** (e.g., tPA)

Yes — **Primary PCI**

Non-ST-Elevation (UA and NSTEMI)

Risk Assessment (e.g., TIMI Score)

Low — **Conservative strategy** (Proceed to cardiac cath only if recurrent angina or predischarge stress test is markedly positive)

High — **Invasive strategy** (Cardiac cath leading to PCI or CABG)

Figure 7.10. Management strategies in acute coronary syndromes (ACS). The measures listed in the top box should be considered in all patients with ACS. In those with STEMI, primary PCI is a preferred approach if it is available within 90 minutes. In UA/NSTEMI, an early invasive intervention is advised if patients present with high-risk features. GP, glycoprotein; LMWH, low molecular weight heparin; PCI, percutaneous coronary intervention.

General in-hospital measures for any patient with ACS include admitting the patient to an intensive care setting where **continuous ECG monitoring** for arrhythmias is undertaken. The patient is initially maintained at **bed rest** to minimize myocardial oxygen demand, while supplemental **oxygen** is provided (by face mask or nasal cannula), if there is any degree of hypoxemia, to improve oxygen supply. Analgesics, such as **morphine**, are administered to reduce chest pain and anxiety and thus further reduce myocardial oxygen needs.

Acute Treatment of Unstable Angina and Non–ST-Elevation Myocardial Infarction

The management of UA and NSTEMI is essentially the same and is therefore discussed as one entity, whereas the approach to STEMI is described later. The primary focus of treatment for UA and NSTEMI consists of *anti-ischemic* medications to restore the balance between myocardial oxygen supply and demand and *antithrombotic* therapy aimed at preventing further growth, and facilitating resolution of, the underlying partially occlusive coronary thrombus.

Anti-ischemic Therapy

The same pharmacologic agents used to decrease myocardial oxygen demand in chronic stable angina are appropriate in UA and NSTEMI but are often administered more aggressively. β-**Blockers** decrease sympathetic drive to the myocardium, thus reducing oxygen demand, and contribute to electrical stability.

This group of drugs reduces the likelihood of progression from UA to MI and lowers mortality rates in patients who present with infarction. In the absence of contraindications (e.g., marked bradycardia, bronchospasm, decompensated heart failure, or hypotension), a β-blocker is usually initiated in the first 24 hours to achieve a target heart rate of approximately 60 beats/min. Such therapy is usually continued indefinitely after hospitalization because of proven long-term mortality benefits following an MI.

Nitrates help bring about anginal relief through venodilation, which lowers myocardial oxygen demand by diminishing venous return to the heart (reduced preload and therefore less wall stress). Nitrates may also improve coronary flow and prevent vaso-spasm through coronary vasodilation. In UA or NSTEMI, nitroglycerin is often initially administered by the sublingual route, followed by a continuous intravenous infusion. In addition to providing symptomatic relief of angina, intravenous nitroglycerin is useful as a vasodilator in patients with ACS accompanied by heart failure or severe hypertension.

Nondihydropyridine **calcium channel antagonists** (i.e., verapamil and diltiazem) exert anti-ischemic effects by decreasing heart rate and contractility and through their vasodilatory properties (see Chapter 6). These agents do not confer mortality benefit to patients with ACS and are reserved for those in whom ischemia persists despite β-blocker and nitrate therapies, or for those with contraindications to β-blocker use. They should *not* be prescribed to patients with LV systolic dysfunction, because clinical trials have shown adverse outcomes in such cases.

Antithrombotic Therapy

The purpose of antithrombotic therapy, including antiplatelet and anticoagulant medications, is to prevent further propagation of the partially occlusive intracoronary thrombus while facilitating its dissolution by endogenous mechanisms.

Antiplatelet Drugs

Aspirin inhibits platelet synthesis of thromboxane A_2, a potent mediator of platelet activation (see Chapter 17), and is one of the most important interventions to reduce mortality in patients with all forms of ACS. It should be administered immediately on presentation and continued indefinitely in patients without contraindications to its use (e.g., allergy or underlying bleeding disorder).

Because aspirin blocks only one pathway of platelet activation and aggregation, other antithrombotic agents have also been studied. **Clopidogrel**, a thienopyridine derivative, blocks activation of the $P2Y_{12}$ ADP receptor on platelets (see Chapter 17). It is recommended as a substitute antiplatelet agent in patients who are allergic to aspirin. Furthermore, the combination of aspirin plus clopidogrel is superior to aspirin alone in reducing cardiovascular mortality, recurrent cardiac events, and stroke in patients with UA or NSTEMI. Thus, clopidogrel is currently recommended for most patients with UA or NSTEMI, except those for whom imminent surgery is planned (because of the increased bleeding risk on such therapy).

Not all patients respond to clopidogrel with similar benefit, as it is a prodrug that requires cytochrome P450-mediated biotransformation to the active metabolite. For example, patients who carry a reduced-function CYP2C19 allele manifest reduced platelet inhibition, and less clinical benefit. Therefore, newer generation platelet $P2Y_{12}$ ADP receptor blockers have been developed without this shortcoming. Of these, **prasugrel**, another thienopyridine derivative, is metabolized more efficiently and has a greater antiplatelet effect. Compared to clopidogrel, it has been shown to further reduce coronary event rates in patients with ACS who undergo percutaneous coronary intervention (PCI), but with an increased bleeding risk.

The **glycoprotein (GP) IIb/IIIa receptor antagonists** (which include the monoclonal antibody *abciximab* and the small molecules *eptifibatide* and *tirofiban*) are potent antiplatelet agents that block the final common pathway of platelet aggregation (see Chapter 17). These agents are effective in reducing adverse coronary events in patients undergoing PCI. In patients presenting with UA or NSTEMI, their benefit is manifest primarily in those at the highest risk of complications (e.g., the presence of elevated serum troponin levels or recurrent episodes of chest pain). Thus, Gp IIb/IIIa receptor antagonist therapy is prescribed to patients at greatest risk and is usually administered at the time of PCI.

Anticoagulant Drugs

Intravenous **unfractionated heparin (UFH)** has long been standard anticoagulant therapy for UA and NSTEMI. It binds to antithrombin, which greatly increases the potency of that plasma protein in the inactivation of clot-forming thrombin. UFH additionally inhibits coagulation factor Xa, slowing thrombin formation and thereby further impeding clot development. In patients with UA or NSTEMI, UFH improves cardiovascular outcomes and reduces the likelihood of progression from UA to MI. It is administered as a weight-based bolus, followed by continuous intravenous infusion. Because of a high degree of pharmacodynamic variability, its anticoagulant effect must be monitored, and its dose adjusted, through serial measurements of the serum activated partial thromboplastin time (aPTT). It is the least expensive of the anticoagulant drugs in this section.

To overcome the pharmacologic shortcomings of UFH, **low molecular weight heparins (LMWHs)** were developed. Like UFH, LMWHs interact with antithrombin but preferentially inhibit coagulation factor Xa. They provide a more predictable pharmacologic response than UFH. As a result, LMWHs are easier to use, prescribed as one or two daily subcutaneous injections based on the patient's weight. Unlike UFH, repeated monitoring of blood tests and dosage adjustments are not generally necessary. In clinical trials in patients with UA or NSTEMI, the LMWH *enoxaparin* (see Chapter 17) has demonstrated reduced death and ischemic event rates compared with UFH.

Two other types of anticoagulants have also been shown to be beneficial in UA and NSTEMI and are sometimes used in place of UFH or LMWHs: (1) the subcutaneously administered factor Xa inhibitor **fondaparinux** (see Chapter 17) is similar to the LMWH enoxaparin at reducing cardiac adverse events but with less bleeding complications and (2) the intravenous direct thrombin inhibitor **bivalirudin** (see Chapter 17) yields superior clinical outcomes compared to the combination of UFH plus a GP IIb/IIIa receptor antagonist in patients with UA or NSTEMI treated with an early invasive strategy, primarily due to a reduced incidence of bleeding. The choice of anticoagulant for an individual patient often depends on whether an initial conservative versus invasive approach is followed.

Conservative Versus Early Invasive Management of UA and NSTEMI

Many patients with UA or NSTEMI stabilize following institution of the therapies described in the previous section, while others progress to a more severe form of ACS. There is currently no definitive way to predict which direction a patient will take or to quickly determine which individuals have such severe underlying CAD that coronary revascularization is warranted. These uncertainties have led to two therapeutic strategies in UA/NSTEMI: (1) an early invasive approach, in which urgent cardiac catheterization is performed and coronary revascularization undertaken as indicated, or (2) a conservative approach, in which the patient is managed with medications (as detailed in the previous section) and undergoes angiography only if ischemic episodes spontaneously recur or if the results of a subsequent stress test indicate substantial residual inducible ischemia. The conservative approach offers the advantage of avoiding costly and potentially risky invasive procedures. Conversely, an early invasive strategy allows rapid identification and definitive treatment (i.e., revascularization) for those with critical coronary disease.

In general, an early invasive approach is recommended to patients with refractory angina, with complications such as shock or ventricular arrhythmias, or those with the most concerning clinical features. Risk assessment algorithms consider such features and help identify patients at high likelihood of a poor outcome. One commonly used tool is the **Thrombolysis in Myocardial Infarction (TIMI) risk score** that employs seven variables to predict a patient's risk level:

1. Age >65 years old
2. ≥3 risk factors for coronary artery disease (as described in Chapter 5)

3. Known coronary stenosis of ≥50% by prior angiography

4. ST segment deviations on the ECG at presentation

5. At least two anginal episodes in prior 24 hours

6. Use of aspirin in prior 7 days (i.e., implying resistance to aspirin's effect)

7. Elevated serum troponin or CK-MB

Clinical studies have confirmed that a patient's TIMI risk score predicts the likelihood of death or subsequent ischemic events, such that an early invasive strategy is recommended in patients with higher scores (≥3). If an early invasive approach is adopted, the patient should undergo angiography within 24 hours.

Acute Treatment of ST-Elevation Myocardial Infarction

In contrast to UA and NSTEMI, the culprit artery in STEMI is typically *completely* occluded. Thus, to limit myocardial damage, the major focus of acute treatment is to achieve prompt reperfusion of the jeopardized myocardium using either fibrinolytic drugs or percutaneous coronary mechanical revascularization. These approaches reduce the extent of myocardial necrosis and greatly improve survival. To be effective, they must be undertaken as soon as possible; the earlier the intervention occurs, the greater the amount of myocardium that can be salvaged. Decisions about therapy must be made within minutes of a patient's assessment, based on the history and electrocardiographic findings, often before serum markers of necrosis would be expected to rise.

In addition, as is the case in UA and NSTEMI, specific medications should be initiated promptly to prevent further thrombosis and to restore the balance between myocardial oxygen supply and demand. For example, antiplatelet therapy with **aspirin** decreases mortality rates and rates of reinfarction after STEMI. It should be administered immediately on presentation (by chewing a tablet to facilitate absorption) and continued orally daily thereafter. Intravenous **UFH** is typically infused to help maintain patency of the coronary vessel and is an important adjunct to modern fibrinolytic regimens. **β-Blockers** reduce myocardial oxygen demand and lower the risk of recurrent ischemia, arrhythmias, and reinfarction. In the absence of contraindications (e.g., asthma, hypotension, or significant bradycardia), an oral β-blocker should be administered to achieve a heart rate of 50 to 60 beats/min. Intravenous blocker therapy should be reserved for patients who are hypertensive at presentation, as that route of administration has otherwise been associated with an increased risk of cardiogenic shock in STEMI. **Nitrate** therapy, usually intravenous nitroglycerin, is used to help control ischemic pain and also serves as a beneficial vasodilator in patients with heart failure or severe hypertension.

Fibrinolytic Therapy

Fibrinolytic drugs accelerate lysis of the occlusive intracoronary thrombus in STEMI, thereby restoring blood flow and limiting myocardial damage. This section does *not* pertain to patients with UA or NSTEMI, as such individuals *do not* benefit from fibrinolytic therapy.

Currently used fibrinolytic agents include recombinant tissue-type plasminogen activator **(alteplase, tPA)**, **reteplase (rPA)**, and **tenecteplase (TNK-tPA)**. Streptokinase, one of the earliest studied fibrinolytics, is now only rarely used in the United States. Each drug functions by stimulating the natural fibrinolytic system, transforming the inactive precursor plasminogen into the active protease plasmin, which lyses fibrin clots. Although the intracoronary thrombus is the target, plasmin has poor substrate specificity and can degrade other proteins, including fibrin's precursor fibrinogen. As a result, bleeding is the most common complication of these drugs. However, unlike the older agent streptokinase, the newer drugs bind preferentially to fibrin in a formed thrombus (i.e., the intracoronary clot), thereby generating plasmin locally at that site, with less interference of coagulation in the general circulation (Fig. 7.11). Nonetheless, bleeding remains the most important risk with all fibrinolytic agents.

rPA and TNK-tPA are derivatives of tPA with longer half-lives. Their main advantage

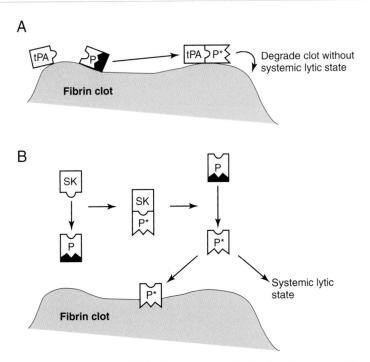

Figure 7.11. Examples of fibrinolytic agents used in ST-elevation myocardial infarction. A. Tissue plasminogen activator (tPA) cleaves fibrin-bound plasminogen (P) to form active plasmin (P*), which degrades the fibrin clot. The selectivity of tPA for fibrin-bound P results in localized thrombolysis and minimizes generalized systemic fibrinolysis. TNK-tPA and rPA (see text) act similarly to tPA but can be administered as boluses, thus simplifying drug administration. **B.** The older fibrinolytic streptokinase (SK) combines with fibrin-bound and circulating plasminogen to form an active complex, which in turn activates additional plasminogen molecules. The lack of selectivity for fibrin-bound plasminogen results in more of a systemic lytic state.

is that they can be administered as IV boluses, which is more convenient and less prone to incorrect administration than the continuous intravenous infusion necessary for tPA.

Administration of fibrinolytic agents in the early hours of an acute STEMI restores blood flow in most (70% to 80%) coronary occlusions and significantly reduces the extent of tissue damage. Improved artery patency translates into substantially increased survival rates and fewer postinfarction complications. The rapid initiation of fibrinolysis is crucial: patients who receive therapy within 2 hours of the onset of symptoms of STEMI have *half* the mortality rate of those who receive it after 6 hours.

Successful reperfusion is marked by the relief of chest pain, return of the ST segments to baseline, and earlier-than-usual peaking of serum markers of necrosis, such as cardiac-specific troponins and CK-MB. During reperfusion, transient arrhythmias are common and do not usually require treatment. To prevent immediate vessel reocclusion after successful thrombolysis, antithrombotic regimens are administered, as described in the next section.

Because the major risk of thrombolysis is bleeding, contraindications to such therapy include situations in which *necessary* fibrin clots within the circulation would be jeopardized (e.g., patients with active peptic ulcer disease or an underlying bleeding disorder, patients who have had a recent stroke, or patients who are recovering from recent surgery). Consequently, approximately 30% of patients may not be suitable candidates for thrombolysis.

Several large-scale comparisons of fibrinolytic agents have been conducted. An early study, the international GUSTO-1 trial found a small postinfarction survival advantage of tPA compared with streptokinase, at the expense of a slightly increased risk of intracranial hemorrhage with tPA. More recent trials compared tPA with the newer agents rPA and TNK-tPA and found similar clinical efficacies for all three agents. The most important message from these trials is that early and sustained patency of the infarct-related coronary artery improves survival. No matter which fibrinolytic is selected, it must be administered as soon as possible, ideally within 30 minutes of the patient's presentation to the hospital.

Adjunctive Antithrombotic Therapies After Fibrinolysis

As previously stated, **aspirin** is a mainstay of therapy in all patients with ACS and is typically initiated on the patient's presentation. Anticoagulants administered with fibrinolytic therapy in STEMI enhance clot lysis and reduce reocclusion rates. Thus, for patients treated with tPA, rPA, or TNK-tPA, adjunctive IV **UFH** should be administered for up to 48 hours. **LMWH** therapy is an alternative to UFH as it has been shown to reduce ischemic complications, but at an increased risk of intracranial hemorrhage in older patients.

The antiplatelet agent **clopidogrel**, administered in combination with aspirin, further reduces mortality and major cardiovascular events in STEMI patients who receive fibrinolytic drugs. Conversely, the antiplatelet GP IIb/IIIa receptor antagonists have not demonstrated a survival benefit in those treated with fibrinolysis and should not be routinely administered to such patients.

Primary Percutaneous Coronary Intervention

An alternative to fibrinolytic therapy in patients with acute STEMI is immediate cardiac catheterization and PCI of the lesion responsible for the infarction. This approach is termed *primary PCI* and involves angioplasty, and usually stenting, of the culprit vessel. Primary PCI is a very effective method for reestablishing coronary perfusion and, in clinical trials performed at highly experienced medical centers, has achieved optimal flow in the infarct-

related artery in more than 95% of patients. Compared with fibrinolytic therapy, primary PCI leads to greater survival with lower rates of reinfarction and bleeding. Therefore, primary PCI is usually the preferred reperfusion approach in acute STEMI, *if* the procedure can be performed by an experienced operator in a rapid fashion (within 90 minutes of hospital presentation). In addition, primary PCI is preferred for patients who have contraindications to fibrinolytic therapy or are unlikely to do well with fibrinolysis, including those who present late (>3 hours from symptom onset to hospital arrival) or are in cardiogenic shock.

Furthermore, "rescue" PCI is recommended for patients initially treated with fibrinolytic therapy who do not demonstrate an adequate response, including expeditious resolution of symptoms and ST segment elevations.

In addition to aspirin and heparin, patients undergoing primary PCI usually receive an intravenous GP IIb/IIIa receptor antagonist in conjunction with the procedure to reduce thrombotic complications (note that the direct thrombin inhibitor bivalirudin can be substituted for the combination of heparin and a GP IIb/IIIa antagonist). For patients who receive coronary stents during PCI, the oral thienopyridines (e.g., clopidogrel) have been shown to reduce the risk of ischemic complications and stent thrombosis. Clopidogrel (or the more potent thienopyridine prasugrel) is therefore continued for a prolonged period (often >12 months), depending on the type of stent placed.

Adjunctive Therapies

Angiotensin-converting enzyme (ACE) inhibitors limit adverse ventricular remodeling and reduce the incidence of heart failure, recurrent ischemic events, and mortality following an MI. Their benefit is additive to that of aspirin and β-blocker therapies, and they have shown favorable improvements especially in higher-risk patients—those with anterior wall infarctions or LV systolic dysfunction.

Cholesterol-lowering **statins** (HMG-CoA reductase inhibitors) reduce mortality rates of patients with coronary artery disease (see Chapter 5). Clinical trials of patients with ACS have demonstrated that it is safe to begin statin therapy early during hospitalization, and that an intensive lipid-lowering regimen, designed to achieve a low-density lipoprotein (LDL) level <70 mg/dL, provides greater protection against subsequent cardiovascular events and death than "standard" targets (i.e., achieving LDL <100 mg/dL). The benefits of statin therapy may extend beyond lipid lowering, because this group of drugs has attributes that can improve endothelial dysfunction, inhibit platelet aggregation, and impair thrombus formation.

In addition to the short-term use of heparin anticoagulation described earlier, a more prolonged course, followed by oral anticoagulation (i.e., warfarin), is appropriate for patients at high risk of thromboembolism—for example, patients with documented intraventricular thrombus (typically identified by echocardiography) or atrial fibrillation and those who have suffered a large acute anterior MI with akinesis of that territory (which is susceptible to thrombus formation because of the stagnant blood flow).

COMPLICATIONS

In UA, the potential complications include death (5% to 10%) or progression to infarction (10% to 20%) over the ensuing days and weeks. Once infarction has transpired, especially STEMI, complications can result from the inflammatory, mechanical, and electrical abnormalities induced by regions of necrosing myocardium (Fig. 7.12). Early complications result from myocardial necrosis itself. Those that develop several days to weeks later reflect the inflammation and healing of necrotic tissue.

Recurrent Ischemia

Postinfarction angina has been reported in 20% to 30% of patients following an MI. This rate has not been reduced by the use of thrombolytic therapy, but it is lower in those who have undergone percutaneous angioplasty or coronary stent implantation as part of early MI management. Indicative of inadequate residual coronary blood flow, it is a poor omen and correlates with an increased risk for reinfarction. Such patients

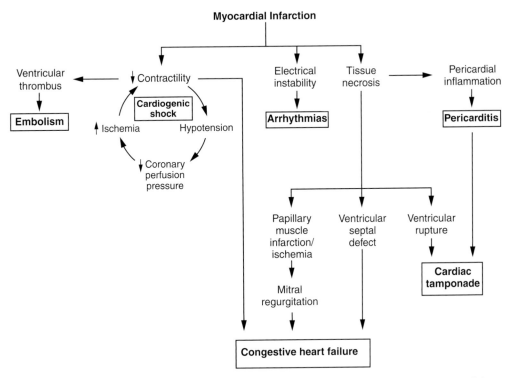

Figure 7.12. Complications of MI. Infarction may result in decreased contractility, electrical instability, and tissue necrosis, which can lead to the indicated sequelae.

Table 7.6. Arrhythmias in Acute Myocardial Infarction

Rhythm	Cause
Sinus bradycardia	• ↑Vagal tone • ↓SA nodal artery perfusion
Sinus tachycardia	• Pain and anxiety • Heart failure • Volume depletion • Chronotropic drugs (e.g., dopamine)
APBs, atrial fibrillation	• Heart failure • Atrial ischemia
VPBs, VT, VF	• Ventricular ischemia • Heart failure
AV block (1°, 2°, 3°)	• IMI: ↑vagal tone and ↓AV nodal artery flow • AMI: extensive destruction of conduction tissue

AMI, anterior myocardial infarction; APBs, atrial premature beats; AV, atrioventricular; IMI, inferior myocardial infarction; SA, sinoatrial; VPBs, ventricular premature beats; VF, ventricular fibrillation; VT, ventricular tachycardia.

usually require urgent cardiac catheterization, often followed by revascularization by percutaneous techniques or coronary artery bypass surgery.

Arrhythmias

Arrhythmias occur frequently during acute MI and are a major source of mortality prior to hospital arrival. Fortunately, modern coronary care units are highly attuned to the detection and treatment of rhythm disturbances; thus, once a patient is hospitalized, arrhythmia-associated deaths are uncommon. Mechanisms that contribute to arrhythmogenesis after MI include the following (Table 7.6):

1. Anatomic interruption of blood flow to structures of the conduction pathway (e.g., sinoatrial node, atrioventricular node, and bundle branches); the normal perfusion of pertinent components of the conduction system is summarized in Table 7.7.

2. Accumulation of toxic metabolic products (e.g., cellular acidosis) and abnormal transcellular ion concentrations owing to membrane leaks.

3. Autonomic stimulation (sympathetic and parasympathetic).

4. Administration of potentially arrhythmogenic drugs (e.g., dopamine).

Table 7.7. Blood Supply of the Conduction System

Conduction Pathway	Primary Arterial Supply
SA node	• RCA (70% of patients)
AV node	• RCA (85% of patients)
Bundle of His	• LAD (septal branches)
RBB	• Proximal portion by LAD • Distal portion by RCA

LBB
  Left anterior fascicle
  Left posterior fascicle
	
	• LAD
	• LAD and PDA

AV, atrioventricular; LAD, left anterior descending coronary artery; LBB, left bundle branch; PDA, posterior descending artery; RBB, right bundle branch; RCA, right coronary artery; SA, sinoatrial.

Ventricular Fibrillation

Ventricular fibrillation (rapid, disorganized electrical activity of the ventricles) is largely responsible for sudden cardiac death during the course of acute MI. Most fatal episodes occur before hospital arrival, a trend that can be impacted by increasing availability of automatic external defibrillators in public places. Episodes of ventricular fibrillation that occur during the first 48 hours of MI are often related to transient electrical instability, and the long-term prognosis of survivors of such events is not adversely affected. However, ventricular fibrillation occurring later than 48 hours after the acute MI usually reflects severe LV dysfunction and is associated with high subsequent mortality rates.

Ventricular ectopic beats, ventricular tachycardia, and ventricular fibrillation during an acute MI arise from either reentrant circuits or enhanced automaticity of ventricular cells (see Chapter 11). Ventricular ectopic beats are common and usually not treated unless the beats become consecutive, multifocal, or frequent. Cardiac care unit personnel are proficient at arrhythmia detection and institution of treatment should more malignant ventricular arrhythmias develop. Therapy for ventricular arrhythmias is described in Chapter 12.

Supraventricular Arrhythmias

Supraventricular arrhythmias are also common in acute MI. *Sinus bradycardia* results from either excessive vagal stimulation or sinoatrial nodal ischemia, usually in the setting of an inferior wall MI. *Sinus tachycardia* occurs frequently and may result from pain and anxiety, heart failure, drug administration (e.g., dopamine), or intravascular volume depletion. Because sinus tachycardia increases myocardial oxygen demand and could exacerbate ischemia, identifying and treating its cause are important. *Atrial premature beats* and *atrial fibrillation* (see Chapter 12) may result from atrial ischemia or atrial distention secondary to LV failure.

Conduction Blocks

Conduction blocks (atrioventricular nodal block and bundle branch blocks) develop commonly in acute MI. They may result from ischemia or necrosis of conduction tracts, or in the case of atrioventricular blocks, may develop transiently because of increased vagal tone. Vagal activity may be increased because of stimulation of afferent fibers by the inflamed myocardium or as a result of generalized autonomic activation in association with the pain of an acute MI.

Myocardial Dysfunction

Congestive Heart Failure

Acute cardiac ischemia results in impaired ventricular contractility (systolic dysfunction) and increased myocardial stiffness (diastolic dysfunction), both of which may lead to symptoms of heart failure. In addition, ventricular remodeling, arrhythmias, and acute mechanical complications of MI (described later in the chapter) may culminate in heart failure. Signs and symptoms of such decompensation include dyspnea, pulmonary rales, and a third heart sound (S_3). Treatment consists of standard heart failure therapy, which typically includes diuretics for relief of volume overload, and ACE inhibitor and β-blocker therapies for long-term mortality benefit (see Chapter 9). In addition, for patients with post-MI heart failure and an LV ejection fraction <40%, an aldosterone antagonist (spironolactone or eplerenone—described in Chapter 9) should be considered, as clinical trials have shown that such therapy further improves survival and reduces rehospitalization rates. However, when an aldosterone antagonist is prescribed along with an ACE inhibitor, the serum potassium level should be carefully monitored to prevent hyperkalemia.

Cardiogenic Shock

Cardiogenic shock is a condition of severely decreased cardiac output and hypotension (systolic blood pressure <90 mm Hg) with inadequate perfusion of peripheral tissues that develops when more than 40% of the LV mass has infarcted. It may also follow certain severe mechanical complications of MI described later. Cardiogenic shock is self-perpetuating because (1) hypotension leads to decreased coronary perfusion, which exacerbates ischemic damage, and (2) decreased stroke volume increases LV size and therefore augments myocardial oxygen demand (see Fig. 7.12). Cardiogenic shock occurs in up to 10% of patients after MI, and the mortality rate is >70%. Early cardiac catheterization and revascularization can improve the prognosis.

Patients in cardiogenic shock require intravenous inotropic agents (e.g., dobutamine) to increase cardiac output and, once the blood pressure has improved, arterial vasodilators to reduce the resistance to LV contraction. Patients are often stabilized by the placement of an **intra-aortic balloon pump**. Inserted into the aorta through a femoral artery, the pump consists of an inflatable, flexible chamber that expands during diastole to increase intra-aortic pressure, thus augmenting perfusion of the coronary arteries. During systole, it deflates to create a "vacuum" that serves to reduce the afterload of the left ventricle, thus aiding the ejection of blood into the aorta and improving cardiac output and peripheral tissue perfusion.

If more extensive and prolonged hemodynamic support is required, a **percutaneous left ventricular assist device (LVAD)** can be placed. Using cannulae inserted via the femoral vessels, a motor located outside of the body pumps oxygenated blood from the LA or the LV (depending on the model) to the aorta and its branches, bypassing or "assisting" the LV.

Right Ventricular Infarction

Approximately one third of patients with infarction of the LV inferior wall also develop necrosis of portions of the right ventricle, because the same coronary artery (usually the right coronary) perfuses both regions in most patients. The resulting abnormal contraction and decreased compliance of the right ventricle lead to signs of right-sided heart failure (e.g., jugular venous distention) out of proportion to signs of left-sided failure. In addition, profound hypotension may result when right ventricular dysfunction impairs blood flow through the lungs, leading to the left ventricle becoming underfilled. In this setting, intravenous volume infusion serves to correct hypotension, often guided by hemodynamic

measurements via a transvenous pulmonary artery catheter (see Chapter 3).

Mechanical Complications

Mechanical complications following MI result from cardiac tissue ischemia and necrosis.

Papillary Muscle Rupture

Ischemic necrosis and rupture of an LV papillary muscle may be rapidly fatal because of acute severe mitral regurgitation, as the valve leaflets lose their anchoring attachments. *Partial* rupture, with more moderate regurgitation, is not immediately lethal but may result in symptoms of heart failure or pulmonary edema. Because it has a more precarious blood supply, the posteromedial LV papillary muscle is more susceptible to infarction than the anterolateral one.

Ventricular Free Wall Rupture

An infrequent but deadly complication, rupture of the LV free wall through a tear in the necrotic myocardium may occur within the first 2 weeks following MI. It is more common among women and patients with a history of hypertension. Hemorrhage into the pericardial space owing to LV free wall rupture results in rapid cardiac tamponade, in which blood fills the pericardial space and severely restricts ventricular filling (see Chapter 14). Survival is rare.

On occasion, a **pseudoaneurysm** results if rupture of the free wall is incomplete and held in check by thrombus formation that "plugs" the hole in the myocardium. This situation is the cardiac equivalent of a time bomb, because subsequent complete rupture into the pericardium and tamponade could follow. If detected (usually by imaging studies), surgical repair may prevent an otherwise disastrous outcome.

Ventricular Septal Rupture

This complication is analogous to LV free wall rupture, but the abnormal flow of blood is not directed across the LV wall into the pericardium. Rather, blood is shunted across the ventricular septum from the left ventricle to the right ventricle, usually precipitating congestive heart failure because of subsequent volume overload of the pulmonary capillaries. A loud systolic murmur at the left sternal border, representing transseptal flow, is common in this situation. Although each results in a systolic murmur, ventricular septal rupture can be differentiated from acute mitral regurgitation by the location of the murmur (see Fig. 2.11), by Doppler echocardiography, or by measuring the O_2 saturation of blood in the right-sided heart chambers through a transvenous catheter. The O_2 content in the right ventricle is abnormally higher than that in the right atrium if there is shunting of oxygenated blood from the left ventricle across the septal defect.

True Ventricular Aneurysm

A late complication of MI, a true ventricular aneurysm occurs weeks to months after the acute infarction. It develops as the ventricular wall is weakened, but not perforated, by the phagocytic clearance of necrotic tissue, and it results in a localized outward bulge (dyskinesia) when the residual viable heart muscle contracts. Unlike the pseudoaneurysm described earlier, a true aneurysm does not involve communication between the LV cavity and the pericardium, so that rupture and tamponade do not develop. Potential complications of LV aneurysm include (1) thrombus formation within this region of stagnant blood flow, serving as a source of emboli to peripheral organs; (2) ventricular arrhythmias associated with the stretched myofibers; and (3) heart failure resulting from reduced forward cardiac output, because some of the LV stroke volume is "wasted" by filling the aneurysm cavity during systole.

Clues to the presence of an LV aneurysm include persistent ST segment elevations on the ECG weeks after an acute ST-elevation MI and a bulge at the LV border on chest radiography. The abnormality can be confirmed by echocardiography.

Pericarditis

Acute pericarditis may occur in the early (in-hospital) post-MI period as inflammation extends from the myocardium to the adjacent pericardium. Sharp pain, fever, and a pericardial friction rub are typically present in this situation and help distinguish pericarditis from the discomfort of recurrent myocardial ischemia (see Chapter 14). The symptoms usually promptly respond to aspirin therapy. Anticoagulants are relatively contraindicated in MI complicated by pericarditis to avoid hemorrhage from the inflamed pericardial lining. The frequency of MI-associated pericarditis has declined since the introduction of acute reperfusion strategies, because those approaches limit the extent of myocardial damage and inflammation.

Dressler Syndrome

Dressler syndrome is another uncommon form of pericarditis that can occur over the weeks following an MI. The cause is unclear, but an immune process directed against damaged myocardial tissue is suspected to play a role. The syndrome is heralded by fever, malaise, and sharp, pleuritic chest pain typically accompanied by leukocytosis, an elevated erythrocyte sedimentation rate, and a pericardial effusion. Similar to other forms of acute pericarditis, Dressler syndrome generally responds to aspirin or other nonsteroidal anti-inflammatory therapies.

Thromboembolism

Stasis of blood flow in regions of impaired LV contraction after an MI may result in intracavity thrombus formation, especially when the infarction involves the LV apex, or when a true aneurysm has formed. Subsequent thromboemboli can result in infarction of peripheral organs (e.g., a cerebrovascular event [stroke] caused by embolism to the brain).

RISK STRATIFICATION AND MANAGEMENT FOLLOWING MYOCARDIAL INFARCTION

The most important predictor of post-MI outcome is the extent of LV dysfunction. Other features that portend adverse outcomes include early recurrence of ischemic symptoms, a large volume of residual myocardium still at risk because of severe underlying coronary disease, and high-grade ventricular arrhythmias.

To identify patients at high risk for complications who may benefit from cardiac catheterization and revascularization, exercise treadmill testing is often performed (unless the patient has already undergone catheterization and corrective percutaneous revascularization for the presenting coronary syndrome). Patients with significantly abnormal results, or those who demonstrate an early spontaneous recurrence of angina, are customarily referred for cardiac catheterization to define their coronary anatomy.

Standard postdischarge therapy includes aspirin, a β-blocker, and an HMG-CoA reductase inhibitor (statin) to achieve an LDL value of <70 mg/dL. ACE inhibitors are prescribed to patients who have LV contractile dysfunction; an aldosterone antagonist should also be considered in those with heart failure symptoms. Rigorous attention to underlying cardiac risk factors, such as smoking, hypertension, and diabetes, is mandatory, and a formal exercise rehabilitation program often speeds convalescence.

Patients who have an LV ejection fraction of ≤30% after MI are at high risk of sudden cardiac death and are candidates for prophylactic placement of an implantable cardioverter-defibrillator. Current guidelines recommend postponing such implantation for at least 40 days post-MI because clinical trials have not shown a survival benefit at earlier stages.

SUMMARY

1. ACS include UA, NSTEMI, and STEMI. Most ACS episodes are precipitated by an intracoronary thrombus at the site of atherosclerotic plaque. Plaque rupture is the usual trigger for thrombus formation through activation of platelets and the coagulation cascade. Atherosclerosis-induced endothelial dysfunction contributes to the process by producing decreased amounts of vasodilators and antithrombotic mediators.

2. Distinctions among types of ACS are based on the severity of ischemia and whether myocardial necrosis results. STEMI is associated with an occlusive thrombus and severe ischemia with necrosis. ACS without ST elevation (NSTEMI and UA) usually result from partially occlusive thrombi with less intense ischemia. Compared with UA, the insult in NSTEMI is of sufficient magnitude to cause some myocardial necrosis.

3. ACS result in biochemical and mechanical changes that impair systolic contraction, decrease myocardial compliance, and predispose to arrhythmias. Infarction initiates an inflammatory response that clears necrotic tissue and leads to scar formation. Transient severe ischemia without infarction can cause "stunned" myocardium, a condition of contractile dysfunction that persists beyond the period of ischemia, with subsequent gradual recovery of function.

4. The diagnosis of specific ACS relies on the patient's history, ECG abnormalities, and appearance of specific biomarkers in the serum (e.g., cardiac troponins).

5. Acute treatment of UA and NSTEMI includes anti-ischemic therapy to restore balance between myocardial oxygen supply and demand (e.g., β-blockers, nitrates) and antithrombotic therapy to facilitate resolution of the intracoronary thrombus (aspirin, an anticoagulant [e.g., IV heparin, LMWH], an ADP receptor antagonist [e.g., clopidogrel], and possibly a GP IIb/IIIa receptor antagonist). Statin therapy is usually indicated. Early coronary angiography, with subsequent coronary revascularization, is beneficial in high-risk patients.

6. Acute treatment for STEMI includes early reperfusion strategies with fibrinolytic drugs or percutaneous catheter-based interventions. Other important measures include antiplatelet therapy (aspirin, clopidogrel), an anticoagulant, a β-blocker, and sometimes nitrate therapy. A statin and an ACE inhibitor are frequently appropriate.

7. Potential complications of infarction include arrhythmias (e.g., ventricular tachycardia and fibrillation), atrioventricular blocks, and bundle branch blocks. Cardiogenic shock or congestive heart failure may develop because of ventricular dysfunction or the development of mechanical complications (e.g., acute mitral regurgitation or ventricular septal defect). Wall motion

abnormalities of the affected segment may predispose to thrombus formation.

8. Standard pharmacologic therapy following discharge from the hospital includes measures to reduce the risks of thrombosis (aspirin and clopidogrel), recurrent ischemia (a β-blocker), progressive atherosclerosis (cholesterol-lowering therapy, usually a statin), and adverse ventricular remodeling (an ACE inhibitor, especially if LV dysfunction is present). Systemic anticoagulation with warfarin is indicated if an intraventricular thrombus, a large akinetic segment, or atrial fibrillation is present.

9. Post-ACS risk stratification can identify patients at high risk of recurrent ischemia, reinfarction, or death. Impaired LV function, high-grade ventricular arrhythmias, and ischemic changes during exercise testing all portend unfavorable outcomes and warrant further investigation and treatment.

Acknowledgments

The authors thank Frederick Schoen, MD, for his helpful suggestions. Contributors to the previous editions of this chapter were Haley Naik, MD; J.G. Fletcher, MD; Anurag Gupta, MD; Marc S. Sabatine, MD; William Carlson, MD; Patrick T. O'Gara, MD; and Leonard S. Lilly, MD.

Additional Reading

Anderson JL, Adams CD, Antman EM, et al. ACC/AHA 2007 guidelines for the management of patients with unstable angina/non ST-elevation myocardial infarction: executive summary: a report of the American College of Cardiology/American Heart Association Task Force on Practice Guidelines. *Circulation*. 2007;116:803–877.

Bonaca MP, Steg PG, Feldman LJ, et al. Antithrombotics in acute coronary syndromes. *J Am Coll Cardiol*. 2009;54:969–984.

Giugliano RP, Braunwald E. The year in non-ST-segment elevation acute coronary syndrome. *J Am Coll Cardiol*. 2008;52:1095–1103.

Hillis LD, Lange RA. Optimal management of acute coronary syndromes. *N Engl J Med*. 2009;360:2237–2240.

Krumholz HM, Wang Y, Chen J, et al. Reduction in acute myocardial infarction mortality in the United States: risk-standardized mortality rates from 1995–2006. *JAMA*. 2009;302:767–773.

Kumar A, Cannon CP. Acute coronary syndromes: diagnosis and management, parts I and II. *Mayo Clin Proc*. 2009;84:917–938, 1021–1036.

Kushner FG, Hand M, Smith SC Jr, et al. Focused updates: ACC/AHA guidelines for the management of patients with ST-elevation myocardial infarction (updating the 2004 guideline and 2007 focused update) and ACC/AHA/SCAI guidelines on percutaneous coronary intervention (updating the 2005 guideline and 2007 focused update): a report of the American College of Cardiology Foundation/American Heart Association Task Force on Practice Guidelines. *Circulation*. 2009;120:2271–2306.

Mega JL, Close SL, Wiviott SD, et al. Cytochrome p-450 polymorphisms and response to clopidogrel. *N Engl J Med*. 2009;360:354–362.

Mehta SR, Granger CB, Boden WE, et al. Early versus delayed invasive intervention in acute coronary syndromes. *N Engl J Med*. 2009;360:2165–2175.

Myerburg RJ. Implantable cardioverter-defibrillators after myocardial infarction. *N Engl J Med*. 2008;359:2245–2253.

Valvular Heart Disease

Christopher A. Miller
Patrick T. O'Gara
Leonard S. Lilly

This chapter describes the pathophysiologic abnormalities in patients with common valvular heart diseases. Each of the conditions is discussed separately because unifying principles do not govern the behavior of all stenotic or regurgitant valves. Effective patient management requires accurate identification of the valvular lesion, a determination of its severity, and a clear understanding of the pathophysiologic consequences and natural history of the condition.

The evaluation of a patient with a suspected valvular lesion begins at the bedside with a careful history and physical examination from which the trained clinician can usually identify the type of abnormalities that are present. The severity of the valve lesions can then be further assessed from the electrocardiogram, chest radiograph, echocardiogram, and, in some cases, cardiac magnetic resonance imaging. In selected patients, additional investigation with exercise testing or cardiac catheterization may be necessary to define fully the significance of the condition and guide therapy.

RHEUMATIC FEVER

Acute rheumatic fever (ARF) was once among the most common causes of valvular heart disease, but its incidence has waned considerably in the past half-century in industrialized societies. In the 1940s, the yearly incidence exceeded 200,000 cases in the United States, whereas the disease is now rare. The decline of this condition immediately preceded or coincided with the introduction of penicillin, as well as with the improvement of general health care and the relief from overcrowding.

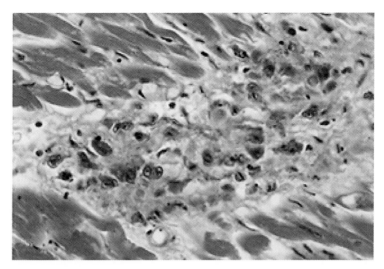

Figure 8.1. Histopathologic appearance of an Aschoff body in acute rheumatic carditis. Mononuclear inflammatory cells surround a center of focal necrosis. (Courtesy of Dr. Frederick J. Schoen, Brigham and Women's Hospital, Boston.)

Although occasional local outbreaks occur, a major resurgence has not been seen in this country. Nevertheless, in developing parts of the world, ARF continues to be a scourge with fulminant consequences.

ARF is an inflammatory condition that primarily involves the heart, skin, and connective tissues. It is a complication of upper respiratory tract infections caused by group A streptococci and mainly occurs in children and young adults. During epidemics, approximately 3% of patients with acute streptococcal pharyngitis develop ARF 2 to 3 weeks after the initial throat infection. Although the pathogenesis remains unknown, it does not involve direct bacterial infection of the heart. Some proposed mechanisms include the elaboration of a toxin by the streptococci or autoimmune cross-reactivity between bacterial and cardiac antigens.

Pathologically in ARF, carditis (i.e., cardiac inflammation) may afflict all three layers of the heart (pericardium, myocardium, and endocardium). Histopathologic examination often demonstrates the **Aschoff body** (Fig. 8.1), an area of focal fibrinoid necrosis surrounded by inflammatory cells, including lymphocytes, plasma cells, and macrophages, that later resolve to form fibrous scar tissue. The most devastating sequelae result from in-flammatory involvement of the valvular endo-cardium, which leads to chronic rheumatic heart disease characterized by permanent deformity and impairment of one or more cardiac valves. Symptoms of valvular dysfunction, however, generally do not become manifest until 10 to 30 years after ARF has subsided. This latency period may be considerably shorter with the more aggressive disease observed in developing countries.

The most common presenting symptoms of ARF are chills, fever, fatigue, and migratory arthralgias. The cardinal symptoms and clinical manifestations of the disease that establish the diagnosis are known as the **Jones criteria** (Table 8.1). During the acute episode, carditis may be associated with tachycardia, decreased left ventricular contractility, a pericardial friction rub, a transient murmur of mitral or aortic regurgitation, or a mid-diastolic murmur at the cardiac apex (termed the Carey–Coombs murmur). These transient murmurs likely reflect turbulent flow across inflamed valve leaflets. Treatment of the acute episode includes the use of high-dose aspirin to reduce inflammation, penicillin to eliminate residual streptococcal infection, and therapy for complications such as congestive heart failure and pericarditis.

During the chronic phase of this condition, stenosis or regurgitation of cardiac valves is

Table 8.1. Jones Criteria for Diagnosis of Rheumatic Fever[a]

Major criteria
Carditis
Polyarthritis
Sydenham chorea (involuntary movements)
Erythema marginatum (skin rash with advancing edge and clearing center)
Subcutaneous nodules

Minor criteria
Migratory arthralgias
Fever
Increased acute phase reactants (ESR, CRP, leukocytosis)
Prolonged PR interval on electrocardiogram

Evidence of streptococcal infection
Antistreptolysin O antibodies
Positive throat culture for streptococci group A

[a]Diagnosis requires evidence of streptococcal infection and either: two major criteria, or one major plus two minor criteria.
ESR, erythrocyte sedimentation rate; *CRP,* C-reactive protein.

common, most often affecting the mitral valve. Forty percent of patients with rheumatic heart disease will develop mitral stenosis. An additional 25% will develop aortic stenosis or regurgitation in addition to the mitral abnormality. Infrequently, the tricuspid valve is affected as well.

Recurrences of ARF in affected patients can incite further cardiac damage. Therefore, individuals who have experienced ARF should receive low-dose penicillin prophylaxis at least until early adulthood, by which time exposure and susceptibility to streptococcal infections have diminished.

MITRAL VALVE DISEASE

Mitral Stenosis

Etiology

The most common cause of mitral stenosis (MS) is rheumatic fever. Approximately 50% of patients with symptomatic MS provide a history of ARF occurring, on average, 20 years before presentation. These patients display typical rheumatic deformity of the valve on echocardiographic and pathologic examina-

tions as described below. Other rare causes of MS (less than 1%) include congenital stenosis of the mitral valve leaflets, prominent calcification extending from the mitral annulus onto the leaflets in elderly patients, or endocarditis with very large vegetations that obstruct the valve orifice.

Pathology

Acute and recurrent inflammation produces the typical pathologic features of rheumatic MS. These include fibrous thickening and calcification of the valve leaflets, fusion of the commissures (the borders where the leaflets meet), and thickening and shortening of the chordae tendineae.

Pathophysiology

In early diastole in the normal heart, the mitral valve opens and blood flows freely from the left atrium (LA) into the left ventricle (LV), such that there is a negligible pressure difference between the two chambers. In MS, however, there is obstruction to blood flow across the valve such that emptying of the LA is impeded and there is an abnormal pressure gradient between the LA and LV (Figs. 8.2 and 8.3). As a result, the left atrial pressure is higher than normal, a necessary feature for blood to be propelled forward across the obstructed valve. The cross-sectional area of a normal mitral valve orifice is 4 to 6 cm^2. Hemodynamically significant MS becomes apparent when the valve area is reduced to less than 2 cm^2. Although left ventricular pressures are usually normal in MS, impaired filling of the chamber across the narrowed mitral valve may reduce LV stroke volume and cardiac output.

The high left atrial pressure in MS is passively transmitted to the pulmonary circulation, resulting in increased pulmonary venous and capillary pressures (see Fig. 8.2). This elevation of hydrostatic pressure in the pulmonary vasculature may cause transudation of plasma into the lung interstitium and alveoli. The patient may therefore experience dyspnea and other symptoms of congestive heart failure. In severe cases, significant elevation of pulmonary venous pressure leads to the opening of collateral

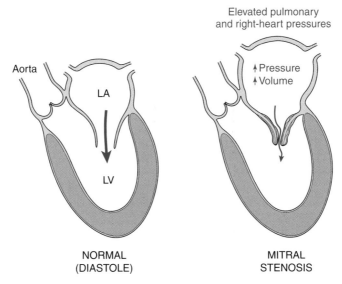

Figure 8.2. Pathophysiology of mitral stenosis. In the normal heart, blood flows freely from the left atrium (LA) into the left ventricle (LV) during diastole. In mitral stenosis, there is obstruction to LA emptying. Thus, the LA pressure increases, which in turn elevates pulmonary and right-heart pressures.

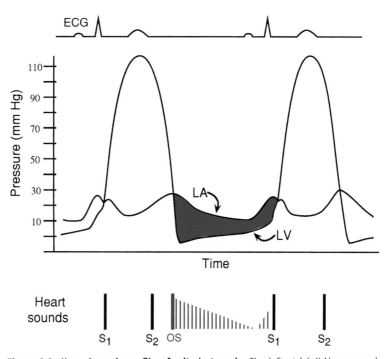

Figure 8.3. Hemodynamic profile of mitral stenosis. The left atrial (LA) pressure is elevated, and there is a pressure gradient (shaded area) between the LA and left ventricle (LV) during diastole. Compare with schematic of normal tracing (see Fig. 2.1). Abnormal heart sounds are present: There is a diastolic opening snap (OS) that corresponds to the opening of the mitral valve, followed by a decrescendo murmur. There is accentuation of the murmur just before S_1 owing to the increased pressure gradient when the LA contracts (presystolic accentuation).

channels between the pulmonary and bronchial veins. Subsequently, the high pulmonary vascular pressures may rupture a bronchial vein into the lung parenchyma, resulting in coughing up of blood (hemoptysis).

The elevation of left atrial pressure in MS can result in two distinct forms of pulmonary hypertension: passive and reactive. Most patients with MS exhibit *passive* pulmonary hypertension, related to the backward transmission of the elevated LA pressure into the pulmonary vasculature. This actually represents an "obligatory" increase in pulmonary artery pressure that develops to preserve forward flow in the setting of increased left atrial and pulmonary venous pressures. Additionally, approximately 40% of patients with MS demonstrate *reactive* pulmonary hypertension with medial hypertrophy and intimal fibrosis of the pulmonary arterioles. Reactive pulmonary hypertension serves a "beneficial" role because the increased arteriolar resistance impedes blood flow into the engorged pulmonary capillary bed and thus reduces capillary hydrostatic pressure (thereby "protecting" the pulmonary capillaries from even higher pressures). However, this benefit is at the cost of decreased blood flow through the pulmonary vasculature and elevation of the right-sided heart pressures, as the right ventricle pumps against the increased resistance. Chronic elevation of right ventricular pressure leads to hypertrophy and dilatation of that chamber and ultimately to right-sided heart failure.

Chronic pressure overload of the LA in MS leads to left atrial enlargement. Left atrial dilatation stretches the atrial conduction fibers and may disrupt the integrity of the cardiac conduction system, resulting in *atrial fibrillation* (a rapid irregular heart rhythm; see Chapter 12). Atrial fibrillation contributes to a decline in cardiac output in MS because the increased heart rate shortens diastole. This reduces the time available for blood to flow across the obstructed mitral valve to fill the LV, and, at the same time, further augments the elevated left atrial pressure.

The relative stagnation of blood flow in the dilated LA in MS, especially when combined with the development of atrial fibrillation, predisposes to intra-atrial thrombus formation. Thromboemboli to peripheral organs may follow, leading to devastating complications such as cerebrovascular occlusion (stroke). Thus, MS patients who develop atrial fibrillation require chronic anticoagulation therapy.

Clinical Manifestations and Evaluation

Presentation

The natural history of MS is variable. The 10-year survival of untreated patients after onset of symptoms is 50% to 60%. Survival exceeds 80% in asymptomatic or minimally symptomatic patients at 10 years. Longevity is much more limited for patients with advanced symptoms and is dismal for those who develop significant pulmonary hypertension, with a mean survival less than 3 years.

The clinical presentation of MS depends largely on the degree of reduction in valve area. The more severe the stenosis, the greater the symptoms related to elevation of left atrial and pulmonary venous pressures. The earliest manifestations are those of dyspnea and reduced exercise capacity. In mild MS, dyspnea may be absent at rest; however, it develops on exertion as LA pressure rises with the exercise-induced increase in blood flow through the heart and faster heart rate (i.e., decreased diastolic filling time). Other conditions and activities that increase heart rate and cardiac blood flow and, therefore, precipitate or exacerbate symptoms of MS, include fever, anemia, hyperthyroidism, pregnancy, rapid arrhythmias such as atrial fibrillation, exercise, emotional stress, and sexual intercourse.

With more severe MS (i.e., a smaller valve area), dyspnea occurs even at rest. Increasing fatigue and more severe signs of pulmonary congestion, such as orthopnea and paroxysmal nocturnal dyspnea, occur. With advanced MS and pulmonary hypertension, signs of right-sided heart failure ensue, including jugular venous distention, hepatomegaly, ascites, and peripheral edema. Compression of the recurrent laryngeal nerve by an enlarged pulmonary artery or LA may cause hoarseness.

Less often, the diagnosis of MS is heralded by one of its complications: atrial fibrillation, thromboembolism, infective endocarditis, or hemoptysis, as described in the earlier section on pathophysiology.

Examination

On examination, there are several typical findings of MS. Palpation of the left anterior chest may reveal a right ventricular "tap" in patients with increased right ventricular pressure. Auscultation discloses a loud S_1 (the first heart sound, which is associated with mitral valve closure) in the early stages of the disease. The increased S_1 results from the high pressure gradient between the atrium and ventricle, which keeps the mobile portions of the mitral valve leaflets widely separated throughout diastole; at the onset of systole, ventricular contraction abruptly slams the leaflets together from the relatively wide position, causing the closure sound to be more prominent (see Chapter 2). In late stages of the disease, the intensity of S_1 may normalize or become reduced as the valve leaflets thicken, calcify, and become immobile.

A main feature of auscultation in MS is a high-pitched "opening snap" (OS) that follows S_2. The OS is thought to result from the sudden tensing of the chordae tendineae and stenotic leaflets on opening of the valve. The interval between S_2 and the OS relates inversely to the severity of MS. That is, the more severe the MS, the higher the LA pressure and the earlier the valve is forced open in diastole. The OS is followed by a low-frequency decrescendo murmur (termed a *diastolic rumble*) caused by turbulent flow across the stenotic valve during diastole (see Fig. 8.3). The duration, but not the intensity, of the diastolic murmur relates to the severity of MS. The more severe the stenosis, the longer it takes for the LA to empty and for the gradient between the LA and LV to dissipate. Near the end of diastole, contraction of the LA causes the pressure gradient between the LA and LV to rise again (see Fig. 8.3); therefore, the murmur briefly becomes louder (termed *presystolic accentuation*). This final accentuation of the murmur does not occur if atrial fibrillation has developed because there is no effective atrial contraction in that situation. Murmurs caused by other valvular lesions are often found concurrently in patients with MS. For example, mitral regurgitation (discussed later in this chapter) frequently coexists with MS. Additionally, right-sided heart failure caused by severe MS may induce tricuspid regurgitation as a result of right

ventricular enlargement. A diastolic decrescendo murmur along the left sternal border may be present owing to coexistent aortic regurgitation (because of rheumatic involvement of the aortic leaflets) or pulmonic regurgitation (because of MS-induced pulmonary hypertension).

The *electrocardiogram* in MS routinely shows left atrial enlargement and, if pulmonary hypertension has developed, right ventricular hypertrophy. Atrial fibrillation may be present. The *chest radiograph* reveals left atrial enlargement, pulmonary vascular redistribution, interstitial edema, and Kerley B lines resulting from edema within the pulmonary septae (see Chapter 3). With the development of pulmonary hypertension, right ventricular enlargement and prominence of the pulmonary arteries also appear.

Echocardiography is of major diagnostic value in MS. It reveals thickened mitral leaflets and abnormal fusion of their commissures with restricted separation during diastole. Left atrial enlargement can be assessed, and if present, intra-atrial thrombus may be visualized. The mitral valve area can be measured directly on cross-sectional views or calculated from Doppler echocardiographic velocity measurements. Patients can be stratified into groups of disease severity based partly on the mitral valve area. A normal mitral valve orifice measures between 4 and 6 cm^2. A reduced mitral valve area of <2 cm^2 correlates with mild MS, and a valve area of 1.1 to 1.5 cm^2 correlates with moderate MS. Severe MS is defined by a valve area of <1.0 cm^2. Although cardiac catheterization is not necessary to confirm the diagnosis of MS, it is sometimes performed to calculate the valve area by direct hemodynamic measurements and to clarify whether significant mitral regurgitation, pulmonary hypertension, or coronary artery disease is present.

Treatment

Diuretics are prescribed to treat symptoms of vascular congestion in MS. If atrial fibrillation has developed, a β-blocker, a calcium channel antagonist with negative chronotropic properties (verapamil or diltiazem), or digoxin may be used to slow the rapid ventricular rate and thereby improve diastolic LV filling. Chronic anticoagulation therapy to prevent thromboembolism is recommended for patients with MS and atrial fibrillation, and for those in whom emboli have already occurred.

If symptoms of MS persist despite diuretic therapy and control of rapid heart rates, or if significant PA hypertension is present, mechanical correction of the stenosis is warranted. *Percutaneous balloon mitral valvuloplasty* is the treatment of choice for MS in appropriately selected patients. During this procedure, a balloon catheter is advanced from the femoral vein into the right atrium, across the atrial septum (by intentionally creating a small septal defect there), and through the narrowed mitral valve orifice. The balloon is then rapidly inflated, thereby "cracking" open the fused commissures. The procedure is safest and most effective in the absence of complicating features, such as mitral regurgitation, extensive valve or subvalvular calcification, or atrial thrombus. The results of this procedure in randomized trials compare favorably with those of surgical treatment in anatomically appropriate patients. Approximately 5% of patients undergoing balloon mitral valvuloplasty are left with a residual atrial septal defect. Less frequent complications include cerebral emboli at the time of valvuloplasty, cardiac perforation, or the creation of mitral

regurgitation requiring subsequent surgical replacement. The estimated event-free survival 7 years after valvuloplasty is 67% to 76%.

Surgical options are undertaken for correcting MS in individuals whose anatomy is not ideal for balloon valvuloplasty. These techniques include *open mitral commissurotomy* (an operation in which the stenotic commissures are separated under direct visualization) and, in severe disease, mitral valve replacement. Open mitral valve commissurotomy is effective, and restenosis occurs in fewer than 20% of patients over 10 to 20 years of follow-up.

Mitral Regurgitation

Etiology

Normal closure of the mitral valve during systole requires the coordinated action of each component of the valve apparatus. Therefore, mitral regurgitation (MR) may result from structural abnormalities of the mitral annulus, the valve leaflets, the chordae tendineae, or the papillary muscles (Fig. 8.4). For example, myxomatous degeneration of the valve (the etiology of mitral valve prolapse) causes MR because enlarged, redundant leaflets bow excessively into the LA during systole rather than opposing each other

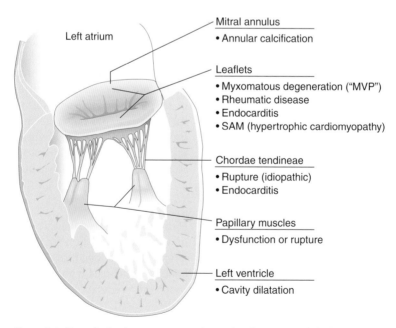

Figure 8.4. The mitral valve apparatus and associated common etiologies of mitral regurgitation. MVP, mitral valve prolapse; SAM, systolic anterior motion.

normally. Infective endocarditis can result in MR because of leaflet perforation or rupture of infected chordae. Rheumatic fever may lead to MS, as already discussed, or primarily MR if excessive shortening of the chordae tendineae and retraction of the leaflets occur. Hypertrophic obstructive cardiomyopathy (see Chapter 10) is associated with abnormal systolic anterior motion of the anterior mitral leaflet, which prevents normal valve closure and can result in significant MR. Calcification of the mitral annulus can occur with normal aging, but this is more common among patients with hypertension, diabetes, or end-stage renal disease. Such calcification impairs the normal movement of the annulus and immobilizes the basal portion of the valve leaflets, interfering with their excursion and systolic closure.

Primary (idiopathic) rupture of chordae tendineae is associated with severe acute valvular incompetence. Ischemic heart disease may scar or cause transient dysfunction of a papillary muscle, interfering with valve closure. Marked left ventricular enlargement of any cause results in MR because of two mechanisms that interfere with mitral leaflet closure: (1) the spatial separation between the papillary muscles is augmented and (2) the mitral annulus is stretched to an increased diameter.

During the 1990s, the commonly used weight-loss drug combination of fenfluramine and phentermine was, in some patients, associated with the development of thickened plaques on the cardiac valves. These patients were prone to develop MR, as well as aortic regurgitation and tricuspid valve disease. Thus, that drug combination is no longer used.

Pathophysiology

In MR, a portion of the left ventricular stroke volume is ejected backward into the low-pressure LA during systole (Fig. 8.5). As a result, the forward cardiac output (into the aorta) is less than the LV's total output (forward flow plus backward leak). Therefore, the direct consequences of MR include (1) an elevation of the left atrial volume and pressure, (2) a reduction of forward cardiac output, and (3) a volume-related stress on the LV because the regurgitated volume returns to the LV in diastole along with the normal pulmonary venous return. To meet normal circulatory

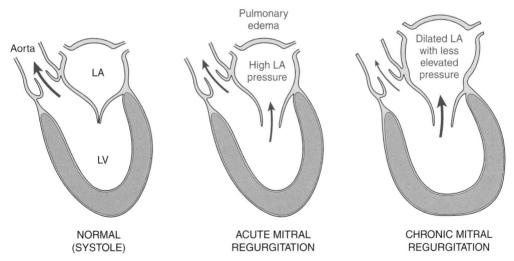

Figure 8.5. Pathophysiology of mitral regurgitation. In the normal heart, left ventricular (LV) contraction during systole forces blood exclusively through the aortic valve into the aorta; the closed mitral valve prevents regurgitation into the left atrium (LA). In mitral regurgitation (MR), a portion of LV output is forced backward into the LA, so that forward cardiac output into the aorta is reduced. In *acute* MR, the LA is of normal size and is relatively noncompliant, such that the LA pressure rises significantly and pulmonary edema may result. In *chronic* MR, the LA has enlarged and is more compliant, so that the LA pressure is less elevated and pulmonary congestive symptoms are less common. The LV enlargement and the eccentric hypertrophy result from the chronically elevated volume load.

needs and to eject the additional volume, LV stroke volume must rise. This increase is accomplished by the Frank–Starling mechanism (see Chapter 9), whereby the elevated LV diastolic volume augments myofiber stretch and stroke volume with each contraction. The subsequent hemodynamic consequences of MR vary depending on the degree of regurgitation and how long it has been present.

The severity of MR and the ratio of forward cardiac output to backward flow are dictated by five factors: (1) the size of the mitral orifice during regurgitation, (2) the systolic pressure gradient between the LV and LA, (3) the systemic vascular resistance opposing forward LV blood flow, (4) the left atrial compliance, and (5) the duration of regurgitation with each systolic contraction.

The *regurgitant fraction* in MR is defined as follows:

$$\frac{\text{Volume of MR}}{\text{Total LV stroke volume}}$$

and this ratio rises whenever the resistance to aortic outflow is increased (i.e., blood follows the path of least resistance). For example, high systemic blood pressure or the presence of aortic stenosis will increase the regurgitant fraction. The extent to which left atrial pressure rises in response to the regurgitant volume is determined by the left atrial compliance. Compliance is a measure of the chamber's pressure–volume relationship, reflecting the ease or difficulty with which the chamber can be filled (see Table 9.1).

In *acute MR* (e.g., owing to sudden rupture of chordae tendineae), left atrial compliance undergoes little immediate change. Because the LA is a relatively stiff chamber, its pressure increases substantially when it is suddenly exposed to the regurgitant volume (see Fig. 8.5). This elevated pressure serves to prevent further regurgitation; however, the high pressure is also transmitted backward to the pulmonary circulation. Therefore, acute MR can result in rapid pulmonary congestion and edema, a medical emergency.

In acute MR, the LA pressure, or the pulmonary capillary wedge pressure (an indirect measurement of LA pressure; see Chapter 3),

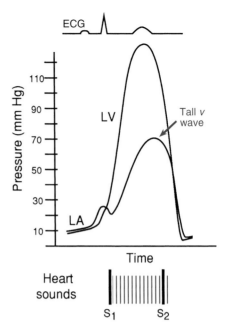

Figure 8.6. Hemodynamic profile of mitral regurgitation (MR). A large systolic v wave is noted in the left atrial (LA) pressure tracing. A holosystolic murmur is present in chronic MR (as shown here), beginning at the first heart sound (S_1) and continuing through the second heart sound (S_2). In severe acute MR, the systolic murmur may actually have a decrescendo quality, reflecting rapid equilibration of LV and LA pressures owing to the relatively reduced LA compliance. ECG, electrocardiogram; LV, left ventricle.

demonstrates a prominent v wave (often referred to as a "cv" wave when it is so prominent that it merges with the preceding c wave), reflecting the increased LA filling during systole (Fig. 8.6). Additionally, as in MS, pulmonary artery and right-heart pressures passively rise such that forward flow through the heart is maintained.

In acute MR, the LV accommodates the increased volume load returning from the LA according to the Frank–Starling relationship. The result is a compensatory increase in the LV stroke volume, such that at the end of each systolic contraction, LV volume remains normal in the nonfailing heart. Systolic emptying of the ventricle is facilitated in MR by the reduced total impedance to LV contraction (i.e., the afterload is lower than normal), since a portion of the LV output is directed into the relatively low-impedance LA, rather than into the higher-pressure aorta as in normal outflow.

In contrast to the acute situation, the more gradual development of *chronic MR* (e.g., owing to rheumatic valve disease) permits the LA to undergo compensatory changes that lessen the effects of regurgitation on the pulmonary circulation (see Fig. 8.5). In particular, the LA dilates and its compliance increases such that the chamber is able to accommodate a larger volume without a substantial increase in pressure. Left atrial dilatation is therefore adaptive in that it prevents significant increases in pulmonary vascular pressures. However, this adaptation occurs at the cost of reduced forward cardiac output, because the compliant LA becomes a preferred low-pressure "sink" for left ventricular ejection, compared with the greater impedance of the aorta. Consequently, as progressively larger fractions of blood regurgitate into the LA, the main symptoms of chronic MR become those of low forward cardiac output (e.g., weakness and fatigue). In addition, chronic left atrial dilatation predisposes to the development of atrial fibrillation.

Thus, major pathophysiologic differences between acute and chronic MR relate to a great extent on left atrial size and compliance (see Fig. 8.5):

Acute MR: Normal LA size and compliance → High LA pressure → High pulmonary venous pressure → Pulmonary congestion and edema

Chronic MR: Increased LA size and compliance → More normal LA and pulmonary venous pressures, but lower forward cardiac output

In chronic MR, the LV also undergoes gradual compensatory dilatation in response to the volume load, through eccentric hypertrophy (see Chapter 9). Compared with acute MR, the resulting increased ventricular compliance accommodates the augmented filling volume with relatively normal diastolic pressures. Forward output in chronic MR is preserved to near-normal levels for an extended period by maintaining a high stroke volume via the Frank–Starling mechanism. Over years, however, chronic volume overload results in

deterioration of systolic ventricular function, a decline in forward output, and symptoms of heart failure.

Clinical Manifestations and Evaluation

Presentation

As should be clear from the pathophysiology discussion, patients with acute MR usually present with symptoms of pulmonary edema (see Chapter 9). The symptoms of *chronic* MR are predominantly due to low cardiac output, especially during exertion, and consist of fatigue and weakness. Patients with severe MR or those who develop LV contractile dysfunction often complain of dyspnea, orthopnea, and/or paroxysmal nocturnal dyspnea. In severe chronic MR, symptoms of right-heart failure (e.g., increased abdominal girth, peripheral edema) may develop as well.

Examination

The physical examination of a patient with chronic MR typically reveals an apical holosystolic (also termed *pansystolic*) murmur that radiates to the axilla (see Fig. 8.6). This description, accurate for rheumatic MR, has some exceptions. For example, when ischemic papillary muscle dysfunction interferes with normal mitral valve closure, the regurgitant jet may be directed toward the anterior left atrial wall, immediately posterior to the aorta. In this setting, the murmur may be best heard along the left sternal edge or in the aortic area (see Chapter 2) and could be confused with the murmur of aortic stenosis (AS). Fortunately, the distinction between the systolic murmur of MR and that of AS can be made by simple bedside maneuvers. If the patient is instructed to clench the fists, systemic vascular resistance will increase, and the severity of MR and its murmur will intensify, whereas the murmur of AS will not. Even more helpful in this distinction is the effect of varying cardiac cycle length (the time between consecutive heart beats) on the intensity of the systolic murmur. In a patient with atrial fibrillation or with frequent premature beats, the LV fills to a degree that directly depends on the preceding cycle length (i.e., a longer cycle length permits greater left ventricular filling). The systolic murmur of AS becomes louder in the beat after a long cycle length because even small pressure gradients are amplified as more blood is ejected across the reduced aortic orifice. In MR, however, the intensity of the murmur does not vary significantly because the change in the LV-to-LA pressure gradient is minimally affected by alterations in the cycle length.

In patients with severe *acute* MR, the systolic murmur is often different, reflecting the underlying pathophysiology. In this case, the murmur may have a *decrescendo* quality, reflecting the rapid equilibration between LV and LA pressures in systole caused by the relatively reduced LA compliance.

In addition to the systolic murmur, a common finding in chronic MR is the presence of an S_3, which reflects increased volume returning to the LV in early diastole (see Chapter 2). In chronic MR, the palpated cardiac apical impulse is often laterally displaced toward the axilla because of LV enlargement.

The *chest radiograph* may display pulmonary edema in acute MR but in chronic asymptomatic MR more likely demonstrates left ventricular and atrial enlargement, without pulmonary congestion. Calcification of the mitral annulus may be seen if that is the cause of the MR. In chronic MR, the *electrocardiogram* typically demonstrates left atrial enlargement and signs of left ventricular hypertrophy. *Echocardiography* can often identify the structural cause of MR and grade its severity by color Doppler analysis. Left ventricular size and function (usually vigorous in the "compensated" heart because of the increased stroke volume) can be observed. *Cardiac catheterization and angiography* is useful for identifying a coronary ischemic cause (i.e., papillary muscle dysfunction) and for grading the severity of MR. The characteristic hemodynamic finding is a large v wave on the pulmonary capillary wedge pressure (reflecting LA pressure) tracing.

Natural History and Treatment

The natural history of chronic MR is related to its underlying cause. For example, in rheumatic heart disease, the course is one of very slow progression with a 15-year survival rate of 70%. On the other hand, abrupt worsening of chronic MR of any cause can occur with superimposed complications, such as rupture of chordae tendineae or endocarditis, and can result in an immediate life-threatening situation.

Medical therapy of MR involves augmenting forward cardiac output while reducing regurgitation into the LA and relieving pulmonary congestion. In acute MR with heart failure, treatment includes intravenous diuretics to relieve pulmonary edema and vasodilators (e.g., intravenous sodium nitroprusside) to reduce the resistance to forward flow and augment forward cardiac output. In chronic MR, vasodilators are less useful and indicated only for the treatment of accompanying hypertension or LV systolic dysfunction, because these drugs have not been shown to delay the need for surgical correction.

Because chronic MR produces continuous left ventricular volume overload, it can slowly result in left ventricular contractile impairment and, ultimately, heart failure. Mitral valve surgery should be performed before this deterioration occurs. *Mitral valve repair* (reconstruction of the native valve) is currently the preferred operative technique for appropriately selected patients. In the past, the operative mortality and the drawbacks associated with the use of prosthetic valves were motivations for delaying surgery as long as possible. Studies showed that survival after *mitral valve replacement* was not clearly better than the natural history of the disease, even though symptomatic improvement was the rule. Fortunately, mitral repair preserves native valve tissue, is associated with less impairment of postoperative LV function, and eliminates many of the problems of artificial valves.

Mitral repair involves the reconstruction of parts of the valve responsible for the regurgitation. For example, a perforated leaflet may be patched with transplanted autologous pericardium, or ruptured chordae may be reattached to a papillary muscle. In patients who undergo a repair operation, the postoperative survival rate appears to be better than the natural history of MR and has provided impetus toward earlier surgical intervention.

The operative mortality rate is approximately 2% to 4% for mitral valve repair and 5% to 7% for mitral replacement. These rates are higher if concurrent coronary artery bypass grafting is performed. In general, mitral valve repair is more often appropriate for younger patients with myxomatous involvement of the mitral valve, and mitral replacement is more often undertaken in older patients with more extensive valve pathology.

Mitral Valve Prolapse

Mitral valve prolapse (MVP) is a common and usually asymptomatic billowing of the mitral leaflets into the LA during ventricular systole, sometimes accompanied by MR (Fig. 8.7). Other names for this condition include *floppy mitral valve, myxomatous mitral valve,* or *Barlow syndrome.* MVP may be inherited as a primary autosomal dominant disorder with variable penetrance or may occur as a part of other connective tissue diseases, such as Marfan syndrome or Ehlers–Danlos syndrome. Pathologically, the valve leaflets, particularly the posterior leaflet,

are enlarged, and the normal dense collagen and elastin matrix of the valvular fibrosa is fragmented and replaced with loose myxomatous connective tissue. Additionally, in more severe lesions, elongated or ruptured chordae, annular enlargement, or thickened leaflets may be present. A recent rigorous echocardiographic study indicated that MVP occurs in about 2% of the population and is more common among women, especially those with thin, lean bodies.

MVP is often asymptomatic, but affected individuals may describe chest pain or palpitations because of associated arrhythmias. Most often it is identified on routine physical examination by the presence of a midsystolic click and late systolic murmur heard best at the cardiac apex. The midsystolic click is thought to correspond to the sudden tensing of the involved mitral leaflet or chordae tendineae as the leaflet is forced back toward the LA; the murmur corresponds to regurgitant flow through the incompetent valve. The click and murmur are characteristically altered during dynamic auscultation at the bedside:

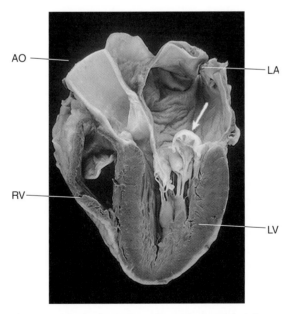

Figure 8.7. Mitral valve prolapse. Long axis view of the left ventricle (LV) demonstrates myxomatous, elongated appearance of the mitral valve with prolapse of the posterior leaflet *(arrow)* into the left atrium (LA). AO, aorta; RV, right ventricle. (From Schoen FJ. The heart. In: Kumar V, Abbas A, Fausto N, eds. *Robbins and Cotran Pathologic Basis of Disease.* 7th ed. Philadelphia: Elsevier Saunders; 2005:592. With permission requested.)

maneuvers that increase the volume of the LV (e.g., sudden squatting, which increases venous return) delay the occurrence of prolapse in systole and cause the click and murmur to occur later (i.e., further from S_1). Conversely, if the volume of blood in the LV is decreased (e.g., on sudden standing), prolapse occurs more readily and the click and murmur occur earlier in systole (closer to S_1).

Confirmation of the diagnosis is obtained by *echocardiography,* which demonstrates posterior displacement of one or both mitral leaflets into the LA during systole. The *electrocardiogram* and *chest radiograph* are usually normal unless chronic MR has resulted in left atrial and left ventricular enlargement.

The clinical course of MVP is most often benign. Treatment consists of reassurance about the usually good prognosis and monitoring for the development of progressive MR. Occasionally, rupture of myxomatous chordae in this condition can cause sudden, severe regurgitation and pulmonary edema. Other rare complications include infective endocarditis, peripheral emboli owing to microthrombus formation behind the redundant valve tissue, and atrial or ventricular arrhythmias.

AORTIC VALVE DISEASE

Aortic Stenosis

Etiology

Aortic stenosis (AS) is often caused by *age-related degenerative calcific changes* of the valve, formerly termed *senile AS.* Calcific changes that progress to AS may also develop in patients with *congenitally deformed aortic valves* (about 1% to 2% of the population is born with an abnormal bicuspid aortic valve). Most patients who present with AS after the age of 65 have the age-related form, whereas younger patients usually have calcification of a congenitally bicuspid valve. AS may also result from chronic *rheumatic valve disease,* although the prevalence of this condition has decreased dramatically in recent decades in the United States. Approximately 95% of patients who are found to have rheumatic AS have coexisting rheumatic involvement of the mitral valve.

Pathology

The pathologic appearance in AS is dependent on its etiology. In age-related degenerative AS, the classic teaching is that the cumulative "wear and tear" of valve motion over many years leads to endothelial and fibrous damage, causing calcification of an otherwise normal trileaflet valve. However, there is also evolving evidence of a common etiology with atherosclerotic vascular disease. Studies have shown that, as in atherosclerosis, the valve tissue of patients with this form of AS display cellular proliferation, inflammation, lipid accumulation, and increased margination of macrophages and T lymphocytes.

In the case of a congenitally deformed valve, years of turbulent flow across the valve disrupt the endothelium and collagen matrix of the leaflets, resulting in gradual calcium deposition. In rheumatic AS, endocardial inflammation leads to organization and fibrosis of the valve, and ultimately fusion of the commissures and the formation of calcified masses within the aortic cusps.

Pathophysiology

In AS, blood flow across the aortic valve is impeded during systole (Fig. 8.8). When the valve orifice area is reduced by more than 50% of its normal size, significant elevation of left ventricular pressure is necessary to drive blood into the aorta (Fig. 8.9).

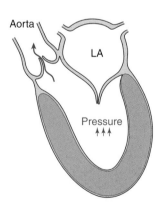

Figure 8.8. Pathophysiology of aortic stenosis (AS). The impediment to left ventricular (LV) outflow in AS results in elevated LV pressures and secondary ventricular hypertrophy.

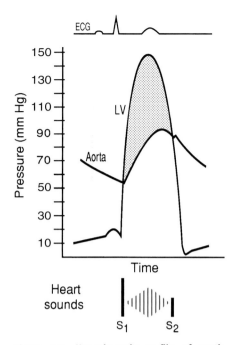

Figure 8.9. Hemodynamic profile of aortic stenosis. A systolic pressure gradient (shaded area) is present between the left ventricle (LV) and aorta. The second heart sound (S_2) is diminished in intensity, and there is a crescendo–decrescendo systolic murmur that does not extend beyond S_2. ECG, electrocardiogram.

Table 8.2. Median Survival Time in Symptomatic Severe Aortic Stenosis	
Clinical Symptoms	*Median Survival*
Angina	5 years
Syncope	3 years
Congestive heart failure	2 years
Atrial fibrillation	6 months

Derived from Ross J Jr, Braunwald E. Aortic stenosis. *Circulation.* 1968;38(suppl v):61.

Since AS develops over a chronic course, the LV is able to compensate initially by undergoing concentric hypertrophy in response to the high systolic pressure it must generate. Such hypertrophy serves an important role in reducing ventricular wall stress (remember from Chapter 6 that wall stress = $(P \times r) \div 2h$, in which h represents wall thickness); however, it also reduces the compliance of the ventricle. The resulting elevation of diastolic LV pressure also causes the LA to hypertrophy in order to fill the "stiff" LV. Whereas left atrial contraction contributes only a small portion of the left ventricular stroke volume in normal individuals, it may provide more than 25% of the stroke volume to the stiffened LV in AS patients. Thus, left atrial hypertrophy is beneficial, and the loss of effective atrial contraction (e.g., development of atrial fibrillation) can cause marked clinical deterioration.

Three major manifestations occur in patients with advanced AS: (1) angina, (2) exertional syncope, and (3) congestive heart failure, all of which can be explained on the basis of the underlying pathophysiology. Each manifestation, in order, heralds an increasingly ominous prognosis (Table 8.2).

AS may result in *angina* because it creates a substantial imbalance between myocardial oxygen supply and demand. Myocardial oxygen *demand* is increased in two ways. First, the muscle mass of the hypertrophied LV is increased, requiring greater-than-normal perfusion. Second, wall stress is increased because of the elevated systolic ventricular pressure. In addition, AS reduces myocardial oxygen *supply* because the elevated left ventricular diastolic pressure reduces the coronary perfusion pressure gradient between the aorta and the myocardium.

AS may cause *syncope* during exertion. Although left ventricular hypertrophy allows the chamber to generate a high pressure and maintain a normal cardiac output at rest, the ventricle cannot significantly increase its cardiac output during exercise because of the fixed stenotic aortic orifice. In addition, exercise leads to vasodilatation of the peripheral muscle beds. Thus, the combination of peripheral vasodilatation and the inability to augment cardiac output contributes to decreased cerebral perfusion pressure and, potentially, loss of consciousness on exertion.

Finally, AS can result in symptoms of *heart failure*. Early in the course of AS, an abnormally increased left atrial pressure occurs primarily at the end of diastole, when the LA contracts into the thickened noncompliant LV. As a result, the mean left atrial pressure and the pulmonary venous pressure are not greatly affected early in the disease. However, with progression of the stenosis, the LV may develop contractile dysfunction because of the insurmountably high afterload, leading to increased left ventricular diastolic volume and pressure. The accompanying marked elevation of LA and pulmonary venous pressures incites pulmonary alveolar congestion and the symptoms of heart failure.

The normal aortic valve cross-sectional area is 3 to 4 cm^2. When the valve area is reduced to less than 2 cm^2, a pressure gradient between the LV and aorta first appears (mild AS). Moderate AS is characterized by a valve area of 1.0 to 1.5 cm^2. When the aortic valve area is reduced to less than 1.0 cm^2, severe valve obstruction is said to be present.

Clinical Manifestations and Evaluation

Presentation

Angina, syncope, and congestive heart failure may appear after many asymptomatic years of slowly progressive valve stenosis. Once these symptoms develop, they confer a significantly decreased survival if surgical correction of AS is not undertaken (see Table 8.2).

Examination

Physical examination often permits accurate detection and estimation of the severity of AS. The key features of advanced AS include (1) a coarse late-peaking systolic ejection murmur and (2) a weakened (*parvus*) and delayed (*tardus*) upstroke of the carotid artery pulsations owing to the obstructed LV outflow. Other common findings on cardiac examination include the presence of an S_4 (because of atrial contraction into the "stiff" LV) and reduced intensity, or complete absence, of the aortic component of the second heart sound (see Fig. 8.9).

On the *electrocardiogram*, left ventricular hypertrophy is common in advanced AS, but *echocardiography* is a more sensitive technique to assess LV wall thickness. The transvalvular pressure gradient and aortic valve area can be calculated by Doppler echocardiography (see Chapter 3). *Cardiac catheterization* is sometimes used to confirm the severity of AS and to define the coronary anatomy, because concurrent coronary artery bypass surgery is often necessary at the time of aortic valve replacement in patients with coexisting coronary disease.

Natural History and Treatment

The natural history of severe, symptomatic, uncorrected AS is very poor. Data from the Mayo Clinic indicate that the 1-year survival rate is 57% for patients with advanced disease. Effective treatment requires replacement of the valve.

Aortic valve replacement (AVR) is indicated when patients with severe AS develop symptoms, or when there is evidence of progressive LV dysfunction in the absence of symptoms. The left ventricular ejection fraction almost always increases after valve replacement, even in patients with impaired preoperative left ventricular function. The effect of AVR on the natural history of AS is dramatic, as the 10-year survival rate rises to approximately 60%.

Unlike its successful role in mitral stenosis, percutaneous valvuloplasty has been disappointing in the treatment of AS in adults. Although balloon dilatation of the aortic valve orifice can fracture calcified commissures leading to some immediate relief of outflow obstruction, up to 50% of patients develop restenosis within 6 months. Valvuloplasty is occasionally a suitable option for patients who are poor surgical candidates or as a temporizing measure in patients too ill to proceed directly to valve replacement. Valvuloplasty is also sometimes effective in young patients with congenitally bicuspid valves.

Mild, asymptomatic AS has a slow rate of progression such that over a 20-year period, only 20% of patients will progress to severe or symptomatic disease. Appropriate therapy for asymptomatic AS includes caution in the use of medications that could result in hypotension in this condition (e.g., vasodilators, diuretics, nitroglycerin). There is no current effective therapy for slowing the actual progression of aortic stenosis. Given the similar risk factors that lead to both atherosclerosis and calcific aortic stenosis, ongoing research trials are testing whether statin therapy administered to patients with mild AS might retard worsening over time.

Table 8.3. Causes of Aortic Regurgitation

Abnormalities of valve leaflets

1. Congenital (bicuspid valve)
2. Endocarditis
3. Rheumatic

Dilatation of aortic root

1. Aortic aneurysm (inflammation; connective tissue disease, e.g., Marfan syndrome)
2. Aortic dissection
3. Annuloaortic ectasia
4. Syphilis

Aortic Regurgitation

Etiology

Aortic regurgitation (AR), also termed *aortic insufficiency*, may result from (1) diseases of the aortic leaflets or (2) dilatation of the aortic root. The most common causes of AR are listed in Table 8.3.

Pathophysiology

In AR, abnormal regurgitation of blood from the aorta into the LV occurs during diastole. Therefore, with each contraction, the LV must pump that regurgitant volume *plus* the normal amount of blood entering from the LA. Hemodynamic compensation relies on the Frank–Starling mechanism to augment stroke volume. Factors influencing the severity of AR are analogous to those of MR: (1) the size of the regurgitant aortic orifice, (2) the pressure gradient across the aortic valve during diastole, and (3) the duration of diastole.

As in MR, the hemodynamic abnormalities and symptoms differ in acute and chronic AR (Fig. 8.10). In *acute AR*, the LV is of normal size and relatively noncompliant. Thus, the volume load of regurgitation causes the LV diastolic pressure to rise substantially. The sudden high diastolic LV pressure is transmitted to the LA and pulmonary circulation, often producing dyspnea and pulmonary edema. Thus, severe acute AR is usually a surgical emergency, requiring immediate valve replacement.

In *chronic AR*, the LV undergoes compensatory adaptation in response to the longstanding regurgitation. AR subjects the LV primarily to volume overload but also to an excessive pressure load; therefore, the ventricle compensates through chronic dilatation (eccentric

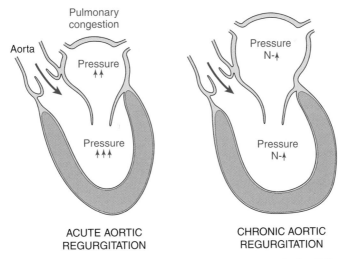

ACUTE AORTIC
REGURGITATION

CHRONIC AORTIC
REGURGITATION

Figure 8.10. Pathophysiology of acute and chronic aortic regurgitation (AR). Abnormal regurgitation of blood from the aorta into the left ventricle (LV) is shown in each schematic drawing *(long arrows)*. In acute AR, the LV is of normal size and relatively low compliance, such that its diastolic pressure rises significantly; this pressure increase is reflected back to the left atrium (LA) and pulmonary vasculature, resulting in pulmonary congestion or edema. In chronic AR, adaptive LV and LA enlargement have occurred, such that a greater volume of regurgitation can be accommodated with less of an increase in diastolic LV pressure, so that pulmonary congestion is less likely. N, normal.

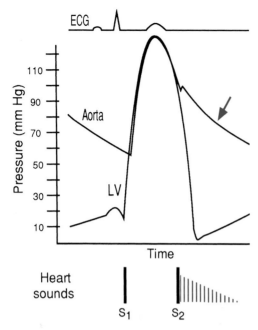

Figure 8.11. Hemodynamic profile of aortic regurgitation. During diastole, the aortic pressure falls rapidly *(arrow)*, and left ventricular (LV) pressure rises as blood regurgitates from the aorta into the LV. A diastolic decrescendo murmur, beginning at the second heart sound (S₂), corresponds with the abnormal regurgitant flow. ECG, electrocardiogram.

Compensatory left ventricular dilatation and hypertrophy are generally adequate to meet the demands of chronic AR for many years, during which affected patients are asymptomatic. Gradually, however, progressive remodeling of the LV occurs, resulting in systolic dysfunction. This causes decreased forward cardiac output as well as an increase in left atrial and pulmonary vascular pressures. At that point, the patient develops symptoms of heart failure.

Clinical Manifestations and Assessment

Presentation

Common symptoms of chronic AR include dyspnea on exertion, fatigue, decreased exercise tolerance, and the uncomfortable sensation of a forceful heartbeat associated with the high pulse pressure.

Examination

Physical examination may show bounding pulses and other stigmata of the widened pulse pressure (Table 8.4), in addition to a hyperdynamic LV impulse and a blowing murmur of

hypertrophy, with replication of sarcomeres in series—see Chapter 9) and, to a lesser degree, increased thickness. Over time, the dilatation increases the compliance of the LV and allows it to accommodate a larger regurgitant volume with less of an increase in diastolic pressure, reducing the pressure transmitted into the LA and pulmonary circulation. However, by accommodating the large regurgitant volume, the aortic (and therefore systemic arterial) diastolic pressure drops substantially. The combination of a high LV stroke volume (and therefore high systolic arterial pressure) with a reduced aortic diastolic pressure produces a widened *pulse pressure* (the difference between arterial systolic and diastolic pressures), a hallmark of chronic AR (Fig. 8.11). As a result of the decreased aortic diastolic pressure, the coronary artery perfusion pressure falls, potentially reducing myocardial oxygen supply. This, coupled with the increase in LV size (which causes increased wall stress and myocardial oxygen demand), can produce angina, even in the absence of atherosclerotic coronary disease.

Table 8.4. Physical Findings Associated with Widened Pulse Pressure in Chronic Aortic Regurgitation	
Name	*Description*
Bisferiens pulse	Double systolic impulse in carotid or brachial artery
Corrigan pulse	"Water-hammer" pulses with marked distention and collapse
de Musset sign	Head-bobbing with each systole
Duroziez sign	To-and-fro murmur heard over femoral artery with light compression
Hill sign	Popliteal systolic pressure more than 60 mm Hg greater than brachial systolic pressure
Müller sign	Systolic pulsations of the uvula
Quincke sign	Capillary pulsations visible at lip or proximal nail beds
Traube sign	"Pistol-shot" sound auscultated over the femoral artery

AR in early diastole along the left sternal border (see Fig. 8.11). It is best heard with the patient leaning forward, after exhaling. In addition, a low-frequency mid-diastolic rumbling sound may be auscultated at the cardiac apex in some patients with severe AR. Known as the *Austin Flint murmur*, it is thought to reflect turbulence of blood flow through the *mitral* valve during diastole owing to downward displacement of the mitral anterior leaflet by the regurgitant stream of AR. It can be distinguished from the murmur of mitral stenosis by the absence of an OS or presystolic accentuation of the murmur.

In chronic AR, the *chest radiograph* shows an enlarged left ventricular silhouette. This is usually absent in acute AR, in which pulmonary vascular congestion is the more likely finding. *Doppler echocardiography* can identify and quantify the degree of AR and often can identify its cause. *Cardiac catheterization* with contrast angiography is useful for evaluation of left ventricular function, quantification of the degree of AR, and assessment of coexisting coronary artery disease.

Treatment

Data from natural history studies indicate that clinical progression of patients with asymptomatic chronic AR and normal LV contractile function is very slow. Therefore, asymptomatic patients are monitored with periodic examinations and assessment of LV function, usually by serial echocardiography. Patients with asymptomatic severe AR and preserved LV function may benefit from afterload reducing vasodilators (e.g., a calcium channel blocker or an angiotensin-converting enzyme inhibitor) when hypertension is present (systolic blood pressure > 140 mm Hg). Such agents do not prolong the compensated stage of chronic AR in the absence of high blood pressure.

Symptomatic patients, or asymptomatic patients with severe AR and impaired LV contractile function (i.e., an ejection fraction <0.50), should be offered surgical correction to prevent progressive deterioration. Studies of patients with AR show that without surgery, death usually occurs within 4 years after the development of angina or 2 years after the onset of heart failure symptoms.

TRICUSPID VALVE DISEASE

Tricuspid Stenosis

Tricuspid stenosis (TS) is rare and is usually a long-term consequence of rheumatic fever. The OS and diastolic murmur of TS are similar to those of MS, but the murmur is heard closer to the sternum and it intensifies on inspiration because of increased right-heart blood flow. In TS, the neck veins are distended and show a large *a* wave as a result of right atrial contraction against the stenotic tricuspid valve orifice. Patients may develop abdominal distention and hepatomegaly owing to passive venous congestion. Surgical therapy is usually required (valvuloplasty or valve replacement).

Tricuspid Regurgitation

Tricuspid regurgitation (TR) is usually *functional* rather than structural; that is, it most commonly results from right ventricular enlargement (e.g., owing to pressure or volume overload) rather than from primary valve disease. Among patients with rheumatic mitral stenosis, 20% also have significant TR (of whom 80% have functional TR because of pulmonary hypertension with right ventricular enlargement, and 20% have "organic" TR resulting from rheumatic involvement of the tricuspid valve). A rare cause of TR is *carcinoid syndrome,* in which a type of neuroendocrine tumor (usually in the small bowel or appendix, with metastases to the liver) releases serotonin metabolites into the bloodstream. These metabolites are thought to be responsible for the formation of endocardial plaques in the right side of the heart. Involvement of the tricuspid valve immobilizes the leaflets, often resulting in substantial TR and, less often, TS.

The most common physical signs of TR are prominent *v* waves in the jugular veins and a pulsatile liver because of regurgitation of right ventricular blood into the systemic veins. The systolic murmur of TR is heard at the lower-left sternal border. It is often soft but becomes louder on inspiration. Doppler echocardiography readily detects TR and can quantify it. The treatment of functional TR is directed at the conditions responsible for the elevated right ventricular size or pressure, and diuretic therapy; surgical repair of the valve is indicated in severe cases.

PULMONIC VALVE DISEASE

Pulmonic Stenosis

Pulmonic stenosis (PS) is rare, and its cause is almost always congenital deformity of the valve. Carcinoid syndrome, described in the previous section, is another rare etiology, in which encasement and immobilization of the valve leaflets can occur.

Severe cases of PS are associated with a peak systolic pressure gradient of greater than 80 mm Hg, moderate disease with a gradient of 40 to 80 mm Hg, and mild PS is said to be present when the transvalvular gradient is less than 40 mm Hg. Only patients with moderate to severe gradients are symptomatic. In such cases, transcatheter balloon valvuloplasty is usually effective therapy.

Pulmonic Regurgitation

Pulmonic regurgitation most commonly develops in the setting of severe pulmonary hypertension and results from dilatation of the valve ring by the enlarged pulmonary artery. Auscultation reveals a high-pitched decrescendo murmur along the left sternal border that is often indistinguishable from AR (the two conditions are easily differentiated by Doppler echocardiography).

PROSTHETIC VALVES

The patient who undergoes valve replacement surgery often benefits dramatically from hemodynamic and symptomatic improvement but also acquires a new set of potential complications related to the valve prosthesis itself. Because all available valve substitutes have certain limitations, valve replacement surgery is not a true "cure."

The first successful valve replacements took place in the 1960s. Currently available valve substitutes include mechanical and biologic (derived from animal or human tissue) devices (Fig. 8.12). Older mechanical valves included a ball-in-cage design, with a bulky shape that often left a significant valvular gradient and occasionally produced intravascular hemolysis from red blood cell trauma. This valve type, however, had an impressive record of durability, with some models functioning well for more than 30 years. Newer mechanical valves, such as bileaflet prostheses, provide a lower profile and superior hemodynamics with no apparent sacrifice of durability. One example is the St. Jude prosthesis, a hinged bileaflet

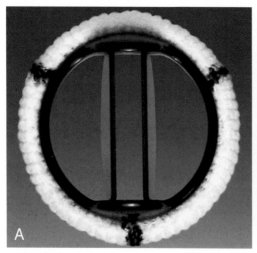
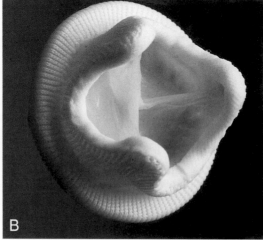

Figure 8.12. Examples of prosthetic heart valves. A. St. Jude mechanical bileaflet valve in the open position. (Courtesy of St. Jude Medical, Inc., St. Paul, MN.) **B.** A bioprosthetic aortic valve with leaflets in the closed position. (Courtesy of Medtronic, Inc., Minneapolis, MN.)

valve consisting of two Pyrolyte carbon discs that open opposite one another (see Fig. 8.12). mechanical valves, while durable, present foreign thrombogenic surfaces to the circulating blood and require lifelong anticoagulation to prevent thromboembolism.

The most commonly used bioprostheses are made from glutaraldehyde-fixed porcine valves secured in a support frame. In addition, bovine pericardium and human homograft (aortic valves harvested and cryopreserved from cadavers) prostheses are used. Bioprosthetic valves have limited durability compared with mechanical valves, and structural failure occurs in up to 50% of valves at 15 years. Failure rates vary greatly depending on the position of the valve. For example, bioprosthetic valves in the mitral position deteriorate more rapidly than those in the aortic position. This is likely because the mitral valve is forced closed during systolic contraction, resulting in greater leaflet stress than that experienced by aortic prostheses that close during diastolic relaxation.

The principal causes of bioprosthetic valve failure over time are leaflet tears and calcification. Conversely, the main advantage of bioprostheses is that they display a very low rate of thromboembolism and do not require long-term anticoagulation therapy. For patients with aortic valve endocarditis, aortic homograft replacements are especially useful because they have very low rates of subsequent infection.

Common to all types of valve replacement is the risk of infective endocarditis (discussed in the next section), which occurs at an incidence of 1% to 2% per patient per year. If endocarditis occurs in the first 60 days after valve surgery, the mortality rate is exceedingly high (50% to 80%). If endocarditis occurs later, mortality rates range from 20% to 50%. Reoperation is usually required if endocarditis involves a mechanical prosthesis, because an adjacent abscess is almost always present (the organism cannot infect the prosthetic material itself). Some cases of bioprosthetic valve endocarditis respond to antibiotic therapy alone.

Given their respective advantages and disadvantages, the mortality and complication rates of mechanical and bioprosthetic valves are similar for the first 10 years after replacement. In 20-year follow-up of long-term, randomized, controlled trials, mechanical valves have been shown to be superior to bioprosthetic valves in event-free survival, except for bleeding complications related to the required anticoagulation therapy. Therefore, the decision about which type of prosthesis to use in a patient often centers on (1) the patient's expected lifespan in comparison to the functional longevity of the valve, (2) risk-versus-benefit considerations of chronic anticoagulation therapy, and (3) patient and surgeon preferences. Mechanical valves are often recommended for younger patients and for those who will be tolerant of, and compliant with, anticoagulant therapy. Bioprosthetic valves are suitable choices for patients of 65 years or older and for patients with contraindications to chronic anticoagulation.

INFECTIVE ENDOCARDITIS

Infection of the endocardial surface of the heart, including the cardiac valves, can lead to extensive tissue damage and is often fatal. Infective endocarditis (IE) carries an overall 6-month mortality rate of 20% to 25%, even with appropriate therapy, and a 100% mortality rate if it is not recognized and treated correctly.

There are three clinically useful ways to classify IE: (1) by clinical course, (2) by host substrate, or (3) by the specific infecting microorganism. In the first classification scheme, IE is termed **acute bacterial endocarditis (ABE)** when the syndrome presents as an acute, fulminant infection, and a highly virulent and invasive organism such as *Staphylococcus aureus* is causal. Because of the aggressiveness of the responsible microorganism, ABE may occur on previously healthy heart valves. When IE presents with a more insidious clinical course, it is termed **subacute bacterial endocarditis (SBE),** and less virulent organisms such as streptococci viridans are involved. SBE most frequently occurs in individuals with prior underlying valvular damage.

The second means of classification of IE is according to the host substrate: (1) native valve endocarditis, (2) prosthetic valve endocarditis, or (3) endocarditis in the setting of intravenous drug abuse. Of these, native valve endocarditis accounts for 60% to 80% of patients. Different microorganisms and clinical courses are associated with each of these categories. For example, the skin contaminant *Staphylococcus epidermidis* is a common cause of prosthetic valve endocarditis, but that is rarely the case when endocarditis occurs on a native heart valve. Intravenous drug users have a propensity for endocarditis of the right-sided heart valves.

The third classification of IE is according to the specific infecting microorganism (e.g., *S. aureus* endocarditis). Although the remainder of this discussion focuses on the endocarditis syndromes based on clinical course, it is important to recognize that all three classifications of IE are used.

Pathogenesis

The pathogenesis of endocarditis requires several conditions: (1) endocardial surface injury, (2) thrombus formation at the site of injury, (3) bacterial entry into the circulation, and (4) bacterial adherence to the injured endocardial surface. The first two conditions provide an environment favorable to infection, whereas the latter two permit implantation of the organism on the endocardial surface. The most common cause of endothelial injury is turbulent blood flow resulting from pre-existing valvular disease; approximately 75% of patients with endocarditis have evidence of underlying structural or hemodynamic abnormalities (Table 8.5). Endothelial injury may also be incited by foreign material within the circulation, such as indwelling venous catheters or prosthetic heart valves.

Once an endocardial surface is injured, platelets adhere to the exposed subendocardial connective tissue and initiate the formation of a sterile thrombus (termed a *vegetation*) through fibrin deposition. This process is referred to as *nonbacterial thrombotic endocarditis* (NBTE). NBTE makes the endocardium more hospitable to microbes in two ways. First, the fibrin-platelet deposits provide a surface for adherence by bacteria. Second, the fibrin covers adherent organisms and protects them from host defenses by inhibiting chemotaxis and migration of phagocytes.

When NBTE is present, the delivery of microorganisms in the bloodstream to the injured

Table 8.5. Cardiac Lesions That Predispose to Endocarditis

Rheumatic valvular disease
Other acquired valvular lesions
  Calcific aortic stenosis
  Aortic regurgitation
  Mitral regurgitation
  Mitral valve prolapse (if murmur auscultated or detected by Doppler)
Hypertrophic obstructive cardiomyopathy
Congenital heart disease
  Ventricular septal defect
  Patent ductus arteriosus
  Tetralogy of Fallot
  Aortic coarctation
  Bicuspid aortic valve
  Pulmonic stenosis
Surgically implanted intravascular hardware
  Prosthetic heart valves
  Pulmonary-systemic vascular shunts
  Ventriculoatrial shunts for hydrocephalus

surface can lead to IE. Three factors determine the ability of an organism to induce IE: (1) access to the bloodstream, (2) survival of the organism in the circulation, and (3) adherence of the bacteria to the endocardium. Bacteria can be introduced into the bloodstream whenever a mucosal or skin surface harboring an organism is traumatized, such as from the mouth during dental procedures or from the skin during illicit intravenous drug use. However, while transient bacteremia is a relatively common event, only microorganisms suited for survival in the circulation and able to adhere to the platelet–fibrin mesh overlying the endocardial defect will cause IE. For example, gram-positive organisms account for approximately 90% of cases of endocarditis, largely because of their resistance to destruction in the circulation by complement and their particular tendency to adhere to endothelial and platelet surface proteins. The ability of certain streptococcal species to produce dextran, a bacterial cell wall component that adheres to thrombus, correlates with their inciting endocarditis. Table 8.6 lists the infectious agents reported to be the most common causes of endocarditis in modern tertiary centers; staphylococci and streptococci are the

Table 8.6. Microbiology of Infective Endocarditis in Tertiary Centers	
Organism	Incidence (%)
Staphylococci	
S. aureus	31.6
Coagulase-negative	10.5
Streptococci	
Viridans	18.0
Enterococci	10.6
S. bovis	6.5
Other streptococci	5.1
Other organisms (e.g., gram-negative bacteria, fungi)	8.7
Culture negative or polymicrobial	~9.4

Derived from Fowler VG Jr, Miro JM, Hoen B, et al. *Staphylococcus aureus* endocarditis: a consequence of medical progress. *JAMA.* 2005; 293:3012–3021.

most frequent. It is important to recognize that in more rural communities with a low prevalence of intravenous drug abuse, the percentage of viridans streptococcal infections tends to be greater than that of *S. aureus.*

Once organisms adhere to the injured surface, they may be protected from phagocytic activity by the overlying fibrin. The organisms are then free to multiply, which enlarges the infected vegetation. The latter provides a source for continuous bacteremia and can lead to several complications, including (1) mechanical cardiac injury, (2) thrombotic or septic emboli, and (3) immune injury mediated by antigen–antibody deposition. For example, local extension of the infection within the heart can result in progressive valvular damage, abscess formation, or erosion into the cardiac conduction system. Portions of a vegetation may embolize systemically, often to the central nervous system, kidneys, or spleen, and incite infection or infarction of the target organs. Each of these is a potentially fatal complication. Additionally, immune complex deposition can result in glomerulonephritis, arthritis, or vasculitis.

The epidemiology of IE has evolved in recent decades, as bacteria resistant to antibiotics have become ubiquitous in the hospital setting and have spread into the community. Antibiotic resistant strains such as methicillin-resistant *S. aureus* and vancomycin-resistant enterococci

have become more common and are associated with increased mortality rates from IE.

Clinical Manifestations

A patient with *acute* IE is likely to report an explosive and rapidly progressive illness with high fever and shaking chills. In contrast, *subacute* IE presents less dramatically with low-grade fever often accompanied by nonspecific constitutional symptoms such as fatigue, anorexia, weakness, myalgia, and night sweats. These symptoms are not specific for IE and could easily be mistaken for influenza or an upper respiratory tract infection. Thus, the diagnosis of subacute IE requires a high index of suspicion. A history of a valvular lesion or other condition known to predispose to endocarditis is helpful. A thorough history should also inquire about intravenous drug use, recent dental procedures, or other potential sources of bacteremia.

Cardiac examination may reveal a murmur representing the underlying valvular pathology that predisposed the patient to IE, or a *new* murmur of valvular insufficiency owing to IE-induced damage. The development of right-sided valvular lesions (e.g., tricuspid regurgitation), although rare in normal hosts, is particularly common in endocarditis associated with intravenous drug abuse. Serial examination in ABE may be especially useful because changes in a particular murmur (i.e., worsening regurgitation) over time may correspond with rapidly progressive valvular damage. During the course of endocarditis, severe valvular damage may result in signs of heart failure.

Other physical findings that may appear in IE are those associated with septic embolism or immune complex deposition. Central nervous system emboli are seen in up to 40% of patients, often resulting in new neurologic findings on physical examination. Injury to the kidneys, of embolic or immunologic origin, may manifest as flank pain, hematuria, or renal failure. Lung infarction (septic pulmonary embolism) or infection (pneumonia) is particularly common in endocarditis that involves the right-sided valves.

Embolic infarction and seeding of the vasa vasorum of arteries can cause localized aneurysm formation (termed a *mycotic aneurysm*) that weakens the vessel wall and may rupture. Mycotic aneurysms may be found in the aorta, viscera, or peripheral organs, and are particularly dangerous in cerebral vessels, because rupture there can result in fatal intracranial hemorrhage.

Skin findings resulting from septic embolism or immune complex vasculitis are often collectively referred to as *peripheral stigmata* of endocarditis. For example, petechiae may appear as tiny, circular, red-brown discolorations on mucosal surfaces or skin. *Splinter hemorrhages*, the result of subungual microemboli, are small, longitudinal hemorrhages found beneath nails. Other peripheral stigmata of IE, which are now rarely encountered, include painless, flat, irregular discolorations found on the palms and soles called *Janeway lesions*; tender, pea-sized, erythematous nodules found primarily in the pulp space of the fingers and toes termed *Osler nodes*; and

emboli to the retina that produce *Roth spots*, microinfarctions that appear as white dots surrounded by hemorrhage.

The systemic inflammatory response produced by the infection is responsible for fever and splenomegaly as well as for a number of laboratory findings, including an elevated white blood cell count with a leftward shift (increase in proportion of neutrophils and immature granulocytes), an elevated erythrocyte sedimentation rate or C-reactive protein level, and in approximately 50% of cases, an elevated serum rheumatoid factor.

The *electrocardiogram* may help identify extension of the infection into the cardiac conduction system, manifest by various degrees of heart block or new arrhythmias. *Echocardiography* is used to visualize vegetations, valvular dysfunction, and associated abscess formation. Echocardiographic assessment can consist of transthoracic echocardiography (TTE)

Table 8.7. Modified Duke Criteria for Diagnosis of Infective Endocarditis (IE)[a]

Major Criteria	Minor Criteria

I. Positive blood culture, defined as either A or B
  A. Typical microorganism for IE from two separate blood cultures
    1. Streptococci viridans, *S. bovis,* HACEK group; or
    2. *Staphylococcus aureus* or enterococci, in the absence of a primary focus
  B. Microorganisms consistent with IE from persistently positive blood cultures
    1. Blood cultures drawn >12 hours apart, or
    2. All of three, or most of four separate cultures drawn at least 1 hour apart
    3. Single positive blood culture for *Coxiella burnetii* or antiphase I IgG antibody titer >1:800
II. Evidence of endocardial involvement, defined as A or B
  A. Echocardiogram positive for endocarditis:
    1. Oscillating intracardiac mass, or
    2. Myocardial abscess, or
    3. New partial detachment of prosthetic valve
  B. New valvular regurgitation
	Predisposing cardiac condition or intravenous drug use
	Fever (≥38.0°C)
	Vascular phenomena (septic arterial or pulmonary emboli, mycotic aneurysm, intracranial hemorrhage, conjunctival hemorrhage, Janeway lesions)
	Immunologic phenomena (glomerulonephritis, Osler nodes, Roth spots, rheumatoid factor)
	Positive blood cultures not meeting major criteria or serologic evidence of infection with organism consistent with IE

[a]Clinical diagnosis of definitive endocarditis requires two major criteria, one major plus three minor criteria, or five minor criteria.
HACEK, *Haemophilus* spp., *Actinobacillus actinomycetemcomitans, Cardiobacterium hominis, Eikenella* spp. and *Kingella kingae.*
Derived from Li JS, Sexton DJ, Mick N, et al. Proposed modifications to the Duke criteria for the diagnosis of infective endocarditis. *Clin Infect Dis.* 2000;30:633–638.

or transesophageal echocardiography (TEE), as described in Chapter 3. TTE is useful in detecting large vegetations and has the advantage of being noninvasive and easy to obtain. However, while the *specificity* of TTE for vegetations is high, the *sensitivity* for finding vegetations is less than 60%. TEE, on the other hand, is much more sensitive (>90%) for the detection of small vegetations and can be particularly useful for the evaluation of infection involving prosthetic valves.

Central to the diagnosis and appropriate treatment of endocarditis is the identification of the responsible microorganism by blood culture. Once positive culture results are obtained, treatment can be tailored to the causative organism according to its antibiotic sensitivities. A specific etiologic agent will be identified approximately 95% of the time. However, blood cultures may fail to grow the responsible organism if antibiotics have already been administered or if the organism has unusual growth requirements.

Even after a careful history, examination, and evaluation of laboratory data, the diagnosis of IE can be elusive. Therefore, attempts have been made to standardize the diagnosis, resulting in the now widely used Duke criteria (Table 8.7). By this standard, the diagnosis of endocarditis rests on the presence of either two major criteria, one major and three minor criteria, or five minor criteria.

Treatment of endocarditis entails 4 to 6 weeks of high-dose intravenous antibiotic therapy. Although empiric broad-spectrum antibiotics may be used initially (after blood cultures are obtained) in patients who are severely ill or hemodynamically unstable, specific, directed therapy is preferable once the causative microorganism has been identified. Surgical intervention, usually with valve replacement, is indicated for patients with persistent bacteremia despite appropriate antibiotic therapy, for those with severe valvular dysfunction leading to heart failure, and for individuals who develop myocardial abscesses or experience recurrent thromboembolic events.

An additional essential concept is *prevention* of endocarditis by administering antibiotics to certain susceptible individuals before invasive procedures that are likely to result in bacteremia. Recently, the American Heart Association issued major changes in the recommendations for such prevention. According to the newest guidelines, antibiotic prophylaxis is indicated only for individuals with cardiac conditions that place them at the highest risk for developing an adverse outcome from IE (Table 8.8). Furthermore, the types of procedures requiring prophylactic treatment have been updated and simplified (Table 8.9).

Table 8.8. Cardiac Conditions for Which Antibiotic Prophylaxis is Reasonable[a]

1. Presence of a prosthetic heart valve, or prior valve repair with prosthetic material
2. Prior history of endocarditis
3. Certain congenital heart diseases (CHD)
   - Unrepaired cyanotic CHD (described in Chapter 16)
   - Completely repaired congenital heart defects with prosthetic material, during the first 6 months after the procedure (i.e., prior to protective endothelialization)
   - Repaired CHD with residual defects adjacent to the site of prosthetic material (which inhibits endothelialization)
4. Cardiac transplant recipients who develop cardiac valve abnormalities

[a]The conditions on this list have the highest risk of adverse outcomes from endocarditis. Note that antimicrobial prophylaxis is no longer recommended for patients with bicuspid aortic valve, acquired aortic or mitral valve disease, or hypertrophic cardiomyopathy.

Derived from Wilson W, et al. Prevention of infective endocarditis: guidelines from the American Heart Association: a guideline from the American Heart Association Rheumatic Cardiovascular Disease in the Young, and the Council on Clinical Cardiology, Council on Cardiovascular Surgery and Anesthesia, and the Quality of Care and Outcomes Research Interdisciplinary Working Group. *Circulation.* 2007;116:1736–1754.

Table 8.9. Procedures That Warrant Endocarditis Prophylaxis for Patients in Table 8.8

1. Dental procedures that involve manipulation of gingival tissue, periapical region of teeth, or perforation of the oral mucosa
2. Upper respiratory tract procedures, *only if* involves incision or biopsy of mucosa (e.g., tonsillectomy, bronchoscopy with biopsy)
3. Genitourinary or gastrointestinal procedures, *only if* infections of those systems are present
4. Procedures on *infected* skin, skin structures, or musculoskeletal tissue

Table 8.10. Summary of Major Valvular Conditions

Valve Lesion	Causes	Symptoms	Physical Findings	Murmur Diagram
Mitral stenosis (MS)	Sequelae of rheumatic fever	Symptoms of left-sided (and later right-sided) heart failure[a]	• Loud S_1 (in early MS) • Opening snap • Diastolic rumble (loudest in left lateral decubitus position)	S_1 ... S_2 OS
Mitral regurgitation (MR)	*Acute:* • Endocarditis • Ruptured chordae • Papillary muscle dysfunction *Chronic:* • Rheumatic • Mitral prolapse • Calcified annulus • LV dilatation	*Acute:* • Pulmonary edema *Chronic:* • Symptoms of left-sided heart failure[a] and low cardiac output (e.g., fatigue)	• Holosystolic murmur at apex (may be decrescendo in *acute* MR) • Murmur accentuated by clenching the fists	S_1 S_2
Aortic stenosis (AS)	• Degenerative calcific • Congenital • Rheumatic	• Chest pain • Syncope • Dyspnea on exertion	• *Carotids:* delayed upstroke and decreased volume • *Palpation:* suprasternal thrill • *Auscultation:* Soft A_2 Systolic ejection-type murmur (loudest at upper-right sternal border)	S_1 S_2
Aortic regurgitation (AR)	• Congenital (e.g., bicuspid valve) • Endocarditis • Rheumatic • Aortic root dilatation	• Dyspnea on exertion • Chest pain (sometimes)	• Wide pulse pressure • Bounding pulses • Early diastolic decrescendo murmur (heard best at end expiration, with patient leaning forward)	S_1 S_2

[a]Symptoms of left-sided heart failure include exertional dyspnea, orthopnea, paroxysmal nocturnal dyspnea; symptoms of right-sided heart failure include peripheral edema, abdominal bloating, and right upper quadrant tenderness (hepatic enlargement).

A_2, aortic component of second heart sound; LV, left ventricular; S_1, first heart sound; S_2, second heart sound.

SUMMARY

Valvular heart disease can be a significant source of disability and mortality. From simple bedside observations to complex hemodynamic measurements, much has been learned about the pathophysiology of these conditions. A summary of the important findings associated with major valve lesions is presented in Table 8.10.

Acknowledgments

Contributors to the previous editions of this chapter were Mia M. Edwards, MD; Edward Chan, MD; Elia Duh, MD; Stephen K. Frankel, MD; Brian Stidham, MD; Patrick Yachimski, MD; John A. Bittl, MD; and Leonard S. Lilly, MD.

Additional Reading

Bonow RO, Carabello BA, Chatterjee K, et al. 2008 Focused update incorporated into the ACC/AHA 2006 guidelines for the management of patients with valvular heart disease: a report of the American College of Cardiology/American Heart Association Task Force on Practice Guidelines. *Circulation.* 2008;118:e523–e661.

Cawley PJ, Maki JH, Otto CM. Cardiovascular magnetic resonance imaging for valvular heart disease. *Circulation.* 2009;119:468–478.

Gerber MA, Baltimore RS, Eaton CB, et al. Prevention of rheumatic fever and diagnosis and treatment of acute streptococcal pharyngitis. *Circulation.* 2009;119:1541–1551.

Habib G, Hoen B, Tomos P, et al. Guidelines on the prevention, diagnosis, and treatment of infective endocarditis (new version 2009); The Task Force on the Prevention, Diagnosis, and Treatment of Infective Endocarditis of the European Society of Cardiology. *Eur Heart J.* 2009;30:2369–2413.

Murdoch DR, Corey GR, Hoen B, et al. Clinical presentation, etiology, and outcome of infective endocarditis in the 21st century. *Arch Intern Med.* 2009;169:463–473.

Nishimura RA, Carabello BA, Faxon DP, et al. ACC/AHA 2008 guideline update on valvular heart disease: focused update on infective endocarditis: a report of the American College of Cardiology/American Heart Association Task Force on Practice Guidelines: endorsed by the Society of Cardiovascular Anesthesiologists, Society for Cardiovascular Angiography and Interventions, and Society of Thoracic Surgeons. *Circulation.* 2008; 118:887–896.

O'Gara P, Braunwald E. Valvular heart disease. In: Fauci AS, Braunwald E, Kasper DL, et al. *Harrison's Principles of Internal Medicine.* 17th ed. New York: McGraw-Hill; 2008:1465–1480.

Stassano P, Di Tommaso L, Monaco M, et al. Aortic valve replacement: a prospective randomized evaluation of mechanical versus biological valves in patients 55 to 70 years. *J Am Coll Cardiol.* 2009;54:1862–1868.

Stout KK, Verrier ED. Acute valvular regurgitation. *Circulation.* 2009;119:3232–3241.

Verma S, Mesana TG. Mitral-valve repair for mitral-valve prolapse. *N England J Med.* 2009;361: 2261–2269.

Weisse AB. The surgical treatment of mitral stenosis: the first heart operation. *Am J Cardiol.* 2009; 103: 143–147.

Wilson W, Taubert KA, Gewitz M, et al. Prevention of infective endocarditis: guidelines from the American Heart Association: a guideline from the American Heart Association Rheumatic Fever, Endocarditis, and Kawasaki Disease Committee, Council on Cardiovascular Disease in the Young, and the Council on Clinical Cardiology, Council on Cardiovascular Surgery and Anesthesia, and the Quality of Care and Outcomes Research Interdisciplinary Working Group. *Circulation.* 2007;116:1736–1754.

Heart Failure

Neal Anjan Chatterjee
Michael A. Fifer

The heart normally accepts blood at low filling pressures during diastole and then propels it forward at higher pressures in systole. Heart failure is present when *the heart is unable to pump blood forward at a sufficient rate to meet the metabolic demands of the body* (forward failure), *or is able to do so only if the cardiac filling pressures are abnormally high* (backward failure), *or both.* Although conditions outside the heart may cause this definition to be met through inadequate tissue perfusion (e.g.,

severe hemorrhage) or increased metabolic demands (e.g., hyperthyroidism), in this chapter, only *cardiac* causes of heart failure are considered.

Heart failure may be the final and most severe manifestation of nearly every form of cardiac disease, including coronary atherosclerosis, myocardial infarction, valvular diseases, hypertension, congenital heart disease, and the cardiomyopathies. More than 500,000 new cases are diagnosed each year in the United States, where the current prevalence is approximately 5 million. The number of patients with heart failure is increasing, not only because the population is aging, but also because of interventions that prolong survival after damaging cardiac insults such as myocardial infarction. As a result, heart failure now accounts for more than 12 million medical office visits annually and is the most common diagnosis of hospitalized patients aged 65 and older.

Heart failure most commonly results from conditions of impaired left ventricular function. Thus, this chapter begins by reviewing the physiology of normal myocardial contraction and relaxation.

PHYSIOLOGY

Experimental studies of isolated cardiac muscle segments have revealed several important principles that can be applied to the intact heart. As a muscle segment is stretched apart, the relation between its length and the tension it passively develops is curvilinear, reflecting its intrinsic elastic properties (Fig. 9.1A, lower curve). If the muscle is first passively stretched and then stimulated to contract while its ends are held at fixed positions (termed an *isometric* contraction), the total tension (the sum of active plus passive tension) generated by the fibers is proportional to the length of the muscle at the time of stimulation (see Fig. 9.1A, upper curve). That is, stretching the muscle before stimulation optimizes the overlap and interaction of myosin and actin filaments, increasing the number of cross bridges and the force of contraction. Stretching cardiac muscle fibers also increases the sensitivity of the myofilaments to calcium, which further augments force development.

This relationship between the initial fiber length and force development is of great importance in the intact heart: within a physiologic range, the larger the ventricular volume during diastole, the more the fibers are stretched before stimulation and the greater the force of the next contraction. This is the basis of the **Frank–Starling relationship**, the observation that ventricular output increases in relation to the **preload** (the stretch on the myocardial fibers before contraction).

A second observation from isolated muscle experiments arises when the fibers are not tethered at a fixed length but are allowed to shorten during stimulation against a fixed load (termed the **afterload**). In this situation (termed an *isotonic* contraction), the final length of the muscle at the end of contraction is determined by the magnitude of the load but is *independent* of the length of the muscle before stimulation (see Fig. 9.1B). That is, (1) the tension generated by the fiber is equal to the fixed load; (2) the greater the load opposing contraction, the less the muscle fiber can shorten; (3) if the fiber is stretched to a longer length before stimulation but the afterload is kept constant, the muscle will shorten a greater distance to attain the same final length at the end of contraction; and (4) the maximum tension that can be produced during isotonic contraction (i.e., using a load sufficiently great such that the muscle is just unable to shorten) is the same as the force produced by an isometric contraction at that initial fiber length.

This concept of afterload is also relevant to the intact heart: the pressure generated by the ventricle, and the size of the chamber at the end of each contraction depend on the load against which the ventricle contracts, but are independent of the stretch on the myocardial fibers before contraction.

A third key experimental observation relates to myocardial **contractility**, which accounts for changes in the force of contraction independent of the initial fiber length and afterload. Contractility reflects chemical and hormonal influences on cardiac contraction, such as exposure to catecholamines. When contractility is enhanced pharmacologically (e.g., by a norepinephrine infusion), the relation between initial fiber length and force developed during contraction is shifted upward (see Fig. 9.1C) such that a greater total tension develops with isometric contraction at any given preload. Similarly, when contractility is augmented and the cardiac muscle is allowed to shorten against a fixed afterload, the fiber contracts to a greater extent and achieves a shorter

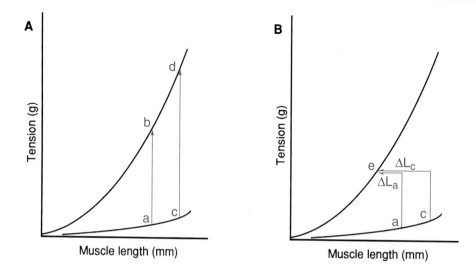

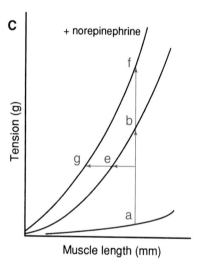

Figure 9.1. Physiology of normal cardiac muscle segments. A. Passive *(lower curve)* and total *(upper curve)* length–tension relations for isolated cat papillary muscle. Lines *ab* and *cd* represent the force developed during isometric contractions. Initial passive muscle length *c* is longer (i.e., has been stretched more) than length *a* and therefore has a greater passive tension. When the muscle segments are stimulated to contract, the muscle with the longer initial length generates greater total tension (point *d* vs. point *b*). **B.** If the muscle fiber preparation is allowed to shorten against a fixed load, the length at the end of the contraction is dependent on the load but not the initial fiber length; stimulation at point *a* or *c* results in the same final fiber length (*e*). Thus, the muscle that starts at length *c* shortens a greater distance (ΔL_c) than the muscle at length *a* (ΔL_a). **C.** The uppermost curve is the length–tension relation in the presence of the positive inotropic agent norepinephrine. For any given initial length, an isometric contraction in the presence of norepinephrine generates greater force (point *f*) than one in the absence of norepinephrine (point *b*). When contracting against a fixed load, the presence of norepinephrine causes greater muscle fiber shortening and a smaller final muscle length (point *g*) compared with contraction in the absence of the inotropic agent (point *e*). (Adapted from Downing SE, Sonnenblick EH. Cardiac muscle mechanics and ventricular performance: force and time parameters. *Am J Physiol.* 1964;207:705–715.)

final fiber length compared with the baseline state. At the molecular level, enhanced contractility is likely related to an increased cycling rate of actin–myosin cross-bridge formation.

Determinants of Contractile Function in the Intact Heart

In a healthy person, cardiac output is matched to the body's total metabolic need. Cardiac output (CO) is equal to the product of stroke volume (SV, the volume of blood ejected with each contraction) and the heart rate (HR):

$$CO = SV \times HR$$

The three major determinants of stroke volume are preload, afterload, and myocardial contractility, as shown in Figure 9.2.

Preload

The concept of preload (Table 9.1) in the intact heart was described by physiologists Frank and Starling a century ago. In experimental preparations, they showed that within physiologic limits, the more a normal ventricle is

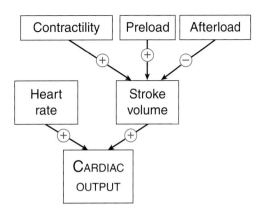

Figure 9.2. **Key mediators of cardiac output.** Determinants of the stroke volume include contractility, preload, and afterload. Cardiac output = Heart rate × Stroke volume.

distended (i.e., filled with blood) during diastole, the greater the volume that is ejected during the next systolic contraction. This relationship is illustrated graphically by the Frank–Starling curve, also known as the ventricular function curve (Fig. 9.3). The graph relates a measurement of cardiac performance (such as cardiac output or stroke volume) on the vertical axis as a function of preload on the horizontal axis. As described earlier, the

Table 9.1. Terms Related to Cardiac Performance	
Term	**Definition**
Preload	The ventricular wall tension at the end of diastole. In clinical terms, it is the stretch on the ventricular fibers just before contraction, often approximated by the end-diastolic volume or end-diastolic pressure.
Afterload	The ventricular wall tension during contraction; the resistance that must be overcome for the ventricle to eject its content. Often approximated by the systolic ventricular (or arterial) pressure.
Contractility (inotropic state)	Property of heart muscle that accounts for changes in the strength of contraction, independent of the preload and afterload. Reflects chemical or hormonal influences (e.g., catecholamines) on the force of contraction.
Stroke volume (SV)	Volume of blood ejected from the ventricle during systole. SV = End-diastolic volume − End-systolic volume.
Ejection fraction (EF)	The fraction of end-diastolic volume ejected from the ventricle during each systolic contraction (normal range = 55% to 75%). EF = Stroke volume ÷ End-diastolic volume.
Cardiac output (CO)	Volume of blood ejected from the ventricle per minute. CO = SV × Heart rate.
Compliance	Intrinsic property of a chamber that describes its pressure–volume relationship during filling. Reflects the ease or difficulty with which the chamber can be filled. Strict definition: Compliance = Δ Volume ÷ Δ Pressure.

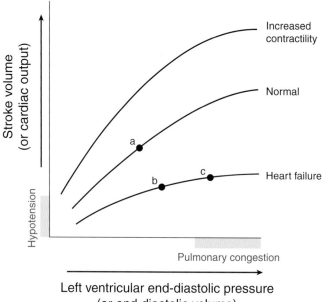

Figure 9.3. Left ventricular (LV) performance (Frank–Starling) curves relate preload, measured as LV end-diastolic volume (EDV) or pressure (EDP), to cardiac performance, measured as ventricular stroke volume or cardiac output. On the curve of a normal heart *(middle line)*, cardiac performance continuously increases as a function of preload. States of increased contractility (e.g., norepinephrine infusion) are characterized by an augmented stroke volume at any level of preload *(upper line)*. Conversely, decreased LV contractility (commonly associated with heart failure) is characterized by a curve that is shifted downward *(lower line)*. Point *a* is an example of a normal person at rest. Point *b* represents the same person after developing systolic dysfunction and heart failure (e.g., after a large myocardial infarction): stroke volume has fallen, and the decreased LV emptying results in elevation of the EDV. Because point *b* is on the ascending portion of the curve, the elevated EDV serves a compensatory role because it results in an increase in subsequent stroke volume, albeit much less than if operating on the normal curve. Further augmentation of LV filling (e.g., increased circulating volume) in the heart failure patient is represented by point *c*, which resides on the relatively flat part of the curve: stroke volume is only slightly augmented, but the significantly increased EDP results in pulmonary congestion.

preload can be thought of as the amount of myocardial stretch at the end of diastole, just before contraction. Measurements that correlate with myocardial stretch, and that are often used to indicate the preload on the horizontal axis, are the ventricular end-diastolic volume (EDV) or end-diastolic pressure (EDP). Conditions that decrease intravascular volume, and thereby reduce ventricular preload (e.g., dehydration or severe hemorrhage), result in a smaller EDV and hence a reduced stroke volume during contraction. Conversely, an increased volume within the left ventricle during diastole (e.g., a large intravenous fluid infusion) results in a greater-than-normal stroke volume.

Afterload

Afterload (see Table 9.1) in the intact heart reflects the resistance that the ventricle must overcome to empty its contents. It is more formally defined as the ventricular wall stress that develops during systolic ejection. Wall stress (σ), like pressure, is expressed as force per unit area, and for the left ventricle, may be estimated from Laplace's relationship:

$$\sigma = \frac{P \times r}{2h}$$

where P is ventricular pressure, r is ventricular chamber radius, and h is ventricular wall thickness. Thus, ventricular wall stress rises in response to a higher pressure load (e.g., hypertension) or an increased chamber size (e.g., a dilated left ventricle). Conversely, as would be expected from LaPlace's relationship, an increase in wall thickness (h) serves a compensatory role in *reducing* wall stress, because the force is distributed over a greater mass per unit surface area of ventricular muscle.

Contractility (also termed "Inotropic State")

In the intact heart, as in the isolated muscle preparation, contractility accounts for changes in myocardial force for a given set of preload and afterload conditions, resulting from chemical and hormonal influences. By relating a measure of ventricular performance (stroke volume or cardiac output) to preload (left ventricular end-diastolic pressure or volume), each Frank–Starling curve is a reflection of the heart's current inotropic state (see Fig. 9.3). The effect on stroke volume by an alteration in preload is reflected by a change in position along a particular Frank–Starling curve. Conversely, a change in contractility actually shifts the entire curve in an upward or downward direction. Thus, when contractility is enhanced pharmacologically (e.g., by an infusion of norepinephrine), the ventricular performance curve is displaced upward such that at any given preload, the stroke volume is increased. Conversely, when a drug that reduces contractility is administered, or the ventricle's contractile function is impaired (as in certain types of heart failure), the curve shifts in a downward direction, leading to reductions in stroke volume and cardiac output at any given preload.

Pressure–Volume Loops

Another useful graphic display to illustrate the determinants of cardiac function is the

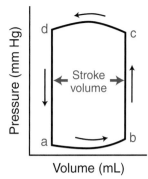

Figure 9.4. **Example of a normal left ventricular (LV) pressure–volume loop.** At point *a*, the mitral valve opens. During diastolic filling of the LV (line *ab*), the volume increases in association with a gradual rise in pressure. When ventricular contraction commences and its pressure exceeds that of the left atrium, the mitral valve (MV) closes (point *b*) and isovolumetric contraction of the LV ensues (the aortic valve is not yet open, and no blood leaves the chamber), as shown by line *bc*. When LV pressure rises to that in the aorta, the aortic valve (AV) opens (point *c*) and ejection begins. The volume within the LV declines during ejection (line *cd*), but LV pressure continues to rise until ventricular relaxation commences, then it begins to lessen. At point *d*, the LV pressure during relaxation falls below that in the aorta, and the AV closes, leading to isovolumetric relaxation (line *da*). As the LV pressure falls further, the mitral valve reopens (point *a*). Point *b* represents the end-diastolic volume (EDV) and pressure, and point *d* is the end-systolic volume (ESV) and pressure. Stroke volume is the difference between the EDV and ESV.

ventricular pressure–volume loop, which relates changes in ventricular volume to corresponding changes in pressure throughout the cardiac cycle (Fig. 9.4). In the left ventricle, filling of the chamber begins after the mitral valve opens in early diastole (point *a*). The curve between points *a* and *b* represents diastolic filling. As the volume increases during diastole, it is associated with a small rise in pressure, in accordance with the passive length–tension properties or **compliance** (see

Table 9.1) of the myocardium, analogous to the lower curve in Figure 9.1A for an isolated muscle preparation.

Next, the onset of left ventricular systolic contraction causes the ventricular pressure to rise. When the pressure in the left ventricle (LV) exceeds that of the left atrium (point *b*), the mitral valve is forced to close. As the pressure continues to increase, the ventricular volume does not immediately change, because the aortic valve has not yet opened; therefore, this phase is called **isovolumetric contraction.** When the rise in ventricular pressure reaches the aortic diastolic pressure, the aortic valve is forced to open (point *c*) and ejection of blood into the aorta commences. During ejection, the volume within the ventricle decreases, but its pressure continues to rise until ventricular relaxation begins. The pressure against which the ventricle ejects (afterload) is represented by the curve *cd*. Ejection ends during the relaxation phase, when the ventricular pressure falls below that of the aorta and the aortic valve closes (point *d*).

As the ventricle continues to relax, its pressure declines while its volume remains constant because the mitral valve has not yet opened (this phase is known as **isovolumetric relaxation**). When the ventricular pressure falls below that of the left atrium, the mitral valve opens again (point *a*) and the cycle repeats.

Note that point *b* represents the pressure and volume at the end of diastole, whereas point *d* represents the pressure and volume at the end of systole. The difference between the EDV and end-systolic volume (ESV) represents the quantity of blood ejected during contraction (i.e., the stroke volume).

Changes in any of the determinants of cardiac function are reflected by alterations in the pressure–volume loop. By analyzing the effects of a change in an individual parameter (preload, afterload, or contractility) on the pressure–volume relationship, the resulting modifications in ventricular pressure and stroke volume can be predicted (Fig. 9.5).

Alterations in Preload

If afterload and contractility are held constant but preload is caused to increase (e.g.,

by administration of intravenous fluid), left ventricular EDV rises. This increase in preload augments the stroke volume via the Frank–Starling mechanism such that the ESV achieved is the same as it was before increasing the preload. This means that the normal left ventricle is able to adjust its stroke volume and effectively empty its contents to match its diastolic filling volume, as long as contractility and afterload are kept constant.

Although end-diastolic volume and end-diastolic pressure are often used interchangeably as markers of preload, the relationship between filling volume and pressure (i.e., ventricular compliance; see Table 9.1) largely governs the extent of ventricular filling. If ventricular compliance is reduced (e.g., in severe LV hypertrophy), the slope of the diastolic filling curve (segment *ab* in Fig. 9.4) becomes steeper. A "stiff" or poorly compliant ventricle reduces the ability of the chamber to fill during diastole, resulting in a lower-than-normal ventricular end-diastolic volume. In this circumstance, the stroke volume will be reduced while the end-systolic volume remains unchanged.

Alterations in Afterload

If preload and contractility are held constant and afterload is augmented (e.g., in high-impedance states such as hypertension or aortic stenosis), the pressure generated by the left ventricle during ejection increases. In this situation, more ventricular work is expended in overcoming the resistance to ejection and less fiber shortening takes place. As shown in Figure 9.5B, an increase in afterload results in a higher ventricular systolic pressure and a greater-than-normal LV end-systolic volume. Thus, in the setting of increased afterload, the ventricular stroke volume (EDV–ESV) is reduced.

The dependence of the end-systolic volume on afterload is approximately linear: the greater the afterload, the higher the end-systolic volume. This relationship is depicted in Figure 9.5 as the **end-systolic pressure–volume relation (ESPVR)** and is analogous to the total tension curve in the isolated muscle experiments described earlier.

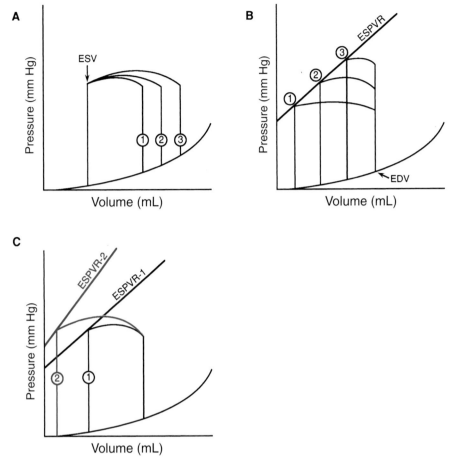

Figure 9.5. **The effect of varying preload, afterload, and contractility on the pressure–volume loop.**
A. When arterial pressure (afterload) and contractility are held constant, sequential increases (lines 1, 2, and 3) in preload (measured in this case as end-diastolic volume [EDV]) are associated with loops that have progressively higher stroke volumes but a constant end-systolic volume (ESV). **B.** When the preload (EDV) and contractility are held constant, sequential increases (points 1, 2, and 3) in arterial pressure (afterload) are associated with loops that have progressively lower stroke volumes and higher end-systolic volume end-systolic volume. There is a nearly linear relationship between the afterload and ESV, termed the end-systolic pressure–volume relation (ESPVR). **C.** A positive inotropic intervention shifts the end-systolic pressure–volume relation upward and leftward from ESPVR-1 to ESPVR-2, resulting in loop 2, which has a larger stroke volume and a smaller end-systolic volume than the original loop 1.

Alterations in Contractility

The slope of the ESPVR line on the pressure-volume loop graph is a function of cardiac contractility. In conditions of increased contractility, the ESPVR slope becomes steeper; that is, it shifts upward and toward the left. Hence, at any given preload or afterload, the ventricle empties more completely (the stroke volume increases) and results in a smaller-than-normal end-systolic volume (see Fig. 9.5C). Conversely, in situations of reduced contractility, the ESPVR line shifts downward, consistent with a decline in stroke volume and a higher end-systolic volume. Thus, the end-systolic volume is *dependent* on the afterload against which the ventricle contracts and the inotropic state, but is *independent* of the end-diastolic volume prior to contraction.

The important physiologic concepts in this section are summarized here:

1. Ventricular stroke volume is a function of preload, afterload, and contractility. SV

rises when there is an increase in preload, a decrease in afterload, or augmented contractility.

2. Ventricular end-diastolic volume (or end-diastolic pressure) is used as a representation of preload. The end-diastolic volume is influenced by the chamber's compliance.

3. Ventricular end-systolic volume depends on the afterload and contractility but not on the preload.

PATHOPHYSIOLOGY

Chronic heart failure may result from a wide variety of cardiovascular insults. The etiologies can be grouped into those that (1) impair ventricular contractility, (2) increase afterload, or (3) impair ventricular relaxation and filling (Fig. 9.6). Heart failure that results from an abnormality of ventricular emptying (due to impaired contractility or

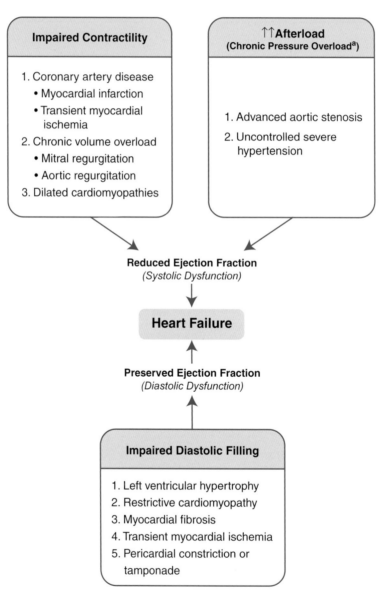

Figure 9.6. **Conditions that cause left-sided heart failure through impairment of ventricular systolic or diastolic function.** [a]Note that in chronic stable stages the conditions in this box may instead result in heart failure with *preserved* EF, due to compensatory ventricular hypertrophy and increased diastolic stiffness (diastolic dysfunction).

greatly excessive afterload) is termed *systolic dysfunction*, whereas heart failure caused by abnormalities of diastolic relaxation or ventricular filling is termed *diastolic dysfunction*. However, there is much overlap, and many patients demonstrate both systolic and diastolic abnormalities. As a result, it is now common to categorize heart failure patients into two general categories, based on the left ventricular ejection fraction (EF), a measure of cardiac performance (see Table 9.1): (1) **heart failure with reduced EF** (i.e., primarily systolic dysfunction) and (2) **heart failure with preserved EF** (i.e., primarily diastolic dysfunction). In the United States, approximately one half of patients with heart failure fall into each of these categories.

Heart Failure with Reduced EF

In states of systolic dysfunction, the affected ventricle has a diminished capacity to eject blood because of impaired myocardial contractility or pressure overload (i.e., excessive afterload). Loss of contractility may result from destruction of myocytes, abnormal myocyte function, or fibrosis. Pressure overload impairs ventricular ejection by significantly increasing resistance to flow.

Figure 9.7A depicts the effects of systolic dysfunction due to impaired contractility on the pressure–volume loop. The ESPVR is shifted downward such that systolic emptying ceases at a higher-than-normal end-systolic volume. As a result, the stroke volume falls. When normal pulmonary venous return is added to the increased end-systolic volume that has remained in the ventricle because of incomplete emptying, the diastolic chamber volume increases, resulting in a higher-than-normal end-diastolic volume and pressure. While that increase in preload induces a compensatory rise in stroke volume (via the Frank–Starling mechanism), impaired contractility and the reduced ejection fraction cause the end-systolic volume to remain elevated.

During diastole, the persistently elevated LV pressure is transmitted to the left atrium (through the open mitral valve) and to the pulmonary veins and capillaries. An elevated pulmonary capillary hydrostatic pressure, when sufficiently high (usually >20 mm Hg), results in the transudation of fluid into the pulmonary

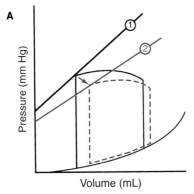 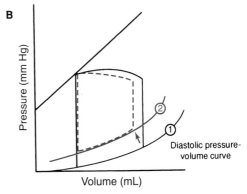

Figure 9.7. The pressure–volume loop in systolic and diastolic dysfunction. A. The normal pressure–volume loop *(solid line)* is compared with one demonstrating systolic dysfunction *(dashed line)*. In systolic dysfunction caused by decreased cardiac contractility, the end-systolic pressure–volume relation is shifted downward and rightward (from line 1 to line 2). As a result, the end-systolic volume (ESV) is increased *(arrow)*. As normal venous return is added to that greater-than-normal ESV, there is an obligatory increase in the end-diastolic volume (EDV) and pressure (preload), which serves a compensatory function by partially elevating stroke volume toward normal via the Frank–Starling mechanism. **B.** The pressure–volume loop of diastolic dysfunction resulting from increased stiffness of the ventricle *(dashed line)*. The passive diastolic pressure–volume curve is shifted upward (from line 1 to line 2) such that at any diastolic volume, the ventricular pressure is higher than normal. The result is a decreased EDV *(arrow)* because of reduced filling of the stiffened ventricle at a higher-than-normal end-diastolic pressure.

interstitium and symptoms of pulmonary congestion.

Heart Failure with Preserved EF

Patients who exhibit heart failure with preserved EF frequently demonstrate abnormalities of ventricular diastolic function: either impaired early diastolic relaxation (an active, energy-dependent process), increased stiffness of the ventricular wall (a passive property), or both. Acute myocardial ischemia is an example of a condition that *transiently* inhibits energy delivery and diastolic relaxation. Conversely, left ventricular hypertrophy, fibrosis, or restrictive cardiomyopathy (see Chapter 10) causes the LV walls to become *chronically* stiffened. Certain pericardial diseases (cardiac tamponade and pericardial constriction, as described in Chapter 14) present an external force that limits ventricular filling and represent potentially reversible forms of diastolic dysfunction. The effect of impaired diastolic function is reflected in the pressure–volume loop (see Fig. 9.7B): in diastole, filling of the ventricle occurs at higher-than-normal pressures because the lower part of the loop is shifted upward as a result of reduced chamber compliance. Patients with diastolic dysfunction often manifest signs of vascular congestion because the elevated diastolic pressure is transmitted retrograde to the pulmonary and systemic veins.

Right-Sided Heart Failure

Whereas the physiologic principles mentioned above may be applied to both right-sided and left-sided heart failure, there are distinct differences in function between the two ventricles. Compared with the left ventricle, the right ventricle (RV) is a thin-walled, highly compliant chamber that accepts its blood volume at low pressures and ejects against a low pulmonary vascular resistance. As a result of its high compliance, the RV has little difficulty accepting a wide range of filling volumes without significant changes in its filling pressures. Conversely, the RV is quite susceptible to failure in situations that present a sudden increase in afterload, such as acute pulmonary embolism.

Table 9.2. Examples of Conditions That Cause Right-Sided Heart Failure
Cardiac causes
Left-sided heart failure
Pulmonic valve stenosis
Right ventricular infarction
Pulmonary parenchymal diseases
Chronic obstructive pulmonary disease
Interstitial lung disease (e.g., sarcoidosis)
Adult respiratory distress syndrome
Chronic lung infection or bronchiectasis
Pulmonary vascular diseases
Pulmonary embolism
Primary pulmonary hypertension

The most common cause of right-sided heart failure is actually the presence of left-sided heart failure (Table 9.2). In this situation, excessive afterload confronts the right ventricle because of the elevated pulmonary vascular pressures that result from LV dysfunction. *Isolated* right-heart failure is less common and usually reflects increased RV afterload owing to diseases of the lung parenchyma or pulmonary vasculature. Right-sided heart disease that results from a primary pulmonary process is known as *cor pulmonale*, which may lead to symptoms of right-heart failure.

When the right ventricle fails, the elevated diastolic pressure is transmitted retrograde to the right atrium with subsequent congestion of the systemic veins, accompanied by signs of right-sided heart failure as described below. Indirectly, isolated right-heart failure may also influence left-heart function: the decreased right ventricular output reduces blood return to the LV (i.e., diminished preload), causing left ventricular stroke volume to decline.

COMPENSATORY MECHANISMS

Several natural compensatory mechanisms are called into action in patients with heart failure that buffer the fall in cardiac output and help preserve sufficient blood pressure to perfuse vital organs. These compensations

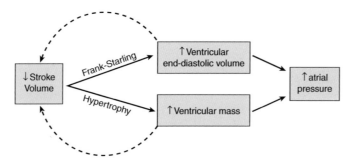

Figure 9.8. **Compensatory mechanisms in heart failure.** Both the Frank–Starling mechanism (which is invoked by the rise in ventricular end-diastolic volume) and myocardial hypertrophy (in response to pressure or volume overload) serve to maintain forward stroke volume *(dashed lines)*. However, the chronic rise in EDV by the former and increased ventricular stiffness by the latter passively augment atrial pressure, which may in turn result in clinical manifestations of heart failure (e.g., pulmonary congestion in the case of left-sided heart failure).

include (1) the Frank–Starling mechanism, (2) neurohormonal alterations, and (3) the development of ventricular hypertrophy and remodeling (Fig. 9.8).

Frank–Starling Mechanism

As shown in Figure 9.3, heart failure caused by impaired left ventricular contractile function causes a downward shift of the ventricular performance curve. Consequently, at a given preload, stroke volume is decreased compared with normal. The reduced stroke volume results in incomplete chamber emptying, so that the volume of blood that accumulates in the ventricle during diastole is higher than normal (see Fig. 9.3, point *b*). This increased stretch on the myofibers, acting via the Frank–Starling mechanism, induces a greater stroke volume on subsequent contraction, which helps to empty the enlarged left ventricle and preserve forward cardiac output (see Fig 9.8).

This beneficial compensatory mechanism has its limits, however. In the case of severe heart failure with marked depression of contractility, the curve may be nearly flat at higher diastolic volumes, reducing the augmentation of cardiac output achieved by the increased chamber filling. Concurrently in such a circumstance, marked elevation of the end-diastolic volume and pressure (which is transmitted retrograde to the left atrium,

pulmonary veins, and capillaries) may result in pulmonary congestion and edema (see Fig. 9.3, point *c*).

Neurohormonal Alterations

Several important neurohormonal compensatory mechanisms are activated in heart failure in response to the decreased cardiac output (Fig. 9.9). Three of the most important involve (1) the adrenergic nervous system, (2) the renin–angiotensin–aldosterone system, and (3) increased production of antidiuretic hormone (ADH). In part, these mechanisms serve to increase systemic vascular resistance, which helps to maintain arterial perfusion to vital organs, even in the setting of a reduced cardiac output. That is, because blood pressure (BP) is equal to the product of cardiac output (CO) and total peripheral resistance (TPR),

$$BP = CO \times TPR$$

a rise in TPR induced by these compensatory mechanisms can nearly balance the fall in CO and, in the early stages of heart failure, maintain fairly normal BP. In addition, neurohormonal activation results in salt and water retention, which in turn increases intravascular volume and left ventricular preload, maximizing stroke volume via the Frank–Starling mechanism.

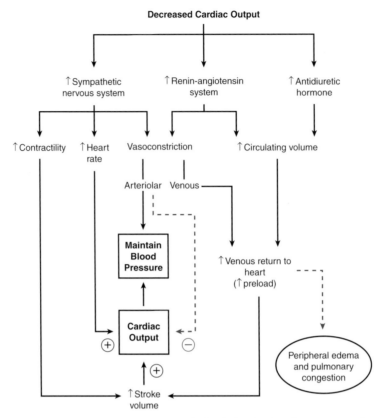

Figure 9.9. Compensatory neurohormonal stimulation develops in response to the reduced forward cardiac output and blood pressure of heart failure. Increased activity of the sympathetic nervous system, renin–angiotensin–aldosterone system, and antidiuretic hormone serve to support the cardiac output and blood pressure *(boxes)*. However, adverse consequences of these activations *(dashed lines)* include an increase in afterload from excessive vasoconstriction (which may then impede cardiac output) and excess fluid retention, which contributes to peripheral edema and pulmonary congestion.

Although the acute effects of neurohormonal stimulation are compensatory and beneficial, chronic activation of these mechanisms often ultimately proves deleterious to the failing heart and contributes to a progressive downhill course, as described later.

Adrenergic Nervous System

The fall in cardiac output in heart failure is sensed by baroreceptors in the carotid sinus and aortic arch. These receptors decrease their rate of firing in proportion to the fall in BP, and the signal is transmitted by the 9th and 10th cranial nerves to the cardiovascular control center in the medulla. As a result, sympathetic outflow to the heart and peripheral circulation is increased, and parasympathetic tone is diminished. There are three immediate consequences (see Fig. 9.9): (1) an increase in heart rate, (2) augmentation of ventricular contractility, and (3) vasoconstriction caused by stimulation of α-receptors on the systemic veins and arteries.

The increased heart rate and ventricular contractility directly augment cardiac output (see Fig. 9.2). Vasoconstriction of the venous and arterial circulations is also initially beneficial. *Venous* constriction augments blood return to the heart, which increases preload and raises stroke volume through the Frank–Starling mechanism, as long as the ventricle is operating on the ascending portion of its ventricular performance curve. *Arteriolar* constriction increases the peripheral vascular resistance and therefore helps to maintain blood pressure (BP = CO × TPR). The regional distribution of α-receptors is such that during sympathetic stimulation, blood flow is redistributed to vital organs (e.g., heart and brain) at the expense of the skin, splanchnic viscera, and kidneys.

Renin–Angiotensin–Aldosterone System

This system is also activated early in patients with heart failure (see Fig. 9.9), mediated by increased renin release. The main stimuli for renin secretion from the juxtaglomerular cells of the kidney in heart failure patients include (1) decreased renal artery perfusion pressure secondary to low cardiac output, (2) decreased salt delivery to the macula densa of the kidney owing to alterations in intrarenal hemodynamics, and (3) direct stimulation of juxtaglomerular β_2-receptors by the activated adrenergic nervous system.

Renin is an enzyme that cleaves circulating angiotensinogen to form angiotensin I, which is then rapidly cleaved by endothelial cell-bound angiotensin-converting enzyme (ACE) to form angiotensin II (AII), a potent vasoconstrictor (see Chapter 13). Increased AII constricts arterioles and raises total peripheral resistance, thereby serving to maintain systemic blood pressure. In addition, AII acts to increase intravascular volume by two mechanisms: (1) at the hypothalamus, it stimulates thirst and therefore water intake; and (2) at the adrenal cortex, it acts to increase aldosterone secretion. The latter hormone promotes sodium reabsorption from the distal convoluted tubule of the kidney into the circulation (see Chapter 17), serving to augment intravascular volume. The rise in intravascular volume increases left ventricular preload and thereby augments cardiac output via the Frank–Starling mechanism in patients on the ascending portion of the ventricular performance curve (see Fig. 9.3).

Antidiuretic Hormone

Secretion of this hormone (also termed *vasopressin*) by the posterior pituitary is increased in many patients with heart failure, presumably mediated through arterial baroreceptors, and

by increased levels of AII. ADH contributes to increased intravascular volume because it promotes water retention in the distal nephron. The increased intravascular volume serves to augment left ventricular preload and cardiac output. ADH also appears to contribute to systemic vasoconstriction.

Although each of these neurohormonal alterations in heart failure is *initially* beneficial, continued activation ultimately proves harmful. For example, the increased circulating volume and augmented venous return to the heart may *worsen* engorgement of the lung vasculature, exacerbating congestive pulmonary symptoms. Furthermore, the elevated arteriolar resistance increases the afterload against which the failing left ventricle contracts and may therefore *impair* stroke volume and reduce cardiac output (see Fig. 9.9). In addition, the increased heart rate augments metabolic demand and can therefore further reduce the performance of the failing heart. Continuous sympathetic activation results in downregulation of cardiac β-adrenergic receptors and upregulation of inhibitory G proteins, contributing to a decrease in the myocardium's sensitivity to circulating catecholamines and a *reduced* inotropic response.

Chronically elevated levels of AII and aldosterone have additional detrimental effects. They provoke the production of cytokines (small proteins that mediate cell–cell communication and immune responses), activate macrophages, and stimulate fibroblasts, resulting in fibrosis and adverse remodeling of the failing heart.

Because the undesired consequences of chronic neurohormonal activation eventually outweigh their benefits, much of today's pharmacologic therapy of heart failure is designed to moderate these "compensatory" mechanisms, as examined later in the chapter.

Natriuretic Peptides

In contrast to the ultimately adverse consequences of the neurohormonal alterations described in the previous section, the natriuretic peptides are natural "beneficial" hormones secreted in heart failure in response to increased intracardiac pressures. The best studied of these are atrial natriuretic peptide (ANP) and B-type natriuretic peptide (BNP). ANP is stored in atrial cells and is released in response to atrial distention. BNP is not detected in normal hearts but is produced when ventricular myocardium is subjected to hemodynamic stress (e.g., in heart failure or during myocardial infarction). Recent studies have shown a close relationship between serum BNP levels and the clinical severity of heart failure.

Actions of the natriuretic peptides are mediated by specific natriuretic receptors and are largely opposite to those of the other hormone systems activated in heart failure. They result in excretion of sodium and water, vasodilatation, inhibition of renin secretion, and antagonism of the effects of AII on aldosterone and vasopressin levels. Although these effects are beneficial to patients with heart failure, they are usually not sufficient to fully counteract the vasoconstriction and volume-retaining effects of the other activated hormonal systems.

Other Peptides

Among other peptides that are generated in heart failure is **endothelin-1**, a potent vasoconstrictor, derived from endothelial cells lining the vasculature (see Chapter 6). In patients with heart failure, the plasma concentration of endothelin-1 correlates with disease severity and adverse outcomes. Drugs designed to inhibit endothelin receptors (and therefore blunt adverse vasoconstriction) improve LV function in heart failure patients, but long-term clinical benefits have not been demonstrated.

Ventricular Hypertrophy and Remodeling

Ventricular hypertrophy and remodeling are important compensatory processes that develop over time in response to hemodynamic burdens. Wall stress (as defined earlier) is often increased in developing heart failure because of either LV dilatation (increased chamber radius) or the need to generate high systolic pressures to overcome excessive afterload (e.g., in aortic stenosis or hypertension). A sustained increase in wall stress (along with neurohormonal and cytokine alterations) stimulates the development of myocardial hypertrophy and deposition of extracellular matrix. This increased mass of muscle fibers serves as a compensatory mechanism that helps to maintain contractile force and *counteracts* the elevated ventricular wall stress (recall that wall thickness is in the denominator of the Laplace wall stress formula). However, because of the increased stiffness of the hypertrophied wall, these benefits come at the expense of higher-than-normal diastolic ventricular pressures, which are transmitted to the left atrium and pulmonary vasculature (see Fig. 9.8).

The pattern of compensatory hypertrophy and remodeling that develops depends on whether the ventricle is subjected to chronic volume or pressure overload. Chronic chamber dilatation owing to *volume* overload (e.g., chronic mitral or aortic regurgitation) results in the synthesis of new sarcomeres in *series* with the old, causing the myocytes to elongate. The radius of the ventricular chamber therefore enlarges, doing so in proportion to the increase in wall thickness, and is termed **eccentric hypertrophy**. Chronic *pressure* overload (e.g., caused by hypertension or aortic stenosis) results in the synthesis of new sarcomeres in *parallel* with the old (i.e., the myocytes thicken), termed **concentric hypertrophy**. In this situation, the wall thickness increases without proportional chamber dilatation, and wall stress may therefore be reduced substantially.

Such hypertrophy and remodeling help to reduce wall stress and maintain contractile force, but ultimately, ventricular function may decline, allowing the chamber to dilate out of proportion to wall thickness. When this occurs, the excessive hemodynamic burden on the contractile units produces a downward spiral of deterioration with progressive heart failure symptomatology.

MYOCYTE LOSS AND CELLULAR DYSFUNCTION

Impairment of ventricular function in heart failure may result from the actual loss of myocytes and/or impaired function of living myocytes. The loss of myocytes may result from cellular *necrosis* (e.g., from myocardial infarction or exposure to cardiotoxic drugs such as doxorubicin) or *apoptosis* (programmed cell death). In apoptosis, genetic instructions activate intracellular pathways that cause the cell to fragment and undergo phagocytosis by other cells, without an inflammatory response. Implicated triggers of apoptosis in heart failure include elevated catecholamines, AII, inflammatory cytokines, and mechanical strain on the myocytes owing to the augmented wall stress.

Even viable myocardium in heart failure is abnormal at the ultrastructural and molecular levels. Mechanical wall stress, neurohormonal activation, and inflammatory cytokines, such as tumor necrosis factor α (TNF-α), are believed to alter the genetic expression of contractile proteins, ion channels, catalytic enzymes, surface receptors, and secondary messengers in the myocyte. Experimental evidence has demonstrated such changes at the subcellular level that affect intracellular calcium handling by the sarcoplasmic reticulum, decrease the responsiveness of the myofilaments to calcium, impair excitation–contraction coupling, and alter cellular energy production. Cellular mechanisms currently considered the most important contributors to dysfunction in heart failure include: (1) a reduced cellular ability to maintain calcium homeostasis, and/or (2) changes in the production, availability, and utilization of high-energy phosphates. However, the exact subcellular alterations that result in heart failure have not yet been unraveled, and this area remains one of the most active in cardiovascular research.

PRECIPITATING FACTORS

Many patients with heart failure remain asymptomatic for extended periods either because the impairment is mild or because cardiac dysfunction is balanced by the compensatory mechanisms described earlier. Often clinical manifestations are precipitated by circumstances that increase the cardiac workload and tip the balanced state into one of decompensation.

Common precipitating factors are listed in Table 9.3. For example, conditions of increased metabolic demand such as fever or infection may not be matched by a sufficient increase in output by the failing heart, so that symptoms of cardiac

Table 9.3. Factors That May Precipitate Symptoms in Patients with Chronic Compensated Heart Failure

Increased metabolic demands
  Fever
  Infection
  Anemia
  Tachycardia
  Hyperthyroidism
  Pregnancy
Increased circulating volume (increased preload)
  Excessive sodium content in diet
  Excessive fluid administration
  Renal failure
Conditions that increase afterload
  Uncontrolled hypertension
  Pulmonary embolism (increased right ventricular afterload)
Conditions that impair contractility
  Negative inotropic medications
  Myocardial ischemia or infarction
  Excessive ethanol ingestion
Failure to take prescribed heart failure medications
Excessively slow heart rate

insufficiency are precipitated. Tachyarrhythmias precipitate heart failure by decreasing diastolic ventricular filling time and by increasing myocardial oxygen demand. Excessively *low* heart rates directly cause a drop in cardiac output (remember, cardiac output = stroke volume × heart rate). An increase in salt ingestion, renal dysfunction, or failure to take prescribed diuretic medications may increase the circulating volume, thus promoting systemic and pulmonary congestion. Uncontrolled hypertension depresses systolic function because of excessive afterload. A large pulmonary embolism results in both hypoxemia (and therefore decreased myocardial oxygen supply) and a substantial increase in right ventricular afterload. Ischemic insults (i.e., myocardial ischemia or infarction), ethanol ingestion, or negative inotropic medications (e.g., large doses of β-blockers and certain calcium channel blockers) can all depress myocardial contractility and precipitate symptoms in the otherwise compensated congestive heart failure patient.

CLINICAL MANIFESTATIONS

The clinical manifestations of heart failure result from impaired forward cardiac output and/or elevated venous pressures, and relate to the ventricle that has failed (Table 9.4). A patient may present with the chronic progressive symptoms of heart failure described here or, in certain cases, with sudden decompensation of left-sided heart function (e.g., acute pulmonary edema, as described later in the chapter).

Symptoms

The most prominent manifestation of chronic left ventricular failure is *dyspnea* (breathlessness) on exertion. Controversy regarding the cause of this symptom has centered on whether it results primarily from pulmonary venous congestion, or from decreased forward cardiac output. A pulmonary venous pressure that exceeds approximately 20 mm Hg leads to transudation of fluid into the pulmonary interstitium and congestion of the lung parenchyma. The resulting reduced pulmonary compliance increases the work of breathing to move the same volume of air. Moreover, the excess fluid in the interstitium compresses the walls of the bronchioles and alveoli, increasing the resistance to airflow and requiring greater effort of respiration. In addition, juxtacapillary receptors (J receptors) are stimulated and mediate rapid shallow breathing. The heart failure patient can also suffer from dyspnea even in the absence of pulmonary congestion, because reduced blood flow to overworked respiratory muscles and accumulation of lactic acid may also contribute to that sensation. Heart failure may initially cause dyspnea only on exertion, but more severe dysfunction results in symptoms at rest as well.

Other manifestations of low forward output in heart failure may include *dulled mental status* because of reduced cerebral perfusion and *impaired urine output* during the day because of decreased renal perfusion. The latter often gives way to increased urinary frequency at night (*nocturia*) when, while supine, blood flow is redistributed to the kidney, promoting renal perfusion and diuresis. Reduced skeletal muscle perfusion may result in *fatigue* and *weakness.*

Other congestive manifestations of heart failure include *orthopnea, paroxysmal nocturnal dyspnea (PND),* and *nocturnal cough.* Orthopnea is the sensation of labored breathing while lying flat and is relieved by sitting upright. It results from the redistribution of intravascular blood from the gravity-dependent portions of the body (abdomen and lower extremities) toward the lungs after lying down. The degree of orthopnea is generally assessed by the number of pillows on which the patient sleeps to avoid breathlessness. Sometimes, orthopnea is so significant that the patient may try to sleep upright in a chair.

PND is severe breathlessness that awakens the patient from sleep 2 to 3 hours after retiring to bed. This frightening symptom results from the gradual reabsorption into the circulation of

Table 9.4. Common Symptoms and Physical Findings in Heart Failure	
Symptoms	*Physical Findings*
Left-sided	
Dyspnea	Diaphoresis (sweating)
Orthopnea	Tachycardia, tachypnea
Paroxysmal nocturnal dyspnea	Pulmonary rales
Fatigue	Loud P_2
	S_3 gallop (in systolic dysfunction)
	S_4 gallop (in diastolic dysfunction)
Right-sided	
Peripheral edema	Jugular venous distention
Right upper quadrant discomfort	Hepatomegaly
(because of hepatic enlargement)	Peripheral edema

Table 9.5. New York Heart Association Classification of Chronic Heart Failure	
Class	**Definition**
I	No limitation of physical activity.
II	Slight limitation of activity. Dyspnea and fatigue with moderate exertion (e.g., walking upstairs quickly).
III	Marked limitation of activity. Dyspnea with minimal exertion (e.g., slowly walking upstairs).
IV	Severe limitation of activity. Symptoms are present even at rest.

lower extremity interstitial edema after lying down, with subsequent expansion of intravascular volume and increased venous return to the heart and lungs. A nocturnal cough is another symptom of pulmonary congestion and is produced by a mechanism similar to orthopnea. Hemoptysis (coughing up blood) may result from rupture of engorged bronchial veins.

In right-sided heart failure, the elevated systemic venous pressures can result in *abdominal discomfort* because the liver becomes engorged and its capsule stretched. Similarly, *anorexia* (decreased appetite) and nausea may result from edema within the gastrointestinal tract. *Peripheral edema*, especially in the ankles and feet, also reflects increased hydrostatic venous pressures. Because of the effects of gravity, it tends to worsen while the patient is upright during the day and is often improved by morning after lying supine at night. Even before peripheral edema develops, the patient may note an unexpected *weight*

gain resulting from the accumulation of interstitial fluid.

The symptoms of heart failure are commonly graded according to the New York Heart Association (NYHA) classification (Table 9.5), and patients may shift from one class to another, in either direction, over time. A newer system classifies patients according to their stage in the temporal course of heart failure (Table 9.6). In this system, progression is in only one direction, from Stage A to Stage D, reflecting the typical sequence of heart failure manifestations in clinical practice.

Physical Signs

The physical signs of heart failure depend on the severity and chronicity of the condition and can be divided into those associated with left- or right-heart dysfunction (see Table 9.4). Patients with only mild impairment may appear well. However, a patient with severe chronic heart failure may demonstrate

Table 9.6. Stages of Chronic Heart Failure	
Stage	**Description**
A	Patient who is at risk of developing heart failure but has not yet developed structural cardiac dysfunction (e.g., patient with coronary artery disease, hypertension, or family history of cardiomyopathy).
B	Patient who has structural heart disease associated with heart failure but has not yet developed symptoms.
C	Patient who has current or prior symptoms of heart failure associated with structural heart disease.
D	Patient who has structural heart disease and *marked* heart failure symptoms despite maximal medical therapy and requires advanced interventions (e.g., cardiac transplantation).

Derived from Hunt SA, Baker DW, Chin MH, et al. ACC/AHA guidelines for the evaluation and management of chronic heart failure in the adult: executive summary. *Circulation.* 2001;104:2996–3007.

cachexia (a frail, wasted appearance) owing in part to poor appetite and to the metabolic demands of the increased effort in breathing. In decompensated left-sided heart failure, the patient may appear *dusky* (decreased cardiac output) and *diaphoretic* (sweating because of increased sympathetic nervous activity), and the extremities are cool because of peripheral arterial vasoconstriction. *Tachypnea* (rapid breathing) is common. The pattern of Cheyne–Stokes respiration may also be present in advanced heart failure, characterized by periods of hyperventilation separated by intervals of apnea (absent breathing). This pattern is related to the prolonged circulation time between the lungs and respiratory center of the brain in heart failure that interferes with the normal feedback mechanism of systemic oxygenation. *Sinus tachycardia* (resulting from increased sympathetic nervous system activity) is also common. *Pulsus alternans* (alternating strong and weak contractions detected in the peripheral pulse) may be present as a sign of advanced ventricular dysfunction.

In left-sided heart failure, the auscultatory finding of *pulmonary rales* is created by the "popping open" of small airways during inspiration that had been closed off by edema fluid. This finding is initially apparent at the lung bases, where hydrostatic forces are greatest; however, more severe pulmonary congestion is associated with additional rales higher in the lung fields. Compression of conduction airways by pulmonary congestion may produce coarse rhonchi and wheezing; the latter finding in heart failure is termed *cardiac asthma.*

Depending on the cause of heart failure, palpation of the heart may show that the left ventricular impulse is not focal but diffuse (in dilated cardiomyopathy), sustained (in pressure overload states such as aortic stenosis or hypertension), or lifting in quality (in volume overload states such as mitral regurgitation). Because elevated left-heart filling pressures result in increased pulmonary vascular pressures, the pulmonic component of the second heart sound is often louder than normal. An *early diastolic sound (S$_3$)* is frequently heard in adults with systolic heart failure and is caused by abnormal filling of the dilated chamber (see Chapter 2). A *late diastolic sound (S$_4$)* results

from forceful atrial contraction into a stiffened ventricle and is common in states of decreased LV compliance (diastolic dysfunction). The murmur of *mitral regurgitation* is sometimes auscultated in left-sided heart failure if LV dilatation has stretched the valve annulus and spread the papillary muscles apart from one another, thus preventing proper closure of the mitral leaflets in systole.

In right-sided heart failure, different physical findings may be present. Cardiac examination may reveal a palpable parasternal *right ventricular heave*, representing RV enlargement, or a *right-sided S$_3$* or *S$_4$ gallop*. The murmur of *tricuspid regurgitation* may be auscultated and is due to right ventricular enlargement, analogous to mitral regurgitation that develops in LV dilatation. The elevated systemic venous pressure produced by right-heart failure is manifested by *distention of the jugular veins* as well as *hepatic enlargement* with abdominal right upper quadrant tenderness. *Edema* accumulates in the dependent portions of the body, beginning in the ankles and feet of ambulatory patients and in the presacral regions of those who are bedridden.

Pleural effusions may develop in either left- or right-sided heart failure, because the pleural veins drain into both the systemic and pulmonary venous beds. The presence of pleural effusions is suggested on physical examination by dullness to percussion over the posterior lung bases.

Diagnostic Studies

A normal mean left atrial (LA) pressure is ≤10 mm Hg. If the LA pressure exceeds approximately 15 mm Hg, the chest radiograph shows *upper-zone vascular redistribution*, such that the vessels supplying the upper lobes of the lung are larger than those supplying the lower lobes (see Fig. 3.5). This is explained as follows: when a patient is in the upright position, blood flow is normally greater to the lung bases than to the apices because of the effect of gravity. Redistribution of flow occurs with the development of interstitial and perivascular edema, because such edema is most prominent at the lung bases (where the hydrostatic pressure is the highest), such that the blood vessels in the bases are compressed, whereas flow into the upper lung zones is less affected.

When the LA pressure surpasses 20 mm Hg, interstitial edema is usually manifested on the chest radiograph as indistinctness of the vessels and the presence of *Kerley B lines* (short linear markings at the periphery of the lower lung fields indicating interlobular edema). If the LA pressure exceeds 25 to 30 mm Hg, alveolar pulmonary edema may develop, with opacification of the air spaces. The relationship between LA pressure and chest radiograph findings is modified in patients with *chronic* heart failure because of enhanced lymphatic drainage, such that higher pressures can be accommodated with fewer radiologic signs.

Depending on the cause of heart failure, the chest radiograph may show *cardiomegaly*, defined as a cardiothoracic ratio of greater than 0.5 on the posteroanterior film. A high right atrial pressure also causes enlargement of the azygous vein silhouette. Pleural effusions may be present.

Assays for BNP, described earlier in the chapter, correlate well with the degree of LV dysfunction and prognosis. Furthermore, an elevated serum level of BNP can help distinguish heart failure from other causes of dyspnea, such as pulmonary parenchymal diseases.

The cause of heart failure is often evident from the history, such as a patient who has sustained a large myocardial infarction, or by physical examination, as in a patient with a murmur of valvular heart disease. When the cause is not clear from clinical evaluation, the first step is to determine whether systolic ventricular function is normal or depressed (see Fig. 9.6). Of the several noninvasive tests that can help make this determination, echocardiography is especially useful and readily available (as described in Chapter 3).

PROGNOSIS

The prognosis of heart failure is dismal in the absence of a correctable underlying cause. The 5-year mortality rate following the diagnosis ranges between 45% and 60%, with men having worse outcomes than women. Patients with severe symptoms (i.e., NYHA class III or IV) fare the least well, having a 1-year survival rate of only 40%. The greatest mortality is due to refractory heart failure, but many patients die suddenly, presumably because of associated ventricular arrhythmias. Heart failure patients with preserved EF have similar rates of hospitalization, in-hospital complications, and mortality as those with reduced EF.

Ventricular dysfunction usually begins with an inciting insult, but is a progressive process, contributed to by the maladaptive activation of neurohormones, cytokines, and continuous ventricular remodeling. Thus, it should not be surprising that measures of neurohormonal and cytokine stimulation predict survival in heart failure patients. For example, adverse prognosis correlates with the serum norepinephrine level (marker of sympathetic nervous system activity), serum sodium (reduced level reflects activation of renin–angiotensin–aldosterone system and alterations in intrarenal hemodynamics), endothelin-1, B-type natriuretic peptide, and cytokine TNF-α levels.

Despite the generally bleak prognosis, a heart failure patient's outlook can be substantially improved by specific interventions, as discussed in the following section.

TREATMENT OF HEART FAILURE WITH REDUCED EJECTION FRACTION

There are five main goals of therapy in patients with chronic heart failure and a reduced ejection fraction:

1. *Identification and correction of the underlying condition causing heart failure.* In some patients, this may require surgical repair or replacement of dysfunctional cardiac valves, coronary artery revascularization, aggressive treatment of hypertension, or cessation of alcohol consumption.

2. *Elimination of the acute precipitating cause of symptoms* in a patient with heart failure who was previously in a compensated state. This may include, for example, treating acute infections or arrhythmias, removing sources of excessive salt intake, or eliminating drugs that can aggravate symptomatology (e.g., certain calcium channel blockers, which have a negative inotropic effect, or nonsteroidal anti-inflammatory

drugs, which can contribute to volume retention).

3. *Management of heart failure symptoms:*

  a. *Treatment of pulmonary and systemic vascular congestion.* This is most readily accomplished by dietary sodium restriction and diuretic medications.

  b. *Measures to increase forward cardiac output* and perfusion of vital organs through the use of vasodilators and positive inotropic drugs.

4. *Modulation of the neurohormonal response* to prevent adverse ventricular remodeling in order to slow the progression of LV dysfunction.

5. *Prolongation of long-term survival.* There is strong evidence from clinical trials that longevity is enhanced by specific therapies, as described below.

Diuretics

The mechanisms of action of diuretic drugs are summarized in Chapter 17. By promoting the elimination of sodium and water through the kidney, diuretics reduce intravascular volume and thus venous return to the heart. As a result, the preload of the left ventricle is decreased, and its diastolic pressure falls out of the range that promotes pulmonary congestion (Fig. 9.10, point *b*). The intent is to

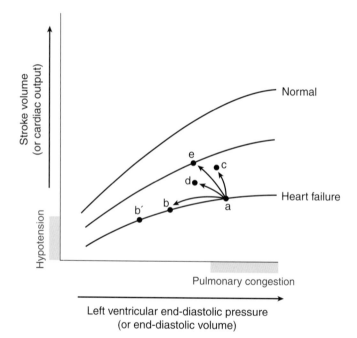

Figure 9.10. The effect of treatment on the left ventricular (LV) Frank–Starling curve in patients who have heart failure with reduced EF. Point *a* represents the failing heart on a curve that is shifted downward compared with normal. The stroke volume is reduced (with blood pressure bordering on hypotension), and the LV end-diastolic pressure (LVEDP) is increased, resulting in symptoms of pulmonary congestion. Therapy with a diuretic or pure venous vasodilator (point *b* on the same Frank–Starling curve) reduces LV pressure without much change in stroke volume (SV). However, excessive diuresis or venous vasodilatation may result in an undesired fall in SV with hypotension (point *b'*). Inotropic drug therapy (point *c*) and arteriolar (or "balanced") vasodilator therapy (point *d*) augment SV, and because of improved LV emptying during contraction, the LVEDP lessens. Point *e* represents the potential added benefit of combining an inotrope and vasodilator together. The middle curve shows one example of how the Frank–Starling relationship shifts upward during inotropic/vasodilator therapy but does not achieve the level of a normal ventricle.

reduce the end-diastolic pressure (and therefore hydrostatic forces contributing to pulmonary congestion) without a significant fall in stroke volume. The judicious use of diuretics does not significantly reduce stroke volume and cardiac output in this setting, because the failing ventricle is operating on the "flat" portion of a depressed Frank–Starling curve. However, overly vigorous diuresis *can* lower LV filling pressures into the steep portion of the ventricular performance curve, resulting in an undesired fall in cardiac output (see Fig. 9.10, point *b'*). Thus, diuretics should be used only if there is evidence of pulmonary congestion (rales) or peripheral interstitial fluid accumulation (edema).

Agents that act primarily at the renal loop of Henle (e.g., furosemide, torsemide, and bumetanide) are the most potent diuretics in heart failure. Thiazide diuretics (e.g., hydrochlorothiazide and metolazone) are also useful but are less effective in the setting of decreased renal perfusion, which is often present in this condition.

The potential adverse effects of diuretics are described in Chapter 17. The most important in heart failure patients include overly vigorous diuresis resulting in a fall in cardiac output, and electrolyte disturbances (particularly hypokalemia and hypomagnesemia), which may contribute to arrhythmias.

Vasodilators

One of the most important cardiac advances in the late twentieth century was the introduction of vasodilator therapy for the treatment of heart failure, particularly the class of agents known as ACE inhibitors. As indicated earlier, neurohormonal compensatory mechanisms in heart failure often lead to excessive vasoconstriction, volume retention, and ventricular remodeling, with progressive deterioration of cardiac function. Vasodilator drugs help to reverse these adverse consequences. Moreover, multiple studies have shown that certain vasodilator regimens significantly extend survival in patients with heart failure. The pharmacology of these drugs is described in Chapter 17.

Venous vasodilators (e.g., nitrates) increase venous capacitance, and thereby decrease venous return to the heart and left ventricular preload. Consequently, LV diastolic pressures fall and the pulmonary capillary hydrostatic pressure declines, similar to the hemodynamic effects of diuretic therapy. As a result, pulmonary congestion improves, and as long as the heart failure patient is on the relatively "flat" part of the depressed Frank–Starling curve (see Fig. 9.10), the cardiac output does not fall despite the reduction in ventricular filling pressure. However, venous vasodilatation in a patient who is operating on the steeper part of the curve may result in an undesired fall in stroke volume, cardiac output, and blood pressure.

Pure *arteriolar vasodilators* (e.g., hydralazine) reduce systemic vascular resistance and therefore LV afterload, which in turn permits increased ventricular muscle fiber shortening during systole (see Fig. 9.5B). This results in an augmented stroke volume and is represented on the Frank–Starling diagram as a shift in an upward direction (see Fig. 9.10). Although an arterial vasodilator might be expected to reduce blood pressure—an undesired effect in patients with heart failure who may already be hypotensive—this generally does not happen. As resistance is reduced by arteriolar vasodilatation, a concurrent *rise* in cardiac output usually occurs, such that blood pressure remains constant or decreases only mildly.

Some groups of drugs result in vasodilatation of both the venous and arteriolar circuits ("balanced" vasodilators). Of these, the most important are agents that inhibit the renin–angiotensin–aldosterone system. **ACE inhibitors** (described in Chapters 13 and 17) interrupt the production of AII, thereby modulating the vasoconstriction incited by that hormone in heart failure patients. In addition, because aldosterone levels fall in response to ACE inhibitor therapy, sodium elimination is facilitated, resulting in reduced intravascular volume and improvement of systemic and pulmonary vascular congestion. ACE inhibitors also augment circulating levels of bradykinin (see Chapter 17), which is thought to contribute to beneficial vasodilation in heart failure. As a result of these effects, ACE inhibitors limit maladaptive ventricular remodeling in patients with chronic heart failure and following acute myocardial infarction (see Chapter 7).

Supporting the beneficial hemodynamic and neurohormonal blocking effects of ACE inhibitors, many large clinical trials have shown that these drugs reduce heart failure symptoms, improve stamina, reduce the need for hospitalization, and most importantly, extend survival in patients with heart failure with reduced EF. Thus, ACE inhibitors are standard first-line chronic therapy for patients with LV systolic dysfunction.

The renin–angiotensin–aldosterone system can also be therapeutically inhibited by **angiotensin II receptor blockers (ARBs),** as described in Chapters 13 and 17. Since AII can be formed by pathways other than ACE, ARBs provide a more complete inhibition of the system than ACE inhibitors, through blockade of the actual AII receptor (see Fig. 17.6). Conversely, ARBs do not stimulate the potentially beneficial rise in serum bradykinin. The net result is that the hemodynamic effects of ARBs in heart failure are similar to those of ACE inhibitors, and studies thus far have not shown any superiority of these agents over ACE inhibitors in terms of patient survival. Thus, they are prescribed to heart failure patients mainly when ACE inhibitors are not tolerated (e.g., because of the common side effect of cough).

Chronic therapy using the combination of the venous dilator **isosorbide dinitrate** plus the arteriolar dilator **hydralazine** has also been shown to improve survival in patients with moderate symptoms of heart failure. However, when administration of the ACE inhibitor enalapril was compared with the hydralazine–isosorbide dinitrate (H-ISDN) combination, the ACE inhibitor was shown to produce the greater improvement in survival. Thus, H-ISDN is generally substituted when a patient cannot tolerate ACE inhibitor or ARB therapy (e.g., because of renal insufficiency or hyperkalemia). Of note, H-ISDN has been shown to have particular benefit in certain individuals with heart failure. The African–American Heart Failure trial demonstrated that the addition of H-ISDN to standard heart failure therapy (including a diuretic, β-blocker, ACE inhibitor, or ARB) in black patients with heart failure further improved functional status and survival.

Nesiritide (human recombinant B-type natriuretic peptide) is an intravenous vasodilator drug available for hospitalized patients with decompensated heart failure. It causes rapid and potent vasodilatation, reduces elevated intracardiac pressures, augments forward cardiac output, and lessens the activation of the renin-angiotensin-aldosterone and sympathetic nervous systems. It promotes diuresis, reduces heart failure symptoms, and can be combined with diuretics and positive inotropic drugs. However, it is an expensive drug, and recent evidence has raised questions about its safety. One analysis shows that patients treated with nesiritide are more likely to die over the following month than are those receiving traditional heart failure therapies. Therefore, nesiritide is currently used primarily in patients who have not responded to or cannot tolerate other intravenous vasodilators, such as intravenous nitroglycerin or nitroprusside (see Chapter 17).

Inotropic Drugs

The inotropic drugs include β-adrenergic agonists, digitalis glycosides, and phosphodiesterase inhibitors (see Chapter 17). By increasing the availability of intracellular calcium, each of these drug groups enhances the force of ventricular contraction and therefore shifts the Frank–Starling curve in an upward direction (see Fig. 9.10). As a result, stroke volume and cardiac output are augmented at any given ventricular end-diastolic volume. Therefore, these agents may be useful in treating patients with systolic dysfunction but typically not those with heart failure with preserved EF.

The **β-adrenergic agonists** (e.g., dobutamine and dopamine) are administered intravenously for temporary hemodynamic support in acutely ill, hospitalized patients. Their long-term use is limited by the lack of an oral form of administration and by the rapid development of drug tolerance. The latter refers to the progressive decline in effectiveness during continued administration of the drug, possibly owing to downregulation of myocardial adrenergic receptors. Likewise, the role of **phosphodiesterase inhibitors** (e.g., milrinone) is limited to the intravenous treatment of congestive heart failure in acutely ill patients. Despite the initial promise of effective *oral* phosphodiesterase inhibitors, studies thus far actually demonstrate reduced survival among patients receiving this form of treatment.

One of the oldest forms of inotropic therapy is **digitalis** (see Chapter 17), which can be administered intravenously or orally. Digitalis preparations enhance contractility, reduce cardiac enlargement, improve symptoms, and augment cardiac output in patients with systolic heart failure. Digitalis also increases the sensitivity of the baroreceptors, so that the compensatory sympathetic drive in heart failure is blunted, a desired effect that reduces left ventricular afterload. By slowing AV nodal conduction and thereby reducing the rate of ventricular contractions, digitalis has an added benefit in patients with congestive heart failure who have concurrent atrial fibrillation. Although digitalis can improve symptomatology and reduce the rate of hospitalizations in heart failure patients, it has not been shown to improve long-term survival. Its use is thus limited to patients who remain symptomatic despite other standard therapies or to help slow the ventricular rate if atrial fibrillation is also present. Digitalis is *not* useful in the treatment of heart failure with preserved EF because it does not improve ventricular relaxation properties.

β-Blockers

Historically, β-blockers were contraindicated in patients with systolic dysfunction because the negative inotropic effect of the drugs would be expected to worsen symptomatology. Paradoxically, more recent studies have actually shown that β-blockers have important *benefits* in heart failure, including augmented cardiac output, reduced hemodynamic deterioration, and improved survival. The explanation for this observation remains conjectural but may relate to the drugs' effect on reducing heart rate and blunting chronic sympathetic activation, or to their anti-ischemic properties.

In clinical trials of patients with symptomatic heart failure with reduced EF, β-blockers have been well tolerated in stable patients (i.e., those without recent deterioration of symptoms or active signs of volume overload) and have resulted in improved mortality rates and fewer hospitalizations compared with placebo. Not all β-blockers have been tested in heart failure. Those that have, and have shown benefit in randomized clinical trials include **carvedilol** (a nonselective β_1- and β_2-receptor blocker with weak α-blocking properties) and the β_1-selective **metoprolol** (in a sustained-release formulation). Despite these benefits, β-blockers must be used cautiously in heart failure to prevent acute deterioration due to their potentially negative inotropic effect. Regimens should be started at low dosages and augmented gradually.

Aldosterone Antagonist Therapy

There is evidence that chronic excess of aldosterone in heart failure contributes to cardiac fibrosis and adverse ventricular remodeling. Antagonists of this hormone (which have been used historically as mild diuretics—see Chapter 17) have shown clinical benefit in heart failure patients. For example, in a clinical trial of patients with advanced heart failure who were already taking an ACE inhibitor and diuretics, the aldosterone receptor antagonist **spironolactone** substantially reduced mortality rates and improved heart failure symptoms. **Eplerenone**, a more specific aldosterone receptor inhibitor, has been shown to improve survival of patients with congestive heart failure after an acute myocardial infarction (see Chapter 7). Although aldosterone antagonists are well tolerated in carefully controlled studies, the serum potassium level must be closely monitored to prevent hyperkalemia, especially if there is renal impairment or concomitant ACE inhibitor therapy.

In summary, standard therapy of chronic heart failure with reduced EF should include several drugs, the cornerstones of which are an ACE inhibitor and a β-blocker. An accepted sequence of therapy is to start with an ACE inhibitor, as well as a diuretic if pulmonary or systemic congestive symptoms are present. If the patient is unable to tolerate the ACE inhibitor, then an ARB (or hydralazine plus isosorbide dinitrate) may be substituted. For patients without recent clinical deterioration or volume overload, a β-blocker should be added. Those with advanced heart failure may benefit from the addition of an aldosterone antagonist. For persistent symptoms, digoxin can be prescribed for its hemodynamic benefit.

Additional Therapies

Other therapies sometimes administered to patients with heart failure and reduced EF include (1) chronic **anticoagulation** with warfarin to prevent intracardiac thrombus formation if LV systolic function is severely impaired (a controversial therapy in the absence of other indications for anticoagulation, because this approach has not yet been tested in clinical trials) and (2) **treatment of atrial and ventricular arrhythmias** that frequently accompany chronic heart failure. For example, atrial fibrillation is very common in heart failure, and conversion back to sinus rhythm can substantially improve cardiac output. Ventricular arrhythmias are also frequent in this population and may lead to sudden death. The antiarrhythmic drug that is most effective at suppressing arrhythmias and least likely to *provoke* other dangerous rhythm disorders in heart failure patients is amiodarone. However, studies of amiodarone for treatment of asymptomatic ventricular arrhythmias in heart failure have not shown a consistent survival benefit. In addition, heart failure patients with symptomatic or sustained ventricular arrhythmias, or those with inducible ventricular tachycardia during electrophysiologic testing, benefit more from the insertion of an implantable cardioverter-defibrillator (ICD; see Chapter 11). Based on the results of large-scale randomized trials, ICD implantation is indicated for many patients with chronic ischemic or nonischemic dilated cardiomyopathies and

at least moderately reduced systolic function (e.g., left ventricular ejection fraction ≤35%), regardless of the presence of ventricular arrhythmias, because this approach reduces the likelihood of sudden cardiac death in this population.

Cardiac Resynchronization Therapy

Intraventricular conduction abnormalities with widened QRS complexes (especially left bundle branch block) are common in patients with advanced heart failure. Such abnormalities can actually contribute to cardiac symptoms because of the uncoordinated pattern of right and left ventricular contraction. Advanced pacemakers have therefore been developed that stimulate both ventricles simultaneously, thus resynchronizing the contractile effort. This technique of biventricular pacing, also termed cardiac resynchronization therapy (CRT), has been shown to augment left ventricular systolic function, improve exercise capacity, and reduce the frequency of heart failure exacerbations and mortality. Thus, CRT is appropriate for selected patients with advanced systolic dysfunction (LV ejection fraction ≤35%), a prolonged QRS duration (>120 msec) and continued symptoms of heart failure despite appropriate pharmacologic therapies. Since patients who receive CRT are typically also candidates for an ICD, modern devices combine both functions in a single, small implantable unit.

Cardiac Replacement Therapy

A patient with severe LV dysfunction whose condition remains refractory to maximal medical management may be a candidate for cardiac transplantation. Because of a shortage of donor hearts, only approximately 3,000 transplants are performed worldwide each year, much fewer than the number of patients with refractory heart failure symptoms. Thus, alternative heart support therapies are in selected use and are undergoing further intense development, including ventricular mechanical assist devices and implanted artificial hearts.

TREATMENT OF HEART FAILURE WITH PRESERVED EJECTION FRACTION

The goals of therapy in heart failure with pre-served EF include (1) the relief of pulmonary and systemic congestion, and (2) addressing correctable causes of the impaired diastolic function (e.g., hypertension, coronary artery disease). Diuretics reduce pulmonary conges-tion and peripheral edema but must be used cautiously to avoid under filling of the left ventricle. A stiffened left ventricle relies on higher-than-normal pressures to achieve ad-equate diastolic filling (see Fig. 9.7B) and ex-cessive diuresis could reduce filling and stroke volume (see Fig. 9.10).

Unlike patients with impaired systolic func-tion, β-blockers, ACE inhibitors, and ARBs have no demonstrated mortality benefit in patients with heart failure with preserved EF. Additionally, since contractile function is pre-served, inotropic drugs have no role in this condition.

ACUTE HEART FAILURE

In contrast to the findings of chronic heart fail-ure described to this point, patients with acute heart failure are those who present with urgent and often life-threatening symptomatology. Acute heart failure may develop in a previously asymptomatic patient (e.g., resulting from an acute coronary syndrome [Chapter 7], severe hypertension [Chapter 13], or acute valvular regurgitation [Chapter 8]), or it may complicate chronic compensated heart failure following a precipitating trigger (see Table 9.3). Manage-ment of acute heart failure typically requires hospitalization and prompt interventions.

The classification of patients with acute heart failure, and the approach to therapy, can be tailored based on the presence or absence of two major findings at the bedside: (1) volume overload (i.e., "wet" vs. "dry") as a reflection of elevated LV filling pressures, and (2) signs of decreased cardiac output with reduced tis-sue perfusion ("cold" vs. "warm" extremities). Examples of a "wet" profile, indicative of vol-ume overload, include: pulmonary rales, jugu-lar venous distension, and edema of the lower extremities. Figure 9.11 shows how patients

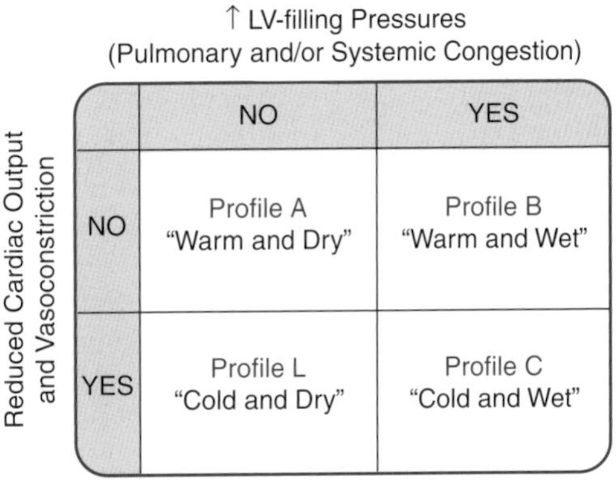

Figure 9.11. **Hemodynamic profiles in acute heart fail-ure.** (Derived from Nohria A, Tsang SW, Fang JC, et al. Clinical assessment identifies hemodynamic profiles that predict outcomes in patients admitted with heart failure. *J Am Coll Cardiol.* 2003;41:1797–1804.)

with acute heart failure can be divided into four profiles based on observations of these parameters.

Profile A indicates normal hemodynamics. Cardiopulmonary symptoms in such patients would be due to factors other than heart fail-ure, such as parenchymal lung disease or tran-sient myocardial ischemia. Profiles B and C are typical of patients with acute pulmonary edema (described below). Those with Profile B have "wet" lungs but preserved ("warm") tissue perfusion. Profile C is more serious; in addition to congestive findings, impaired forward cardiac output results in marked systemic vasoconstriction (e.g., activation of the sympathetic nervous system) and there-fore "cold" extremities. Patients with Profile C have a prognosis worse than those with Pro-file B, who in turn have poorer outcomes than those with Profile A.

Patients with Profile L do not represent an extension of this continuum. Rather, they display "cold" extremities due to low output (hence the label "L") but no signs of vascular congestion. This profile may arise in patients who are actually volume deplete, or those with very limited cardiac reserve in the ab-sence of volume overload (e.g., a patient with a dilated left ventricle and mitral regurgitation who becomes short of breath with activity be-cause of the inability to generate adequate for-ward cardiac output). These profiles of acute heart failure should not be confused with the classification of chronic heart failure (Stages A through D) presented in Table 9.6.

The goals of therapy in acute heart failure are to (1) normalize ventricular filling pressures and (2) restore adequate tissue perfusion. Identification of the patient's profile type guides therapeutic interventions. For example, a patient with Profile B would require diuretic and/or vasodilator therapy for pulmonary edema (described in the next section), and those with Profile C may additionally require intravenous inotropic medications to strengthen cardiac output. Patients with Profile L may require volume expansion. The presence of profile A would prompt a search for contributions to the patient's symptoms other than heart failure.

Acute Pulmonary Edema

A common manifestation of acute left-sided heart failure (e.g., typical of Profiles B and C) is cardiogenic pulmonary edema, in which elevated capillary hydrostatic pressure causes rapid accumulation of fluid within the interstitium and alveolar spaces of the lung. In the presence of normal plasma oncotic pressure, pulmonary edema develops when the pulmonary capillary wedge pressure, which reflects LV diastolic pressure, exceeds approximately 25 mm Hg.

This condition is frequently accompanied by hypoxemia because of shunting of pulmonary blood flow through regions of hypoventilated alveoli. Like other manifestations of acute heart failure, pulmonary edema may appear suddenly in a previously asymptomatic person (e.g., in the setting of an acute myocardial infarction) or in a patient with chronic compensated congestive heart failure following a precipitating event (see Table 9.3). Pulmonary edema is a horrifying experience for the patient, resulting in severe dyspnea and anxiety while struggling to breathe.

On examination, the patient is tachycardic and may demonstrate cold, clammy skin owing to peripheral vasoconstriction in response to increased sympathetic outflow (i.e., Profile C). Tachypnea and coughing of "frothy" sputum represent transudation of fluid into the alveoli. Rales are present initially at the bases and later throughout the lung fields, sometimes accompanied by wheezing because of edema within the conductance airways.

Pulmonary edema is a life-threatening emergency that requires immediate improvement of systemic oxygenation and elimination of the underlying cause. The patient should be seated upright to permit pooling of blood within the systemic veins of the lower body, thereby reducing venous return to the heart. Supplemental oxygen is provided by a face mask. Morphine sulfate is administered intravenously to reduce anxiety and as a venous dilator to facilitate pooling of blood peripherally. A rapidly acting diuretic, such as intravenous furosemide, is administered to further reduce LV preload and pulmonary capillary hydrostatic pressure. Other means of reducing preload include administration of nitrates (often intravenously). Intravenous inotropic drugs (e.g., dopamine—see Chapter 17) may increase forward CO and are used primarily in patients with Profile C. During resolution of the pulmonary congestion and hypoxemia, attention should be directed at identifying and treating the underlying precipitating cause.

An easy-to-remember mnemonic for the principal components of management of pulmonary edema is the alphabetic sequence LMNOP:

Lasix (trade name for furosemide)

Morphine

Nitrates

Oxygen

Position (sit upright)

SUMMARY

1. Heart failure is present when cardiac output fails to meet the metabolic demands of the body or meets those demands only if the cardiac filling pressures are abnormally high. Chronic heart failure may be classified into two categories: (1) heart failure with reduced EF (impaired left ventricular systolic function) and (2) heart failure with preserved EF (e.g., diastolic dysfunction).

2. Compensatory mechanisms in heart failure that initially maintain circulatory function include (1) preload augmentation with increased stroke volume via the Frank–Starling mechanism, (2) activation of neurohormonal systems, and (3) ventricular hypertrophy. However, these compensations eventually become maladaptive, contributing to adverse ventricular remodeling and progressive deterioration of ventricular function.

3. Symptoms of heart failure may be exacerbated by precipitating factors that increase metabolic demand, increase circulating volume, raise afterload, or decrease contractility (summarized in Table 9.3).

4. Treatment of heart failure includes identification of the underlying cause of the condition, elimination of precipitating factors, and modulation of neurohormonal activations. Standard treatment of heart failure patients with reduced EF includes an ACE inhibitor, β-blocker and, as needed, diuretics and inotropic drugs. For patients who do not tolerate an ACE inhibitor, an ARB or the combination of hydralazine plus nitrates can be substituted. The addition of spironolactone should be considered for patients with advanced heart failure. In patients with advanced disease who meet specific criteria, CRT (biventricular pacing) and/or insertion of an ICD should be considered.

5. Therapy for heart failure with preserved EF relies primarily on diuretics and vasodilators to relieve pulmonary congestion. Such therapy must be administered cautiously to avoid excess reduction of preload and hypotension.

6. Acute heart failure can be characterized by, and treatment decisions based on, the presence or absence of (1) elevated left heart filling pressures (wet vs. dry) and (2) reduced systemic tissue perfusion with elevated systemic vascular resistance (i.e., cold vs. warm) as in Figure 9.11.

Acknowledgments

Contributors to the previous editions of this chapter were Ravi V. Shah, MD; Arthur Coday Jr, MD; George S. M. Dyer, MD; Stephen K. Frankel, MD; Vikram Janakiraman, MD; and Michael A. Fifer, MD.

Additional Reading

Braunwald, E. Biomarkers in heart failure. *N Engl J Med.* 2008;358:2148–2159.

Dec GW, ed. *Heart Failure: A Comprehensive Guide to Diagnosis and Treatment.* New York: Marcel Dekker; 2005.

Dickstein K, Cohen-Solal A, Filippatos G, et al. ESC Guidelines for the diagnosis and treatment of acute and chronic heart failure 2008: the Task Force for the Diagnosis and Treatment of Acute and Chronic Heart Failure 2008 of the European Society of Cardiology. *Eur Heart J.* 2008;29:2388–2442.

Hsich EM, Pina IL. Heart failure in women. *J Am Coll Cardiol.* 2009;54:491–498.

Jessup M, Abraham WT, Casey DE, et al. 2009 Focused update: ACCF/AHA guidelines for the diagnosis and management of heart failure in adults: a report of the American College of Cardiology Foundation/ American Heart Association Task Force on Practice Guidelines. *Circulation.* 2009;119:1977–2016.

Maeder MT, Kaye DM. Heart failure with normal left ventricular ejection fraction. *J Am Coll Cardiol.* 2009;53:905–918.

McMurray JJV. Systolic heart failure. *N Engl J Med.* 2010;362:228–238.

Ramani GV, Uber PA, Mehra MR. Chronic heart failure: contemporary diagnosis and management. *Mayo Clin. Proc.* 2010;85:180–195.

Schocken DD, Benjamin EJ, Fonarow GC, et al. Prevention of heart failure: a scientific statement from the American Heart Association councils on epidemiology and prevention, clinical cardiology, cardiovascular nursing, and high blood pressure research; quality of care and outcomes research interdisciplinary working group; and functional genomics and translational biology interdisciplinary working group. *Circulation.* 2008;117:2544–2565.

Triposkiadis F, Karayannis G, Giamouzis G, et al. The sympathetic nervous system in heart failure: physiology, pathophysiology, and clinical implications. *J Am Coll Cardiol.* 2009;54:1747–1762.

Walsh RA., ed. *Molecular Mechanisms of Cardiac Hypertrophy and Failure.* New York: Taylor & Francis; 2005.

Wang J, Nagueh SF. Current perspectives on cardiac function in patients with diastolic heart failure. *Circulation.* 2009;119:1146–1157.

Ware LB, Matthay MA. Acute pulmonary edema. *N Engl J Med.* 2005;353:2788–96.

Wilson SR, Givertz MM, Stewart GC, et al. Ventricular assist devices. *J Am Coll Cardiol.* 2009;54: 1647–1659.

The Cardiomyopathies

Christopher T. Lee
G. William Dec
Leonard S. Lilly

The cardiomyopathies are a group of heart disorders in which the major structural abnormality is limited to the myocardium. These conditions often result in symptoms of heart failure, and although the underlying cause of myocardial dysfunction can sometimes be identified, the etiology frequently remains unknown. Excluded from the classification of this group of diseases is heart muscle impairment resulting from other defined cardiovascular conditions, such as hypertension, valvular disorders, or coronary artery disease.

Cardiomyopathies can be classified into three types based on the anatomic appearance and abnormal physiology of the left ventricle (LV) (Fig. 10.1). **Dilated** cardiomyopathy is characterized by ventricular chamber enlargement with impaired *systolic* contractile function; **hypertrophic** cardiomyopathy, by an abnormally thickened ventricular wall with abnormal *diastolic* relaxation but usually intact systolic function; and **restrictive** cardiomyopathy, by an abnormally stiffened myocardium (because of fibrosis or an infiltrative process) leading to impaired *diastolic* relaxation, but systolic contractile function is normal or near normal.

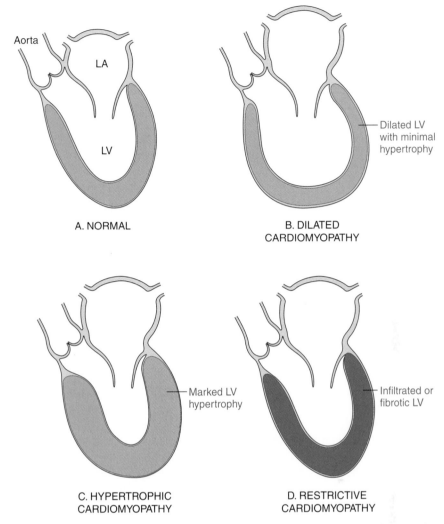

Figure 10.1. Anatomic appearance of the cardiomyopathies (CMPs). A. Normal heart demonstrating left ventricle (LV) and left atrium (LA). **B.** Dilated CMP is characterized by prominent ventricular enlargement with only mildly increased thickness. **C.** Hypertrophic CMP demonstrates significant ventricular hypertrophy, often asymmetrically involving the intraventricular septum. **D.** Restrictive CMP is caused by infiltration or fibrosis of the ventricles, usually without chamber enlargement. LA enlargement is common to all three types of CMP.

DILATED CARDIOMYOPATHY

Etiology

Myocyte damage and cardiac enlargement in dilated cardiomyopathy (DCM) result from a wide spectrum of genetic, inflammatory, toxic, and metabolic causes (Table 10.1). Although most cases are idiopathic (i.e., the cause is undetermined), examples of defined conditions that are associated with DCM include viral myocarditis, chronic excessive alcohol ingestion, the peripartum state, and specific gene mutations.

Acute viral myocarditis generally afflicts young, previously healthy people. Common responsible infecting organisms include coxsackievirus group B, parvovirus B19, and adenovirus, among many others. Viral myocarditis is usually a self-limited illness with full recovery, but for unknown reasons, some patients progress to DCM. It is hypothesized that myocardial destruction and fibrosis result from immune-mediated injury triggered by viral constituents. Nonetheless, immunosuppressive drugs have not been shown to improve

Table 10.1. Examples of Dilated Cardiomyopathies
Idiopathic
Familial (genetic)
Inflammatory
Infectious (especially viral)
Noninfectious
Connective tissue diseases
Peripartum cardiomyopathy
Sarcoidosis
Toxic
Chronic alcohol ingestion
Chemotherapeutic agents (e.g., doxorubicin)
Metabolic
Hypothyroidism
Chronic hypocalcemia or hypophosphatemia
Neuromuscular
Muscular or myotonic dystrophy

the prognosis of this condition. Transvenous right ventricular biopsy during acute myocarditis may demonstrate active inflammation, but specific viral genomic sequences have been demonstrated in only a minority of patients.

Alcoholic cardiomyopathy develops in a small number of people who consume alcoholic beverages excessively and chronically. Although the pathophysiology of the condition is unknown, ethanol is thought to impair cellular function by inhibiting mitochondrial oxidative phosphorylation and fatty acid oxidation. Its clinical presentation and histologic features are similar to those of other dilated cardiomyopathies. Alcoholic cardiomyopathy is important to identify because it is potentially reversible; cessation of ethanol consumption can lead to dramatic improvement of ventricular function.

Peripartum cardiomyopathy is a form of DCM that presents with heart failure symptoms between the last month of pregnancy and up to 6 months postpartum. Risk factors include older maternal age, being African American, and having multiple pregnancies. A unifying etiology of this condition has not yet been identified. Ventricular function returns to normal in approximately 50% of affected women in the months following pregnancy,

but recurrences of DCM with subsequent pregnancies have been reported. Other potentially reversible causes of DCM include other toxin exposures, metabolic abnormalities (such as hypothyroidism), and some inflammatory etiologies, including sarcoidosis and connective tissue diseases.

Several familial forms of DCM have been identified and are believed to be responsible for 20% to 30% of what were once classified as idiopathic DCM. Autosomal dominant, autosomal recessive, X-linked, and mitochondrial patterns of inheritance have been described, leading to defects in contractile force generation, force transmission, energy production, and myocyte viability. Identified mutations occur in genes that code for cardiac cytoskeletal, myofibrillar, and nuclear membrane proteins (Table 10.2).

Pathology

Marked enlargement of all four cardiac chambers is typical of DCM (Fig. 10.2), although sometimes the disease is limited to the left or right side of the heart. The thickness of the ventricular walls may be increased, but chamber dilatation is out of proportion to any concentric hypertrophy. Microscopically, there is evidence of myocyte degeneration with irregular hypertrophy and atrophy of myofibers. Interstitial and perivascular fibrosis is often extensive.

Pathophysiology

The hallmark of DCM is ventricular dilatation with decreased contractile function (Fig. 10.3). Most often in DCM, both ventricles are impaired, but sometimes dysfunction is limited to the LV and even less commonly to the right ventricle (RV).

As ventricular stroke volume and cardiac output decline because of impaired myocyte contractility, two compensatory effects are activated: (1) the Frank–Starling mechanism, in which the elevated ventricular diastolic volume increases the stretch of the myofibers, thereby increasing the subsequent stroke volume; and (2) neurohormonal activation, initially mediated by the sympathetic nervous

Table 10.2. Familial Forms of Dilated and Hypertrophic Cardiomyopathies

Protein	Mutations Identified in Dilated Cardiomyopathy	Mutations Identified in Hypertrophic Cardiomyopathy
Cytoskeletal Proteins		
Desmin	√	
Dystrophin	√	
Myosin-binding protein C	√	√
Sarcoglycans	√	
Titin	√	√
Myofibrillar Proteins		
β-Myosin heavy chain	√	√
Cardiac troponin T	√	√
Cardiac troponin I	√	√
Cardiac troponin C	√	√
α-Tropomyosin	√	√
Essential myosin light chain		√
Cardiac actin	√	√
Nuclear Membrane Protein		
Lamin A/C	√	

system (see Chapter 9). The latter contributes to an increased heart rate and contractility, which help to buffer the fall in cardiac output. These compensations may render the patient asymptomatic during the early stages of ventricular dysfunction; however, as progressive myocyte degeneration and volume overload ensue, clinical symptoms of heart failure develop.

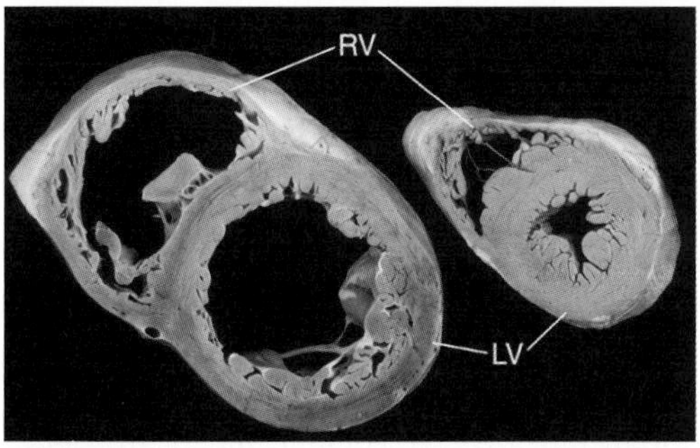

With a persistent reduction of cardiac output, the decline in renal blood flow prompts the kidneys to secrete increased amounts of renin. This activation of the renin-angiotensin-aldosterone axis increases peripheral vascular resistance (mediated through angiotensin II) and intravascular volume (because of increased aldosterone). As described in Chapter 9, these effects are also initially helpful in buffering the fall in cardiac output.

Ultimately, however, the "compensatory" effects of neurohormonal activation prove detrimental. Arteriolar vasoconstriction and increased systemic resistance render it more difficult for the LV to eject blood in the forward direction, and the rise in intravascular volume further burdens the ventricles, resulting in pulmonary and systemic congestion. In addition, chronically elevated levels of angiotensin II and aldosterone directly contribute to pathological myocardial remodeling and fibrosis.

As the cardiomyopathic process causes the ventricles to enlarge over time, the mitral and tricuspid valves may fail to coapt properly in

Figure 10.2. Transverse sections of a normal heart (right) and a heart from a patient with dilated cardiomyopathy (DCM). In the DCM specimen, there is biventricular dilatation without a proportional increase in wall thickness. LV, left ventricle; RV, right ventricle. (Modified from Emmanouilides GC, ed. *Moss and Adams' Heart Disease in Infants, Children, and Adolescents*. 5th ed. Baltimore, MD: Lippincott Williams & Wilkins; 1995:86.)

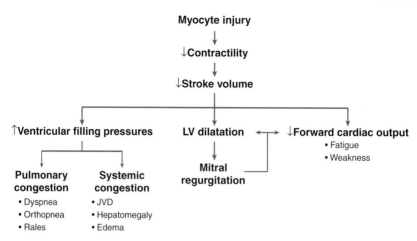

Figure 10.3. **Pathophysiology of dilated cardiomyopathy.** The reduced ventricular stroke volume results in decreased forward cardiac output and increased ventricular filling pressures. The listed clinical manifestations follow. JVD, jugular venous distention.

systole, and valvular regurgitation ensues. This regurgitation has three detrimental consequences: (1) excessive volume and pressure loads are placed on the atria, causing them to dilate, often leading to atrial fibrillation; (2) regurgitation of blood into the left atrium further decreases forward stroke volume into the aorta and systemic circulation; and (3) when the regurgitant volume returns to the LV during each diastole, an even greater volume load is presented to the dilated LV.

Clinical Findings

The clinical manifestations of DCM are those of congestive heart failure. The most common symptoms of low forward cardiac output include fatigue, lightheadedness, and exertional dyspnea associated with decreased tissue perfusion. Pulmonary congestion results in dyspnea, orthopnea, and paroxysmal nocturnal dyspnea, whereas chronic systemic venous congestion causes ascites and peripheral edema. Because these symptoms may develop insidiously, the patient may complain only of recent weight gain (because of interstitial edema) and shortness of breath on exertion.

Physical Examination

Signs of decreased cardiac output are often present and include cool extremities (owing to peripheral vasoconstriction), low arterial pressure, and tachycardia. Pulmonary venous congestion results in auscultatory crackles (rales), and basilar chest dullness to percussion may be present because of pleural effusions. Cardiac examination shows an enlarged heart with leftward displacement of a diffuse apical impulse. On auscultation, a third heart sound (S_3) is common as a sign of poor systolic function. The murmur of mitral valve regurgitation is often present as a result of the significant left ventricular dilatation. If right ventricular heart failure has developed, signs of systemic venous congestion may include jugular vein distention, hepatomegaly, ascites, and peripheral edema. Right ventricular enlargement and contractile dysfunction are often accompanied by the murmur of tricuspid valve regurgitation.

Diagnostic Studies

The *chest radiograph* shows an enlarged cardiac silhouette. If heart failure has developed, then pulmonary vascular redistribution, interstitial and alveolar edema, and pleural effusions are evident (see Fig. 3.5).

The *electrocardiogram (ECG)* usually demonstrates atrial and ventricular enlargement. Patchy fibrosis of the myofibers results in a wide array of arrhythmias, most importantly atrial fibrillation and ventricular tachycardia.

Conduction defects (left or right bundle branch block) occur in most cases. Diffuse repolarization (ST segment and T wave) abnormalities are common. In addition, regions of dense myocardial fibrosis may produce localized Q waves, resembling the pattern of previous myocardial infarction.

Echocardiography is very useful in the diagnosis of DCM. It typically demonstrates four-chamber cardiac enlargement with little hypertrophy and global reduction of systolic contractile function. Mitral and/or tricuspid regurgitation is also frequently visualized.

Cardiac catheterization is often performed to determine whether coexistent coronary artery disease is contributing to the impaired ventricular function. This procedure is most useful diagnostically in patients who have symptoms of angina or evidence of prior myocardial infarction on the ECG. Typically, hemodynamic measurements show elevated right- and left-sided diastolic pressures and diminished cardiac output. In the catheterization laboratory, a transvenous biopsy of the RV is sometimes performed in an attempt to clarify the etiology of the cardiomyopathy.

Cardiac magnetic resonance imaging (described in Chapter 3) is emerging as a promising technique in the evaluation of DCM, particularly for the diagnosis of myocardial inflammation (myocarditis).

Treatment

The goal of therapy in DCM is to relieve symptoms, prevent complications, and improve long-term survival. Thus, in addition to treating any identified underlying cause of DCM, therapeutic considerations include those described in the following sections.

Medical Treatment of Heart Failure

Approaches for the relief of vascular congestion and improvement in forward cardiac output are the same as standard therapies for heart failure (see Chapter 9). Initial therapy typically includes salt restriction and *diuretics,* vasodilator therapy with an *angiotensin-converting enzyme (ACE) inhibitor* or *angiotensin II receptor blocker (ARB),* and a β-*blocker.*

In patients with advanced heart failure, the potassium-sparing diuretic *spironolactone* should be considered. These measures have been shown to improve symptoms and reduce mortality in patients with DCM.

Prevention and Treatment of Arrhythmias

Atrial and ventricular arrhythmias are common in advanced DCM, and approximately 40% of deaths in this condition are caused by ventricular tachycardia or fibrillation. It is important to maintain serum electrolytes (notably, potassium and magnesium) within their normal ranges, especially during diuretic therapy, to avoid provoking serious arrhythmias. Studies have shown that available antiarrhythmic drugs do not prevent death from ventricular arrhythmias in DCM. In fact, when used in patients with poor LV function, many antiarrhythmic drugs may *worsen* the rhythm disturbance. *Amiodarone* is the contemporary antiarrhythmic studied most extensively in patients with DCM. Whereas there is no convincing evidence that it reduces mortality from ventricular arrhythmias in DCM, it is the safest antiarrhythmic for treating atrial fibrillation and other supraventricular arrhythmias in this population. In contrast to antiarrhythmic drugs, the placement of an implantable cardioverter-defibrillator (ICD) *does* reduce arrhythmic deaths in patients with DCM. Therefore, based on large-scale randomized trials, ICD placement is a recommended approach for patients with chronic symptomatic DCM and at least moderately reduced systolic function (e.g., LV ejection fraction ≤35%), regardless of the detection of ventricular arrhythmias.

Many patients with DCM have electrical conduction abnormalities that contribute to dyssynchronous ventricular contraction and reduced cardiac output. Electronic pacemakers capable of stimulating both ventricles simultaneously have been devised to better coordinate systolic contraction as an adjunct to medical therapy (*cardiac resynchronization therapy,* as described in Chapter 9). Demonstrated benefits of this approach include improved quality of life and exercise tolerance as well as decreased hospitalizations for heart failure and reduced mortality, particularly in those with pretreatment left bundle branch block or other conduction abnormalities with a markedly prolonged QRS duration.

Prevention of Thromboembolic Events

Patients with DCM are at increased risk of thromboembolic complications for reasons that include: (1) stasis in the ventricles resulting from poor systolic function, (2) stasis in the atria due to chamber enlargement or atrial fibrillation, and (3) venous stasis because of poor circulatory flow. Peripheral venous or right ventricular thrombus may lead to pulmonary emboli, whereas thromboemboli of left ventricular origin may lodge in any systemic artery, resulting in, for example, devastating cerebral, myocardial, or renal infarctions. The only *definite* indications for systemic anticoagulation in DCM patients are atrial fibrillation, a previous thromboembolic event, or an intracardiac thrombus visualized by echocardiography. However, chronic oral anticoagulation therapy (i.e., warfarin) is often administered to DCM patients who have *severe* depression of ventricular function (e.g., LV ejection fraction <30%) to prevent thromboembolism (be aware that prospective studies are lacking to confirm the effectiveness of this approach in DCM patients who are in sinus rhythm).

Cardiac Transplantation

In suitable patients, cardiac transplantation offers a substantially better 5-year prognosis than the standard therapies for DCM previously described. The current 5- and 10-year survival rates after transplantation are 74% and 55%, respectively. However, the scarcity of donor hearts greatly limits the availability of this technique. As a result, other mechanical options have been explored and continue to undergo experimental refinements, including ventricular assist devices and completely implanted artificial hearts.

Prognosis

Up to one third of patients will experience spontaneous improvement of heart function after the diagnosis of DCM is made. However, the prognosis for patients with persistent DCM who do not undergo cardiac transplantation is poor—the average 5-year survival rate is <50%. Methods to reduce progressive LV dysfunction by early intervention in asymptomatic or minimally symptomatic patients, and the prevention of sudden cardiac death, remain major research goals in the management of this disorder.

HYPERTROPHIC CARDIOMYOPATHY

Hypertrophic cardiomyopathy (HCM) has received notoriety in the lay press because it is the most common cardiac abnormality found in young athletes who die suddenly during vigorous physical exertion. With an incidence of about 1 of 500 in the general population, HCM is characterized by asymmetric (or sometimes global) left ventricular hypertrophy that is not caused by chronic pressure overload (i.e., *not* the result of systemic hypertension or aortic stenosis). Other terms frequently used to describe this disease are "hypertrophic obstructive cardiomyopathy" and "idiopathic hypertrophic subaortic stenosis". In this condition, systolic LV contractile function is vigorous but the thickened muscle is stiff, resulting in impaired ventricular relaxation and high diastolic pressures.

Etiology

HCM is a familial disease in which inheritance follows an autosomal dominant pattern with variable penetrance, and hundreds of mutations in several different genes have been implicated. The proteins encoded by the responsible genes are all part of the sarcomere complex and include β-myosin heavy chain (β-MHC), cardiac troponins, and myosin-binding protein C (see Table 10.2). The incorporation of these mutated peptides into the sarcomere is thought to cause impaired contractile function. The resultant increase in myocyte stress is then hypothesized to lead to compensatory hypertrophy and proliferation of fibroblasts.

The pathophysiology and natural history of familial HCM are quite variable and appear related to particular mutations within the disease-causing gene, rather than the actual gene involved. In fact, it has been shown that the precise genetic mutation determines the age of onset of hypertrophy, the extent and pattern of cardiac remodeling, and the person's risk of developing symptomatic heart failure or sudden death. For example, mutations in the β-MHC gene that alter electrical charge in the encoded protein are associated with worse prognoses than other mutations.

Pathology

Although hypertrophy in HCM may involve any portion of the ventricles, asymmetric hypertrophy of the ventricular septum (Fig. 10.4) is most common (approximately 90% of cases). Less often, the hypertrophy involves the ventricular walls symmetrically or is localized to the apex or midregion of the LV.

Unlike ventricular hypertrophy resulting from hypertension in which the myocytes enlarge uniformly and remain orderly, the histology of HCM is unusual. The myocardial fibers are in a pattern of extensive disarray (Fig. 10.5). Short, wide, hypertrophied fibers are oriented in chaotic directions and are surrounded by numerous cardiac fibroblasts and extracellular matrix. This myocyte disarray and fibrosis are characteristic of HCM

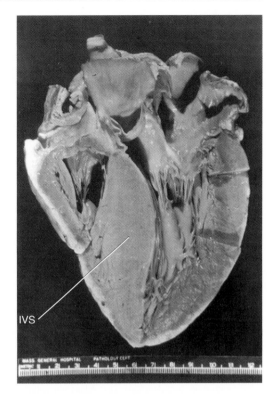

Figure 10.4. Postmortem heart specimen from a patient with hypertrophic cardiomyopathy. Marked left ventricular hypertrophy is present, especially of the interventricular septum (IVS).

and play a role in the abnormal diastolic stiffness and the arrhythmias common to this disorder.

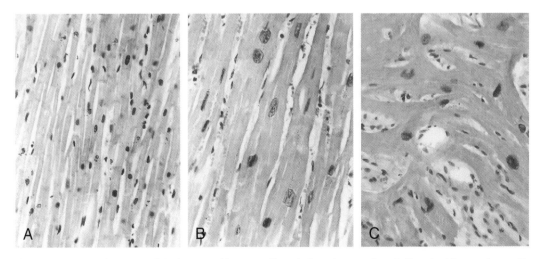

Figure 10.5. Light microscopy of the hypertrophic myocardium. A. Normal myocardium. **B.** Hypertrophic myocytes resulting from pressure overload in a patient with valvular heart disease. **C.** Disordered myocytes with fibrosis in a patient with hypertrophic cardiomyopathy. (Modified from Schoen FJ. *Interventional and Surgical Cardiovascular Pathology: Clinical Correlations and Basic Principles.* Philadelphia, PA: WB Saunders; 1989:181.)

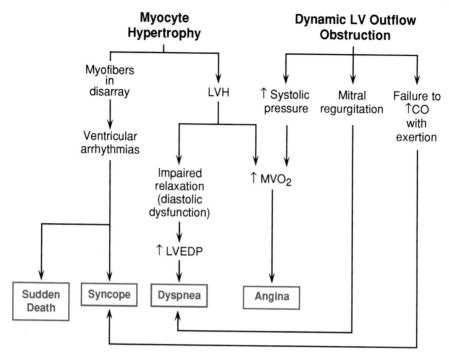

Figure 10.6. Pathophysiology of hypertrophic cardiomyopathy. The disarrayed and hypertrophied myocytes may lead to ventricular arrhythmias (which can cause syncope or sudden death) and impaired diastolic left ventricular (LV) relaxation (which causes elevated LV filling pressures and dyspnea). If dynamic left ventricular outflow obstruction is present, mitral regurgitation often accompanies it (which contributes to dyspnea), and the impaired ability to raise cardiac output with exertion can lead to exertional syncope. The thickened LV wall, and increased systolic pressure associated with outflow tract obstruction, each contribute to increased myocardial oxygen consumption (MVO$_2$) and can precipitate angina. CO, cardiac output; LVEDP, LV end-diastolic pressure; LVH, LV hypertrophy.

Pathophysiology

The predominant feature of HCM is marked ventricular hypertrophy that reduces the compliance and diastolic relaxation of the chamber, such that filling becomes impaired (Fig. 10.6). Patients who have asymmetric hypertrophy of the proximal interventricular septum may display additional findings related to transient obstruction of left ventricular outflow during systole. It is useful to consider the pathophysiology of HCM based on whether such systolic outflow tract obstruction is present.

HCM Without Outflow Tract Obstruction

Although systolic contraction of the LV is usually vigorous in HCM, hypertrophy of the walls results in increased stiffness and impaired relaxation of the chamber. The reduced ventricular compliance alters the normal pressure–volume relationship, causing the passive diastolic filling curve to shift upward (see Fig. 9.7B). The associated rise in diastolic LV pressure is transmitted backward, leading to elevated left atrial, pulmonary venous, and pulmonary capillary pressures. Dyspnea, especially during exertion, is thus a common symptom in this disorder.

HCM With Outflow Obstruction

Approximately one third of patients with HCM manifest systolic outflow tract obstruction. The mechanism of systolic obstruction is thought to involve abnormal motion of the anterior mitral valve leaflet toward the LV outflow tract where the thickened septum protrudes (Fig. 10.7). The process is explained as follows: (1) during ventricular contraction, ejection of blood toward the aortic valve is more rapid than usual, because it must flow through an outflow tract that is narrowed by the thickened septum; (2) this rapid flow creates Venturi

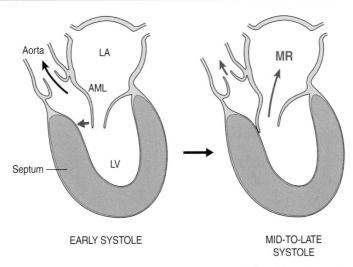

EARLY SYSTOLE

MID-TO-LATE
SYSTOLE

Figure 10.7. Pathophysiology of left ventricular (LV) outflow obstruction and mitral regurgitation in hypertrophic cardiomyopathy. Left panel. The LV outflow tract is abnormally narrowed between the hypertrophied interventricular septum and the anterior leaflet of the mitral valve (AML). It is thought that the rapid ejection velocity along the narrowed tract in early systole draws the AML toward the septum *(small arrow)*. **Right panel.** As the mitral valve anterior leaflet abnormally moves toward, and contacts, the septum, outflow into the aorta is transiently obstructed. Because the mitral leaflets do not coapt normally in systole, mitral regurgitation (MR) also results.

forces that abnormally draw the anterior mitral leaflet toward the septum during contraction; and (3) the anterior mitral leaflet approaches and abuts the hypertrophied septum, causing transient obstruction of blood flow into the aorta.

In patients with outflow obstruction, elevated left atrial and pulmonary capillary wedge pressures result from both the decreased ventricular compliance and the outflow obstruction during contraction. During systolic obstruction, a pressure gradient develops between the main body of the LV and the outflow tract distal to the obstruction (see Fig. 10.7). The elevated ventricular systolic pressure increases wall stress and myocardial oxygen consumption, which can result in angina (see Fig. 10.6). In addition, because obstruction is caused by abnormal motion of the anterior mitral leaflet toward the septum (and therefore *away* from the posterior mitral leaflet), the mitral valve does not close properly during systole, and mitral regurgitation may result. Such regurgitation further elevates left atrial and pulmonary venous pressures and may worsen symptoms of dyspnea, as well

as contribute to the development of atrial fibrillation.

The systolic pressure gradient observed in obstructive HCM is dynamic in that its magnitude varies during the contraction phase and depends, at any given time, on the distance between the anterior leaflet of the mitral valve and the hypertrophied septum. Situations that *decrease* LV cavity size (e.g., reduced venous return because of intravascular volume depletion) bring the mitral leaflet and septum into closer proximity and *promote* obstruction. Conversely, conditions that *enlarge* the LV (e.g., augmented intravascular volume) increase the distance between the anterior mitral leaflet and septum and *reduce* the obstruction. Positive inotropic drugs (which augment the force of contraction) also force the mitral leaflet and septum into closer proximity and contribute to obstruction, whereas negative inotropic drugs (e.g., β-blockers, verapamil) have the opposite effect.

Although dynamic systolic outflow tract obstruction creates impressive murmurs and receives great attention, the symptoms of obstructive HCM appear to primarily stem from the increased LV stiffness and diastolic dysfunction also present in the nonobstructive form.

Clinical Findings

The symptoms of HCM vary widely in different individuals, from none to marked physical limitations. The average age of presentation is the mid-20s.

The most frequent symptom is *dyspnea* owing to elevated diastolic LV (and therefore pulmonary capillary) pressure. This symptom is further exacerbated by the high systolic LV pressure and mitral regurgitation found in patients with outflow tract obstruction.

Angina is often described by patients with HCM, even in the absence of obstructive coronary artery disease. Myocardial ischemia may be contributed to by (1) the high oxygen demand of the increased muscle mass and (2) the narrowed small branches of the coronary arteries within the hypertrophied ventricular wall. If outflow tract obstruction is present, the high systolic ventricular pressure also increases myocardial oxygen demand because of the increased wall stress.

Syncope in HCM may result from cardiac arrhythmias that develop because of the structurally abnormal myofibers. In patients with outflow tract obstruction, syncope may also be induced by exertion, when the pressure gradient is made worse by the increased force of contraction, thereby causing a transient fall in cardiac output. Orthostatic lightheadedness is also common in patients with outflow tract obstruction. This occurs because venous return to the heart is reduced on standing by the gravitational pooling of blood in the lower extremities. The LV thus decreases in size and outflow tract obstruction intensifies, transiently reducing cardiac output and cerebral perfusion.

When arrhythmias occur, symptoms of HCM may be exacerbated. For example, *atrial fibrillation* is not well tolerated because the loss of the normal atrial "kick" further impairs diastolic filling and can worsen symptoms of pulmonary congestion. Of greatest concern, the first clinical manifestation of HCM may be *ventricular fibrillation,* resulting in *sudden cardiac death,* particularly in young adults with HCM during strenuous physical exertion.

Risk factors for sudden death among patients with HCM include a history of syncope, a family history of sudden death, certain high-risk HCM mutations, and extreme hypertrophy of the LV wall (>30 mm in thickness).

Physical Examination

Patients with mild forms of HCM are often asymptomatic and have normal or near-normal physical exams. A common finding is the presence of a fourth heart sound (S_4), generated by left atrial contraction into the stiffened LV (see Chapter 2). The forceful atrial contraction may also result in a palpable presystolic impulse over the cardiac apex (a "double apical impulse").

Other findings are common in patients with systolic outflow obstruction. The carotid pulse rises briskly in early systole but then quickly declines as obstruction to cardiac outflow appears. The characteristic systolic murmur of LV outflow obstruction is rough and crescendo–decrescendo in shape, heard best at the left lower sternal border (because of turbulent flow through the narrowed outflow tract). In addition, as the stethoscope is moved toward the apex, the holosystolic blowing murmur of the accompanying mitral regurgitation may be auscultated. Although the LV outflow obstruction murmur may be soft at rest, bedside maneuvers that alter preload and afterload can dramatically increase its intensity and help differentiate this murmur from other conditions, such as aortic stenosis (Table 10.3).

A commonly used technique in this regard is the *Valsalva maneuver,* produced by asking the patient to "bear down" (technically defined as forceful exhalation with the nose, mouth, and glottis closed). The Valsalva maneuver increases intrathoracic pressure, which decreases venous return to the heart and transiently

Table 10.3. Effect of Maneuvers on Murmurs of Aortic Stenosis and Hypertrophic Cardiomyopathy

	Valsalva	Squatting	Standing
HCM murmur	↑	↓	↑
AS murmur	↓	↑	↓

HCM, hypertrophic cardiomyopathy; AS, aortic stenosis.

reduces LV size. This action brings the hypertrophied septum and anterior leaflet of the mitral valve into closer proximity, creating greater obstruction to forward flow. Thus, during Valsalva, the murmur of HCM *increases* in intensity. In contrast, the murmur of aortic stenosis decreases in intensity during Valsalva because of the reduced flow across the stenotic valve.

Conversely, a change from standing to a *squatting position* suddenly augments venous return to the heart (which increases preload) while simultaneously increasing the systemic vascular resistance. The increased preload raises the stroke volume and therefore causes the murmur of aortic stenosis to become louder. In contrast, the transient increase in LV size during squatting reduces the LV outflow tract obstruction in HCM and softens the intensity of that murmur. Sudden *standing* from a squatting position has the opposite effect on each of these murmurs (see Table 10.3).

Diagnostic Studies

The *ECG* typically shows left ventricular hypertrophy and left atrial enlargement. Prominent Q waves are common in the inferior and lateral leads, representing amplified forces of initial depolarization of the hypertrophied septum directed away from those leads. In some patients, diffuse T wave inversions are present, which can predate clinical, echocardiographic, or other electrocardiographic manifestations of HCM. Atrial and ventricular arrhythmias are frequent, especially atrial fibrillation. Ventricular arrhythmias are particularly ominous because they may herald ventricular fibrillation and sudden death, even in previously asymptomatic patients.

Echocardiography is very helpful in the evaluation of HCM. The degree of LV hypertrophy can be measured and regions of asymmetrical wall thickness readily identified. Signs of left ventricular outflow obstruction may also be demonstrated and include abnormal anterior motion of the mitral valve as it is drawn toward the hypertrophied septum during systole, and partial closure of the aortic valve in midsystole as flow across it is transiently obstructed. Doppler recordings during echocardiography

accurately measure the outflow pressure gradient and quantify any associated mitral regurgitation. Children and adolescents with apparently mild HCM should undergo serial echocardiographic assessment over time, because the degree of hypertrophy may increase during puberty and early adulthood.

Cardiac catheterization is reserved for patients for whom the diagnosis is uncertain or if percutaneous septal ablation (described in the Treatment section) is planned. The major feature in patients with obstruction is the finding of a pressure gradient within the outflow portion of the LV, either at rest or during maneuvers that transiently reduce LV size and promote outflow tract obstruction. Myocardial biopsy at the time of catheterization is not necessary, because histologic findings do not predict disease severity or long-term prognosis.

Finally, genetic testing can be helpful in establishing, or excluding, the diagnosis of HCM in family members of an affected patient when a specific mutation in that family has been identified.

Treatment

β-*Blockers* are standard therapy for HCM because they (1) reduce myocardial oxygen demand by slowing the heart rate and the force of contraction (and therefore diminish angina and dyspnea); (2) lessen any LV outflow gradient during exercise by reducing the force of contraction (allowing the chamber size to increase, thus separating the anterior leaflet of the mitral valve from the ventricular septum); (3) increase passive diastolic ventricular filling time owing to the decreased heart rate; and (4) decrease the frequency of ventricular ectopic beats. Despite their antiarrhythmic effect, β-blockers have *not* been shown to prevent sudden arrhythmic death in this condition.

Calcium channel antagonists can reduce ventricular stiffness and are sometimes useful in improving exercise capacity in patients who fail to respond to β-blockers. Patients who develop pulmonary congestion may benefit from mild diuretic therapy, but these drugs must be administered cautiously to avoid volume depletion; reduced intravascular volume decreases LV size and could exacerbate outflow tract obstruction. Vasodilators (including nitrates) similarly reduce LV size and should be avoided.

Atrial fibrillation is poorly tolerated in HCM and should be controlled aggressively, most commonly with *antiarrhythmic drugs.* Effective and useful antiarrhythmic drugs for atrial fibrillation in HCM include amiodarone and disopyramide (a type IA antiarrhythmic drug that also possesses negative inotropic properties that may help reduce LV outflow tract obstruction; see Chapter 17). Digitalis should be avoided in HCM because its positive inotropic effect increases the force of contraction and can worsen LV outflow tract obstruction.

Sudden cardiac death has a propensity to occur in patients with HCM in association with physical exertion; therefore, strenuous exercise and competitive sports should be avoided. Sudden death in this syndrome is almost always caused by ventricular tachycardia or fibrillation. Although amiodarone may reduce the frequency of ventricular arrhythmias, HCM patients who are at high risk (i.e., a family history of sudden death, extreme hypertrophy with ventricular wall thickness >30 mm, unexplained prior syncopal episodes, history of high-grade ventricular tachyarrythmias) should receive an ICD. ICD therapy is life saving for both primary prevention in such patients, and for HCM patients who have already survived a cardiac arrest.

Some studies have shown clinical improvement when patients with the obstructive form of HCM are treated with a dual-chamber permanent pacemaker, the electrodes of which are placed in the right atrium and RV. The LV outflow gradient may become reduced by this procedure, possibly by altering the normal sequence of ventricular contraction, such that septal–mitral valve apposition becomes less prominent. This technique seems to be useful for only a small percentage of markedly symptomatic patients.

Surgical therapy (*myomectomy*) is considered for patients whose symptoms do not respond adequately to pharmacologic therapy. This procedure involves excision of portions of the hypertrophied septal muscle mass and usually improves outflow tract obstruction, symptoms, and exercise capacity. A less invasive alternative is *percutaneous septal ablation,* performed in the cardiac catheterization laboratory, in which ethanol is injected directly into the first major septal coronary artery (a branch of the left anterior descending artery), causing a small, controlled myocardial infarction. The desired and often achieved result is reduction of septal thickness and improvement in outflow tract obstruction. Randomized trials have not been performed to compare the outcomes of ethanol septal ablation with surgical myomectomy. Thus, while septal ablation is an alternative for persistently symptomatic patients who cannot tolerate an operation, myomectomy remains the standard accepted procedure given its 40+ year history of experience and efficacy.

Theoretically, infective endocarditis could develop in patients with the obstructive form of HCM because of turbulent blood flow through the LV outflow tract and the associated mitral regurgitation. However, that is rare and antibiotic prophylaxis for prevention of endocarditis in this condition is no longer recommended (see Chapter 8).

Finally, genetic counseling should be provided to all patients with HCM. Because it is an autosomal dominant disease, children of affected persons have a 50% chance of inheriting the abnormal gene. First-degree relatives of patients with HCM should be screened by physical examination, electrocardiography, echocardiography, and sometimes genetic testing. Even asymptomatic HCM patients are at risk of complications, including sudden death, and must be evaluated.

Prognosis

The incidence of sudden death in HCM is 2% to 4% per year in adults and 4% to 6% in children and adolescents. It has become clear that different mutations have vastly different phenotypes. Some cause extreme hypertrophy in childhood without any clinical symptoms until the occurrence of sudden death; others present later in life with heart failure symptoms. Most mutations produce only mild hypertrophy and are associated with a normal life expectancy. As the natural histories of specific mutations are better defined, the use and timing of specific therapeutic interventions will likely improve.

RESTRICTIVE CARDIOMYOPATHY

The restrictive cardiomyopathies are less common than DCM and HCM. They are characterized by abnormally rigid (but not necessarily thickened) ventricles with impaired diastolic filling but usually normal, or near-normal, systolic function. This condition results from either (1) fibrosis or scarring of the endomyocardium or (2) infiltration of the myocardium by an abnormal substance (Table 10.4).

The most common recognized cause of restrictive cardiomyopathy in nontropical countries is **amyloidosis.** In this systemic disease, insoluble misfolded amyloid fibrils deposit within tissues, including the heart, causing organ dysfunction. Amyloid deposition is diagnosed histologically by the Congo red stain, which displays amyloid fibrils with a characteristic green birefringence under polarized light.

Amyloid fibrils can pathologically develop from a host of different proteins that distinguish the categories of disease. *Primary amyloidosis* is caused by deposition of immunoglobulin light chain AL fragments secreted by a plasma cell tumor (usually, multiple

myeloma). In contrast, *secondary amyloidosis* is characterized by the presence of AA amyloid (derived from the inflammatory marker serum amyloid A) in a variety of chronic inflammatory conditions, such as rheumatoid arthritis. Less common is *hereditary amyloidosis,* an autosomal dominant condition in which amyloid fibrils form from point mutations in the protein transthyretin (formerly known as prealbumin). *Senile amyloidosis* refers to a condition in the elderly, in which amyloid deposits, derived from transthyretin or other proteins, are found scattered throughout the vascular system, muscles, kidney, and lung. In each form of amyloidosis, cardiac involvement is marked by deposition of extracellular amyloid between myocardial fibers in the atria and ventricles, in the coronary arteries and veins, and in the heart valves.

Clinical manifestations of cardiac involvement are most common in the primary (AL) form of amyloidosis and typically relate to the development of restrictive cardiomyopathy because of the infiltrating amyloid protein. Diastolic dysfunction is the prominent cardiac abnormality; systolic dysfunction may also develop later in the disease. Orthostatic hypotension is present in about 10% of patients, likely contributed to by amyloid deposition in the autonomic nervous system and peripheral blood vessels. Infiltration of amyloid into the cardiac conduction system can cause arrhythmias and conduction impairments, which can result in syncope or sudden death.

Pathophysiology

Reduced compliance of the ventricles in restrictive cardiomyopathy, whether due to infiltration or fibrosis, results in an upward shift of the passive ventricular filling curve (see Fig. 9.7B), leading to abnormally high diastolic pressures. This condition has two major consequences: (1) elevated systemic and pulmonary venous pressures, with signs of right- and left-sided vascular congestion, and (2) reduced ventricular cavity size with decreased stroke volume and cardiac output.

Clinical Findings

It follows from the underlying pathophysiology that signs of left- and right-sided heart

Table 10.4. Examples of Restrictive Cardiomyopathy

Noninfiltrative
Idiopathic
Scleroderma

Infiltrative
Amyloidosis
Sarcoidosis

Storage diseases
Hemochromatosis
Glycogen storage diseases

Endomyocardial disease
Endomyocardial fibrosis
Hypereosinophilic syndrome
Metastatic tumors
Radiation therapy

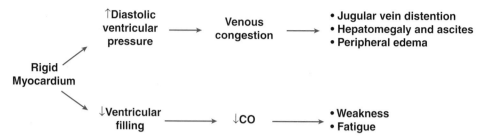

Figure 10.8. Pathophysiology of restrictive cardiomyopathy. The rigid myocardium results in elevated ventricular diastolic pressures and decreased ventricular filling. The resultant symptoms can be predicted from these abnormalities. CO, cardiac output.

failure are expected (Fig. 10.8). Decreased cardiac output is manifested by fatigue and decreased exercise tolerance. Systemic congestion (often more prominent than pulmonary congestion in this syndrome) leads to jugular venous distention, peripheral edema, and ascites with a large, tender liver. Arrhythmias, including atrial fibrillation, are common. Infiltrative etiologies that involve the cardiac conduction system can cause conduction blocks.

Physical Examination

Signs of congestive heart failure are often present, including pulmonary rales, distended neck veins, ascites, and peripheral edema. Similar to constrictive pericarditis (see Chapter 14), jugular venous distention may paradoxically worsen with inspiration (the *Kussmaul sign*) because the stiffened RV cannot accommodate the increased venous return.

Diagnostic Studies

The *chest radiograph* usually shows a normal-sized heart with signs of pulmonary congestion. The *ECG* often displays nonspecific ST and T wave abnormalities; conduction disturbances such as atrioventricular block or a bundle branch block may be present.

The restrictive cardiomyopathies share nearly identical symptoms, physical signs, and hemodynamic profiles with constrictive pericarditis, as described in Chapter 14. However, it is important to distinguish these two entities because constrictive pericarditis is often correctable, whereas interventions for the restrictive cardiomyopathies are more limited.

The most useful diagnostic tools to differentiate restrictive cardiomyopathy from constrictive pericarditis are transvenous endomyocardial biopsy, computed tomography (CT), and magnetic resonance imaging (MRI). For example, in restrictive cardiomyopathy, a transvenous endomyocardial biopsy may demonstrate the presence of infiltrative matter such as amyloid, iron deposits (hemochromatosis), or metastatic tumors. Conversely, CT or MRI scans are useful to identify the thickened pericardium of constrictive pericarditis, a finding that is not expected in restrictive cardiomyopathy.

Treatment

Restrictive cardiomyopathy typically has a very poor prognosis, except when treatment can target an underlying cause. For example, phlebotomy and iron chelation therapy may be helpful in the early stages of hemochromatosis. Symptomatic therapy for all etiologies includes salt restriction and cautious use of diuretics to improve symptoms of systemic and pulmonary congestion. Unlike the dilated cardiomyopathies, vasodilators are not helpful because systolic function is usually preserved. Maintenance of sinus rhythm (e.g., converting atrial fibrillation if it occurs) is important to maximize diastolic filling and forward cardiac output. Some restrictive cardiomyopathies are prone to intraventricular thrombus formation, thus warranting chronic oral anticoagulant therapy. In the case of primary (AL) amyloidosis, chemotherapy followed by autologous bone marrow stem cell transplantation has proved effective in selected patients with early cardiac involvement.

SUMMARY

1. The cardiomyopathies are diseases of heart muscles classified by their pathophysiologic presentation into dilated, hypertrophic, or restrictive types (Table 10.5).

2. Dilated cardiomyopathies are characterized by ventricular dilatation with impaired systolic function. Progressive left ventricular enlargement often leads to symptomatic heart failure, ventricular arrhythmias, and/or embolic complications.

3. HCM is characterized by a thickened LV with impaired diastolic relaxation. Dynamic LV outflow tract obstruction during systole may be present. The most common symptoms are dyspnea and exertional angina. Ventricular arrhythmias may lead to sudden cardiac death.

4. The restrictive cardiomyopathies are uncommon and are characterized by impairment of diastolic ventricular relaxation owing to an infiltrated or fibrotic myocardium. Symptoms of heart failure are typical.

Table 10.5. Summary of the Cardiomyopathies

	Dilated Cardiomyopathy	Hypertrophic Cardiomyopathy	Restrictive Cardiomyopathy
Ventricular morphology	Dilated LV with little concentric hypertrophy	Marked hypertrophy, often asymmetric	Fibrotic or infiltrated myocardium
	LA / LV		
Etiologies	Genetic, infectious, alcoholic, peripartum	Genetic	Amyloidosis, hemochromatosis, scleroderma, radiation therapy
Symptoms	Fatigue, weakness, dyspnea, orthopnea, PND	Dyspnea, angina, syncope	Dyspnea, fatigue
Physical exam	Pulmonary rales, S_3; if RV failure present: JVD, hepatomegaly, peripheral edema	S_4; if outflow obstruction present: systolic murmur loudest at left sternal border, accompanied by mitral regurgitation	Predominantly signs of RV failure: JVD, hepatomegaly, peripheral edema
Pathophysiology	Impaired systolic contraction	Impaired diastolic relaxation; LV systolic function vigorous, often with dynamic obstruction	"Stiff" LV with impaired diastolic relaxation but usually normal systolic function
Cardiac size on chest radiograph	Enlarged	Normal or enlarged	Usually normal
Echocardiogram	Dilated, poorly contractile LV	LV hypertrophy, often more pronounced at septum; systolic anterior movement of MV with mitral regurgitation	Usually normal systolic contraction; "speckled" appearance in infiltrative disorders

LV, left ventricle; PND, paroxysmal nocturnal dyspnea; RV, right ventricle; JVD, jugular venous distension; MV, mitral valve.

Acknowledgments

The authors thank Frederick Schoen, MD, for providing pathology specimens. Contributors to the previous editions of this chapter were Marc N. Wein, MD; Yi-Bin Chen, MD; Kay Fang, MD; David Grayzel, MD; G. William Dec, MD; and Leonard S. Lilly, MD.

Additional Reading

Cooper L. Myocarditis. *N Engl J Med*. 2009;360: 1526–1538.

Fifer MA, Vlahakes GJ. Management of symptoms in hypertrophic cardiomyopathy. *Circulation*. 2008;117:429–439.

Friedrich MG, Sechtem U, Schulz-Menger J, et al. Cardiovascular magnetic resonance in myocarditis: a JACC white paper. *J Am Coll Cardiol*. 2009;53:1475–1487.

Hershberger RE, Lindenfeld J, Mestroni L, et al. Genetic evaluation of cardiomyopathy. *J Card Fail*. 2009;15:83–97.

Ho CY, Seidman CE. A contemporary approach to hypertrophic cardiomyopathy. *Circulation*. 2006; 113:e858–e862.

Maron BJ, Spirito P, Shen WK, et al. Implantable cardioverter-defibrillators and prevention of sudden cardiac death in hypertrophic cardiomyopathy. *JAMA*. 2007;298:405–412.

Maron BJ, Towbin JA, Thiene G, et al. Contemporary definitions and classification of the cardiomyopathies: an American Heart Association scientific statement from the Council on Clinical Cardiology, Heart Failure and Transplantation Committee; Quality of Care and Outcomes Research and Functional Genomics and Translational Biology Interdisciplinary Working Groups; and Council on Epidemiology and Prevention. *Circulation*. 2006;113:1807–1816.

Schultz JC, Hilliard AA, Cooper LT, et al. Diagnosis and treatment of viral myocarditis. *Mayo Clin Proc*. 2009;84:1001–1009.

Selvanayagam JB, Hawkins PN, Paul B, et al. Evaluation and management of the cardiac amyloidosis. *J Am Coll Cardiol*. 2007;50: 2101–2110.

Silwa K, Fett J, Elkayam U. Peripartum cardiomyopathy. *Lancet*. 2006;38:687–693.

Yazdani K, Maraj S, Amanullah AM. Differentiating constrictive pericarditis from restrictive cardiomyopathy. *Rev Cardiovasc Med*. 2005;6:61–71.

Mechanisms of Cardiac Arrhythmias

Ranliang Hu
William G. Stevenson
Gary R. Strichartz
Leonard S. Lilly

NORMAL IMPULSE FORMATION
Ionic Basis of Automaticity
Native and Latent Pacemakers
Overdrive Suppression
Electrotonic Interactions

ALTERED IMPULSE FORMATION
Alterations in Sinus Node Automaticity
Escape Rhythms
Enhanced Automaticity of Latent Pacemakers
Abnormal Automaticity
Triggered Activity

ALTERED IMPULSE CONDUCTION
Conduction Block
Unidirectional Block and Reentry

PHYSIOLOGIC BASIS OF ANTIARRHYTHMIC THERAPY
Bradyarrhythmias
Tachyarrhythmias

Normal cardiac function relies on the flow of electric impulses through the heart in an exquisitely coordinated fashion. Abnormalities of the electric rhythm are known as *arrhythmias* (also termed *dysrhythmias*) and are among the most common clinical problems encountered. The presentations of arrhythmias range from common benign palpitations to very severe symptoms of low cardiac output and death; therefore, a thorough understanding of these disorders is important to the daily practice of medicine.

Abnormally slow rhythms are termed *bradycardias* (or *bradyarrhythmias*). Fast rhythms are known as *tachycardias* (or *tachyarrhythmias*). Tachycardias are further characterized as *supraventricular* when they involve the atrium or AV node, and designated *ventricular* when they originate from the His-Purkinje system or ventricles. This chapter describes the mechanisms by which such arrhythmias develop, followed by a general description of their management. Chapter 12 summarizes specific rhythm disorders and how to recognize and treat them.

Disorders of heart rhythm result from alterations of **impulse formation, impulse conduction,** or both. This chapter first addresses how abnormalities of impulse formation and conduction occur, and under what circumstances they cause arrhythmias. Figure 11.1 provides an organizational schema for this presentation.

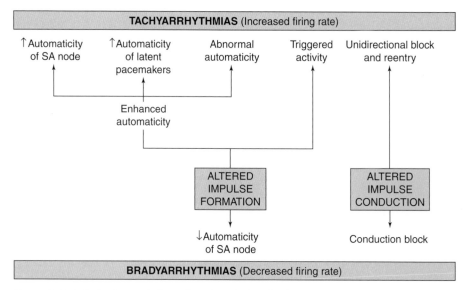

Figure 11.1. Arrhythmias result from alterations in impulse formation and/or impulse conduction. Tachyarrhythmias result from enhanced automaticity, unidirectional block with reentry, or triggered activity. Bradyarrhythmias result from decreased automaticity or conduction block. SA, sinoatrial.

NORMAL IMPULSE FORMATION

As described in Chapter 1, electric impulse formation in the heart arises from the intrinsic automaticity of specialized cardiac cells. **Automaticity** refers to a cell's ability to depolarize itself to a threshold voltage to generate a *spontaneous* action potential. Although atrial and ventricular myocytes do not have this property under normal conditions, the cells of the specialized conducting system do possess natural automaticity and are therefore termed **pacemaker cells.** The specialized conducting system includes the sinoatrial (SA) node, the atrioventricular (AV) nodal region, and the ventricular conducting system. The latter is composed of the bundle of His, the bundle branches, and the Purkinje fibers. In *pathologic* situations, myocardial cells outside the conducting system may also acquire automaticity.

Ionic Basis of Automaticity

Cells with natural automaticity do not have a static resting voltage. Rather, they inherently display gradual depolarization during phase 4 of the action potential (Fig. 11.2). If this spontaneous diastolic depolarization reaches the threshold condition, an action potential upstroke is generated. An important ionic current largely responsible for phase 4 spontaneous depolarization is known as the **pacemaker current (I_f).** The channels that carry this current are activated by hyperpolarization (increasingly negative voltages) and mainly conduct sodium ions. I_f channels begin to open when the membrane voltage becomes more negative than approximately -50 mV and are *different* from the fast sodium channels responsible for rapid phase 0 depolarization in ventricular and atrial myocytes. The inward flow of Na^+ through these slow channels, driven by its concentration gradient and the negative intracellular potential, depolarizes the membrane toward threshold.

In the pacemaker cells of the SA node, alterations in three other ionic currents also contribute to phase 4 gradual depolarization: (1) a slow inward calcium current, carried mostly by L-type Ca^{++} channels that become activated at voltages reached near the end of phase 4, (2) a progressive decline of an *outward* potassium current, and (3) an additional inward sodium current mediated by activation of the sodium—calcium exchanger by calcium release from the sarcoplasmic reticulum (SR). The latter mechanism, driven by oscillatory release of calcium from the SR, has been referred to as the "calcium clock."

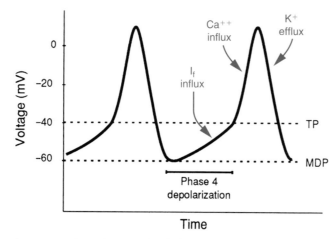

Figure 11.2. **The action potential (AP) of a pacemaker cell (e.g., from the sinus node).** Notice the slow phase 4 depolarization, largely caused by the I_f (pacemaker) current through slow Na^+ channels, which drives the cell to threshold (potential of approximately -40 mV). The upstroke of the AP is caused by the slow inward current of Ca^+ ions. Inactivation of the calcium channels and K^+ wefflux through potassium channels are responsible for repolarization. MDP, maximum negative diastolic potential; TP, threshold potential.

When the membrane potential of a pacemaker cell reaches the threshold condition, the upstroke of the action potential is generated. In contrast to the phase 0 upstroke of cells in the Purkinje system, that of cells in the sinus and AV nodes is much slower (see Fig. 11.2). The reason for the difference is that the membrane potential determines the proportion of fast sodium channels that are in a resting state capable of depolarization, compared with an inactivated state. The number of available (or resting-state) fast sodium channels increases as the resting membrane potential becomes more negative. Because sinus and AV nodal cells have *less negative* maximum diastolic membrane voltages (-50 to -60 mV) than do Purkinje cells (-90 mV), a greater proportion of the fast sodium channels is inactivated in these pacemaker cells. Thus, the action potential upstroke relies to a greater extent on a *calcium* current (through the relatively slower opening of Ca^{++} channels) and has a less rapid rate of rise than cells of the Purkinje system or ventricular myocardium. The repolarization phase of pacemaker cells depends on inactivation of the calcium channels and the opening of voltage-gated potassium channels that permit efflux of potassium from the cells.

Native and Latent Pacemakers

The distinct populations of automatic cells in the specialized conduction pathway have different intrinsic rates of firing. These rates are determined by three variables that influence how fast the membrane potential reaches the threshold condition: (1) the rate (i.e., the slope) of phase 4 spontaneous depolarization, (2) the maximum negative diastolic potential, and (3) the threshold potential. A more negative maximum diastolic potential, or a less negative threshold potential, slows the rate of impulse initiation because it takes longer to reach the threshold value (Fig. 11.3). Conversely, the greater the I_f, the steeper the slope of phase 4 and the faster the cell depolarizes. The size of I_f depends on the number and kinetics of the individual pacemaker channels through which this current flows.

Since all healthy myocardial cells are electrically connected by gap junctions, an action potential generated in one part of the myocardium will ultimately spread to all other regions. When an impulse arrives at a cell that is not yet close to threshold, current from the depolarized cell will bring the adjacent cell's membrane potential to the threshold level so that it will fire (regardless of how close its

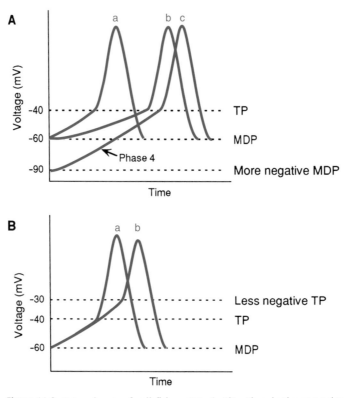

Figure 11.3. Determinants of cell firing rates. A. Alterations in the pacemaker current (I_f) and in the magnitude of the maximum diastolic potential (MDP) alter the cell firing rate. (a) The normal action potential (AP) of a pacemaker cell. (b) Reduced I_f renders the slope of phase 4 less steep; thus, the time required to reach threshold potential (TP) is increased. (c) The MDP is more negative; therefore, the time required to reach TP is increased. **B.** Alterations in TP change the firing rate of the cell. Compared with the normal TP (a), the TP in b is less negative; thus, the duration of time to achieve threshold is increased, and the firing rate decreases.

intrinsic I_f has brought it to threshold). Thus, the pacemaker cells with the fastest rate of depolarization set the heart rate. In the normal heart, the dominant pacemaker is the *sinoatrial node*, which at rest initiates impulses at a rate of 60 to 100 bpm. Because the sinus node rate is faster than that of the other tissues that possess automaticity, its repeated discharges prevent spontaneous firing of other potential pacemaker sites.

The SA node is known as the **native pacemaker** because it normally sets the heart rate. Other cells within the specialized conduction system harbor the potential to act as pacemakers if necessary, and are therefore called **latent pacemakers** (or **ectopic pacemakers**). In contrast to the SA node, the AV node and the bundle of His have intrinsic firing rates of 50 to 60 bpm, and cells of the Purkinje system have rates of

approximately 30 to 40 bpm. These latent sites may initiate impulses and take over the pacemaking function if the SA node slows or fails to fire, or if conduction abnormalities block the normal wave of depolarization from reaching them.

Overdrive Suppression

Not only does the cell population with the fastest intrinsic rhythm preempt all other automatic cells from spontaneously firing, it also directly *suppresses* their automaticity. This phenomenon is called overdrive suppression. Cells maintain their trans-sarcolemmal ion distributions because of the continuously active Na^+K^+-ATPase pump that extrudes three Na^+ ions from the cell in exchange for two K^+ ions transported in (Fig. 11.4). Because its net transport effect is one positive charge in the outward

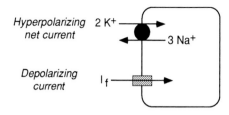

Figure 11.4. Competition between the depolarizing pacemaker current (I_f) and the Na^+K^+-ATPase pump, which produces a hyperpolarizing current. The Na^+K^+-ATPase pump transports three positive charges outside the cell for every two it pumps in. The hyperpolarizing current acts to suppress automaticity by antagonizing I_f and contributes to overdrive suppression in cells that are stimulated more rapidly than their intrinsic firing rate.

direction, the Na^+K^+-ATPase pump creates a *hyperpolarizing* current (i.e., it tends to make the inside of the cell *more negative*). As the cell potential becomes increasingly negative, additional time is required for spontaneous phase 4 depolarization to reach the threshold voltage (see Fig. 11.3A), and therefore the rate of spontaneous firing is decreased. Although the hyperpolarizing current moves the membrane away from threshold, pacemaker cells firing at their own intrinsic rate have an I_f current sufficiently large to overcome this hyperpolarizing influence (see Fig. 11.4).

The hyperpolarizing current *increases* when a cell is forced to fire faster than its intrinsic pacemaker rate. The more frequently the cell is depolarized, the greater the quantity of Na^+ ions that enter the cell per unit time. As a result of the increased intracellular Na^+, the Na^+K^+-ATPase pump becomes more active, thereby tending to restore the normal transmembrane Na^+ gradient. This increased pump activity provides a larger hyperpolarizing current, opposing the depolarizing current I_f, and further decreases the rate of spontaneous depolarization. Thus, overdrive suppression decreases a cell's automaticity when that cell is driven to depolarize faster than its intrinsic discharge rate.

Electrotonic Interactions

In addition to overdrive suppression, *anatomic connections* between pacemaker and nonpacemaker cells are important in determining how adjacent cells suppress latent pacemaker foci.

Myocardial cells in the ventricle and Purkinje system repolarize to a resting potential of approximately -90 mV, whereas pacemaker cells in the sinus and AV nodes repolarize to a maximum diastolic potential of about -60 mV. When these two cell types are adjacent to one another, they are *electrically coupled* through low-resistance gap junctions concentrated in their intercalated discs. This coupling results in a compromise of electric potentials owing to electrotonic current flow between the cells, causing relative *hyperpolarization* of the pacemaker cell and relative *depolarization* of the nonpacemaker cell (Fig. 11.5). The hyperpolarizing current in the coupled pacemaker cell competes with I_f and causes the slope of phase 4 diastolic depolarization to be less steep, thereby reducing the cell's automaticity. Electrotonic effects may be particularly important in suppressing automaticity in the AV node (via connections between atrial myocytes and AV nodal cells) and in the distal Purkinje fibers (which are coupled to nonautomatic ventricular myocardial cells). In contrast, cells in the center of the SA node are less tightly coupled to atrial myocytes; thus, their automaticity is less subject to electrotonic interactions.

Decoupling of normally suppressed cells, such as those in the AV node (e.g., by ischemic damage), may reduce the inhibitory electrotonic influence and *enhance* automaticity, producing ectopic rhythms by the latent pacemaker tissue.

ALTERED IMPULSE FORMATION

Arrhythmias may arise from altered impulse formation at the SA node or from other sites, including the specialized conduction pathways or regions of cardiac muscle. The main abnormalities of impulse initiation that lead to arrhythmias are (1) **altered automaticity** (of the sinus node or latent pacemakers within the specialized conduction pathway), (2) **abnormal automaticity** in atrial or ventricular myocytes, and (3) **triggered activity**.

Alterations in Sinus Node Automaticity

The rate of impulse initiation by the sinus node, as well as by the latent pacemakers of

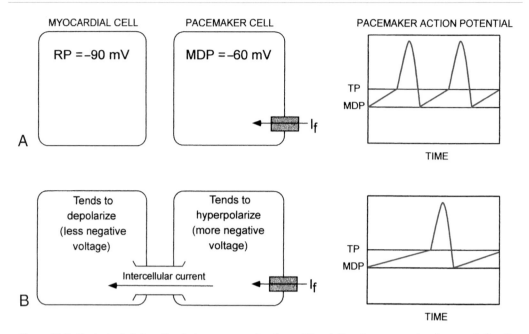

Figure 11.5. **Electrotonic interaction between pacemaker (e.g., AV nodal) and nonpacemaker (myocardial) cells.** **A.** When pacemaker cells are not coupled to myocardial cells, they have a maximum negative potential (MDP) of approximately −60 mV, whereas myocardial cells have a resting potential (RP) of approximately −90 mV. **B.** When pacemaker cells and myocytes are neighbors, they may be connected electrically by gap junctions in their intercalated discs (e.g., in the AV node). In this situation, electric current flows between the pacemaker cell and the myocardial cell, tending to hyperpolarize the former and depolarize the latter, driving their membrane potentials closer to one another. The hyperpolarizing current opposes I_f of the pacemaker cell, such that the slope of phase 4 depolarization is less steep and therefore cellular automaticity is suppressed. If a disease state impairs coupling between cells, the influence of surrounding myocytes on the pacemaker cell is reduced, allowing I_f to depolarize to threshold more readily and enhancing automaticity. TP, threshold potential.

the specialized conducting system, is regulated primarily by neurohumoral factors.

Increased Sinus Node Automaticity

The most important modulator of normal sinus node automaticity is the autonomic nervous system. Sympathetic stimulation, acting through β_1-adrenergic receptors, increases the open probability of the pacemaker channels (Fig. 11.6), through which I_f can flow. The increase in I_f leads to a steeper slope of phase 4 depolarization, causing the SA node to reach threshold and fire earlier than normal and the heart rate to increase.

In addition, sympathetic stimulation shifts the action potential threshold to more negative voltages by increasing the probability that voltage-sensitive Ca^{++} channels are capable of opening (recall that calcium carries the current of phase 0 depolarization in pacemaker cells). Therefore, diastolic depolarization reaches

the threshold potential earlier. Sympathetic activity thus increases sinus node automaticity both by increasing the rate of pacemaker depolarization via I_f and by causing the action potential threshold to become more negative. Examples of this normal physiologic effect occur during exercise or emotional stress, when sympathetic stimulation appropriately increases the heart rate.

Decreased Sinus Node Automaticity

Normal decreases in SA node automaticity are mediated by reduced sympathetic stimulation and by increased activity of the parasympathetic nervous system. Whereas activation of the sympathetic nervous system has a major role in increasing the heart rate during times of stress, the parasympathetic nervous system is the major controller of the heart rate at rest.

Cholinergic (i.e., parasympathetic) stimulation via the vagus nerve acts at the SA node

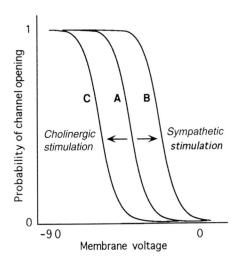

Figure 11.6. Effect of sympathetic and parasympathetic (cholinergic) stimulation on pacemaker current channels. The channels through which the pacemaker current (I_f) flows are voltage gated, opening at more negative membrane potentials. At any given voltage, there exists a probability between 0 and 1 that a specific channel will be open. Compared with normal baseline behavior *(curve A)*, sympathetic stimulation *(curve B)* or treatment with anticholinergic drugs shifts this probability to a higher value for any given level of membrane voltage, thus increasing the number of open channels and the rate at which the cell will fire. *Curve C* shows that parasympathetic stimulation (or treatment with β-blockers) has the opposite effect, decreasing the probability of a channel being open, and therefore inhibiting depolarization.

to reduce the probability of pacemaker channels being open (see Fig. 11.6). Thus, I_f and the slope of phase 4 depolarization are reduced, and the intrinsic firing rate of the cell is slowed. In addition, the probability of the Ca^{++} channels being open is decreased, such that the action potential threshold increases to a more positive potential. Furthermore, cholinergic stimulation increases the probability of acetylcholine-sensitive K^+ channels being open at rest. Positively charged K^+ ions exit through these channels, producing an outward current that drives the diastolic potential to become more negative. The overall effect of reduced I_f, a more negative maximum diastolic potential, and a less negative threshold level is a slowing of the intrinsic firing rate and therefore a reduced heart rate.

It follows that the use of pharmacologic agents that modify these effects of the autonomic nervous system will also affect the firing rate of the SA node. For example, β-receptor blocking drugs ("β-blockers") antagonize the β-adrenergic sympathetic effect; therefore, they *decrease* the rate of phase 4 depolarization of the SA node and slow the heart rate. Conversely, atropine, an anticholinergic (antimuscarinic) drug, has the opposite effect: by blocking parasympathetic activity, the rate of phase 4 depolarization *increases* and the heart rate accelerates.

Escape Rhythms

If the sinus node becomes suppressed and fires less frequently than normal, the site of impulse formation often shifts to a latent pacemaker within the specialized conduction pathway. An impulse initiated by a latent pacemaker because the SA node rate has slowed is called an **escape beat.** Persistent impairment of the SA node will allow a continued series of escape beats, termed an **escape rhythm.** Escape rhythms are protective in that they prevent the heart rate from becoming pathologically slow when SA node firing is impaired.

As discussed in the previous section, suppression of sinus node activity may occur because of increased parasympathetic tone. Different regions of the heart have different sensitivities to parasympathetic (vagal) stimulation. The SA node and the AV node are most sensitive to such an influence, followed by atrial tissue. The ventricular conducting system is the least sensitive. Therefore, moderate parasympathetic stimulation slows the sinus rate and allows the pacemaker to shift to the AV node. However, very strong parasympathetic stimulation suppresses excitability at both the SA node and AV node, and may therefore result in the emergence of a ventricular escape pacemaker.

Enhanced Automaticity of Latent Pacemakers

Another means by which a latent pacemaker can assume control of impulse formation is if it develops an intrinsic rate of depolarization *faster* than that of the sinus node. Termed an **ectopic beat,** the impulse is *premature* relative to the normal rhythm, whereas an escape beat is *late* and terminates a pause caused by a slowed sinus rhythm. A sequence of similar ectopic beats is called an **ectopic rhythm.**

Ectopic beats may arise in several circumstances. For example, high catecholamine concentrations can enhance the automaticity of latent pacemakers, and if the resulting rate of depolarization exceeds that of the sinus node, then an ectopic rhythm will develop. Ectopic beats are also commonly induced by hypoxemia, ischemia, electrolyte disturbances, and certain drug toxicities (such as digitalis, as described in Chapter 17).

Abnormal Automaticity

Cardiac tissue injury may lead to pathologic changes in impulse formation whereby myocardial cells *outside* the specialized conduction system acquire automaticity and spontaneously depolarize. Although such activity may appear similar to impulses originating from latent pacemakers within the specialized conduction pathways, these ectopic beats arise from cells that do not usually possess automaticity. If the rate of depolarization of such cells exceeds that of the sinus node, they transiently take over the pacemaker function and become the source of an abnormal ectopic rhythm.

Because these myocardial cells have few or no activated pacemaker channels, they do not normally carry I_f. How injury allows such cells to spontaneously depolarize has not been fully elucidated. However, when myocytes become injured, their membranes become "leaky." As such, they are unable to maintain the concentration gradients of ions, and the resting potential becomes less negative (i.e., the cell partially depolarizes). When a cell's membrane potential is reduced to a value less negative than -60 mV, gradual phase 4 depolarization can be demonstrated even among nonpacemaker cells. This spontaneous depolarization probably results from a very slowly inactivating calcium current and a decrease in the outward potassium current that normally acts to repolarize the cell.

Triggered Activity

Under certain conditions, an action potential can "trigger" abnormal depolarizations that result in extra heart beats or rapid arrhythmias. This process may occur when the first action potential leads to oscillations of the membrane voltage known as *afterdepolarizations*. Unlike the *spontaneous* activity seen when enhanced automaticity occurs, this type of automaticity is *stimulated* by a preceding action potential. As illustrated in Figures 11.7 and 11.8, there are two types of afterdepolarizations depending on their timing after the inciting action potential: *early* afterdepolarizations occur during the repolarization phase of the inciting beat, whereas *delayed* afterdepolarizations occur shortly after repolarization has been completed. In either case, abnormal action potentials are triggered if the afterdepolarization reaches a threshold voltage.

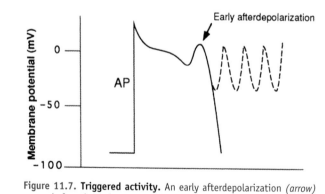

Figure 11.7. **Triggered activity.** An early afterdepolarization *(arrow)* occurs before the action potential (AP) has fully repolarized. Repetitive afterdepolarizations *(dashed curve)* may produce a rapid sequence of triggered action potentials and hence a tachyarrhythmia.

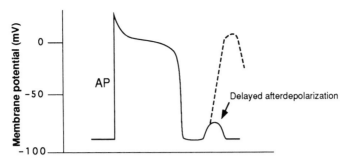

Figure 11.8. Triggered activity. A delayed afterdepolarization *(arrow)* arises after the cell has fully repolarized. If the delayed afterdepolarization reaches the threshold voltage, a propagated action potential (AP) is triggered *(dashed curve)*.

Early afterdepolarizations are changes of the membrane potential in the positive direction that interrupt normal repolarization (see Fig 11.7). They can occur either during the plateau of the action potential (phase 2) or during rapid repolarization (phase 3). Early afterdepolarizations are more likely to develop in conditions that prolong the action potential duration (and therefore the electrocardiographic QT interval), as may occur during therapy with certain drugs (see Chapter 17) and in the inherited long-QT syndromes (see Chapter 12).

The ionic current responsible for an early afterdepolarization depends on the membrane voltage at which the triggered event occurs. If the early afterdepolarization occurs during phase 2 of the action potential, when most of the Na^+ channels are in an inactivated state, the upstroke of the triggered beat relies mostly on an inward Ca^{++} current. If, however, the afterdepolarization occurs during phase 3 (when the membrane voltage is more negative), there is partial recovery of the inactivated Na^+ channels, which then contribute more to the current underlying the triggered beat.

An early afterdepolarization-triggered action potential can be self-perpetuating and lead to a series of depolarizations (see Fig. 11.7). Early afterdepolarizations appear to be the initiating mechanism of the polymorphic ventricular tachycardia known as torsades de pointes, which is described in Chapter 12.

Delayed afterdepolarizations may appear shortly after repolarization is complete (see Fig. 11.8). They most commonly develop in states of *high intracellular calcium*, as may be present with digitalis intoxication (see Chapter 17), or during marked catecholamine stimulation. It is thought that intracellular Ca^{++} accumulation causes the activation of chloride currents or of the $Na^+–Ca^{++}$ exchanger that results in brief inward currents that generate the delayed afterdepolarization.

As with early afterdepolarizations, if the amplitude of the delayed afterdepolarization reaches a threshold voltage, an action potential will be generated. Such action potentials can be self-perpetuating and lead to tachyarrhythmias. Some idiopathic ventricular tachycardias that occur in otherwise structurally normal hearts are likely due to this mechanism, as are atrial and ventricular tachycardias associated with digitalis toxicity (see Chapter 17).

ALTERED IMPULSE CONDUCTION

Alterations in impulse conduction also lead to arrhythmias. Conduction blocks generally slow the heart rate (bradyarrhythmias); however, under certain circumstances, the process of reentry (described later) can ensue and produce abnormal fast rhythms (tachyarrhythmias).

Conduction Block

A propagating impulse is blocked when it encounters a region of the heart that is electrically unexcitable. Conduction block can be either transient or permanent and may be unidirectional (i.e., conduction proceeds when the involved region is stimulated from one direction, but not when stimulated from the opposite direction, as described below) or bidirectional (conduction is blocked in both directions). Various conditions may cause conduction block, including ischemia, fibrosis, inflammation, and certain drugs. When conduction block occurs because a propagating impulse encounters cardiac cells that are still refractory (from a previous depolarization), the block is said to be *functional*. A propagating impulse that arrives later may be conducted. For example, antiarrhythmic drugs that prolong action potential duration tend to produce functional conduction block. When conduction block is caused by a barrier imposed by fibrosis or scarring that replaces myocytes, conduction block is *fixed*.

Conduction block within the specialized conducting system of the AV node or the His-Purkinje system prevents normal propagation of the cardiac impulse from the sinus node to more distal sites. This atrioventricular block (AV block) removes the normal overdrive suppression that keeps latent pacemakers in the His-Purkinje system in check. Thus, conduction block usually results in emergence of escape beats or escape rhythms, as the more distal sites assume the pacemaker function.

AV block is common and a major reason for implantation of a permanent pacemaker, as discussed in Chapter 12.

Unidirectional Block and Reentry

A common mechanism by which altered impulse conduction leads to tachyarrhythmias is termed **reentry.** During such a rhythm, an electric impulse circulates repeatedly around a reentry path, recurrently depolarizing a region of cardiac tissue.

During normal cardiac conduction, each electric impulse that originates in the SA node travels in an orderly, sequential fashion through the rest of the heart, ultimately depolarizing all the myocardial fibers. The refractory period of each cell prevents immediate reexcitation from adjacent depolarized cells, so that the impulse stops when all of the heart muscle has been excited. However, conduction blocks that prevent rapid depolarization of parts of the myocardium can create an environment conducive to continued impulse propagation and reentry, as illustrated in Figure 11.9.

The figure depicts electric activity as it flows through a branch point anywhere within the conduction pathways. Panel A shows propagation of a normal action potential. At point *x*, the impulse reaches two parallel pathways (α and β) and travels down each into the more distal conduction tissue. In the normal heart, the α and β pathways have similar conduction velocities and refractory periods such that the wave fronts that pass through them may collide in the distal conduction tissue and extinguish each other.

Panel B shows what happens if conduction is blocked in one limb of the pathway. In this example, the action potential is obstructed when it encounters the β pathway from above and therefore propagates only down the α tract into the distal tissue. As the impulse continues to spread, it encounters the distal end of the β pathway (at point *y*). If the tissue in the distal β tract is also unable to conduct, the impulse simply continues to propagate into the deeper tissues and reentry does not occur. However, if the impulse at point *y* is able to propagate retrogradely (backward) into pathway β, one of the necessary conditions for reentry has been met.

When an action potential can conduct in a retrograde direction in a conduction pathway, whereas it had been prevented from doing so in the forward direction, **unidirectional block** is said to be present. Unidirectional block tends to occur in regions where the refractory periods of adjacent cells are heterogeneous, such that some cells recover before others. In addition, unidirectional block may occur in states of cellular dysfunction, and in regions where fibrosis has altered the myocardial structure.

As shown in panel C of Figure 11.9, if the impulse is able to propagate retrogradely up the β pathway, it will again arrive at point *x*. At that time, if the α pathway has not yet repolarized from the previous action potential that had occurred moments earlier, that limb is refractory to repeat stimulation and the returning impulse simply stops there.

However, panel D illustrates what happens if the velocity of retrograde conduction

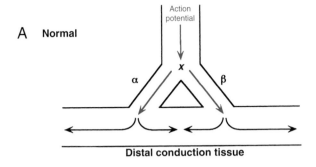

A   Normal

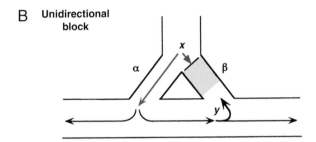

B   Unidirectional block

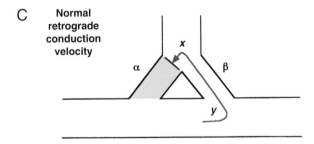

C   Normal retrograde conduction velocity

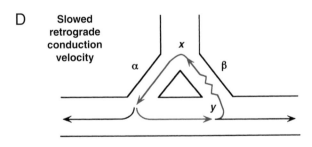

D   Slowed retrograde conduction velocity

Figure 11.9. **Mechanism of reentry. A.** Normal conduction. When an action potential (AP) reaches a branch in the conduction pathway (point *x*), the impulse travels down both fibers (α and β) to excite distal conduction tissue. **B.** Unidirectional block. Forward passage of the impulse is blocked in the β pathway but proceeds normally down the α pathway. When the impulse reaches point *y*, if retrograde conduction of the β pathway is intact, the AP can enter β from below and conduct in a retrograde fashion. **C.** When point *x* is reached again, if the α pathway has not had sufficient time to repolarize, then the impulse stops. **D.** However, if conduction through the retrograde pathway is sufficiently slow *(jagged line)*, it reaches point *x* after the α pathway has recovered. In that circumstance, the impulse is able to excite the α pathway again and a reentrant loop is formed.

in the diseased β path is not normal but *slower than normal.* In that case, sufficient time may elapse for the α pathway to repolarize before the returning impulse reaches point *x* from the β limb. Then the invading impulse is able to stimulate the α pathway once again, and the cycle repeats itself. This circular stimulation can continue indefinitely, and each pass of the impulse through the loop excites cells of the distal conduction tissue, which propagates to the rest of the myocardium, at an abnormally high rate resulting in a tachyarrhythmia.

For the mechanism of reentry to occur, the propagating impulse must continuously encounter excitable tissue. Thus, the time it takes for the impulse to travel around the reentrant loop must be greater than the time required for recovery (the refractory period) of the tissue, and this must be true for each point in the circuit. If the conduction time is shorter than the recovery time, the impulse will encounter refractory tissue and stop. Because normal conduction velocity in ventricular myocytes is approximately 50 cm/sec and their average effective refractory period is about 0.2 sec, a reentry path circuit would need to be at least 10 cm long for reentry to occur in a normal ventricle. However, with *slower* conduction velocities, a shorter reentry circuit is possible. Most clinical cases of reentry occur within small regions of tissue because the conduction velocity within the reentrant loop is, in fact, abnormally slow.

In summary, the two critical conditions for reentry are (1) unidirectional block and (2) slowed conduction through the reentry path. These conditions commonly occur in regions where fibrosis has developed, such as infarction scars. In some cases, reentry occurs over an anatomically fixed circuit or path, such as AV reentry using an accessory pathway (as discussed in the following section). Reentry around distinct anatomic pathways usually appears as a *monomorphic tachycardia* on the electrocardiogram (ECG); that is, in the case of ventricular tachycardia, each QRS has the same appearance as the preceding and subsequent QRS complexes. This is because the reentry path is the same from beat to beat, producing a stable, regular tachycardia. This is the most common mechanism of ventricular tachycardia associated with areas of ventricular scar, as from a prior myocardial infarction.

Other types of reentry do not require a stable, fixed path. For example, one form can occur in electrically heterogeneous myocardium, in which waves of reentrant excitation spiral through the tissue, continually changing direction. These so-called "spiral waves" can be initiated when a wave front of depolarization encounters a broad region of functional block, which could be refractory from a preceding wave front, or be poorly excitable tissue due to myocardial ischemia or be under the influence of certain antiarrhythmic medications. Forward propagation of the wave front is asymmetrically blocked by this region, as the remainder of the front proceeds around the block. As the region repolarizes and becomes excitable again, parts of the wave front then spread retrogradely through it and continue in a spiral path following in the wake of the depolarization that had just passed. Unlike an anatomically fixed reentrant tract, the center of the spiral wave can move through the myocardium and even split into two or more reentry waves. In the ventricles, the resulting tachycardia has a continually changing QRS appearance producing *polymorphic ventricular tachycardia*. If such activation is rapid and very disorganized, no distinct QRS complexes will be discernable and the rhythm is *ventricular fibrillation* (as described in Chapter 12).

Accessory Pathways and the Wolff–Parkinson–White Syndrome

The concept of reentry is dramatically illustrated by the **Wolff–Parkinson–White (WPW) syndrome.** In the normal heart, the impulse generated by the SA node propagates through atrial tissue to the AV node, where expected slower conduction causes a short delay before continuing on to the ventricles. However, approximately 1 in 1,500 people has the WPW syndrome and is born with an additional connection between an atrium and ventricle. Termed an accessory pathway or bypass tract, this connection allows conduction between the atria and ventricles to bypass the AV node. The most common type of accessory pathway consists of microscopic fibers that span the AV groove somewhere along the mitral or tricuspid annuli (known as a *bundle of Kent*), as shown in Figure 11.10.

Because accessory pathway tissue conducts impulses faster than the AV node, stimulation of the ventricles during sinus rhythm begins earlier than normal, and the PR interval of the ECG is therefore *shortened* (usually <0.12 sec, or <3 small boxes). In this situation, the ventricles are said to be "preexcited." However, the accessory pathway connects to ventricular myocardium rather than to the Purkinje

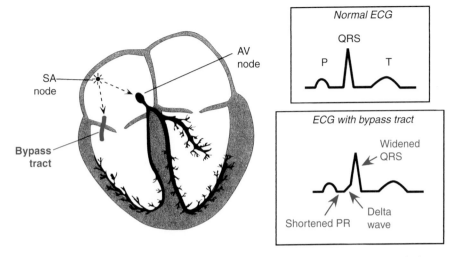

Figure 11.10. Accessory pathway (also termed a bypass tract). Example of an atrioventricular bypass tract (bundle of Kent), shown schematically, which can conduct impulses from the atrium directly to the ventricles, bypassing the AV node. The ECG demonstrates a short PR interval and a "delta wave" caused by early excitation of the ventricles via the accessory pathway. ECG, electrocardiogram; SA, sinoatrial.

system, such that the subsequent spread of the impulse through the ventricles from that site is slower than usual. In addition, because *normal* conduction over the AV node proceeds concurrently, ventricular depolarization represents a combination of the electric impulse traveling via the accessory tract *and* that conducted through the normal conduction pathway. As a result, the QRS complex in patients with WPW is wider than normal and demonstrates an abnormally slurred initial upstroke, known as a *delta wave* (Fig. 11.10).

During sinus rhythm, simultaneous conduction through the accessory pathway and AV node creates an interesting ECG appearance but causes no symptoms. The presence of the abnormal pathway, however, creates an ideal condition for reentry because the refractory period of the pathway is usually different from that of the AV node. An appropriately timed abnormal impulse (e.g., a premature beat) may encounter block in the accessory pathway but conduct through the AV node, or vice versa. If the propagating impulse then finds that the initially blocked pathway has recovered (unidirectional block), it can conduct in a retrograde direction up to the atrium and then down the other pathway back to the ventricles. Thus, a large anatomic loop is established, with the accessory pathway serving as

one limb and the normal conduction pathway through the AV node as the other. The clinical characteristics of the WPW syndrome, including the types of reentrant tachycardia associated with it, are described in Chapter 12.

The mechanisms of altered impulse formation and conduction form the basis of all common arrhythmias, both abnormally slow rhythms (bradyarrhythmias) and abnormally fast ones (tachyarrhythmias). Table 11.1 lists the underlying mechanisms and examples of their commonly associated rhythm disturbances.

PHYSIOLOGIC BASIS OF ANTIARRHYTHMIC THERAPY

Appropriate treatment of a rhythm disorder depends on its severity and its likely mechanism. When an arrhythmia produces severe hypotension or cardiac arrest, it must be immediately terminated to restore effective cardiac function. Therapy for termination may include electric cardioversion (an electric "shock") for tachycardias, cardiac pacing for bradycardias, or administration of medications.

Additional therapy to prevent recurrences is guided by the etiology of the rhythm

Table 11.1. Mechanisms of Arrhythmia Development

Abnormality	Mechanism	Examples
Bradyarrhythmias		
Altered impulse formation		
• Decreased automaticity	Decreased phase 4 depolarization (e.g., parasympathetic stimulation)	Sinus bradycardia
Altered impulse conduction		
• Conduction blocks	Ischemic, anatomic, or drug-induced impaired conduction	First-, second-, and third-degree AV blocks
Tachyarrhythmias		
Altered impulse formation		
• Enhanced automaticity		
Sinus node	Increased phase 4 depolarization (e.g., sympathetic stimulation)	Sinus tachycardia
AV node		AV junctional tachycardia
Ectopic focus	Acquires phase 4 depolarization	Ectopic atrial tachycardia and some forms of VT
• Triggered activity		
Early afterdepolarization	Prolonged action potential duration	Torsades de pointes
Delayed afterdepolarization	Intracellular calcium overload (e.g., digitalis toxicity)	APBs, VPBs, digitalis-induced arrhythmias, "idiopathic" VT
Altered impulse conduction		
• Reentry	Unidirectional block plus slowed conduction	
Anatomical		Atrial flutter, AV nodal reentrant tachycardia, VT related to ventricular scar tissue
Functional		Atrial fibrillation, polymorphic VT, ventricular fibrillation

AV, atrioventricular; APB, atrial premature beat; VPB, ventricular premature beat; VT, ventricular tachycardia.

disturbance. Correctable factors that contribute to abnormal impulse formation and conduction (such as ischemia or electrolyte abnormalities) should be corrected. If there is a risk of recurrent arrhythmia, medications that alter automaticity, conduction and/or refractoriness may be administered. Sometimes, catheter or surgical ablation of conduction pathways is undertaken to physically disrupt the region responsible for the arrhythmia. Other advanced options include implantation of a permanent pacemaker for serious bradyarrhythmias or an internal cardioverter-defibrillator (ICD) to automatically terminate malignant tachyarrhythmias should they recur. The following sections summarize the common therapeutic modalities, and Chapter 12 describes how they are used to address specific rhythm disorders.

Bradyarrhythmias

Not all slow heart rhythms require specific treatment. For those that do, pharmacologic therapy can increase the heart rate acutely, but the effect is transient. Electronic pacemakers are used when more sustained therapy is needed.

Pharmacologic Therapy

Pharmacologic therapy of bradyarrhythmias modifies the autonomic input to the heart in one of two ways:

1. *Anticholinergic drugs* (i.e., antimuscarinic agents such as atropine). Vagal stimulation reduces the rate of sinus node depolarization (which slows the heart rate) and decreases conduction through the AV node, through the release of acetylcholine onto muscarinic receptors. Anticholinergic drugs competitively bind to muscarinic receptors and thereby reduce the vagal effect. This results in an increased heart rate and enhanced AV nodal conduction.

2. β_1-*Receptor agonists* (e.g., isoproterenol). Mimicking the effect of endogenous catecholamines, these drugs increase heart rate and speed AV nodal conduction.

Atropine and isoproterenol are administered intravenously. Although these drugs are useful in managing certain slow heart rhythms emergently, it is not practical to continue them over the long term to treat persistent bradyarrhythmias.

Electronic Pacemakers

Electronic pacemakers apply repeated electric stimulation to the heart to initiate depolarizations at a desired rate, thereby assuming control of the rhythm. Pacemakers may be installed on a temporary or a permanent basis. Temporary units are used to stabilize patients who are awaiting implantation of a permanent pacemaker or to treat transient bradyarrhythmias, such as those caused by reversible drug toxicities.

There are two types of **temporary pacemakers.** *External* transthoracic pacemakers deliver electric pulses to the patient's chest through large adhesive electrodes placed on the skin. The advantage of this technique is that it can be applied rapidly. Unfortunately, because the current used must be sufficient to initiate a cardiac depolarization, it stimulates thoracic nerves and skeletal muscle, which can be quite uncomfortable. Therefore, this form of pacing is usually used only on an emergency basis until another means of treating the arrhythmia can be implemented.

The other option for temporary pacing is a *transvenous* unit. In this case, an electrode-tipped catheter is inserted percutaneously into the venous system, passed into the heart, and connected to an external power source (termed a pulse generator). Electric pulses are applied directly to the heart through the electrode catheter, which is typically placed in the right ventricle or right atrium. This type of pacing is not painful and can be effective for days. There is, however, a risk of infection and/or thrombosis associated with the catheter.

Permanent pacemakers are more sophisticated than the temporary variety. Various configurations can sense and capture the electric activity of the atria and/or ventricles. One or more wires (known as leads) with pacing electrodes are passed through an axillary or subclavian vein into the right ventricle or right atrium, or through the coronary sinus into a cardiac vein (to stimulate the left ventricle). The pulse generator, similar in size to two silver dollars stacked on top of one another, is connected to the leads and then implanted under the skin, typically in the infraclavicular region. The pacemaker battery typically lasts about 10 years.

Modern permanent pacemakers sense cardiac activity and pace only when needed. They incorporate complex functions to track the patient's normal heart rate and can stimulate beats automatically in response to activity. They can also record useful data, such as whether fast rates have been sensed (that might indicate a tachyarrhythmia), the amount of pacing that has been required, and other parameters of pacemaker function. An external radio frequency programming device is used to "interrogate" the pacemaker to obtain the recorded information and to adjust the pacing functions.

Although the most common indications for permanent pacemakers are bradyarrhythmias, pacemakers that incorporate a left ventricular pacing lead are also used to improve cardiac performance in some patients with heart failure (*cardiac resynchronization therapy*—see Chapter 9).

Tachyarrhythmias

The treatment of tachyarrhythmias is directed at (1) protection of the patient from the consequences of the arrhythmia and (2) the specific mechanism responsible for the abnormal rhythm. Pharmacologic agents and cardioversion/defibrillation are commonly used approaches, but innovative electric devices and transvenous catheter–based techniques to intentionally damage (ablate) arrhythmia-causing tissue have revolutionized treatment of these disorders.

Pharmacologic Therapy

Pharmacologic management of tachyarrhythmias is directed against the underlying mechanism (abnormal automaticity, reentrant circuits, or triggered activity). Many antiarrhythmic drugs are available and the choice of which to use relies on the cause of the specific arrhythmia. From consideration of the arrhythmia mechanisms presented in this chapter, the following strategies emerge.

Desired Drug Effects to Eliminate Rhythms Caused by Increased Automaticity:

1. Reduce the slope of phase 4 spontaneous depolarization of the automatic cells
2. Make the diastolic potential more negative (hyperpolarize)
3. Make the threshold potential less negative

Desired Antiarrhythmic Effects to Interrupt Reentrant Circuits:

1. Decrease conduction in the reentry circuit to the point that conduction fails, thus stopping the reentry impulse
2. Increase the refractory period within the reentrant circuit so that a propagating impulse finds tissue within the loop unexcitable and the impulse stops
3. Suppress premature beats that can initiate reentry

Desired Drug Effects to Eliminate Triggered Activity:

1. Shorten the action potential duration (to prevent early afterdepolarizations)
2. Correct conditions of calcium overload (to prevent delayed afterdepolarizations)

Drugs used to achieve these goals modulate the action potential through interactions with ion channels, surface receptors, and transport pumps. Many drugs have multiple effects and may attack arrhythmias through more than one mechanism. The commonly used antiarrhythmic drugs and their actions are described in Chapter 17.

It is extremely important to recognize that in addition to suppressing arrhythmias, these drugs have the potential to *aggravate* or provoke certain rhythm disturbances. This undesired consequence is referred to as **proarrhythmia** and is a major limitation of contemporary antiarrhythmic drug therapy. For example, antiarrhythmic agents that act therapeutically to prolong the action potential duration can, as an undesired effect, cause early afterdepolarizations, the mechanism underlying the polymorphic ventricular tachycardia known as torsades de pointes (see Chapter 12). In addition, most agents used to treat tachyarrhythmias have the potential to aggravate bradyarrhythmias, and all antiarrhythmics have potentially toxic noncardiac side effects. These shortcomings have led to an increased reliance on nonpharmacologic treatment options, as described in the following sections.

Vagotonic Maneuvers

Many tachycardias involve transmission of impulses through the AV node, a structure that is sensitive to vagal modulation. Vagal tone can be transiently increased by a number of bedside maneuvers, and performing these may slow conduction, which terminates some reentrant tachyarrhythmias. For example, **carotid sinus massage** is performed by rubbing firmly for a few seconds over the carotid sinus, located at the bifurcation of the internal and external carotid arteries on either side of the neck. This maneuver stimulates the baroreceptor reflex (see Chapter 13), which elicits the desired increase in vagal tone and withdrawal of sympathetic tone. This maneuver should be performed on only one carotid sinus at a time (to prevent interference with brain perfusion) and is best avoided in patients with known atherosclerosis involving the carotid arteries.

Electric Cardioversion and Defibrillation

Cardioversion and defibrillation involve the application of an electric shock to terminate a tachycardia. A shock with sufficient energy depolarizes the bulk of excitable myocardial tissue, interrupts reentrant circuits, establishes electric homogeneity, and allows the sinus node (the site of fastest spontaneous discharge) to regain pacemaker control. Tachyarrhythmias that are caused by reentry can usually be terminated by this procedure, whereas arrhythmias due to abnormal automaticity may simply persist.

External cardioversion is used to terminate supraventricular tachycardias or organized ventricular tachycardias. It is performed by briefly sedating the patient and then placing two large electrode paddles (or adhesive electrodes) against the chest on either side of the heart. The electric discharge is electronically *synchronized* to occur at the time of a QRS complex (i.e., when ventricular depolarization occurs). This prevents the possibility of discharge during the T-wave, when a shock can induce reentry (leading to ventricular fibrillation) because regions of myocardium are in different phases of depolarization and recovery.

External defibrillation is performed to terminate ventricular fibrillation, employing the same equipment as that used for cardioversion. However, during fibrillation, there is no organized QRS complex on which to synchronize the electric discharge, so it is delivered using the "asynchronous" mode of the device.

Implantable Cardioverter Defibrillators

ICDs automatically terminate dangerous ventricular arrhythmias using *internal* cardioversion/defibrillation, or by way of a special type of artificial pacing. These devices are implanted, in a manner similar to that of permanent pacemakers, in patients at high risk of sudden cardiac death from ventricular arrhythmias. The device continuously monitors cardiac activity, and if the heart rate exceeds a certain programmable threshold for a specified time, the ICD delivers an appropriate intervention, such as an electric shock. Internal cardioversion or defibrillation requires substantially less energy

than external defibrillation but is still painful if the patient is conscious.

The majority of monomorphic ventricular tachycardias can be terminated by an ICD with a rapid burst of electric impulses, termed *antitachycardia pacing (ATP)*, rather than a shock. The goal is to artificially pace the heart at a rate faster than the tachycardia to prematurely depolarize a portion of a reentrant circuit, thereby rendering it refractory to further immediate stimulation. Consequently, when a reentrant impulse returns to the zone that has already been depolarized by the device, it encounters unexcitable tissue, it cannot propagate further, and the circuit is broken. An advantage of the ATP technique is that, unlike internal cardioversion, it is painless. However, ATP is not effective for terminating ventricular fibrillation, a situation in which the device is programmed to deliver an electric shock instead.

Catheter Ablation

If an arrhythmia originates from a distinct anatomical reentry circuit or an automatic focus, electrophysiologic mapping techniques can be used to localize the region of myocardium or conduction tissue responsible for the disturbance. It is then often possible to ablate the site via a catheter that applies radiofrequency current to heat and destroy the tissue. Such procedures have revolutionized the management of patients with many types of tachycardias, because they often offer a permanent therapeutic solution that spares patients from prolonged antiarrhythmic drug therapy. Additionally, for patients with ICDs and recurrent ventricular tachycardias causing defibrillator shocks, ablation is often effective in reducing the frequency of episodes.

SUMMARY

1. Arrhythmias result from disorders of impulse formation, impulse conduction, or both.
2. Bradyarrhythmias develop because of decreased impulse formation (e.g., sinus bradycardia) or decreased impulse conduction (e.g., AV nodal conduction blocks).

3. Tachyarrhythmias result from increased automaticity (of the SA node, latent pacemakers, or abnormal myocardial sites), triggered activity, or reentry.

4. Bradyarrhythmias are usually treated with drugs that accelerate the rate of sinus node discharge and enhance AV nodal conduction (atropine, isoproterenol) or electronic pacemakers.

5. Pharmacologic therapy for tachyarrhythmias is directed at the mechanism responsible for the rhythm disturbance. For refractory tachyarrhythmias, or in emergency situations, electric cardioversion or defibrillation is used. Catheter-based ablative techniques are useful for long-term control of certain tachyarrhythmias. ICDs are lifesaving devices implanted in patients at high risk of sudden cardiac death because of ventricular tachyarrhythmias.

Chapter 12 describes the diagnosis and management of the most common arrhythmias. Additional reading suggestions are listed at the end of that chapter. Chapter 17 describes commonly used antiarrhythmic drugs.

Acknowledgments

Contributors to the previous editions of this chapter were Hillary K. Rolls, MD; Wendy Armstrong, MD; Nicholas Boulis, MD; Jennifer E. Ho, MD; Mark S. Sabatine, MD; Elliott M. Antman, MD; Leonard I. Ganz, MD; Gary R. Strichartz, PhD; and Leonard S. Lilly, MD.

Clinical Aspects of Cardiac Arrhythmias

Ranliang Hu
William G. Stevenson
Leonard S. Lilly

BRADYARRHYTHMIAS

Sinoatrial Node
Escape Rhythms
Atrioventricular Conduction System

TACHYARRHYTHMIAS

Supraventricular Arrhythmias
Ventricular Arrhythmias

Chapter 11 presented the mechanisms by which abnormal heart rhythms develop. This chapter describes how to recognize and treat such disorders. Table 12.1 categorizes the common arrhythmias considered in this chapter.

There are five basic questions to consider when confronted with a patient with an abnormal heart rhythm, as detailed in the sections that follow:

1. Identification: What is arrhythmia?
2. Pathogenesis: What is the underlying mechanism?
3. Precipitating factors: What conditions provoke it?
4. Clinical presentation: What symptoms and signs accompany the arrhythmia?
5. Treatment: What to do about it?

BRADYARRHYTHMIAS

The normal resting heart rate, resulting from repetitive depolarization of the sinus node,

ranges from 60 to 100 bpm. Bradyarrhythmias are rhythms in which the heart rate is <60 bpm. They arise from disorders of impulse formation or impaired impulse conduction, as discussed in Chapter 11.

Sinoatrial Node

Sinus Bradycardia

Sinus bradycardia (Fig. 12.1) is a slowing of the normal heart rhythm, as a result of decreased firing of the sinoatrial (SA) node, to a rate <60 bpm. Sinus bradycardia at rest or during sleep is normal and a benign finding in many people. Conversely, pathologic sinus bradycardia can result from either intrinsic SA node disease or extrinsic factors that affect the node. Depressed intrinsic automaticity can be caused by aging or any disease process that affects the atrium, including ischemic heart disease or cardiomyopathy. Extrinsic factors that suppress SA nodal activity include medications (e.g., β-blockers and certain calcium channel blockers) and metabolic causes (e.g., hypothyroidism).

Table 12.1. Common Arrhythmias

Location	Bradyarrhythmias	Tachyarrhythmias
SA node	Sinus bradycardia Sick sinus syndrome	Sinus tachycardia
Atria		Atrial premature beats Atrial flutter Atrial fibrillation Paroxysmal supraventricular tachycardias Focal atrial tachycardia Multifocal atrial tachycardia
AV node	Conduction blocks Junctional escape rhythm	Paroxysmal reentrant tachycardias (AV or AV nodal)
Ventricles	Ventricular escape rhythm	Ventricular premature beats Ventricular tachycardia Torsades de pointes Ventricular fibrillation

AV, atrioventricular; SA, sinoatrial.

Highly trained athletes often have elevated vagal tone, which results in physiologic and asymptomatic resting sinus bradycardia. Transient periods of high vagal tone can also occur in individuals as a reflex response to pain or fear, resulting in inappropriate sinus bradycardia.

Mild sinus bradycardia is usually asymptomatic and does not require treatment. However, a pronounced reduction of the heart rate can produce a fall in cardiac output with fatigue, light-headedness, confusion, or syncope. In such cases, any extrinsic provocative factors should be corrected, and specific therapy, as described in the next section, may be needed.

Sick Sinus Syndrome

Intrinsic SA node dysfunction that causes periods of inappropriate bradycardia is known as sick sinus syndrome (SSS). This condition often produces symptoms of dizziness, confusion, or syncope. Patients with this syndrome (or any cause of symptomatic sinus bradycardia) can be treated with intravenous anticholinergic drugs (e.g., atropine) or β-adrenergic agents (e.g., isoproterenol), which transiently accelerate the heart rate. If the problem is chronic and not corrected by removal of aggravating factors, placement of a permanent pacemaker is required.

SSS is common in elderly patients, who are also susceptible to supraventricular tachycardias (SVTs), most commonly atrial fibrillation (AF). This combination is known as the **bradycardia–tachycardia syndrome** (Fig. 12.2) and is thought to result from atrial fibrosis that impairs function of the SA node and predisposes to AF and flutter. During the tachyarrhythmia, overdrive suppression of the SA node occurs, and when the tachycardia terminates, a period of profound sinus bradycardia may ensue. Treatment generally requires the combination of antiarrhythmic drug therapy to suppress the tachyarrhythmias plus a permanent pacemaker to prevent bradycardia.

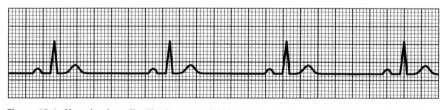

Figure 12.1. Sinus bradycardia. The P wave and QRS complexes are normal but the rate is <60 bpm.

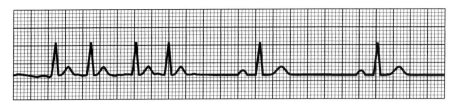

Figure 12.2. **Bradycardia–tachycardia syndrome.** A brief irregular tachycardia is followed by slow sinus node discharge.

Escape Rhythms

Cells in the atrioventricular (AV) node and His–Purkinje system are capable of automaticity but typically have slower firing rates than the sinus node and are therefore suppressed during normal sinus rhythm. However, if SA node activity becomes impaired or if there is conduction block of the impulse from the SA node, escape rhythms can emerge from the more distal latent pacemakers (Fig. 12.3).

Junctional escape beats arise from the AV node or proximal bundle of His. They are characterized by a normal, narrow QRS complex, and when they occur in sequence (termed a **junctional escape rhythm**), appear at a rate of 40 to 60 bpm. The QRS complexes are not preceded by normal P waves because the impulse originates below the atria. However, *retrograde* P waves may be observed as an impulse propagates from the more distal pacemaker backward to the atrium. Retrograde P waves typically *follow* the QRS complex and are *inverted* (negative deflection on the electrocardiogram [ECG]) in limb leads II, III,

and aVF, indicating activation of the atria from the inferior direction.

Ventricular escape rhythms are characterized by even slower rates (30 to 40 bpm) and *widened* QRS complexes. The complexes are wide because the ventricles are not depolarized by the normal rapid simultaneous conduction over the right and left bundle branches but rather from a more distal point in the conduction system. The morphology that the QRS shows depends on the site of origin of the escape rhythm. For example, an escape rhythm originating from the left bundle branch will cause a right bundle branch block QRS pattern, because the impulse depolarizes the left ventricle first and then spreads more slowly through the right ventricle (RV). Conversely, an escape rhythm originating in the right bundle branch causes the QRS to appear with a left bundle branch block configuration. Escape rhythms that originate more distally, in the ventricular myocardium itself, are characterized by even wider QRS complexes because such impulses are conducted outside the rapidly propagating Purkinje fibers.

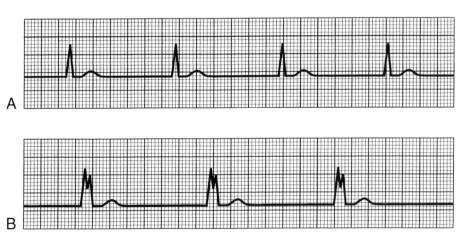

Figure 12.3. **Escape rhythms.** No P waves are evident. **A.** Junctional escape rhythm with normal-width QRS complexes. **B.** Wide QRS complexes typical of a ventricular escape rhythm.

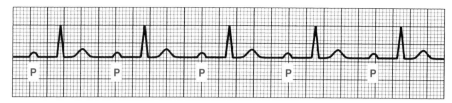

Figure 12.4. **First-degree AV block.** The PR interval is prolonged.

Junctional and ventricular escape rhythms are protective backup mechanisms that maintain a heart rate and cardiac output when the sinus node or normal AV conduction fails. The clinical findings and treatment of bradycardia associated with escape rhythms are identical to those of SSS described earlier.

Atrioventricular Conduction System

The AV conduction system includes the AV node, bundle of His, and the left and right bundle branches. Impaired conduction between the atria and ventricles can result in three degrees (types) of AV conduction block.

First-Degree AV Block

First-degree AV block, shown in Figure 12.4, indicates prolongation of the normal delay between atrial and ventricular depolarization, such that the PR interval is lengthened (>0.2 sec, which is >5 small boxes on the ECG). In this situation, the 1:1 relationship between P waves and QRS complexes is preserved. The impairment of conduction is usually within the AV node itself and can be caused by a transient reversible influence or a structural defect. *Reversible* causes include heightened vagal tone, transient AV nodal ischemia, and drugs that depress conduction through the AV node, including β-blockers, certain calcium channel antagonists, digitalis, and other antiarrhythmic medications. *Structural* causes of first-degree AV block include myocardial infarction and chronic degenerative diseases of the conduction system, which commonly occur with aging.

Generally, first-degree AV block is a benign, asymptomatic condition that does not require treatment. However, it can indicate disease in the AV node associated with susceptibility to higher degrees of AV block if drugs are administered that further impair AV conduction, or if the conduction disease progresses.

Second-Degree AV Block

Second-degree AV block is characterized by *intermittent failure* of AV conduction, resulting in some P waves not followed by a QRS complex. There are two forms of second-degree AV block. In **Möbitz type I** block (also termed **Wenckebach** block), shown in Figure 12.5, the degree of AV delay gradually increases with each beat until an impulse is completely blocked, such that a QRS does not follow a P wave for a single beat. Therefore, the ECG shows a progressive increase in the PR interval from one beat to the next until a single QRS complex is absent, after which the PR interval shortens to its initial length, and the cycle starts anew. Möbitz type I block almost always results from impaired conduction in the AV node (rather than more distally

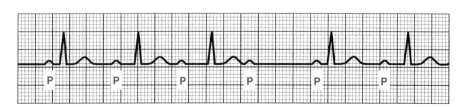

Figure 12.5. **Second-degree AV block: Möbitz type I (Wenckebach).** The P-wave rate is constant, but the PR interval progressively lengthens until a QRS is completely blocked (after fourth P wave).

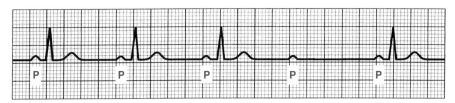

Figure 12.6. Second-degree AV block: Möbitz type II. A QRS complex is blocked (after the fourth P wave) without gradual lengthening of the preceding PR intervals. While the QRS width in this example is normal, it is often widened in patients with Möbitz type II block.

in the conduction system). It is usually benign and may be seen in children, trained athletes, and people with high vagal tone, particularly during sleep. It may also occur during an acute myocardial infarction because of increased vagal tone or ischemia of the AV node, but the block is usually temporary. Treatment is typically not necessary, but in symptomatic cases, administration of intravenous atropine or isoproterenol usually improves AV conduction transiently. Placement of a permanent pacemaker is required for a symptomatic block that does not resolve spontaneously or persists despite the correction of aggravating factors.

Möbitz type II second-degree AV block is characterized by the sudden intermittent loss of AV conduction, *without* preceding gradual lengthening of the PR interval (Fig. 12.6). The block may persist for two or more beats (i.e., two sequential P waves not followed by QRS complexes), in which case it is known as **high-grade** AV block (Fig. 12.7). Möbitz type II block is usually caused by conduction block beyond the AV node (in the bundle of His or more distally in the Purkinje system), and the QRS pattern often is widened in a pattern of right or left bundle branch block. This type of block may arise from extensive myocardial infarction involving the septum or from chronic degeneration of the His–Purkinje system. It usually indicates severe disease and is more

dangerous than Möbitz type I block. Möbitz type II may progress to third-degree block without warning; therefore, treatment with a pacemaker is usually warranted, even in asymptomatic patients.

Third-Degree AV Block

Third-degree AV block, also termed **complete heart block** (Fig. 12.8), is present when there is complete failure of conduction between the atria and ventricles. In adults, the most common causes are acute myocardial infarction and chronic degeneration of the conduction pathways with age. Third-degree AV block electrically disconnects the atria and ventricles; there is no relationship between the P waves and QRS complexes because the atria depolarize in response to SA node activity, while a more distal escape rhythm drives the ventricles independently. Thus, the P waves "march out" at a rate that is not related to the intervals at which QRS complexes appear. Depending on the site of the escape rhythm, the QRS complexes may be of normal width and occur at 40 to 60 bpm (originating from the AV node) or may be widened and occur at slower rates (originating from the His–Purkinje system). As a result of the slow rate, patients frequently experience light-headedness or syncope. Permanent pacemaker therapy is almost always necessary.

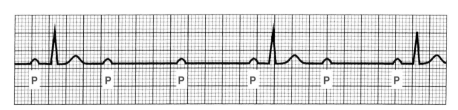

Figure 12.7. High-grade AV block. Sequential QRS complexes are blocked (after the second and third P waves).

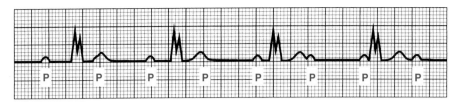

Figure 12.8. Third-degree AV block. The P wave and QRS rhythms are independent of one another. The QRS complexes are widened as they originate within the distal ventricular conduction system, not at the bundle of His. The second and fourth P waves are superimposed on normal T waves.

The term **AV dissociation** is a general description that refers to any situation in which the atria and ventricles beat independently, without any direct relationship between P waves and QRS complexes. Third-degree AV block is one example of AV dissociation.

TACHYARRHYTHMIAS

When the heart rate is >100 bpm for three beats or more, a tachyarrhythmia is present. Tachyarrhythmias result from one of the three mechanisms: enhanced automaticity, reentry, or triggered activity (see Chapter 11). Tachy-arrhythmias are categorized into those that arise *above* the ventricles (supraventricular) and those that arise *within* the ventricles.

Supraventricular Arrhythmias

Figure 12.9 presents a schema to help organize the common supraventricular tachyarrythmias presented in this section.

Sinus Tachycardia

Sinus tachycardia is characterized by an SA node discharge rate >100 bpm (typically 100

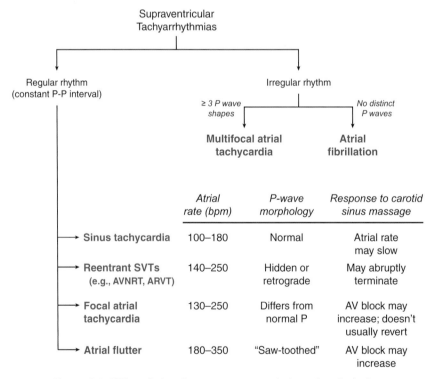

	Atrial rate (bpm)	P-wave morphology	Response to carotid sinus massage
Sinus tachycardia	100–180	Normal	Atrial rate may slow
Reentrant SVTs (e.g., AVNRT, ARVT)	140–250	Hidden or retrograde	May abruptly terminate
Focal atrial tachycardia	130–250	Differs from normal P	AV block may increase; doesn't usually revert
Atrial flutter	180–350	"Saw-toothed"	AV block may increase

Figure 12.9. Differentiation of common supraventricular tachyarrhythmias.

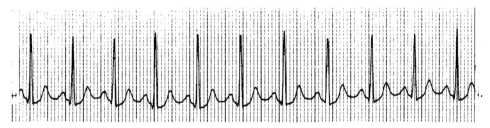

Figure 12.10. **Sinus tachycardia.** The P wave and QRS complexes are normal, but the rate is >100 bpm.

to 180 bpm) with normal P waves and QRS complexes (Fig. 12.10). This rhythm most often results from increased sympathetic and/or decreased vagal tone. Sinus tachycardia is an appropriate physiologic response to exercise. However, it may also result from sympathetic stimulation in pathologic conditions, including fever, hypoxemia, hyperthyroidism, hypovolemia, and anemia. In disease states, sinus tachycardia is usually a sign of the severity of the primary pathophysiologic process and treatment should be directed at the underlying cause.

Atrial Premature Beats

Atrial premature beats (APBs) are common in healthy as well as diseased hearts (Fig. 12.11). They originate from automaticity or reentry in an atrial focus outside the SA node and are often exacerbated by sympathetic stimulation. APBs are usually asymptomatic but may cause palpitations. On the ECG, an APB appears as an earlier-than-expected P wave with an *abnormal shape* (the impulse does not arise from the SA node, resulting in abnormal conduction through the atria). The QRS complex that follows the P wave is usually normal, resembling the QRS during sinus rhythm, because ventricular conduction is not impaired. However, if the abnormal atrial focus fires

very soon after the previous beat, the impulse may encounter an AV node that is refractory to excitation, resulting in a blocked impulse that does not conduct to the ventricles. The premature P wave is then *not* followed by a QRS complex and is termed a *blocked APB*. Similarly, if the ectopic focus fires just a bit later in diastole, it may conduct through the AV node but encounter portions of the His–Purkinje system that are still refractory. As a result, the impulse is conducted through those territories and to the ventricular myocytes more slowly than normal, producing QRS complexes that are abnormally wide (termed an APB with *aberrant conduction*).

APBs require treatment only if they are symptomatic. Because caffeine, alcohol, and adrenergic stimulation (e.g., emotional stress) can all predispose to APBs, it is important to address these factors. β-Blockers are the initial preferred pharmacologic treatment if needed.

Atrial Flutter

Atrial flutter is characterized by rapid, regular atrial activity at a rate of 180 to 350 bpm (Fig. 12.12). Many of these fast impulses reach the AV node during its refractory period and do not conduct to the ventricles, resulting in a slower ventricular rate, often an even fraction

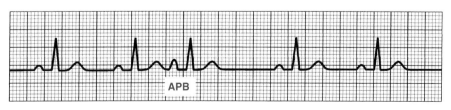

Figure 12.11. **Atrial premature beat (APB).** The P wave occurs earlier than expected, and its shape is abnormal.

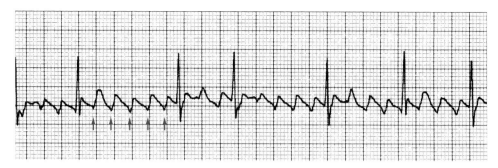

Figure 12.12. Atrial flutter is typified by rapid "saw-toothed" atrial activity *(arrows)*.

of the atrial rate. Thus, if the atrial rate is 300 bpm and 2:1 block occurs at the AV node (i.e., every other atrial impulse finds the AV node refractory), the ventricular rate is 150 bpm. Because vagal maneuvers (e.g., carotid sinus massage) decrease AV nodal conduction, they increase the degree of block, temporarily slowing the ventricular rate, which allows better visualization of the underlying atrial activity. In general, atrial flutter is caused by reentry over a large anatomically fixed circuit. In the common form of atrial flutter, this circuit is the atrial tissue along the tricuspid valve annulus: the circulating depolarization wave propagates up the interatrial septum, across the roof and down the free wall of the right atrium and finally along the floor of the right atrium between the tricuspid valve annulus and inferior vena cava. Because large parts of the atrium are depolarized throughout the cycle, P waves often have a sinusoidal or "sawtooth" appearance. Large flutter circuits can occur in other parts of the right or left atrium as well, usually associated with areas of atrial scarring from disease, prior heart surgery, or ablation procedures.

Atrial flutter generally occurs in patients with preexisting heart disease. It may be paroxysmal and transient, persistent (lasting for days or weeks), or permanent. Symptoms of atrial flutter depend on the accompanying ventricular rate. If the rate is <100 bpm, the patient may be asymptomatic. Conversely, faster rates often cause palpitations, dyspnea, or weakness. Paradoxically, antiarrhythmic medications that reduce the rate of atrial flutter by slowing conduction in the atrium may paradoxically make the rhythm more

dangerous by allowing the AV node more time to recover between impulses. In this situation, the AV node may begin to conduct in a 1:1 fashion, producing very rapid ventricular rates. For example, a patient with atrial flutter at a rate of 280 bpm and 2:1 conduction block at the AV node would have a ventricular rate of 140 bpm. If the atrial rate then slows to 220 bpm, the AV node may be able to recover sufficiently between depolarizations to conduct every atrial impulse, causing the ventricular rate to *accelerate* to 220 bpm. In patients with limited cardiac reserve, this acceleration may result in a profound reduction of cardiac output and hypotension. Atrial flutter also predisposes to atrial thrombus formation.

Several approaches to the treatment of atrial flutter are available:

1. For symptomatic patients with recent-onset atrial flutter, the most expeditious therapy is electrical cardioversion to restore sinus rhythm. This technique is also used to revert chronic atrial flutter that has not responded to other approaches.

2. Flutter can be terminated by rapid atrial stimulation (burst pacing) using a temporary or permanent pacemaker (see Chapter 11). This procedure can be used when temporary atrial pacing wires are already present, as in the days following cardiac surgery. In addition, certain types of permanent pacemakers and implanted defibrillators can be programmed to perform burst pacing automatically when atrial flutter occurs.

3. Patients without an immediate need for cardioversion can begin pharmacologic

therapy. First, the ventricular rate is slowed by drugs that increase AV block: β-blockers, calcium channel blockers (e.g., verapamil, diltiazem), or digoxin. Once the rate is effectively slowed, attempts are made to restore sinus rhythm using antiarrhythmic drugs that slow conduction or prolong the refractory period of the atrial myocardium (class IA, IC, or III agents; see Chapter 17). Should these drugs fail to convert the rhythm, electrical cardioversion can be undertaken. Once sinus rhythm has been restored, class IA, IC, or III antiarrhythmic drugs may be administered chronically to prevent recurrences.

4. When chronic therapy is required to prevent recurrences, catheter ablation is often a better alternative than pharmacologic approaches. In this method, an electrode catheter is inserted into the femoral vein, passed via the inferior vena cava to the right atrium, and used to localize and cauterize (ablate) part of the reentrant loop to permanently interrupt the flutter circuit.

Atrial Fibrillation

AF is a chaotic rhythm with an atrial rate so fast (350 to 600 discharges/min) that distinct P waves are not discernible on the ECG (Fig. 12.13). As with atrial flutter, many of the atrial impulses encounter refractory tissue at the AV node, allowing only some of the depolarizations to be conducted to the ventricles in a very irregular fashion (indicated by a characteristic "irregularly irregular" rhythm). The average ventricular rate in untreated AF is approximately 140 to 160 bpm. Because discrete P waves are not visible on the ECG, the baseline shows low-amplitude undulations punctuated by QRS complexes and T waves.

The mechanism of AF probably involves multiple wandering reentrant circuits within the atria, and in some patients, the rhythm repetitively shifts between fibrillation and atrial flutter. When fibrillation is paroxysmal (i.e., sudden, unpredictable episodes), it is often initiated by rapid firing of foci in sleeves of atrial muscle that extend into the pulmonary veins. To sustain AF, a minimum number of reentrant circuits is needed, and an enlarged atrium increases the potential for this to occur. Thus, AF is often associated with right or left atrial enlargement. Accordingly, diseases that increase atrial pressure and size promote AF, including heart failure, hypertension, coronary artery disease, and pulmonary disease. Thyrotoxicosis and alcohol consumption can precipitate AF in some people.

AF is a potentially dangerous arrhythmia because: (1) rapid ventricular rates may compromise cardiac output, resulting in hypotension and pulmonary congestion (especially in patients with a hypertrophied or "stiff" left ventricle in whom the loss of normal atrial contraction can significantly reduce left ventricular filling and stroke volume), and (2) the absence of organized atrial contraction promotes blood stasis in the atria, increasing the risk of thrombus formation, particularly in the left atrial appendage. Embolization of left atrial thrombi is an important cause of stroke. Thus, treatment of AF considers three aspects of the arrhythmia: (1) ventricular rate control, (2) consideration of methods to restore sinus rhythm, and (3) assessment of the need for anticoagulation to prevent thromboembolism.

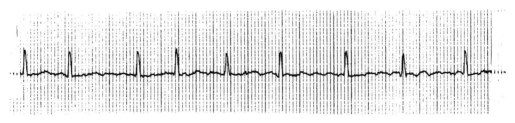

Figure 12.13. Atrial fibrillation is characterized by chaotic atrial activity without organized P waves and by irregularity of the ventricular (QRS) rate.

Antiarrhythmic drug treatment of AF is similar to that of atrial flutter. β-Blockers or certain Ca^{++} channel antagonists (diltiazem, verapamil) are administered to promote block at the AV node and to reduce the ventricular rate. Digitalis is less effective for this purpose, although it may be useful in patients with accompanying impairment of ventricular contractile function. For those who remain symptomatic despite adequate rate control, conversion to sinus rhythm is usually attempted, as described in the next paragraph. AF that has been present for more than 48 hours may predispose to atrial thrombus formation, and systemic anticoagulation (for at least 3 weeks) is usually warranted prior to cardioversion to reduce the risk of thromboembolism. Alternatively, a transesophageal echocardiogram can be performed to evaluate for the presence of thrombus; if none is found, cardioversion may proceed directly, with minimum thromboembolic risk.

Cardioversion to sinus rhythm can be attempted *chemically* by administration of class IA, IC, or III antiarrhythmic drugs (see Chapter 17). Alternatively, *electrical cardioversion* can be undertaken. Following successful conversion to sinus rhythm, antiarrhythmic drugs are often continued in an attempt to prevent recurrences. Note that these drugs have the capacity to cause serious, sometimes lethal, side effects (see Chapter 17). Thus, in patients with *asymptomatic* AF, it is often appropriate to simply control the ventricular rate and continue anticoagulation therapy chronically, rather than to pursue cardioversion. Such an approach is supported by clinical trials of AF that have assessed long-term clinical outcomes.

Because the efficacies and toxicities of antiarrhythmic drugs have been disappointing, nonpharmacologic options for the management of AF have been devised. For example, the surgical *maze procedure* places multiple incisions in the left and right atria to prevent the formation of reentry circuits and is sometimes performed in patients who undergo cardiac surgery for coronary artery or valve disease who also have AF. A less invasive approach is *percutaneous catheter ablation*. In this approach, areas of the left atrium around the pulmonary veins are cauterized to interrupt potential reentry circuits and foci that initiate AF. It requires extensive catheter manipulation and ablation in the left atrium, and risks of the procedure includes stroke from systemic thromboembolism and cardiac perforation that can cause tamponade. Thus, catheter ablation for AF is usually reserved for patients who remain symptomatic despite pharmacologic approaches.

When sinus rhythm cannot be maintained and the heart rate cannot be controlled adequately with medications, *catheter ablation of the AV node* is another available procedure. This method intentionally creates complete heart block as a means to permanently slow the ventricular rate. As a consequence, a permanent pacemaker is also required to generate an adequate ventricular rate.

Paroxysmal Supraventricular Tachycardias

Paroxysmal supraventricular tachycardias (PSVTs) are manifested by (1) sudden onset and termination, (2) atrial rates between 140 and 250 bpm, and (3) narrow (normal) QRS complexes (Fig. 12.14), unless *aberrant conduction*

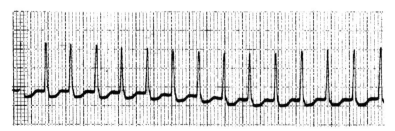

Figure 12.14. Paroxysmal supraventricular tachycardia caused by AV nodal reentry. Retrograde P waves in this example occur simultaneously with, and are "hidden" in, the QRS complexes.

is present, as summarized later. The mechanism of PSVTs is most often reentry involving the AV node, atrium, or an accessory pathway between an atrium and ventricle. Enhanced automaticity and triggered activity in the atrium or AV node are less common causes.

AV Nodal Reentrant Tachycardia

Atrioventricular nodal reentrant tachycardia (AVNRT) is the most common form of PSVT in adults. In the normal heart, the AV node is a lobulated structure that consists of a compact portion and several atrial extensions. The latter constitute two (or more) potential pathways for conduction through the AV node (Fig. 12.15). In some people, these extensions conduct at different velocities, providing both slow- and fast-conducting pathways. The fast pathway is characterized by a rapid conduction velocity, whereas the slow pathway demonstrates slower conduction but typically has a shorter refractory period than the fast pathway. Thus, although the fast pathway conducts rapidly, it takes longer to recover between impulses compared with the slow pathway. Normally, a stimulus arriving at the AV node travels down both pathways, but the impulse traveling down the fast pathway reaches the bundle of His first. By the time the impulse traversing the slow pathway reaches the bundle of His, it encounters refractory tissue and is extinguished. Thus, under normal conditions, only the fast pathway impulse makes its way forward to the ventricles (see Fig. 12.15A).

In contrast, consider what happens when an APB spontaneously occurs (Fig. 12.15B). Because the refractory period of the fast pathway is relatively long, an APB would find that pathway unexcitable and unable to conduct the impulse. However, the impulse *is* able to conduct over the slow pathway (which *is* excitable because it has a shorter refractory period than the fast pathway and has already repolarized when the APB arrives). By the time this impulse travels down the slowly conducting pathway and reaches the compact portion of the AV node, the distal end of the fast pathway may have had time to repolarize, and the impulse is able to propagate both distally (to the bundle of His and ventricles) *and* backward to

the atria, up the fast pathway in a retrograde direction. On reaching the atria, the impulse can then circulate back down the slow pathway, completing the reentrant loop and initiating tachycardia as this sequence repeats. Thus, the fundamental conditions for reentry in AVNRT in this example are transient unidirectional block in the fast pathway (an APB encountering refractory tissue) and relatively slow conduction through the other pathway.

The ECG in AVNRT shows a regular tachycardia with normal-width QRS complexes. P waves may not be apparent, because retrograde atrial depolarization typically occurs simultaneously with ventricular depolarization. Thus, the retrograde P wave and QRS are inscribed at the same time and the P is typically "hidden" in the QRS complex. When P waves *are* visible, they are superimposed on the terminal portion of the QRS complex and inverted (negative deflection) in limb leads II, III, and aVF because of the caudocranial direction of atrial activation.

Rarely, the reentrant loop revolves in the reverse direction, with anterograde conduction down the fast pathway and retrograde conduction up the slow pathway. This is known as *uncommon AVNRT* and, unlike the more common rhythm, results in clearly visible retrograde P waves following the QRS complex on the ECG.

AVNRT often presents in teenagers or young adults. It is usually well tolerated but causes palpitations that many patients find frightening, and rapid tachycardias can cause lightheadedness or shortness of breath. In elderly patients or those with underlying heart disease, more severe symptoms may result, such as syncope, angina, or pulmonary edema.

Acute treatment of AVNRT is aimed at terminating reentry by impairing conduction in the AV node. Transient increases in vagal tone produced by the Valsalva maneuver or carotid sinus massage (see Chapter 11) may block AV conduction, terminating the tachycardia. The most rapidly effective pharmacologic treatment is intravenous adenosine, which impairs AV nodal conduction and often aborts the reentrant rhythm (see Chapter 17). Other drug options include intravenous calcium channel antagonists (verapamil and diltiazem) or β-blockers.

Most patients with AVNRT have infrequent episodes that terminate with vagal maneuvers

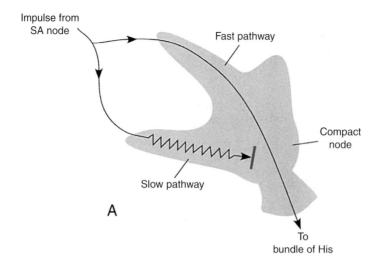

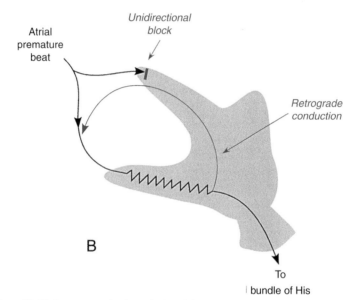

Figure 12.15. Common mechanism of AV nodal reentry. In most patients, the AV node (gray region in the drawing) is a lobulated structure consisting proximally of several atrial extensions and distally of a compact node portion. **A.** In patients with AV nodal reentry, two functionally distinct tracts exist within the AV node (termed the slow and fast pathways). The slow pathway conducts slowly and has a short refractory period, whereas the fast pathway conducts more rapidly but has a long refractory period. Impulses from above conduct down both pathways; because the fast pathway impulse reaches the distal common pathway first, it continues to the bundle of His. Conversely, the slow pathway impulse arrives later and encounters refractory tissue. **B.** An atrial premature beat arrives at the entrance of the two pathways. The fast pathway is still refractory from the preceding beat and the impulse is blocked, but the slow pathway has repolarized and is able to conduct. When the impulse reaches the distal portion of the fast pathway after traveling down the slower pathway, the fast pathway has repolarized and is able to conduct the impulse in a retrograde direction (exemplifying unidirectional block). The impulse can then travel through the atrium and back to the slow pathway, and a reentrant loop is initiated.

and do not require other specific interventions. Frequent symptomatic episodes, particularly when requiring visits to the emergency department for treatment, warrant preventive therapy: oral β-blockers, calcium channel blockers, or digoxin are often successful for this purpose. Catheter ablation of the slow AV nodal pathway is also an effective option but is associated with a small risk (<2%) of heart block owing to unintended damage to the fast AV nodal pathway, a complication that requires permanent pacemaker implantation. Chronic class IA or IC antiarrhythmic drugs are also effective, but are often less desirable than catheter ablation, because of associated potential drug toxicities.

Atrioventricular Reentrant Tachycardias

Atrioventricular reentrant tachycardias (AVRTs) are similar to AVNRTs except that in the former, one limb of the reentrant loop is constituted by an accessory pathway (*bypass tract*), rather than by separate fast and slow pathways within the AV node itself. As described in Chapter 11, an accessory pathway is an abnormal band of myocytes that spans the AV groove and connects atrial to ventricular tissue separately from the normal conduction system (see Fig. 11.10). Approximately 1 in 1,500 people has such a pathway.

Accessory pathways allow an impulse to conduct from atrium to ventricle (anterograde conduction), from ventricle to atrium (retrograde conduction), or in both directions. Depending on the characteristics of the pathway, one of two characteristic entities can result: (1) the ventricular pre-excitation syndrome, or (2) PSVT resulting from a concealed accessory pathway. Some pathways do not conduct impulses at rates sufficient to cause tachycardias and cause no symptoms at all.

Ventricular Pre-excitation Syndrome

In patients with ventricular pre-excitation (also termed Wolff–Parkinson–White [WPW] syndrome; see Chapter 11), atrial impulses can pass in an anterograde direction to the ventricles through both the AV node *and* the accessory pathway. Because conduction through the accessory pathway is usually faster than that via the AV node, the ventricles are stimulated *earlier* than by normal conduction over the AV node. During sinus rhythm, activation of the ventricle from the accessory pathway causes a characteristic ECG appearance: (1) the PR interval is short (<0.12 sec) because ventricular stimulation begins earlier than normal through the accessory pathway, (2) the QRS has a slurred rather than a sharp upstroke (referred to as a *delta wave*) because the initial ventricular activation by the accessory pathway is slower than activation over the Purkinje system, and (3) the QRS complex is widened because it represents fusion of two excitation wave fronts through the ventricles, one from the accessory pathway and one from the normal His–Purkinje system (Figs. 12.16 and 12.17).

Patients with WPW syndrome are predisposed to PSVTs because the accessory pathway provides a potential limb of a reentrant loop. The most common PSVT in these patients is **orthodromic** AVRT. During this tachycardia, an impulse travels *anterogradely* down the AV node to the ventricles and then *retrogradely* up the accessory tract back to the atria (see Fig. 12.17B). Because the ventricles in this situation are depolarized exclusively via the normal conduction system (through the AV node and the bundle of His), there is no delta wave during the tachycardia and the width of the QRS is usually normal. Retrograde P waves are often visible

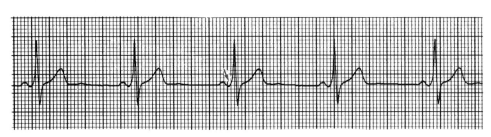

Figure 12.16. Wolff–Parkinson–White syndrome. The delta wave *(arrow)* indicates pre-excitation of the ventricles. Note the shortened PR interval.

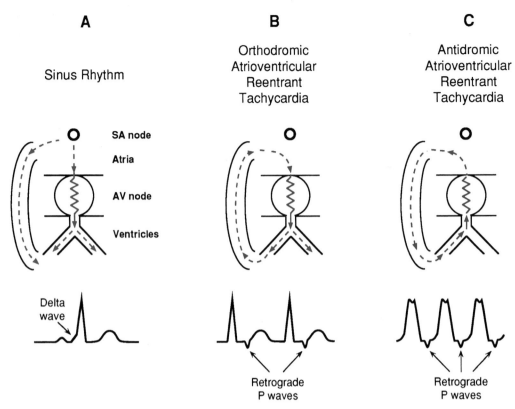

A

Sinus Rhythm

B

Orthodromic
Atrioventricular
Reentrant
Tachycardia

C

Antidromic
Atrioventricular
Reentrant
Tachycardia

SA node

Atria

AV node

Ventricles

Delta
wave

Retrograde
P waves

Retrograde
P waves

Figure 12.17. Wolff–Parkinson–White syndrome. A. During normal sinus rhythm, the shortened PR interval, delta wave, and widened QRS complex indicate fusion of ventricular activation via the AV node and accessory pathway. **B.** An atrial premature beat can trigger an orthodromic atrioventricular reentrant tachycardia, in which impulses are conducted anterogradely down the AV node and retrogradely up the accessory pathway. Retrograde P waves are visible immediately after the QRS complex. There is no delta wave because anterograde ventricular stimulation passes exclusively through the AV node. **C.** Antidromic atrioventricular reentrant tachycardia in which impulses are conducted anterogradely down the accessory tract and retrogradely up the AV node. The QRS complex is very widened because the ventricles are stimulated by abnormal conduction through the accessory pathway. SA, sinoatrial.

soon after each QRS complex because the atria are stimulated from below via retrograde conduction through the accessory pathway.

In fewer than 10% of patients with AVRT involving an accessory pathway, the reentrant arrhythmia travels in the opposite direction. Impulses travel *anterogradely* down the accessory pathway and *retrogradely* up the AV node (see Fig. 12.17C). Termed **antidromic** AVRT, its ECG pattern is characterized by a *wide* QRS complex because the ventricles are activated entirely from anterograde conduction over the accessory pathway. From the ECG alone, such antidromic tachycardia is difficult to distinguish from ventricular tachycardia (described later in the chapter).

A third type of arrhythmia encountered in patients with WPW syndrome is anterograde conduction over the accessory pathway when AF or atrial flutter is present. Some accessory pathways have short refractory periods that allow faster rates of ventricular stimulation than does the AV node. Thus, during AF or atrial flutter, ventricular rates as fast as 300 bpm may result. Such rates are poorly tolerated and can lead to ventricular fibrillation and cardiac arrest, even in a young, otherwise healthy patient.

Pharmacologic management of arrhythmias in patients with the WPW syndrome requires greater caution than those with AVNRTs. Although digitalis, β-blockers, and certain calcium channel blockers are effective at blocking conduction through the AV node, they do *not* slow conduction over most accessory pathways. Sometimes these drugs actually *shorten* the refractory period of the accessory pathway, thus *speeding* conduction. Therefore, the drugs could precipitate even faster ventricular rates (and hemodynamic collapse) when administered to patients with WPW syndrome who develop AF or flutter. In contrast, sodium channel blockers (specifically, class IA and IC antiarrhythmics) and some class III antiarrhythmic drugs slow conduction and prolong the refractory period of accessory pathways as well as the AV node; therefore, these are the preferred pharmacologic agents for this condition.

When a patient with WPW presents with a wide QRS tachycardia, acute therapy depends on the patient's tolerance of the arrhythmia. If accompanied by hemodynamic collapse, immediate cardioversion is required. Conversely, if the patient is hemodynamically stable, intravenous administration of procainamide (a class IA agent that slows conduction in the accessory pathway) or ibutilide (a class III agent that prolongs refractoriness in the accessory pathway) will often terminate the arrhythmia.

Patients who have WPW with symptomatic arrhythmias should generally undergo an invasive electrophysiologic study and have radiofrequency catheter ablation of the accessory pathway. Ablation abolishes conduction over the pathway, curing the condition. If this procedure is not an option, chronic oral therapy should include a drug that slows accessory pathway conduction (i.e., a class IA, IC, or III agent).

The **Lown–Ganong–Levine syndrome** is also characterized by a short PR interval, but a normal, narrow QRS complex (i.e., no delta wave during sinus rhythm). It used to be considered a form of pre-excitation, but most patients just have enhanced conduction through the normal AV node, thus shortening the PR interval. When PSVT occurs in these patients, it is usually simply due to AV nodal reentry.

Concealed Accessory Pathways

Accessory pathways do not always result in ECG findings of ventricular pre-excitation (i.e., short PR, delta wave). Many are capable of only *retrograde* conduction. In this case, during sinus rhythm, the ventricles are depolarized normally through the AV node alone and the ECG is normal (i.e., the accessory pathway is *concealed*). However, because the accessory pathway is capable of retrograde conduction, it can form a limb of a reentrant circuit under appropriate circumstances and result in orthodromic AVRT.

Management of patients with tachycardia involving a concealed accessory pathway is the same as for patients with AVNRT. Because the reentrant circuit travels anterogradely down the AV node, vagal maneuvers and drugs that interrupt conduction over the AV node (e.g., adenosine, verapamil, diltiazem, and β-blockers) can terminate the tachycardia. Another option for recurrent episodes is catheter ablation of the accessory pathway, which is curative in most patients.

Focal Atrial Tachycardia

Focal atrial tachycardia (AT) results from either automaticity of an atrial ectopic site, or reentry. The ECG has the appearance of sinus tachycardia, with a P wave before each QRS complex, but the P-wave morphology is different from that of sinus rhythm, indicating depolarization of the atrium from an abnormal site. The arrhythmia can be paroxysmal and of limited duration, or it can persist. Short, asymptomatic bursts of atrial tachycardia are commonly observed on 24-hour ECG recordings, even in otherwise healthy people.

Atrial tachycardia can be caused by digitalis toxicity and is also aggravated by elevated sympathetic tone (e.g., during exertion or periods of illness). Initial treatment includes correction of any contributing factors. Unlike AVNRT or AVRT, vagal maneuvers (such as carotid sinus massage) may have no effect on atrial discharges from an ectopic pacemaker focus. However, β-blockers, calcium channel blockers, and class IA, IC, and III antiarrhythmic drugs can be effective. Catheter ablation is also a useful option for symptomatic patients.

Multifocal Atrial Tachycardia

In multifocal atrial tachycardia (MAT), the ECG shows an irregular rhythm with multiple (at least three) P-wave morphologies, and the average atrial rate is >100 bpm (Fig. 12.18).

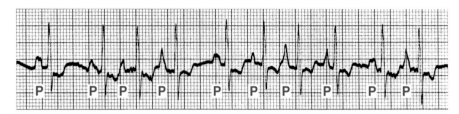

Figure 12.18. Multifocal atrial tachycardia. The rhythm is irregular and each QRS is preceded by a P wave of varying morphology.

An isoelectric (i.e., "flat") baseline between P waves distinguishes MAT from the chaotic baseline of AF. This rhythm is likely caused by either abnormal automaticity in several foci within the atria or triggered activity and occurs most often in the setting of severe pulmonary disease and hypoxemia. Because patients with this rhythm are often critically ill from the underlying disease, the mortality rate is high, and treatment is aimed at the causative disorder. The calcium channel blocker verapamil is often effective at slowing the ventricular rate as a temporizing measure.

Ventricular Arrhythmias

The common ventricular arrhythmias are (1) ventricular premature beats (VPBs), (2) ventricular tachycardia (VT), and (3) ventricular fibrillation (VF). Ventricular arrhythmias are usually more dangerous than supraventricular rhythm disorders and are responsible for many of the approximately 300,000 sudden cardiac deaths that occur every year in the United States.

Ventricular Premature Beats

Similar to APBs, VPBs are common even among healthy people and are often asymptomatic and benign (Fig. 12.19). A VPB arises when an ectopic ventricular focus fires an action potential. On the ECG, a VPB appears as a *widened* QRS complex, because the impulse travels from its ectopic site through the ventricles via slow cell-to-cell connections rather than through the normal rapidly conducting His–Purkinje system. Furthermore, the ectopic beat is not related to a preceding P wave.

VPBs can also occur in repeating patterns. When every alternate beat is a VPB, the rhythm is termed **bigeminy.** When two normal beats precede every VPB, **trigeminy** is present. Consecutive VPBs are referred to as **couplets** (two in a row) or **triplets** (three in a row).

VPBs are not dangerous by themselves, and in patients without heart disease, they confer no added risk of a life-threatening arrhythmia. They can, however, be an indication of an underlying cardiac disorder and take on added significance in that case. For example, in patients with structural heart disease, VPBs generally increase in frequency in relation to the severity of depressed ventricular contractility. They have been associated with an increased risk of sudden death in patients with heart failure or prior myocardial infarction.

In otherwise healthy persons, treatment of VPBs mainly involves reassurance and, if needed, symptomatic control using β-blockers. In patients with advanced structural heart disease with features that place them at risk of life-threatening ventricular arrhythmias,

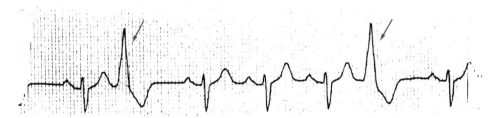

Figure 12.19. Ventricular premature beats *(arrows)*.

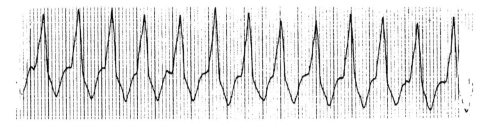

Figure 12.20. **Monomorphic ventricular tachycardia.**

placement of an implantable cardioverter-defibrillator (ICD) is typically recommended.

Ventricular Tachycardia

VT is a series of three or more VPBs (Fig. 12.20). VT is divided arbitrarily into two categories. If it persists for more than 30 sec, produces severe symptoms such as syncope, or requires termination by cardioversion or administration of an antiarrhythmic drug, it is designated as **sustained VT;** self-terminating episodes are termed **nonsustained VT.** Both forms of VT are found most commonly in patients with structural heart disease, including myocardial ischemia and infarction, heart failure, ventricular hypertrophy, primary electrical diseases (e.g., long-QT syndromes [LQTS]; see Box 12.1), valvular heart diseases, and congenital cardiac abnormalities.

The QRS complexes of VT are typically wide (>0.12 sec) and occur at a rate of 100 to 200 bpm or sometimes faster. VT is further categorized according to its QRS morphology. When every QRS complex appears the same and the rate is regular, it is referred to as **monomorphic VT** (see Fig. 12.20). Sustained monomorphic VT usually indicates a structural abnormality that supports a reentry circuit, most commonly a region of myocardial scar from an old infarction or cardiomyopathy. Occasionally, sustained monomorphic VT occurs as a result of an ectopic ventricular focus in an otherwise healthy person (referred to as *idiopathic VT*).

When the QRS complexes continually change in shape and the rate varies from beat to beat, the VT is referred to as **polymorphic.** Multiple ectopic foci or a continually changing reentry circuit is the cause. Torsades de pointes (discussed later in the chapter) and acute myocardial ischemia or infarction are the most common causes of polymorphic VT. Rare, inherited predispositions to polymorphic VT and sudden death arise from abnormalities of cardiac ion channels or calcium handling (e.g., the LQTS, the Brugada syndrome, familial catecholaminergic polymorphic VT), as described in Box 12.1. Sustained polymorphic VT usually degenerates to VF.

The symptoms of VT vary depending on the rate of the tachycardia, its duration, and the underlying condition of the heart. Sustained VT can cause low cardiac output resulting in the loss of consciousness (syncope), pulmonary edema, or progress to cardiac arrest. These severe consequences of VT are most likely in patients who have underlying depressed contractile function. Conversely, if sustained VT is relatively slow (e.g., <130 bpm), it may be well tolerated and cause only palpitations.

Distinguishing Monomorphic VT from Supraventricular Tachycardia

VT can usually be distinguished from SVT by the width of the QRS complex: it is routinely wide in the former and narrow (i.e., normal) in the latter. However, under certain circumstances, arrhythmias that originate from sites above the ventricles *can* result in wide QRS complexes and may appear similar to monomorphic VT. This situation is termed *SVT with aberrant ventricular conduction,* or simply *SVT with aberrancy,* and may arise in three scenarios: (1) a patient has an underlying conduction abnormality (e.g., a bundle branch block), such that the QRS is abnormally wide even when in normal sinus rhythm; (2) repetitive rapid ventricular stimulation during

BOX 12.1 Genetic Mutations and Ventricular Arrhythmias

Genetic causes of ventricular arrhythmias occur either in association with various types of structural heart disease or as isolated conditions. Examples of inherited structural disease that can be complicated by life-threatening arrhythmias include **hypertrophic cardiomyopathy** and the **familial dilated cardiomyopathies,** both described in Chapter 10. **Arrhythmogenic right ventricular dysplasia (ARVD;** also called "arrhythmogenic right ventricular cardiomyopathy") is another form of myocardial disease associated with reentrant VT, typically originating from the RV. This condition is characterized by replacement of portions of the RV with adipose and fibrous tissue, and approximately half of patients display a familial pattern with autosomal dominant inheritance. The most common mutations involve genes that encode components of cell membrane desmosomes, which may result in loss of cell-to-cell adhesion, leading to fibrosis or aberrant signaling with proliferation of adipose tissue in the myocardium. ARVD may be suspected on routine ECG by the presence of inverted T waves in leads V_1 through V_3 and occasionally an *epsilon wave,* a terminal notch of the QRS complex in lead V_1 (see arrow in the accompanying figure), which reflects abnormal RV activation. The abnormal

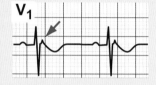

RV morphology can be identified by noninvasive imaging techniques in some patients. Treatment typically includes an ICD because the disease is progressive and VT is common, which can lead to sudden death.

Several other inherited arrhythmic disorders occur in the absence of structural cardiac disease. These occur infrequently but are important because they can cause life-threatening arrhythmias in young, otherwise healthy people without prior warning. The most common of these conditions are (1) the Brugada syndrome, (2) the congenital LQTS, and (3) familial catecholaminergic polymorphic VT.

The **Brugada syndrome** is believed to be responsible for a significant percentage of idiopathic ventricular fibrillation. It is inherited in an autosomal dominant fashion and has been linked in some (but not all) families to mutations in a sodium channel subunit gene *(SCN5A).* A clue to the presence of this syndrome is a specific ECG finding of prominent ST elevation in leads V_1 through V_3 (see accompanying figure). This pattern may be present chronically or intermittently; in the latter case, the syndrome may be unmasked by administering certain antiarrhythmic drugs (e.g., flecainide, procainamide). Brugada syndrome is a potentially lethal condition, and

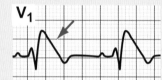

ICD implantation is the most effective way to prevent an arrhythmic death.

The **congenital long-QT syndromes** are associated with prolonged ventricular repolarization (hence the long QT interval), which can lead to life-threatening polymorphic VT (i.e., torsades de pointes). Mutations in a number of different genes result in LQTS (the three most common are listed in the accompanying table) by prolonging the action potential duration. Most identified mutations alter ion channel function to either *enhance* the depolarizing Na^+ current or *impair* the repolarizing K^+ current. Autosomal dominant and recessive patterns of inheritance occur.

Genetic Basis of the Three Most Common Congenital Long-QT Syndromes

Type	Gene (location)	Protein	Mechanism of Prolonged Repolarization	Inheritance
LQT1	*KCNQ1* (11p15)	KvLQT1 (α subunit of I_{Ks} K^+ channel)	$\downarrow$ Outward K^+ current	AD and AR
LQT2	*KCNH2* (7q35)	HERG (α subunit of I_{Kr} K^+ channel)	$\downarrow$ Outward K^+ current	AD
LQT3	*SCN5A* (3p21)	Nav 1.5 (Na^+ channel)	$\uparrow$ Inward Na^+ current	AD

AD, autosomal dominant; AR, autosomal recessive.

Gene penetrance and symptomatology of patients with LQTS is highly variable, even for individuals with the same mutation. The degree of QT prolongation and, in some cases, the patient's gender are predictors of arrhythmic risk when a mutation is present. An affected patient may be asymptomatic and come to medical attention only as a result of the abnormal ECG, or because of a family member with this condition. Others present with syncope or even sudden death caused by torsades de pointes. The most common forms (LQT1 and LQT2) are associated with ventricular arrhythmias during physical exercise (particularly swimming), or emotional stress. Conversely, those with LQT3 are much more likely to experience cardiac events at rest or during sleep.

Other acquired conditions that prolong the QT interval can trigger life-threatening arrhythmias in patients with LQTS, including hypokalemia, hypomagnesemia, hypocalcemia, and several medications (including many antiarrhythmic drugs). Conversely, β-blockers reduce the risk of arrhythmias in many forms of LQTS, even though they do not shorten the QT interval. For patients at high risk of life-threatening arrhythmias, ICD implantation is warranted.

Familial catecholaminergic polymorphic VT, inherited in autosomal dominant and recessive patterns, is marked by VT and/or ventricular fibrillation during exercise or emotional arousal. The mechanism is thought to be triggered activity resulting from delayed afterdepolarizations (described in Chapter 11). Mutations in affected families have been demonstrated in at least two genes involved in intracellular calcium handling, including a missense mutation in the locus that codes for the cardiac ryanodine receptor. β-Blockers are effective for some patients; otherwise, an ICD is implanted.

SVT finds one of the bundle branches refractory (because of insufficient time to recover from the previous depolarization), such that the impulse propagates abnormally through the ventricles, causing the QRS to be distorted and wide; or (3) a patient develops antidromic tachycardia through an accessory pathway (described earlier).

Certain clinical and electrocardiographic features can help to distinguish wide QRS complexes of monomorphic VT from those of supraventricular rhythms with aberrant conduction. In patients with a history of prior myocardial infarction, congestive heart failure, or left ventricular dysfunction, a wide complex tachycardia is more likely to be VT rather than SVT with aberrancy. At the bedside, SVT is more probable if vagal maneuvers (such as carotid sinus massage) affect the rhythm (see Fig. 12.9).

Electrocardiographically, a *supraventricular* tachyarrhythmia is more likely if the morphology of the QRS at the rapid rate is similar to that on the patient's ECG tracing obtained while in sinus rhythm (i.e., the complex is widened because of an underlying bundle branch block). Conversely, VT is more likely if (1) there is no relationship between the QRS complexes and any observed P waves (AV dissociation) or (2) the QRS complexes in each of the chest leads (V_1 through V_6) have a similar appearance, with a dominant positive or negative deflection (i.e., there is "concordance" of the precordial QRS complexes). These features are summarized in Table 12.2. Other morphologic ECG features have been

Table 12.2. Differentiation of Wide Complex Tachycardias	
Supports SVT with Aberrant Conduction	*Supports Ventricular Tachycardia*
QRS morphology same as when in sinus rhythm	History of prior MI or heart failure
	No relationship between P waves and QRS complexes
Rhythm responds to vagal maneuvers (see Fig. 12.9)	Concordance of QRS complexes in the chest leads (V_1–V_6)

MI, myocardial infarction; SVT, supraventricular tachycardia.

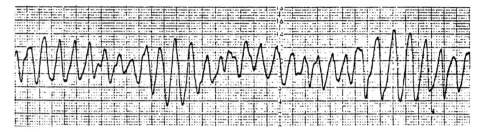

Figure 12.21. Torsades de pointes. The widened polymorphic QRS complexes demonstrate a waxing and waning pattern.

used to distinguish VT from SVT with aberrancy, but the distinction is often very difficult. Most patients with wide QRS tachycardia should be managed as though they have VT until proven otherwise.

Management of Patients with VT

Sustained episodes of VT are dangerous because they can produce syncope or deteriorate into VF, which is fatal if not quickly corrected. Acute treatment usually consists of electrical cardioversion. Intravenous administration of certain antiarrhythmic drugs, such as amiodarone, procainamide, or lidocaine, can be considered if the patient is hemodynamically stable.

After sinus rhythm is restored, a patient who has had sustained VT requires careful evaluation to define whether underlying structural heart disease is present and to correct any aggravating factors, such as myocardial ischemia, electrolyte disturbances, or drug toxicities. Patients who have suffered VT in the setting of structural heart disease have a high risk of recurrence and sudden cardiac death; implantation of an ICD is usually warranted to automatically and promptly terminate future episodes.

Patients who experience VT in the absence of underlying structural heart disease are usually found to have idiopathic VT. This type of arrhythmia tends to originate from foci in the right ventricular outflow tract or in the septal portion of the left ventricle. It is rarely life threatening. β-Blockers, calcium channel blockers, or catheter ablation are commonly effective to control symptomatic episodes of idiopathic VT.

Torsades de Pointes

Torsades de pointes ("twisting of the points") is a form of polymorphic VT that presents as varying amplitudes of the QRS, as if the complexes were "twisting" about the baseline (Fig. 12.21). It can be produced by early afterdepolarizations (triggered activity), particularly in patients who have a *prolonged QT interval.* QT prolongation (which indicates a lengthened action potential duration) can result from electrolyte disturbances (hypokalemia or hypomagnesemia), persistent bradycardia, and drugs that block cardiac potassium currents, including many antiarrhythmic agents (particularly the class III drugs sotalol, ibutilide, and dofetilide and some class I drugs, including quinidine, procainamide, and disopyramide). Many medications administered for noncardiac illnesses can also prolong the QT interval and predispose to torsades de pointes, including erythromycin, phenothiazines, haloperidol, and methadone. A rare group of hereditary ion channel abnormalities produces *congenital* QT prolongation, which can also lead to torsades de pointes (see Box 12.1).

Torsades de pointes is usually symptomatic, causing light-headedness or syncope, but is frequently self-limited. Its main danger results from degeneration into VF. When it is drug or electrolyte induced, correcting the underlying cause abolishes recurrences. In other cases, administration of intravenous magnesium often suppresses repeated episodes. Additional preventive strategies are aimed at shortening the QT interval by increasing the underlying heart rate with intravenous β-adrenergic *stimulating* agents (e.g., isoproterenol) or

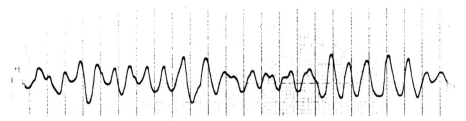

Figure 12.22. **Ventricular fibrillation.**

an artificial pacemaker. When torsades de pointes results from congenital prolongation of the QT interval, *β-blocking* drugs are often the treatment of choice, because sympathetic stimulation actually aggravates the arrhythmia in many such individuals. An implantable defibrillator is often appropriate for these patients.

Ventricular Fibrillation

VF is an immediately life-threatening arrhythmia (Fig. 12.22). It results in disordered, rapid stimulation of the ventricles with no coordinated contractions. The result is essentially cessation of cardiac output and death if not quickly reversed. This rhythm most often occurs in patients with severe underlying heart disease and is the major cause of mortality in acute myocardial infarction.

VF is often initiated by an episode of VT, which degenerates, it is believed, by the breakup of excitation waves into multiple smaller wavelets of reentry that wander through the myocardium. On the ECG, VF is characterized by a chaotic irregular appearance without discrete QRS waveforms.

Untreated, VF rapidly leads to death. The only effective therapy is prompt electrical defibrillation. As soon as the heart has been converted to a safe rhythm, the underlying precipitant of the arrhythmia (e.g., electrolyte imbalances, hypoxemia, or acidosis) should be sought and corrected to prevent further episodes. Intravenous antiarrhythmic drug therapy may be administered to prevent immediate recurrences. If no reversible inciting precipitant is found, survivors of VF usually receive an ICD.

SUMMARY

1. Disorders of impulse formation and conduction result in bradyarrhythmias and tachyarrhythmias. Through careful analysis of the ECG, it is usually possible to distinguish individual rhythm disorders so that appropriate therapy can be administered.

2. When evaluating a patient with a slow heart rhythm (Figs. 12.1–12.8), two key questions should be addressed:
   a. Are P waves present?
   b. What is the relationship between the P waves and the QRS complexes?

3. Differentiation of tachyarrhythmias requires assessment of:
   a. The width of the QRS complex (normal or wide).
   b. The morphology and rate of the P waves.
   c. The relationship between the P waves and the QRS complexes.
   d. The response to vagal maneuvers (see Fig. 12.9).

Each of the ECG texts listed at the end of Chapter 4 provides many additional examples of the rhythm disorders presented in this chapter.

Acknowledgments

Contributors to the previous editions of this chapter were Hillary K. Rolls, MD; Wendy Armstrong, MD; Nicholas Boulis, MD; Jennifer E. Ho, MD; Marc S. Sabatine, MD; Elliott M. Antman, MD; Leonard I. Ganz, MD; William G. Stevenson, MD; and Leonard S. Lilly, MD.

Additional Reading

Crandall MA, Bradley DJ, Packer DL, et al. Contemporary management of atrial fibrillation: update on anticoagulation and invasive management strategies. *Mayo Clin Proc.* 2009;84:643–662.

Delacretaz E. Supraventricular tachycardia. *N Engl J Med.* 2006;354:1039–1051.

Dobrzynski H, Boyett MR, Anderson RH. New insights into pacemaker activity: promoting understanding of sick sinus syndrome. *Circulation.* 2007;115: 1921–1932.

Epstein AE, DiMarco JP, Ellenbogen KA, et al. ACC/AHA/HRS 2008 Guidelines for Device-Based Therapy of Cardiac Rhythm Abnormalities: a report of the American College of Cardiology/American Heart Association Task Force on Practice Guidelines. *Circulation.* 2008; 17:e350–e408.

Nass RD, Aiba T, Tomaselli GF, et al. Mechanisms of disease: ion channel remodeling in the failing ventricle. *Nat Clin Pract Cardiovasc Med.* 2008;5:196–207.

Noseworthy PA, Newton-Cheh C. Genetic determinants of sudden cardiac death. *Circulation.* 2008;118:1854–1863.

Roberts JD, Gollb MH. Impact of genetic discoveries on the classification of lone atrial fibrillation. *J Am Coll Cardiol.* 2010;55:705–712.

Roden DM. Clinical practice. Long-QT syndrome. *N Engl J Med.* 2008;358:169–176.

Shah M, Akar FG, Tomaselli GF. Molecular basis of arrhythmias. *Circulation.* 2005;112:2517–2529.

Thavendiranathan P, Bagai A, Khoo C, et al. Does this patient with palpitations have a cardiac arrhythmia? *JAMA.* 2009;302:2135–2143.

Zipes DP, Camm AJ, Borggrefe M, et al. ACC/AHA/ESC 2006 guidelines for management of patients with ventricular arrhythmias and the prevention of sudden cardiac death. *J Am Coll Cardiol.* 2006;48:e247–e346.

Hypertension

Christopher T. Lee
Gordon H. Williams
Leonard S. Lilly

Approximately 60 million Americans, and 1 billion people throughout the world, have hypertension—a blood pressure high enough to be a danger to their well-being. This number will undoubtedly rise; data from the Framingham Heart Study indicate that 90% of people over age 55 will develop hypertension during their lifetimes. Thus, this condition represents a great public health concern because it is a major risk factor for coronary artery disease, stroke, heart failure, renal disease, and peripheral vascular disease. Surprisingly, more than two thirds of hypertensive persons are either unaware of their elevated blood pressure or are not treated adequately to minimize the cardiovascular risk. Moreover, because elevated blood pressure is usually asymptomatic until an acute cardiovascular event strikes, screening for hypertension is a critical aspect of preventive medicine.

Hypertension is also a scientific problem of unexpected complexity. In approximately 90% of affected patients, the cause of the blood pressure elevation is unknown, a condition termed primary or **essential hypertension (EH)**. Evidence suggests that the causes of EH are multiple and diverse, and considerable insight into those causes can be achieved by studying the normal physiology of blood pressure control, as examined in this chapter.

High blood pressure attributed to a *definable* cause is termed **secondary hypertension.** Although far less common than EH, conditions that cause secondary hypertension are important because many are amenable to permanent cure. Following the discussions of EH

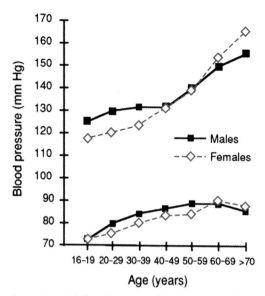

Figure 13.1. Relationship between blood pressure and age (*n* = 1,029). Systolic *(upper curves)* and diastolic *(lower curves)* values are shown. Notice that by age 60, the average systolic pressure of women exceeds that of men. (Modified from Kotchen JM, McKean HE, Kotchen TA. Blood pressure trends with aging. *Hypertension*. 1982;4(suppl 3):111–129.)

and secondary hypertension, this chapter considers the clinical consequences of elevated blood pressure and approaches to treatment.

WHAT IS HYPERTENSION?

Blood pressure values vary widely in the population and tend to increase with age, as illustrated in Figure 13.1. The risk of a vascular complication increases progressively and linearly with higher blood pressure values, so the exact cutoff points to define stages of hypertension are somewhat arbitrary. The currently accepted criteria are listed in Table 13.1.

By this classification, a diastolic pressure consistently ≥90 mm Hg or a systolic pressure ≥140 mm Hg establishes the diagnosis of hypertension. Those with *prehypertension* (systolic 120 to 139 mm Hg or diastolic 80 to 99 mm Hg) have an increased risk of developing definite hypertension over time. Although the emphasis has historically been on the level of *diastolic* pressure, more recent evidence suggests that *systolic* pressure more accurately predicts cardiovascular complications.

HOW IS BLOOD PRESSURE REGULATED?

Hemodynamic Factors

Blood pressure (BP) is the product of cardiac output (CO) and total peripheral resistance (TPR):

$$BP = CO \times TPR$$

And CO is the product of cardiac stroke volume (SV) and heart rate (HR):

$$CO = SV \times HR$$

As described in Chapter 9, SV is determined by (1) cardiac contractility; (2) the venous return to the heart (the preload); and (3) the resistance the left ventricle must overcome to eject blood into the aorta (the afterload).

It follows that at least four systems are directly responsible for blood pressure regulation: the *heart*, which supplies the pumping pressure; the *blood vessel tone*, which largely determines systemic resistance; the *kidney*, which regulates intravascular volume; and *hormones*, which modulate the functions of

Table 13.1. Classification of Blood Pressure in Adults			
Category	*Systolic Pressure (mm Hg)*		*Diastolic Pressure (mm Hg)*
Normal	<120	And	<80
Prehypertension	120–139	Or	80–89
Stage 1 hypertension	140–159	Or	90–99
Stage 2 hypertension	≥160	Or	≥100

Modified from The seventh report of the Joint National Committee on Prevention, Detection, Evaluation, and Treatment of High Blood Pressure. *JAMA*. 2003;289:2560–2572.

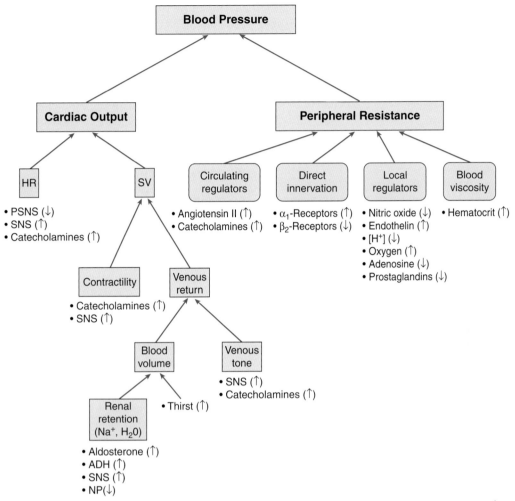

Figure 13.2. Regulation of systemic blood pressure. The small arrows indicate whether there is a stimulatory (↑) or inhibitory (↓) effect on the boxed parameters. ADH, antidiuretic hormone; HR, heart rate; NP, natriuretic peptides; PSNS, parasympathetic nervous system; SNS, sympathetic nervous system; SV, stroke volume.

the other three systems. Figure 13.2 shows how factors related to these systems contribute to CO and TPR.

The renal component of blood pressure regulation deserves special mention, in light of the temptation to view hypertension simply as a cardiovascular problem. No matter how high the CO or TPR, renal excretion has the capacity to completely return blood pressure to normal by reducing intravascular volume. Therefore, the maintenance of chronic hypertension requires renal participation. Transplantation studies have confirmed this point: the implantation of a kidney from a normotensive person into a hypertensive one typically improves the blood pressure. Similarly, surgical placement

of a kidney from a genetically hypertensive rat into a previously normotensive one usually leads to hypertension.

In the presence of normally functioning kidneys, an increase in blood pressure leads to augmented urine volume and sodium excretion, which then returns the blood pressure back to normal. This process, known as *pressure natriuresis*, is blunted in the kidneys of hypertensive patients; thus, higher pressures are required to excrete a given sodium and water load. Current evidence suggests at least two possible reasons for this blunted response. First, microvascular and tubulointerstitial injury within the kidneys of hypertensive patients impairs sodium excretion.

Second, the defect may lie with hormonal factors critical to appropriate renal reactions to the sodium and intravascular volume environment (e.g., the renin–angiotensin system, as described later in the chapter). In contrast to the first possibility, abnormalities of hormonal regulation are amenable to correction with appropriate therapy.

Blood Pressure Reflexes

The cardiovascular system is endowed with feedback mechanisms that continuously monitor arterial pressure: they sense when the pressure becomes excessively high or low and then respond rapidly to those changes. One such mechanism is the **baroreceptor reflex**, which is mediated by receptors in the walls of the aortic arch and the carotid sinuses. The baroreceptors monitor changes in pressure by sensing the stretch and deformation of the arteries. If the arterial pressure rises, the baroreceptors are stimulated, increasing their transmission of impulses to the central nervous system (i.e., the medulla). Negative feedback signals are then sent back to the circulation via the autonomic nervous system, causing the blood pressure to fall back to its baseline level.

The higher the blood pressure rises, the more the baroreceptors are stretched and the greater the impulse transmission rate to the medulla. Signals from the carotid sinus receptors are carried by the glossopharyngeal nerve (cranial nerve IX), whereas those from the aortic arch receptors are carried by the vagus nerve (cranial nerve X). These nerve fibers converge at the tractus solitarius in the medulla, where the baroreceptor impulses *inhibit* sympathetic nervous system outflow and *excite* parasympathetic effects. The net result is (1) a decline in peripheral vascular resistance (i.e., vasodilation) and (2) a reduction in CO (because of a lower HR and reduced force of cardiac contraction). Each of these effects tends to lower arterial pressure back toward its baseline. Conversely, when a *fall* in systemic pressure is sensed by the baroreceptors, fewer impulses are transmitted to the medulla, leading to a reflexive *increase* in blood pressure.

The main effect of the baroreceptor mechanism is to modulate moment-by-moment variations in systemic blood pressure. However, the baroreceptor reflex is not involved in the long-term regulation of blood pressure and does not prevent the development of chronic hypertension. The reason for this is that the baroreceptors constantly reset themselves. After a day or two of exposure to higher-than-baseline pressures, the baroreceptor-firing rate slows back to its control value.

ESSENTIAL HYPERTENSION

Approximately 90% of hypertensive patients have blood pressures that are elevated for no readily definable reason, a condition termed essential hypertension. The diagnosis of EH is one of exclusion; it is the option left to the clinician after considering the causes of secondary hypertension described later in this chapter.

EH is more a description than a diagnosis, indicating only that a patient manifests a specific physical finding (high blood pressure) for which no cause has been found. In all likelihood, different underlying defects are responsible for the elevated pressure in different subpopulations of patients. Because the exact nature of these defects is unknown, to understand EH is to understand the possibilities: what could go wrong with normal physiology to produce chronically elevated blood pressure?

This discussion of EH therefore reflects what is currently known about its epidemiology and genetics, experimental findings, and natural history. The picture that emerges is that EH likely results from multiple defects of blood pressure regulation that interact with environmental stressors. The regulatory defects may be acquired or genetically determined and may be independent of one another. As a result, EH patients exhibit varied combinations of abnormalities and, therefore, have various physiologic bases for their elevated blood pressures.

Epidemiology and Genetics

Heredity appears to play an important role in EH, but definite genetic markers have not been consistently identified. It seems most likely that EH is a complex genetic disorder, involving several loci. Evidence for a hereditary role is suggested by the higher rate of elevated blood pressures among first-degree relatives of hypertensive patients than in the general population. Concordance between identical twins is high and significantly greater than between dizygotic twins. Furthermore, an uneven distribution of EH exists among different racial groups. For example, in most age distributions, blacks are significantly more likely to be hypertensive than persons of other races.

Although no gene has been consistently linked to EH, several loci have demonstrated positive associations. For example, autosomal dominant contributors to elevated blood pressure have been discovered, usually involving defects of renal sodium channels. However, these abnormalities are rare and are thought to be present in only a small fraction of hypertensive patients. Genes regulating the renin–angiotensin–aldosterone axis have been most thoroughly studied in hypertensives because of the central role of this system in determining intravascular volume and vascular tone. Within this group, certain polymorphisms in the gene for *angiotensinogen* confer an increased risk of hypertension. Additionally, polymorphisms in the gene for *alpha-adducin*, a cytoskeletal protein, may be involved in a subgroup of EH patients, possibly by increasing renal tubular sodium absorption. And as described later in the chapter, significant associations exist between hypertension and obesity, insulin resistance, and diabetes. The pathophysiologic and genetic links among these four conditions are areas of very active investigation.

Experimental Findings

Systemic Abnormalities

Multiple defects in blood pressure regulation have been found in EH patients and their relatives. By themselves, or in conjunction with one another, these abnormalities may contribute to chronic blood pressure elevation.

The *heart* can contribute to a high CO-based hypertension owing to sympathetic overactivity. For example, when tested under psychologically stressful conditions, hypertensive patients (and their first-degree relatives) often develop excessive HR acceleration compared with control subjects, suggesting an excessive sympathetic response.

The *blood vessels* may contribute to peripheral vascular resistance–based hypertension by constricting in response to (1) increased sympathetic activity; (2) abnormal regulation of vascular tone by local factors, including nitric oxide, endothelin, and natriuretic factors; or (3) ion channel defects in contractile vascular smooth muscle.

The *kidney* can induce volume-based hypertension by retaining excessive sodium and water as a result of (1) failure to regulate renal blood flow appropriately; (2) ion channel defects (e.g., reduced basolateral Na^+K^+-ATPase), which directly cause sodium retention; or (3) inappropriate hormonal regulation. For example, the renin–angiotensin–aldosterone axis is an important hormonal regulator of peripheral vascular resistance. Renin levels in EH patients (compared with those in normotensive persons) are subnormal in 25%, normal in ~60%, and high in 10 to 15%. Because renin secretion should be *suppressed* by high blood pressure, even "normal" levels are inappropriate in hypertensives. Thus, abnormalities of this system's regulation may play a role in some individuals with EH.

Figure 13.3 highlights these and other potential mechanisms of EH. Note that although the heart, blood vessels, and kidneys are the organs ultimately responsible for producing the pressure, primary defects may be located elsewhere as well (e.g., the central nervous system, arterial baroreceptors, and adrenal hormone secretion). Yet, although abnormal regulation at these sites can contribute to elevated blood pressure, it is important to remember that without renal complicity, malfunction of other systems would not produce sustained hypertension, since the normal kidney is capable of eliminating sufficient volume to return the blood pressure to normal.

Insulin Resistance, Obesity, and the Metabolic Syndrome

Recent research has suggested that the hormone insulin may play a role in the development of EH. In many people with hypertension, especially

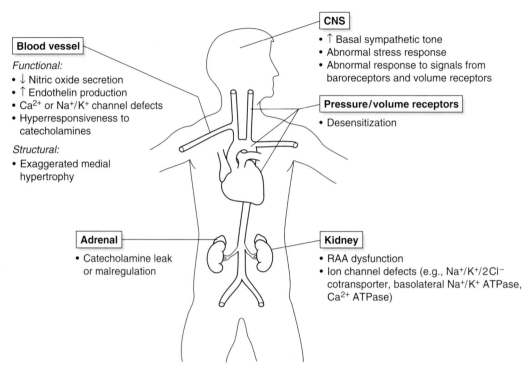

Figure 13.3. Potential primary abnormalities in essential hypertension. These defects are supported by experimental evidence, but their specific contributions to essential hypertension remain unknown. CNS, central nervous system; RAA, renin–angiotensin–aldosterone system.

those who are obese or have type 2 diabetes, there is impaired insulin–dependent transport of glucose into many tissues (termed *insulin resistance*). As a result, serum glucose levels rise, stimulating the pancreas to release additional insulin. Elevated insulin levels may contribute to hypertension via increased sympathetic activation or by stimulation of vascular smooth muscle cell hypertrophy, which increases vascular resistance. Smooth muscle cell hypertrophy may be caused by a direct mitogenic effect of insulin or through enhanced sensitivity to platelet-derived growth factor.

Obesity itself has been directly associated with hypertension. Possible explanations for this relationship include (1) the release of angiotensinogen from adipocytes as substrate for the renin–angiotensin system, (2) augmented blood volume related to increased body mass, and (3) increased blood viscosity caused by adipocyte release of profibrinogen and plasminogen activator inhibitor 1. The current epidemic of obesity has led to a dramatic increase in the number of people

with *metabolic syndrome*. As described in Chapter 5, this condition represents a clustering of atherogenic risk factors, including hypertension, hypertriglyceridemia, low serum high-density lipoprotein (HDL), a tendency toward glucose intolerance, and truncal obesity. Current evidence suggests that insulin resistance is central to the pathogenesis of this clustering.

Natural History

EH characteristically arises after young adulthood. Its prevalence increases with age and more than 60% of Americans older than 60 years are hypertensive. In addition, the hemodynamic characteristics of blood pressure elevation in EH tend to change over time. The systolic pressure increases throughout adult life, while the diastolic pressure rises until about the age of 50 then declines slightly thereafter (see Fig. 13.1). Accordingly, diastolic hypertension is more common in young people, while a substantial number of hypertensive patients over age 50 have isolated

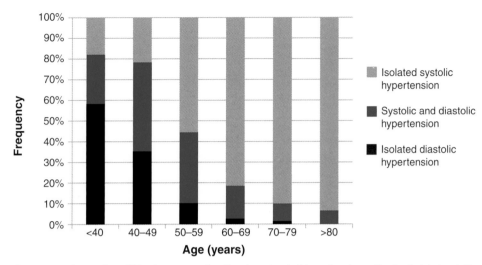

Figure 13.4. Categories of blood pressure elevation in untreated hypertensive patients. Isolated systolic hypertension predominates in patients older than 50 years, primarily as a result of decreased vascular compliance. (Modified from Franklin SS, Jacobs MJ, Wong ND, et al. Predominance of isolated systolic hypertension among middle aged and elderly US hypertensives: analysis based on National Health and Nutrition Examination Survey (NHANES III). *Hypertension.* 2001;37:869–874.)

systolic hypertension with normal diastolic values (see Fig. 13.4).

In younger persons with hypertension, elevated blood pressure tends to be driven by high CO in the setting of relatively normal peripheral vascular resistance, termed the *hyperkinetic* phase of EH (Fig. 13.5). With advancing age, however, the effect of CO declines, perhaps because of the development of left ventricular hypertrophy and its consequent reduced diastolic filling (which in turn reduces SV and CO). Conversely, vascular resistance increases with age due to medial hypertrophy as the vessels adapt

to the prolonged pressure stress. Thus, younger hypertensive patients often display augmented CO as the principal abnormality, and older patients tend to have elevated TPR as the major hemodynamic finding.

In summary, EH is a syndrome that may arise from many potential abnormalities, but it exhibits a characteristic hemodynamic profile and natural history. It is likely that multiple defects, separately inherited or acquired, act together to chronically raise blood pressure. Although we may not understand the precise

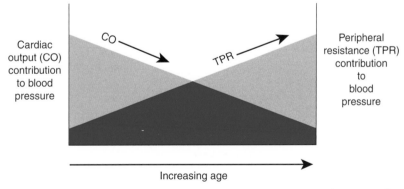

Figure 13.5. Hemodynamic progression of essential hypertension. Schematic representation of the changing contribution of cardiac output (CO) and total peripheral resistance (TPR) as age increases in many patients with essential hypertension.

underlying mechanisms in individual hypertensive patients, we can at least describe what kind of pathophysiology might be at fault.

SECONDARY HYPERTENSION

Although EH dominates the clinical picture, a defined structural or hormonal cause for hypertension may be found in a small percentage of patients. Identification of such cases of secondary hypertension is important because the underlying conditions may require therapy different from that administered for EH and they are often curable. Moreover, if secondary hypertension is left uncontrolled, adaptive cardiovascular changes may develop analogous to those of long-standing EH that could cause the elevated pressures to persist even after the underlying cause is corrected.

Although secondary forms should be considered in the workup of all patients with hypertension, there are clues that a given patient may have one of the correctable conditions (Table 13.2):

1. *Age.* If a patient develops hypertension before age 20 or after age 50 (outside the usual range of EH), secondary hypertension is more likely.

2. *Severity.* Secondary hypertension often causes blood pressure to rise dramatically, whereas most EH patients usually have mild to moderate hypertension.

3. *Onset.* Secondary forms of hypertension often present abruptly in a patient who was previously normotensive, rather than gradually progressing over years as is the usual case in EH.

4. *Associated signs and symptoms.* The process that induces hypertension may give rise to other characteristic abnormalities, identified by the history and physical

Table 13.2. Causes of Hypertension

Type	Percent of Hypertensive Patients	Clinical Clues
Essential	~90%	• Age of onset: 20–50 years • Family history of hypertension • Normal serum K^+, urinalysis
Chronic renal disease	2–4%	• ↑ Creatinine, abnormal urinalysis
Primary aldosteronism	<2%–15% (varies by sensitivity of screening)	• ↓ Serum K^+
Renovascular	1%	• Abdominal bruit • Sudden onset (especially if age >50 or <20) • ↓ Serum K^+
Pheochromocytoma	0.2%	• Paroxysms of palpitations, diaphoresis, and headache • Weight loss • *Episodic* hypertension in one third of patients
Coarctation of the aorta	0.1%	• Blood pressure in arms > legs, or right arm > left arm • Midsystolic murmur between scapulae • Chest x-ray: aortic indentation, rib-notching due to arterial collaterals
Cushing syndrome	0.1%	• "Cushingoid" appearance (e.g., central obesity, hirsutism)

examination. For example, a renal artery *bruit* (swishing sound caused by turbulent blood flow through a stenotic artery) may be heard on abdominal examination in a patient with renal artery stenosis.

5. *Family history.* EH patients often have hypertensive first-degree relatives, whereas secondary hypertension more commonly occurs sporadically.

Patient Evaluation

The usual clinical evaluation of a patient with recently diagnosed hypertension begins with a careful history and physical examination, including a search for clues to the secondary forms. For example, repeated urinary tract infections may suggest the presence of chronic pyelonephritis with renal damage as the cause of hypertension. Excessive weight loss may be an indicator of pheochromocytoma, whereas weight gain may point to the presence of Cushing syndrome. The history also should include an assessment of lifestyle behaviors that may contribute to hypertension, such as excessive alcohol consumption, and the patient's medications should be reviewed because certain drugs (see next section) may elevate blood pressure. Obstructive sleep apnea is commonly associated with hypertension and should be considered particularly in patients who snore and have a history of hypertension refractory to medications.

Laboratory tests commonly performed in the initial evaluation of the hypertensive patient, including general screening for secondary causes, are (1) urinalysis and measurement of the serum concentration of creatinine and blood urea nitrogen to evaluate for renal abnormalities; (2) serum potassium level (abnormally low in renovascular hypertension or aldosteronism); (3) blood glucose level (elevated in diabetes, which is strongly associated with hypertension and renal disease); (4) serum cholesterol, HDL cholesterol, and triglyceride levels, as part of the global vascular risk screen; and (5) an electrocardiogram (for evidence of left ventricular hypertrophy caused by chronic hypertension).

If no abnormalities are found that suggest a secondary form of hypertension, the patient is presumed to have EH and treated accord-ingly. If, however, the patient's blood pressure continues to be elevated despite standard treatments, then more detailed diagnostic testing may be undertaken to search for specific secondary causes.

Exogenous Causes

Several medications can elevate blood pressure. For example, oral contraceptives may cause secondary hypertension in some women. The mechanism is likely related to increased activity of the renin–angiotensin system. Estrogens increase the hepatic synthesis of angiotensinogen, leading to greater production of angiotensin II (Fig. 13.6). Angiotensin II raises blood pressure by several mechanisms, most notably by direct vasoconstriction and by stimulating the adrenal release of aldosterone. The latter hormone causes renal sodium retention and therefore increased intravascular volume.

Other medications that can raise blood pressure include glucocorticoids, cyclosporine (an antirejection drug used in patients with organ transplants), erythropoietin (a hormone that increases bone marrow red blood cell formation and elevates blood pressure by increasing blood viscosity and reversing local hypoxic vasodilatation), and sympathomimetic drugs (which are common in over-the-counter cold remedies). Nonsteroidal anti-inflammatory drugs can contribute to hypertension through dose-related augmentation of sodium and water retention by the kidneys.

Two other substances that may contribute to hypertension are ethanol (i.e., chronic excessive consumption) and cocaine. Both of these are associated with increased sympathetic nervous system activity.

Renal Causes

Given the crucial role of kidney in the control of blood pressure, it is not surprising that renal dysfunction can lead to hypertension. In fact, renal disease contributes to two important endogenous causes of secondary hypertension: renal parenchymal disease, accounting for 2% to 4% of hypertensive patients, and renal arterial stenosis, which accounts for approximately 1%.

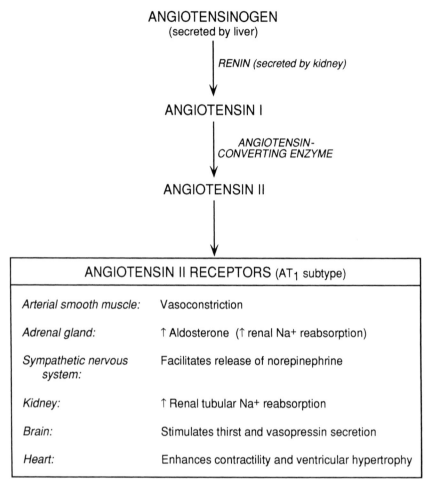

ANGIOTENSINOGEN
(secreted by liver)

RENIN (secreted by kidney)

ANGIOTENSIN I

ANGIOTENSIN-
CONVERTING ENZYME

ANGIOTENSIN II

ANGIOTENSIN II RECEPTORS (AT$_1$ subtype)	
Arterial smooth muscle:	Vasoconstriction
Adrenal gland:	↑ Aldosterone (↑ renal Na$^+$ reabsorption)
Sympathetic nervous system:	Facilitates release of norepinephrine
Kidney:	↑ Renal tubular Na$^+$ reabsorption
Brain:	Stimulates thirst and vasopressin secretion
Heart:	Enhances contractility and ventricular hypertrophy

Figure 13.6. The renin–angiotensin–aldosterone system. Liver-derived angiotensinogen is cleaved in the circulation by renin (of kidney origin) to form angiotensin I (AI). AI is rapidly converted to the potent vasoconstrictor angiotensin II (AII) by angiotensin-converting enzyme. AII also modulates the release of aldosterone from the adrenal cortex. Aldosterone in turn acts to reabsorb Na$^+$ from the distal nephron, resulting in increased intravascular volume. The other listed effects of AII receptor stimulation may also contribute to the development and maintenance of hypertension.

Renal Parenchymal Disease

Parenchymal damage to the kidney can result from diverse pathologic processes. The major mechanism by which injury leads to elevated blood pressure is through increased intravascular volume. Damaged nephrons are unable to excrete normal amounts of sodium and water, leading to a rise in intravascular volume, elevated CO, and hence increased blood pressure.

If renal function is only mildly impaired, blood pressure may stabilize at a level at which the higher systemic pressure (and therefore renal perfusion pressure) enables sodium excretion to balance sodium intake. Conversely, if a patient has end-stage renal failure, the glomerular filtration rate may be so greatly decreased that the kidneys simply cannot excrete sufficient volume, and malignant-range blood pressures may follow. Renal parenchymal disease may further contribute to hypertension even if the glomerular filtration rate is not greatly reduced, through the excessive elaboration of renin.

Renovascular Hypertension

Stenosis of one or both renal arteries leads to hypertension. Although emboli, vasculitis, and external compression of the renal arteries can be responsible, the two most common causes of renovascular hypertension (RH) are atherosclerosis and fibromuscular dysplasia. *Atherosclerotic* lesions arise from extensive plaque formation either within the renal artery or in the aorta at the origin of the renal artery. This form accounts for about two thirds of cases of RH and occurs most commonly in elderly men. In contrast, *fibromuscular* lesions consist of discrete regions of fibrous or muscular proliferation, generally within the arterial media. Fibromuscular dysplasia accounts for one third of cases of RH and characteristically occurs in young women.

The elevated blood pressure in RH arises from reduced renal blood flow to the affected kidney, which responds to the lower perfusion pressure by secreting renin. The latter raises the blood pressure through the subsequent actions of angiotensin II (vasoconstriction) and aldosterone (sodium retention), as shown in Figure 13.6.

The diagnosis of RH is suggested by an abdominal bruit, which can be found in 40% to 60% of patients, or by the presence of unexplained hypokalemia (owing to excessive renal excretion of potassium as a result of elevated aldosterone levels). RH is a correctable form of hypertension that may be treated successfully by percutaneous catheter interventions or surgical reconstruction of the stenosed vessel. Medical therapy, particularly with angiotensin-converting enzyme (ACE) inhibitors, can also be effective initial therapy in patients with *unilateral* renal artery disease. ACE inhibitors negate the hypertensive effects of elevated circulating renin in this situation by impeding the formation of angiotensin II (see Chapter 17). Conversely, this class of drugs should be avoided, or used cautiously, in patients with *bilateral* stenotic lesions. The inhibition of angiotensin II production may excessively reduce intraglomerular pressure and filtration, and worsen renal function, in patients with bilateral disease who already have compromised perfusion to both kidneys.

Mechanical Causes

Coarctation of the Aorta

Coarctation is an infrequent congenital narrowing of the aorta typically located just distal to the origin of the left subclavian artery (see Chapter 16). As a result of the relative obstruction to flow, the blood pressure in the aortic arch, head, and arms is higher than that in the descending aorta and its branches and in the lower extremities. Sometimes the coarctation involves the origin of the left subclavian artery, causing lower pressure in the left arm compared with the right arm.

Hypertension in this condition arises by two mechanisms. First, reduced blood flow to the kidneys stimulates the renin–angiotensin system, resulting in vasoconstriction (via angiotensin II). Second, high pressures proximal to the coarctation stiffen the aortic arch through medial hyperplasia and accelerated atherosclerosis, blunting the normal baroreceptor response to elevated intravascular pressure.

Clinical clues to the presence of coarctation include symptoms of inadequate blood flow to the legs or left arm, such as claudication or fatigue, or the finding of weakened or absent femoral pulses. A midsystolic murmur associated with the stenotic segment of the aorta may be auscultated, especially over the back, between the scapulae. The chest radiograph may show indentation of the aorta at the level of the coarctation. It may also demonstrate a notched appearance of the ribs secondary to the enlargement of collateral intercostal arteries, which shunt blood around the aortic narrowing. Treatment options include angioplasty or surgery to correct the stenosis. However, hypertension may not abate completely after mechanical correction, in part because of persistent desensitization of the arterial baroreceptors.

Endocrine Causes

Circulating hormones play an important role in the control of normal blood pressure, so it should not be surprising that endocrine diseases may cause hypertension. When suspected, the presence of such conditions is evaluated in four ways:

1. History of characteristic signs and symptoms
2. Measurement of hormone levels

3. Assessment of hormone secretion in response to stimulation or inhibition

4. Imaging studies to identify tumors secreting the excessive hormone

Pheochromocytoma

Pheochromocytomas are catecholamine-secreting tumors of neuroendocrine cells (usually in the adrenal medulla) that cause approximately 0.2% of cases of hypertension. The release of epinephrine and norepinephrine by the tumor results in intermittent or chronic vasoconstriction, tachycardia, and other sympathetic-mediated effects. A characteristic presentation consists of paroxysmal rises in blood pressure accompanied by "autonomic attacks" caused by the increased catecholamine levels: severe throbbing headaches, profuse sweating, palpitations, and tachycardia. Although some patients are actually normotensive between attacks, most have sustained hypertension. Ten percent of pheochromocytomas are malignant.

Determination of plasma catecholamine levels, or urine catecholamines and their metabolites (e.g., vanillylmandelic acid and metanephrine), obtained under controlled circumstances, are used to identify this condition. Because some pheochromocytomas secrete only episodically, diagnosis may require measurement of catecholamines immediately following an attack.

Pharmacologic therapy of pheochromocytomas includes the combination of an α-receptor blocker (e.g., phenoxybenzamine) combined with a β-blocker. However, once the tumor is localized by computed tomography, magnetic resonance imaging, or angiography, the definitive therapy is surgical resection. For patients with inoperable disease, treatment consists of α- and β-blockade as well as drugs that inhibit catecholamine biosynthesis (e.g., α-methyltyrosine).

Adrenocortical Hormone Excess

Among the hormones produced by the adrenal cortex are mineralocorticoids and glucocorticoids. Excess of either of these can result in hypertension.

Mineralocorticoids, primarily aldosterone, increase blood volume by stimulating reabsorption of sodium into the circulation by the distal portions of the nephron. This occurs in exchange for potassium excretion into the urine, and the resulting hypokalemia is an important marker of mineralocorticoid excess. *Primary aldosteronism* results either from an adrenal adenoma (termed *Conn syndrome*) or from bilateral hyperplasia of the adrenal glands. While once considered rare, recent data suggest that the frequency of primary aldosteronism may be as high as 10% to 15% among hypertensives, depending on the sensitivity of screening, with a substantial majority having the bilateral hyperplasia form. The diagnosis may be suspected by the presence of hypokalemia and is confirmed by the finding of excessive plasma aldosterone and a suppressed renin level. Therapy includes either surgical removal of the responsible adenoma (if present) or medical management with aldosterone receptor antagonists.

Glucocorticoid-remediable aldosteronism (GRA), an uncommon hereditary (autosomal dominant) form of primary aldosteronism, results from a genetic rearrangement in which aldosterone synthesis abnormally comes under the regulatory control of adrenocorticotropic hormone (ACTH). This condition typically presents as severe hypertension in childhood or young adulthood, as opposed to the more common forms of primary aldosteronism, which are generally diagnosed in the third through sixth decades. Unlike other forms of hypertension, GRA-related blood pressure elevation responds to glucocorticoid therapy, which suppresses ACTH release from the pituitary gland.

Secondary aldosteronism can result from increased angiotensin II production stimulated by rare renin-secreting tumors. More commonly, secondary elevation of aldosterone is a result of augmented circulating angiotensin II in women taking oral contraceptives (which stimulate hepatic production of angiotensinogen, as described earlier) or because of impaired angiotensin II degradation in chronic liver diseases.

Glucocorticoids, such as cortisol, elevate blood pressure when present in excess amounts, likely via blood volume expansion and stimulated synthesis of components of the renin–angiotensin system. In addition, though mineralocorticoids are more potent activators of mineralocorticoid receptors in the renal tubules, excess glucocorticoids may also activate them.

Nearly 80% of patients with *Cushing syndrome*, a disorder of glucocorticoid excess, have some degree of hypertension. These patients often present with classic "cushingoid" features: a characteristic rounded facial appearance, central obesity, proximal muscle weakness, and hirsutism. The cause of the excess glucocorticoids may be either a pituitary ACTH-secreting adenoma, a peripheral ACTH-secreting tumor (either of which causes adrenal cortical hyperplasia), or an adrenal cortisol–secreting adenoma. The diagnosis of Cushing syndrome is confirmed by a 24-hour urine collection for the measurement of cortisol, or by a dexamethasone test, which evaluates whether exogenous glucocorticoids can suppress cortisol secretion.

Thyroid Hormone Abnormalities

Approximately one third of *hyperthyroid* and one fourth of *hypothyroid* patients have significant hypertension. Thyroid hormones exert their cardiovascular effects by (1) inducing sodium–potassium ATPases in the heart and vessels; (2) increasing blood volume; and (3) stimulating tissue metabolism and oxygen demand, with secondary accumulation of metabolites that modulate local vascular tone. Hyperthyroid patients develop hypertension through cardiac hyperactivity with an increase in blood volume. Hypothyroid patients demonstrate predominantly diastolic hypertension and an increase in peripheral vascular resistance. Though the precise mechanism is unclear, the latter effect appears to be mediated by sympathetic and adrenal activation in hypothyroidism.

CONSEQUENCES OF HYPERTENSION

Whatever the cause of blood pressure elevation, the ultimate consequences are similar. High blood pressure itself is generally asymptomatic but can result in devastating effects on many organs, especially the blood vessels, heart, kidney, and retina.

Clinical Signs and Symptoms

In the past, "classic" symptoms of hypertension were considered to include headache, epistaxis (nose bleeds), and dizziness. The usefulness of these symptoms has been called into question, however, by studies that indicate that they are found no more frequently among hypertensive patients than in the general population. Other symptoms, such as flushing, sweating, and blurred vision, do seem more common in the hypertensive population. In general, however, most hypertensive patients are asymptomatic and are diagnosed simply by blood pressure measurement during routine physical examinations.

Several physical signs of hypertension discussed in the following sections result directly from elevated pressure, including left ventricular hypertrophy and retinopathy. In addition, hypertension complicated by atherosclerosis can manifest by arterial bruits, particularly in the carotid and femoral arteries.

Organ Damage Caused by Hypertension

Target organ complications of hypertension reflect the degree of chronic blood pressure elevation. Such organ damage can be attributed to (1) the increased workload of the heart and (2) arterial damage resulting from the combined effects of the elevated pressure itself (weakened vessel walls) and accelerated atherosclerosis (Fig. 13.7). Abnormalities of the vasculature that result from elevated pressure include smooth muscle hypertrophy, endothelial cell dysfunction, and fatigue of elastic fibers. Chronic hypertensive trauma to the endothelium promotes atherosclerosis possibly by disrupting normal protective mechanisms, such as the secretion of nitric oxide. Arteries lined by atherosclerotic plaque may thrombose or may serve as a source of cholesterol emboli that occlude distal vessels, causing organ infarction (such as cerebrovascular occlusion, resulting in stroke). In addition, atherosclerosis of large arteries hinders their elasticity, resulting in

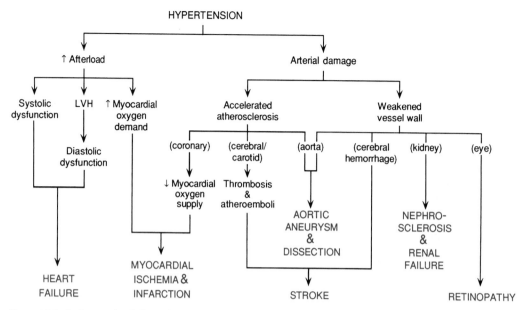

Figure 13.7. **Pathogenesis of the major consequences of arterial hypertension.** LVH, left ventricular hypertrophy.

systolic pressure spikes that can further traumatize endothelium or provoke events such as aneurysm rupture.

The major target organs for the destructive complications of chronic hypertension are the heart, the cerebrovascular system, the aorta and peripheral vascular system, the kidney, and the retina (Table 13.3). Left untreated, ap-

proximately 50% of hypertensive patients die of coronary artery disease or congestive heart failure, about 33% succumb to stroke, and 10% to 15% die from complications of renal failure.

Heart

The major cardiac effects of hypertension relate to the increased afterload against which the heart must contract and accelerated atherosclerosis within the coronary arteries.

Left Ventricular Hypertrophy and Diastolic Dysfunction

The high arterial pressure (heightened afterload) increases the wall tension of the left ventricle, which compensates through hypertrophy. *Concentric hypertrophy* (without dilatation) is the normal pattern of compensation, although conditions that elevate blood pressure by virtue of increased circulating volume (e.g., primary aldosteronism) may instead cause *eccentric* hypertrophy with chamber dilatation (see Chapter 9). Left ventricular hypertrophy (LVH) results in increased stiffness of the left ventricle with diastolic dysfunction, manifested

Table 13.3. Target Organ Damage in Hypertension	
Organ System	*Manifestations*
Heart	• Left ventricular hypertrophy • Heart failure • Myocardial ischemia and infarction
Cerebrovascular	• Stroke
Aorta and peripheral vascular	• Aortic aneurysm and/or dissection • Arteriosclerosis
Kidney	• Nephrosclerosis • Renal failure
Retina	• Arterial narrowing • Hemorrhages, exudates, papilledema

by elevation of LV filling pressures that can result in pulmonary congestion.

Physical findings of LVH may include a heaving LV impulse on chest palpation, indicative of increased muscle mass. It is frequently accompanied by a fourth heart sound, as the left atrium contracts into the stiffened left ventricle (see Chapter 2).

LVH is one of the strongest predictors of cardiac morbidity in hypertensive patients. The degree of hypertrophy correlates with the development of congestive heart failure, angina, arrhythmias, myocardial infarction, and sudden cardiac death.

Systolic Dysfunction

Although LVH initially serves a compensatory role, later in the course of systemic hypertension, the increased LV mass may be insufficient to balance the high wall tension caused by the elevated pressure. As LV contractile capacity deteriorates, findings of systolic dysfunction become evident (i.e., reduced CO and pulmonary congestion). Systolic dysfunction is also provoked by the accelerated development of coronary artery disease with resultant periods of myocardial ischemia.

Coronary Artery Disease

Chronic hypertension is a major contributor to the development of myocardial ischemia and infarction. These complications reflect the combination of accelerated coronary atherosclerosis (decreased myocardial oxygen supply) and the high systolic workload (increased oxygen demand). In addition, hypertensives have a higher incidence of postmyocardial infarction complications such as rupture of the ventricular wall, LV aneurysm formation, and congestive heart failure. In fact, 60% of patients who die of transmural myocardial infarctions have a history of hypertension.

Cerebrovascular System

Hypertension is the major modifiable risk factor for strokes, also termed **cerebrovascular accidents (CVAs)**. Although diastolic pressure is important, it is the magnitude of the systolic pressure that has been most closely linked to CVAs. The presence of isolated systolic hypertension more than doubles a person's risk for this complication.

Hypertension-induced strokes can be hemorrhagic or, more commonly, atherothrombotic. *Hemorrhagic* CVAs result from rupture of microaneurysms induced in cerebral parenchymal vessels by long-standing hypertension. *Atherothrombotic* (also called *thromboembolic*) CVAs arise when portions of atherosclerotic plaque within the carotids or major cerebral arteries, or thrombi that form on those plaques, break off, and embolize to smaller distal vessels. Additionally, intracerebral vessels may be directly occluded by local atherosclerotic plaque rupture and thrombosis.

Occlusion of small penetrating brain arteries can result in multiple tiny infarcts. As these lesions soften and are absorbed by phagocytic cells, small (≤3 mm diameter) cavities form, termed *lacunae.* These lacunar infarctions are seen almost exclusively in patients with long-standing hypertension and are usually localized to the penetrating branches of the middle and posterior circulation of the brain.

The generalized arterial narrowing found in hypertensive patients reduces collateral flow to ischemic tissues and imposes structural requirements for higher perfusion pressure to maintain adequate tissue flow. This leaves the hypertensive patient vulnerable to cerebral infarcts in areas supplied by the distal ends of arterial branches ("watershed" infarcts) if blood pressure should fall suddenly.

Effective treatment of hypertension diminishes the risk of stroke and has contributed to a 50% reduction in deaths attributed to cerebrovascular events in recent decades.

Aorta and Peripheral Vasculature

The accelerated atherosclerosis associated with hypertension may result in plaque formation and narrowing throughout the arterial vasculature. In addition to the coronary arteries, lesions most commonly appear within the aorta and the major arteries to the lower extremities, neck, and brain.

Chronic hypertension may lead to the development of aneurysms, particularly of the abdominal aorta. An **abdominal aortic aneurysm (AAA)** represents prominent dilatation of the vessel, usually located below the level of the renal arteries, contributed to by the mechanical stress of the high pressure on an arterial wall already weakened by medial damage and atherosclerosis (see Chapter 15). Aneurysms greater than 6 cm in diameter have a very high likelihood of rupture within 2 years if not surgically corrected.

Another life-threatening vascular consequence of high blood pressure is **aortic dissection** (see Chapter 15). Elevated blood pressure, especially in the highest ranges, accelerates degenerative changes in the media of the aorta. When the weakened wall is further exposed to high pressure, the intima may tear, allowing blood to dissect into the aortic media and propagate in either direction within the vessel wall, "clipping off" and obstructing major branch vessels along the way (including coronary or carotid arteries). The mortality rate of aortic dissection is greater than 90% unless treated emergently, usually by surgical repair if the proximal aorta is involved. Rigorous control of hypertension is essential.

Kidney

Hypertension-induced kidney disease (nephrosclerosis) is a leading cause of renal failure that results from damage to the organ's vasculature. Histologically, the vessel walls become thickened with a hyaline infiltrate, known as *hyaline arteriolosclerosis* (Fig. 13.8). Greater levels of hypertension can induce smooth muscle hypertrophy and even necrosis of capillary walls, termed *fibrinoid necrosis*. These changes result in reduced vascular supply and

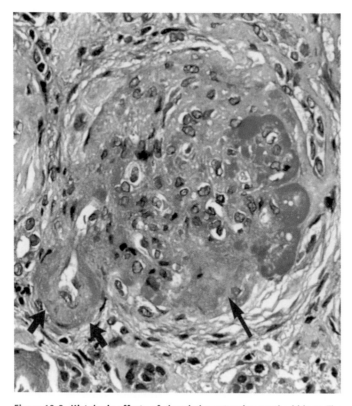

Figure 13.8. Histologic effects of chronic hypertension on the kidney. The arteriolar walls are thickened by hyaline infiltrate *(short arrows)*. The glomeruli*(long arrow)* appear partially sclerosed because of reduced vascular supply. (Courtesy of Dr. Helmut G. Rennke, Brigham and Women's Hospital, Boston, MA.)

subsequent ischemic atrophy of tubules and, to a lesser extent, glomeruli. Because intact nephrons can usually compensate for those damaged by patchy ischemia, mild hypertension rarely leads to renal insufficiency in the absence of other insults to the kidney. However, malignant levels of hypertension can inflict permanent damage leading to chronic renal failure.

One of the consequences of hypertensive renal failure is perpetuation of elevated blood pressure. For example, progressive renal dysfunction compromises the ability of the kidney to regulate blood volume, which contributes further to chronic hypertension.

Retina

The retina is the only location where systemic arteries can be directly visualized by physical examination. High blood pressure induces abnormalities that are collectively termed **hypertensive retinopathy**. Although vision may be compromised when the damage is extensive, more commonly the changes serve as an asymptomatic clinical marker for the severity of hypertension and its duration.

Severe hypertension that is *acute* in onset (e.g., uncontrolled and/or malignant hypertension) may burst small retinal vessels, causing *hemorrhages, exudation of plasma lipids*, and areas of *local infarction*. If ischemia of the optic nerve develops, patients may describe generalized blurred vision. Retinal ischemia caused by hemorrhage leads to more patchy loss of vision. *Papilledema*, or swelling of the optic disk with blurring of its margins, may arise from high intracranial pressure when the blood pressure reaches malignant levels and cerebrovascular autoregulation begins to fail.

Chronically elevated blood pressure results in a different set of retinal findings. Papilledema is absent, but vasoconstriction results in *arterial narrowing*, and medial hypertrophy thickens the vessel wall, which "nicks" (indents) crossing veins. With more severe chronic hypertension, *arterial sclerosis* is evident as an increased reflection of light through the ophthalmoscope (termed "copper" or "silver" wiring). Although these changes are not in themselves of major functional importance,

they indicate that the patient has had long-standing, poorly controlled hypertension.

HYPERTENSIVE CRISIS

A hypertensive crisis is a medical emergency characterized by a severe elevation of blood pressure. In the past, this type of elevation was usually a consequence of inadequate blood pressure treatment. Now a hypertensive crisis is more often caused by an acute hemodynamic insult (e.g., acute renal disease) superimposed on a chronic hypertensive state. As a result of rapid pathologic changes (fibrinoid necrosis) within the blood vessels and kidneys, a spiraling increase in blood pressure evolves. Further volume expansion and vasoconstriction occur as renal perfusion drops and serum renin and angiotensin levels rise.

Severe blood pressure elevation results in increased intracranial pressure, and patients may present with **hypertensive encephalopathy** manifested by headache, blurred vision, confusion, somnolence, and sometimes coma. When hypertension results in acute damage to retinal vessels, **accelerated-malignant hypertension** is said to be present. Funduscopic examination shows the effects of the rapid pressure rise as hemorrhages, exudates, and sometimes papilledema, as described earlier. The increased load on the left ventricle during a hypertensive crisis may precipitate angina (because of increased myocardial oxygen demand) or pulmonary edema.

A hypertensive crisis requires rapid therapy to prevent permanent vascular complications. Correction of blood pressure is generally followed by reversal of the acute pathologic changes, including papilledema and retinal exudation, although renal damage often persists.

TREATMENT OF HYPERTENSION

The therapeutic approach to the hypertensive patient should be influenced by two considerations. First, a single elevated blood pressure measurement does not establish the diagnosis of hypertension because blood pressure varies considerably from day to day. Moreover, blood pressure measurement in the hospital or doctor's office may be affected by the "white coat" effect resulting from patient anxiety. The average of multiple readings taken at two or three office visits and/or in the home provides a more reliable basis for labeling a patient as hypertensive. There is also evidence that automatic ambulatory blood pressure measurements, taken over the course of 24 hours while the patient follows a daily routine, are more predictive of cardiovascular mortality than traditional in-clinic measurements.

Second, although even mild hypertension is a major public health problem because of its high prevalence, for the person with stage 1 hypertension, the risks are small. For example, the additional risk of a stroke is approximately 1 in 850 per year. Hence, observation over time to determine whether the low-level hypertension persists, or whether lifestyle changes can reduce the pressure, is often a recommended alternative to immediate drug therapy. This is especially true in the absence of other cardiovascular risk factors such as smoking, diabetes, or high serum cholesterol. However, for patients with established cardiovascular disease or for those who have other major atherosclerotic risk factors, a more aggressive approach to pharmacologic therapy is usually warranted to reduce the risk burden.

For most hypertensive patients, drug therapy is ultimately the most effective way to prevent future complications, but that should not deter consideration of other beneficial lifestyle changes.

Nonpharmacologic Treatment

Certain lifestyle modifications have been shown to be effective in lowering blood pressure and should be considered in the treatment plan for any patient with hypertension.

Weight Reduction

Studies have consistently found obesity and hypertension to be highly correlated, especially when the obesity is of a central (abdominal) distribution. Blood pressure reduction follows weight loss in a large portion of hypertensive patients who are more than 10% above their ideal weights. Each 10 kg of weight loss is associated with a 5 to 20 mm Hg fall in systolic blood pressure.

Exercise

Sedentary normotensive people have a 20% to 50% higher risk of developing hypertension than their more active peers. Regular aerobic exercise, such as walking, jogging, or bicycling, has been shown to contribute to blood pressure reduction over and above any resulting weight loss. A hypertensive patient who becomes physically conditioned manifests a lower resting HR and reduced levels of circulating catecholamines than before training, suggesting a fall in sympathetic tone.

Diet

In addition to caloric restriction for weight loss, changes in the composition of a patient's diet may be important for blood pressure reduction. For example, a diet high in fruits, vegetables, and low-fat dairy products has been shown to significantly reduce blood pressure.

Sodium

Salt restriction for people with high blood pressure is a controversial issue, but there are several epidemiologic and clinical trials that support the benefit of moderating sodium intake. In normotensive persons, excess salt ingestion is simply excreted by the kidneys, but approximately 50% of patients with EH are found to have blood pressures that vary with sodium intake, suggesting a defect in natriuresis. Sensitivity to sodium levels is more common in African-American and elderly hypertensive patients. Because low-salt diets tend to increase the effectiveness of antihypertensive medications in general, the current recommendation is to limit salt intake to <6 g of sodium chloride (<2.3 g sodium) per day, which is one third less than the average U.S. consumption.

Potassium

Total body potassium content tends to decrease when a person eats a diet low in fruits and vegetables or takes potassium-wasting diuretics.

Potassium deficiency has several theoretical effects that may raise blood pressure and contribute to adverse cardiovascular outcomes, such that dietary supplements are routinely recommended to help replete low serum K^+ levels. There is no convincing evidence that prescribing potassium supplements to a normokalemic hypertensive patient will lower blood pressure.

Alcohol

The chronic excessive intake of alcoholic beverages correlates with high blood pressure and resistance to antihypertensive medications. Moreover, experimental evidence shows that blood pressure (especially systolic) may rise acutely following alcohol consumption. The reason for this link remains incompletely understood, but decreasing chronic alcohol intake has been shown to lower blood pressure.

Other

Low calcium intake and magnesium depletion have been associated with elevated blood pressure, but the responsible mechanisms and the implications for therapy are unclear. Caffeine ingestion transiently increases blood pressure (as much as 5 to 15 mm Hg after two cups of coffee), but routine use does not seem to produce chronic pressure elevation.

Smoking Cessation

Cigarette smoking transiently increases blood pressure, likely because of the effect of nicotine on autonomic ganglia, and is a risk factor for the development of sustained hypertension. In addition, the atherogenic effect of smoking may contribute to the development of renovascular hypertension. Cigarette usage is associated with many other health hazards, and all patients should be discouraged from smoking.

Relaxation Therapy

Blood pressure frequently rises under conditions of stress. In addition, essential hypertensive patients and their relatives often show higher-than-normal basal sympathetic tone and exaggerated autonomic responses to mental stress. Hence, relaxation techniques have been advocated as a method to control hypertension. Available methods include biofeedback and meditation. The effectiveness of such therapy has not been consistently demonstrated in clinical trials and seems to depend on the patient's attitude and long-term compliance.

In summary, nonpharmacologic therapy offers a wide range of options that do not have the expense and potential side effects of prescribed drug use. The effectiveness of these therapies should come as no surprise, given the extent to which environmental factors play a role in hypertension. Therefore, behavior-based interventions are recommended as first-line therapy in any patient whose hypertension is not an immediate danger.

Pharmacologic Treatment

Antihypertensive medications are the standard means to lower chronically elevated blood pressure and are indicated if nonpharmacologic treatment proves inadequate. More than 100 drug preparations are available to treat hypertension, but fortunately the most commonly used medications fall into four classes: diuretics, sympatholytics, vasodilators, and drugs that interfere with the renin–angiotensin system (Table 13.4). The individual actions of these groups on the physiologic abnormalities in hypertension are shown in Figure 13.9. The pharmacology and use of antihypertensive drugs are described in greater detail in Chapter 17.

Diuretics have been in use for many decades to treat hypertension. They reduce circulatory volume, CO, and mean arterial pressure and are most effective in patients with mild to moderate hypertension who have normal renal function. They are especially effective in African-American or elderly persons, who tend to be salt sensitive. In clinical trials, diuretics have reduced the risk of strokes and cardiovascular events in hypertensive patients and are inexpensive compared with other agents. *Thiazide diuretics* (e.g., hydrochlorothiazide) and *potassium-sparing diuretics* (e.g., spironolactone) promote Na^+ excretion in the distal nephron (see Chapter 17). *Loop diuretics*

Table 13.4. Classes of Antihypertensive Medications

Drug Class	Examples (See Chapter 17)	Physiologic Action
Diuretics	Thiazides Potassium-sparing diuretics Loop diuretics	↓ Circulating volume
Sympatholytics	β-Blockers	↓ Heart rate, cardiac contractility and renin secretion
	Combined α- and β-blockers	Same as β-blocker plus vascular smooth muscle relaxation
	Central α₂-agonists	↓ Sympathetic tone
	Peripheral α₁-antagonists	Relaxation of vascular smooth muscle
Vasodilators	Calcium channel blockers	↓ Peripheral vascular resistance
	Direct vasodilators (e.g., hydralazine, minoxidil)	↓ Peripheral vascular resistance
Renin–angiotensin–aldosterone system antagonists	Angiotensin-converting enzyme inhibitors	↓ Peripheral vascular resistance ↓ Sodium retention
	Angiotensin II receptor blockers	
	Direct renin inhibitors	

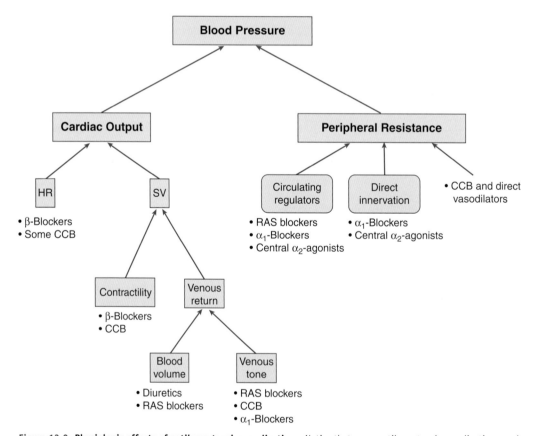

Figure 13.9. Physiologic effects of antihypertensive medications. Notice that some antihypertensive medications work at multiple sites. CCB, calcium channel blockers; HR, heart rate; RAS blockers, renin–angiotensin system blockers (i.e., angiotensin-converting enzyme inhibitors and angiotensin II receptor blockers); SV, stroke volume.

(e.g., furosemide) are generally too potent and their actions too short-lived for use as antihypertensive agents; however, they are useful in lowering blood pressure in patients with renal insufficiency, who often do not respond to other diuretics.

Thiazides, the most commonly used diuretics in hypertension, may result in adverse metabolic side effects, including elevation of serum glucose, cholesterol, and triglyceride levels. In addition, hypokalemia, hyperuricemia, and decreased sexual function are potential side effects. However, when diuretics are prescribed in low dosages, it is often possible to accrue the desired antihypertensive effect while minimizing adverse complications.

Sympatholytic agents include (1) β-blockers, (2) central α-adrenergic agonists, and (3) systemic α-adrenergic-blocking drugs. **β-Blockers** are believed to lower blood pressure through several mechanisms, including (1) reducing CO through a decrease in HR and a mild decrease in contractility and (2) decreasing the secretion of renin (and therefore levels of angiotensin II), which leads to a decrease in TPR. β-Blockers are less effective than diuretics in elderly and African-American hypertensive patients. Adverse effects of β-blockers include bronchospasm (because of bronchiolar β_2-receptor blockade), fatigue, impotence, and hyperglycemia. They may also adversely alter lipid metabolism. Most β-blockers cause an increase in serum triglyceride levels and a decrease in "good" HDL cholesterol levels. However, β-blockers with intrinsic sympathomimetic activity (see Chapter 17) or those with combined α- and β-blocking properties (such as labetalol) do not adversely affect HDL levels.

Centrally acting α_2-adrenergic agonists, such as methyldopa and clonidine, reduce sympathetic outflow to the heart, blood vessels, and kidneys. These are now rarely used owing to their high frequency of side effects (e.g., dry mouth, sedation). Systemic α_1-antagonists, such as prazosin, terazosin, and doxazosin, cause a decrease in TPR through relaxation of vascular smooth muscle. They may be useful for hypertension in some older men because the drugs also improve symptoms of prostatic enlargement. However, they are otherwise not often recommended for treatment of hypertension because a major clinical trial showed that an α_1-antagonist was associated with a greater number of adverse cardiovascular events than a diuretic.

Peripheral **vasodilators** include calcium channel blockers, hydralazine, and minoxidil. **Calcium channel blockers** reduce the influx of Ca^{++} responsible for cardiac and vascular smooth muscle contraction, thus reducing cardiac contractility and TPR (see Chapter 17). Clinical trials in patients with hypertension have shown that calcium channel blockers reduce the risk of myocardial infarction and stroke. Thus, long-acting (i.e., sustained-release drugs taken once a day) members of this group are frequently used to treat hypertension. The shorter-acting calcium channel blocker preparations are no longer used for this purpose; they are less convenient and have actually been associated with adverse cardiovascular outcomes (see Chapter 6).

Hydralazine and *minoxidil* lower blood pressure by directly relaxing vascular smooth muscle of precapillary resistance vessels. However, this action can result in a reflex increase in HR, so that combined β-blocker therapy is frequently necessary. The use of these direct vasodilators in treating hypertension has waned with the advent of newer agents with fewer side effects.

Drugs that interfere with the renin–angiotensin–aldosterone system include ACE inhibitors, angiotensin II receptor blockers, and direct renin inhibitors. **ACE inhibitors** decrease blood pressure by blocking the conversion of angiotensin I to angiotensin II (see Fig. 17.6), thereby reducing the vasopressor effect of angiotensin II and the secretion of aldosterone. As a result, peripheral vascular resistance falls and sodium retention by the kidney declines. An additional antihypertensive effect of ACE inhibitors occurs via an *increase* in the concentration of the circulating vasodilator bradykinin (see Fig. 17.6). ACE inhibitors are important drugs that have been shown to reduce mortality rates in patients following an acute myocardial infarction, in patients with chronic symptomatic systolic heart failure (see Chapter 9), and even in people at high risk for developing cardiovascular disease. The drugs also slow the deterioration of renal function in patients with diabetic nephropathy. The most common side effect of ACE inhibitors is the development of a reversible dry cough (likely related to the increased bradykinin effect); hyperkalemia and azotemia may also occur, as described in Chapter 17.

Angiotensin II receptor blockers (ARBs) block the binding of angiotensin II to its receptors (i.e., subtype AT_1 receptors) in blood vessels and other targets (see Fig. 17.6). By inhibiting the effects of angiotensin II (and thereby causing vasodilatation and reduced secretion of aldosterone), blood pressure falls. In clinical trials, the antihypertensive efficacy of this group is similar to that of ACE inhibitors. They are very well-tolerated drugs, and unlike ACE inhibitors, cough is not a common side effect. Like ACE inhibitors, ARBs have been shown to reduce cardiovascular event rates (including myocardial infarction and stroke) in high-risk patients.

The oral **direct renin inhibitor** aliskiren represents the most recently introduced class of antihypertensive drugs. It reduces levels of angiotensin I and angiotensin II by binding to the proteolytic site of renin, thus inhibiting cleavage of angiotensinogen. Antihypertensive effectiveness is no greater than other drugs that inhibit the rennin–angiotensin–aldosterone axis and long-term effects on cardiovascular event rates are not yet known.

Given the large number of effective antihypertensive drugs available, the choice of which drug to use as initial therapy in an individual patient can seem daunting. Clinical trial data reveal little difference between antihypertensive agents on cardiovascular outcomes in the average hypertensive subject as long as equivalent decreases in blood pressure are achieved. As of this writing, the Joint National Committee on Detection, Evaluation, and Treatment of High Blood Pressure recommends thiazide diuretics as the first-line treatment for uncomplicated hypertension, because of their proven long-term benefits at reducing morbidity and mortality and their low cost. In certain circumstances, or if initial therapy with a diuretic is not sufficient, another type of antihypertensive should be substituted or added (Table 13.5). For example,

Table 13.5. Indications for Specific Antihypertensive Medications

Concurrent Condition	Initial Therapy Drug Classes
Heart failure	Diuretics
	β-blockers
	ACE inhibitors
	Angiotensin II receptor blockers
	Mineralocorticoid receptor antagonists (e.g., spironolactone—see Chapter 9)
Postmyocardial infarction	β-blockers
	ACE inhibitors
	Angiotensin II receptor blockers
	Mineralocorticoid receptor antagonists
Diabetes	ACE inhibitors
	Angiotensin II receptor blockers
	Calcium channel blockers
Chronic kidney disease	ACE inhibitors
	Angiotensin II receptor blockers

ACE, angiotensin-converting enzyme.

an ACE inhibitor would be given prime consideration in patients with concurrent heart failure, diabetes, or LV dysfunction following myocardial infarction. A β-blocker would be an appropriate initial choice in a patient with concurrent ischemic heart disease.

There are some other guiding principles. First, the chosen drug regimen should conform to the patient's specific needs. For example, an anxious young patient in the throes of the hyperkinetic phase of essential hypertension might be treated with a β-blocker, whereas a more effective choice for the same patient many years later, after the pressure becomes more dependent on peripheral vascular resistance, could be a vasodilator (e.g., long-acting calcium channel blocker). Because therapy is likely to continue for many years, consideration of adverse effects and impact of drug therapy on the patient's quality of life are very important.

Another principle of antihypertensive drug therapy concerns the use of multiple agents. The effects of one drug, acting at one physiologic control point, can be defeated by natural compensatory mechanisms. For example, the drop in renal perfusion by a direct vasodilator can activate the renin–angiotensin system, prompting the kidney to retain more volume, thereby blunting the antihypertensive benefit. Combination drug therapy is aimed at preventing such an action by using agents acting at different complementary sites. In this example, a direct vasodilator is often paired with a low-dose diuretic to avoid the undesired volume expansion effect.

In conclusion, hypertension emerges as a tremendously important clinical problem because of its prevalence and potentially devastating consequences. The evaluation and treatment of a patient with hypertension require methodical consideration of the ways in which normal cardiovascular physiology may have gone awry. Because most patients still fall into the idiopathic category of essential hypertension there is still much room for creative thought and research in this area.

SUMMARY

1. Hypertension is defined as a chronic diastolic blood pressure ≥ 90 mm Hg and/or systolic blood pressure ≥ 140 mm Hg.

2. Hypertension is of unknown etiology in the vast majority of patients (EH). Secondary hypertension may arise from diverse causes, including (a) renal abnormalities (e.g., renal parenchymal disease and renal artery stenosis); (b) coarctation of the aorta; and (c) endocrine abnormalities (e.g., pheochromocytoma, primary or secondary aldosteronism, Cushing syndrome, and thyroid abnormalities).

3. Most hypertensive patients remain asymptomatic until complications arise. Potential complications include (a) stroke, (b) myocardial infarction, (c) heart failure, (d) aortic aneurysm and dissection, (e) renal damage, and (f) retinopathy.

4. Treatment of hypertension includes lifestyle and dietary improvements, and pharmacologic therapy. The most commonly used antihypertensive drugs include diuretics, ACE inhibitors, angiotensin receptor blockers, long-acting calcium channel blockers, and β-blockers.

Acknowledgments

Contributors to the previous editions of this chapter were Payman Zamani, MD; Rajeev Malhotra, MD; Rahul Deshmukh, MD; Rajesh S. Magrulkar, MD; Allison McDonough, MD; Peter A. Nigrovic, MD; Thomas J. Moore, MD; Gordon H. Williams; and Leonard S. Lilly, MD.

Additional Reading

Chobanian AV. The hypertension paradox—more uncontrolled disease despite improved therapy. *N Engl J Med.* 2009;361:878–887.

Chobanian AV, Bakris GL, Black HR, et al. The seventh report of the Joint National Committee on Prevention, Detection, Evaluation, and Treatment of High Blood Pressure: the JNC 7 report. *JAMA.* 2003;289:2560–2571.

Cutler JA, Sorlie PD, Wolz M, et al. Trends in hypertension prevalence, awareness, treatment, and control rates in United States adults between 1988–1994 and 1999–2004. *Hypertension.* 2008;52:818–827.

Dolan E, Stanton A, Thijs L, et al. Superiority of ambulatory over clinic blood pressure measurement in predicting mortality. *Hypertension.* 2005;46:156–161.

Ernst ME, Moser M. Use of diuretics in patients with hypertension. *N Engl J Med.* 2009;361: 2153–2164.

Messerli FH, Williams B, Ritz E. Essential hypertension. *Lancet.* 2007;370:591–603.

Raman SV. The hypertensive heart: an integrated understanding informed by imaging. *J Am Coll Cardiol.* 2010;55:91–96.

Shih PA, O'Connor DT. Hereditary determinants of human hypertension: strategies in the setting of genetic complexity. *Hypertension.* 2008;51: 1456–1464.

Wellcome Trust Case Control Consortium. Genome-wide association study of 14,000 cases of seven common diseases and 3,000 shared controls. *Nature.* 2007;447:661–678.

Diseases of the Pericardium

Yin Ren
Leonard S. Lilly

Diseases of the pericardium form a spectrum that ranges from benign, self-limited pericarditis to life-threatening cardiac tamponade. The clinical manifestations of these disorders and the approaches to their management can be predicted from an understanding of pericardial anatomy and pathophysiology, as presented in this chapter.

ANATOMY AND FUNCTION

The pericardium is a two-layered sac that encircles the heart. The inner serosal layer (*visceral pericardium*) adheres to the outer wall of the heart and is reflected back on itself, at the level of the great vessels, to line the tough fibrous outer layer (*parietal pericardium*). A thin film of pericardial fluid slightly separates the two layers and decreases the friction between them.

The pericardium appears to serve three functions: (1) it fixes the heart within the mediastinum and limits its motion, (2) it prevents extreme dilatation of the heart during sudden rises of intracardiac volume, and (3) it may function as a barrier to limit the spread of infection from the adjacent lungs. However, patients with complete absence of the pericardium (either congenitally or after surgical removal) are generally asymptomatic, casting doubt on its actual importance in normal physiology. Yet like the unnecessary appendix, the pericardium can become diseased and cause great harm.

In the healthy heart, intrapericardial pressure varies during the respiratory cycle from −5 mm Hg (during inspiration) to +5 mm Hg (during expiration) and nearly equals the pressure within the pleural space. However, pathologic changes in pericardial stiffness, or the accumulation of fluid within the pericardial sac, may profoundly increase this pressure.

ACUTE PERICARDITIS

The most common affliction of the pericardium is acute pericarditis, which refers to inflammation of its layers. Many disease states and etiologic agents can produce this syndrome (Table 14.1), the most frequent of which are described here.

Etiology

Infectious

Idiopathic and Viral Pericarditis

Acute pericarditis is most often of idiopathic origin, meaning that the actual cause is unknown. However, serologic studies have demonstrated that many such episodes are actually caused by viral infection, especially by echovirus or coxsackievirus group B. Although a viral origin could be confirmed in infected patients by comparing antiviral titers of acute and convalescent serum, this is rarely done in the clinical setting because the patient has usually recovered by the time those results would be available. Thus, idiopathic

Table 14.1. Most Common Causes of Acute Pericarditis

Infectious
  Viral
  Tuberculosis
  Pyogenic bacteria

Noninfectious
  Postmyocardial infarction
  Uremia
  Neoplastic disease
  Radiation-induced
  Connective tissue diseases
  Drug-induced

and viral pericarditis are considered similar clinical entities, and the terms are used interchangeably.

Other viruses known to cause pericarditis include those responsible for influenza, varicella, mumps, hepatitis B, and infectious mononucleosis. Pericarditis is the most common manifestation of cardiovascular disease in patients with AIDS, arising from HIV infection itself or from superimposed tuberculous or other bacterial infections in this immunocompromised population.

Tuberculous Pericarditis

Although tuberculosis remains a worldwide problem, its incidence in the United States is low. It is, however, an important cause of pericarditis in immunosuppressed patients. Tuberculous pericarditis arises from reactivation of the organism in mediastinal lymph nodes, with spread into the pericardium. It can also extend directly from a site of tuberculosis within the lungs, or the organism can arrive at the pericardium by hematogenous dissemination.

Nontuberculous Bacterial Pericarditis (Purulent Pericarditis)

Bacterial pericarditis is a fulminant illness but is rare in otherwise healthy persons; it is most likely to occur in immunocompromised patients, including those with severe burns and malignancies. Pneumococci and staphylococci are responsible most frequently, whereas gram-negative infection occurs less often. Mechanisms by which bacterial invasion of the pericardium develops include (1) perforating trauma to the chest (e.g., stab wound); (2) contamination during chest surgery; (3) extension of an intracardiac infection (i.e., infective endocarditis); (4) extension of pneumonia or a subdiaphragmatic infection; and (5) hematogenous spread from a remote infection.

Noninfectious

Pericarditis Following Myocardial Infarction

There are two forms of pericarditis associated with acute myocardial infarction (MI).

The early type occurs within the first few days after an MI. It likely results from inflammation extending from the epicardial surface of the injured myocardium to the adjacent pericardium; therefore, it is more common in patients with transmural (as opposed to subendocardial) infarctions. The prognosis following acute MI is not affected by the presence of pericarditis; its major importance is in distinguishing it from the pain of recurrent myocardial ischemia. This form of pericarditis occurs in fewer than 5% of patients with acute MI who are treated with acute reperfusion strategies (see Chapter 7) but it is more common in those who are not (and who, therefore, sustain larger infarctions).

The second form of post-MI pericarditis is known as *Dressler syndrome*, which can develop 2 weeks to several months following an acute infarction. Its cause is unknown, but it is thought to be of autoimmune origin, possibly directed against antigens released from necrotic myocardial cells. A clinically similar form of pericarditis may occur weeks to months following heart surgery (termed *postpericardiotomy pericarditis*).

Uremic Pericarditis

Pericarditis is a serious complication of chronic renal failure, but its pathogenesis in this setting is unknown. Studies have shown no correlation between the plasma level of nitrogen waste products and the incidence of pericarditis, and it may even develop in patients during the first few months of dialysis therapy.

Neoplastic Pericarditis

Tumor involvement of the pericardium most commonly results from metastatic spread or local invasion by cancer of the lung, breast, or lymphoma. Primary tumors of the pericardium are rare. Neoplastic effusions are usually large and hemorrhagic and frequently lead to cardiac tamponade, a life-threatening complication described later in the chapter.

Radiation-Induced Pericarditis

Pericarditis may complicate radiation therapy to the thorax (e.g., administered for the treatment of certain tumors), especially if the cumulative dose has exceeded 4,000 centigray. Radiation-induced damage causes a local inflammatory response that can result in pericardial effusions and ultimately fibrosis. Cytologic examination of the pericardial fluid helps to distinguish radiation-induced pericardial damage from that of tumor invasion.

Pericarditis Associated with Connective Tissue Diseases

Pericardial involvement is common in many connective tissue diseases, including systemic lupus erythematosus (SLE), rheumatoid arthritis, and progressive systemic sclerosis. For example, 20% to 40% of patients with SLE experience clinically detectable pericarditis during the course of the disease. Customary treatment of the underlying connective tissue disease usually ameliorates the pericarditis as well.

Drug-Induced Pericarditis

Several pharmaceutical agents have been reported to cause pericarditis as a side effect, often by inducing a systemic lupus-like syndrome (Table 14.2). These drugs include the antiarrhythmic *procainamide* and the vasodilator *hydralazine*. Drug-induced pericarditis usually abates when the causative agent is discontinued.

Table 14.2. Examples of Drug-Induced Pericarditis

Related to drug-induced SLE-like syndrome
  Procainamide
  Hydralazine
  Methyldopa
  Isoniazid
  Phenytoin

Not related to drug-induced SLE-like syndrome
  Anthracycline antineoplastic agents (doxorubicin, daunorubicin)
  Minoxidil

SLE, systemic lupus erythematosus.

Pathogenesis

Similar to other inflammatory processes, pericarditis is characterized by three stages: (1) local *vasodilation* with transudation of protein-poor, cell-free fluid into the pericardial space; (2) *increased vascular permeability*, with leak of protein into the pericardial space; and (3) *leukocyte exudation*, initially by neutrophils, followed later by mononuclear cells.

The leukocytes are of critical importance because they help contain or eliminate the offending infectious or autoimmune agent. However, metabolic products released by these cells may prolong inflammation, cause pain and local cellular damage, and mediate somatic symptoms such as fever. Therefore, the immune response to pericardial injury may significantly contribute to tissue damage and symptomatology.

Pathology

The pathologic appearance of the pericardium depends on the underlying cause and severity of inflammation. **Serous pericarditis** is characterized by scant polymorphonuclear leukocytes, lymphocytes, and histiocytes. The exudate is a thin fluid secreted by the mesothelial cells lining the serosal surface of the pericardium. This likely represents the early inflammatory response common to all types of acute pericarditis.

Serofibrinous pericarditis is the most commonly observed morphologic pattern in patients with pericarditis. The pericardial exudate contains plasma proteins, including fibrinogen, yielding a grossly rough and shaggy appearance (termed "bread and butter" pericarditis). Portions of the visceral and parietal pericardium may become thickened and fused. Occasionally, this process leads to a dense scar that restricts movement and diastolic filling of the cardiac chambers, as described later in the chapter.

Suppurative (or purulent) pericarditis is an intense inflammatory response associated most commonly with bacterial infection. The serosal surfaces are erythematous and coated

Table 14.3. Clinical Features of Acute Pericarditis
Pleuritic chest pain
Fever
Pericardial friction rub
ECG abnormalities

ECG, electrocardiogram.

with purulent exudate. **Hemorrhagic pericarditis** refers to a grossly bloody form of pericardial inflammation and is most often caused by tuberculosis or malignancy.

Clinical Features

History

The most frequent symptoms of acute pericarditis are *chest pain* and *fever* (Table 14.3). The pain may be severe and usually localizes to the retrosternal area and left precordium; it may also radiate to the back and ridge of the left trapezius muscle. What differentiates it from myocardial ischemia or infarction is that the pain of pericarditis is typically sharp, *pleuritic* (it is aggravated by inspiration and coughing), and *positional* (e.g., sitting and leaning forward often lessen the discomfort). *Dyspnea* is common during acute pericarditis but is not exertional and probably results from a reluctance of the patient to breathe deeply because of pleuritic pain.

Patients with idiopathic or viral pericarditis are typically young and previously healthy. Pericarditis of other causes should be suspected in patients with the underlying conditions listed in Table 14.1 who develop the typical sharp, pleuritic chest pains and fever.

Physical Examination

A scratchy pericardial *friction rub* is common in acute pericarditis and is believed to be produced by the movement of the inflamed pericardial layers against one another. Auscultation of the rub is best heard using the diaphragm of the stethoscope with the patient leaning forward while exhaling (which brings the pericardium closer to the chest wall and stethoscope). In its full form, the rub consists of three components, corresponding to the phases of greatest cardiac movement: ventricular contraction, ventricular relaxation, and atrial contraction. Characteristically, the pericardial rub is evanescent, coming and going from one examination to the next.

Diagnostic Studies

The presence of pleuritic, positional chest pain and the characteristic pericardial friction rub implicate the presence of acute pericarditis. However, certain laboratory studies are helpful to confirm the diagnosis and to assess for impending complications.

The *electrocardiogram (ECG)* is abnormal in 90% of patients with acute pericarditis and helps to distinguish it from other forms of cardiac disease, such as an acute MI. The most important ECG pattern, which reflects inflammation of the adjacent myocardium, consists of *diffuse ST segment elevation* in most of the ECG leads, usually with the exception of aVR and V_1 (Fig. 14.1). In addition, *PR segment depression* in several leads is often evident, reflecting abnormal atrial repolarization related to atrial epicardial inflammation. These abnormalities are in contrast to the ECG of acute ST-segment elevation MI, in which the ST segments are elevated only in the leads overlying the region of infarction, and PR depression is not expected.

Blood studies typically reveal signs of acute inflammation, including an increased white blood cell count (usually a mild lymphocytosis in acute viral/idiopathic pericarditis) and elevation of the erythrocyte sedimentation rate. Some patients with acute pericarditis also demonstrate elevated serum cardiac biomarkers (e.g., cardiac troponins), suggesting inflammation of the neighboring myocardium.

Further testing in acute pericarditis often includes *echocardiography* to evaluate for the presence and hemodynamic significance of a pericardial effusion. Additional studies that may be useful in individual cases to define the cause of pericarditis include (1) purified protein derivative (PPD) skin test for tuberculosis, (2) serologic tests (antinuclear antibodies and rheumatoid factor) to screen for connective tissue diseases, and (3) a careful search for malignancy, especially of the lung and breast (physical examination supplemented by chest radiography and mammography). The yield of diagnostic *pericardiocentesis* (removal of pericardial fluid through a needle) in uncomplicated acute pericarditis is low and should be reserved for patients with very large effusions or evidence of cardiac chamber compression, as discussed later in the chapter.

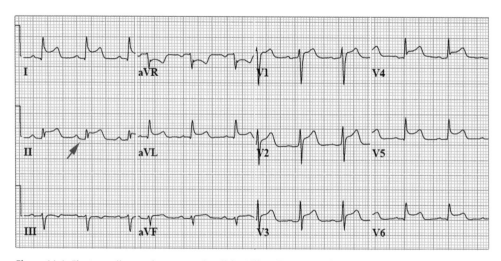

Figure 14.1. Electrocardiogram in acute pericarditis. Diffuse ST segment elevation is present. Also notice depression of the PR segment *(arrow)*.

Treatment

Idiopathic or viral pericarditis is a self-limited disease that usually runs its course in 1 to 3 weeks. Management consists of *rest*, to reduce the interaction of the inflamed pericardial layers, and *pain relief* by analgesic and anti-inflammatory drugs (aspirin, ibuprofen, and other nonsteroidal anti-inflammatory agents). Colchicine, a drug with anti-inflammatory properties usually used to treat gout, may be useful as an additional agent in acute pericarditis. It has been shown to decrease the recurrence rate after an initial episode. Oral corticosteroids are effective for severe or recurrent pericardial pain but should *not* be used in uncomplicated cases because of potentially significant side effects and because even gradual withdrawal of this form of therapy often leads to recurrent symptoms of pericarditis.

The forms of pericarditis related to MI are treated in a similar fashion, with rest and aspirin. Other nonsteroidal anti-inflammatory agents are often avoided immediately following an MI because of experimental evidence linking them to delayed healing of the infarct.

Purulent pericarditis requires more aggressive treatment, including catheter drainage of the pericardium and intensive antibiotic therapy. Nevertheless, even with such therapy, the mortality rate is very high. Tuberculous pericarditis requires prolonged multidrug antituberculous therapy. Pericarditis in the setting of uremia often resolves following intensive dialysis. Neoplastic pericardial disease usually indicates widely metastatic cancer, and therapy is unfortunately only palliative.

PERICARDIAL EFFUSION

Etiology

The normal pericardial space contains 15 to 50 mL of pericardial fluid, a plasma ultrafiltrate secreted by the mesothelial cells that line the serosal layer. A larger volume of fluid may accumulate in association with any of the forms of acute pericarditis previously discussed.

In addition, noninflammatory serous effusions may result from conditions of (1) increased capillary permeability (e.g., severe hypothyroidism); (2) increased capillary hydrostatic pressure (e.g., congestive heart failure); or (3) decreased plasma oncotic pressure (e.g., cirrhosis or the nephrotic syndrome). Chylous effusions may occur in the presence of lymphatic obstruction of pericardial drainage, most commonly caused by neoplasms and tuberculosis.

Pathophysiology

Because the pericardium is a relatively stiff structure, the relationship between its internal volume and pressure is not linear, as shown in curve A in Figure 14.2. Notice that the initial portion of the curve is nearly flat, indicating that at the low volumes normally present within the pericardium, a small increase in volume leads to only a small rise in pressure. However, when the intrapericardial volume expands beyond a critical level (see Fig. 14.2, arrow), a dramatic increase in pressure is incited by the nondistensible sac. At that point, even a minor increase in volume can translate into an enormous compressive force on the heart.

Three factors determine whether a pericardial effusion remains clinically silent or whether symptoms of cardiac compression ensue: (1) the *volume* of fluid, (2) the *rate* at which the fluid accumulates, and (3) the *compliance* characteristics of the pericardium.

A *sudden* increase of pericardial volume, as may occur in chest trauma with intrapericardial hemorrhage, results in marked elevation of pericardial pressure (see Fig. 14.2, steep portion of curve A) and the potential for severe cardiac chamber compression. Even lesser amounts of fluid may cause significant elevation of pressure if the pericardium is pathologically noncompliant and stiff, as may occur in the presence of tumor or fibrosis of the sac. In contrast, if the pericardial effusion accumulates *slowly*, over weeks to months, the pericardium gradually stretches, such that the volume–pressure relationship curve shifts toward the right (see Fig. 14.2, curve B). With this adaptation, the pericardium can accommodate larger volumes without marked elevation of intrapericardial pressure.

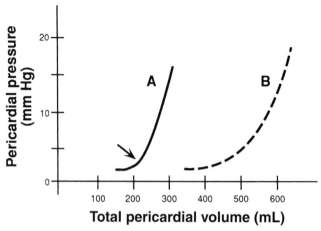

Figure 14.2. **Schematic representation of the volume–pressure relationship of the normal pericardium. A.** At the very lowest levels, a small rise in volume results in a small rise in pressure. However, when the limits of pericardial stretch are reached *(arrow)*, the curve becomes very steep, and a further small rise in intrapericardial volume results in significantly increased pressure. **B.** Chronic slow accumulation of volume allows the pericardium to gradually stretch over time; thus, the curve shifts to the right and much larger volumes are accommodated at lower pressures. (Modified from Freeman GL, LeWinter MM. Pericardial adaptations during chronic dilation in dogs. *Circ Res.* 1984;54:294.)

Clinical Features

A spectrum of possible symptoms is associated with pericardial effusions. For example, the patient with a large effusion may be asymptomatic, may complain of a dull constant ache in the left side of the chest, or may present with findings of cardiac tamponade, as described later in the chapter. In addition, the effusion may cause symptoms resulting from compression of adjacent structures, such as dysphagia (difficult swallowing because of esophageal compression), dyspnea (shortness of breath resulting from lung compression), hoarseness (due to recurrent laryngeal nerve compression), or hiccups (resulting from phrenic nerve stimulation).

On examination (Table 14.4), a large pericardial fluid "insulates" the heart from the chest wall, and the heart sounds may be muffled. In fact, a friction rub that had been present during the acute phase of pericarditis may disappear if a large effusion develops and separates the inflamed layers from one another. Dullness to percussion of the left lung over the angle of the scapula may be present (known as the *Ewart sign*) owing to compressive atelectasis by the enlarged pericardial sac.

Diagnostic Studies

The *chest radiograph* may be normal if only a small pericardial effusion is present. However, if more than approximately 250 mL has accumulated, the cardiac silhouette enlarges in a globular, symmetric fashion. In large effusions, the ECG may demonstrate reduced voltage of the complexes. In the presence of very large effusions, the height of the QRS complex may vary from beat to beat (*electrical alternans*), a result of a constantly changing electrical axis as the heart swings from side to side within the large pericardial volume (Fig. 14.3).

Table 14.4. Clinical Features of Large Pericardial Effusion
Soft heart sounds
Reduced intensity of friction rub
Ewart sign (dullness over posterior left lung)

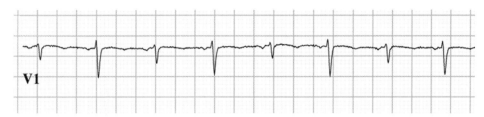

Figure 14.3. **Electrical alternans.** Rhythm strip of lead V_1 showing alternating height of the QRS complex from beat to beat, due to shifting of the cardiac axis as the heart swings within a large pericardial effusion.

One of the most useful laboratory tests in the evaluation of an effusion is *echocardiography* (Fig. 14.4), which can identify pericardial collections as small as 20 mL. This noninvasive technique can quantify the volume of pericardial fluid, determine whether ventricular filling is compromised, and when necessary, help direct the placement of a pericardiocentesis needle.

Treatment

If the cause of the effusion is known, therapy is directed toward the underlying disorder (e.g., intensive dialysis for uremic effusion). If the cause is not evident, the clinical state of the patient determines whether pericardiocentesis (removal of pericardial fluid) should be undertaken. An asymptomatic effusion, even of large volume, can be observed for long periods without specific intervention. However, if serial examination demonstrates a precipitous

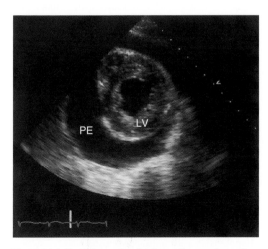

Figure 14.4. **Two-dimensional echocardiogram (parasternal short-axis view) of a pericardial effusion (PE) surrounding the heart.** LV, left ventricle.

rise in pericardial volume or if hemodynamic compression of the cardiac chambers becomes evident, then pericardiocentesis should be performed for therapeutic drainage and for analysis of the fluid.

CARDIAC TAMPONADE

At the opposite end of the spectrum from the asymptomatic pericardial effusion is cardiac tamponade. In this condition, pericardial fluid accumulates under high pressure, compresses the cardiac chambers, and severely limits filling of the heart. As a result, ventricular stroke volume and cardiac output decline, potentially leading to hypotensive shock and death.

Etiology

Any etiology of acute pericarditis (see Table 14.1) can progress to cardiac tamponade, but the most common causes are neoplastic, postviral, and uremic pericarditis. Acute hemorrhage into the pericardium is also an important cause of tamponade, which can result (1) from blunt or penetrating chest trauma, (2) from rupture of the left ventricular (LV) free wall following MI (see Chapter 7), or (3) as a complication of a dissecting aortic aneurysm (see Chapter 15).

Pathophysiology

As a result of the surrounding tense pericardial fluid, the heart is compressed, and *the diastolic pressure within each chamber becomes elevated and equal to the pericardial pressure*. The pathophysiologic consequences of this are illustrated in Figure 14.5. Because the compromised cardiac chambers cannot accommodate

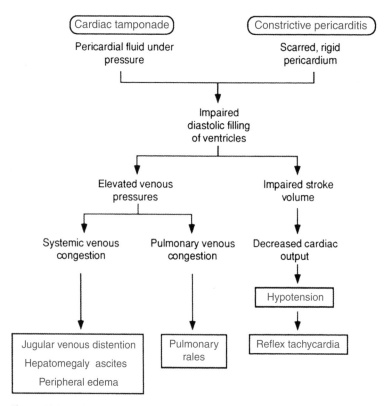

Figure 14.5. Pathophysiology of cardiac tamponade and constrictive pericarditis. The symptoms and signs *(boxes)* arise from impaired diastolic filling of the ventricles in both conditions.

normal venous return, the systemic and pulmonary venous pressures rise. The increase of systemic venous pressure results in signs of right-sided heart failure (e.g., jugular venous distention), whereas elevated pulmonary venous pressure leads to pulmonary congestion. In addition, reduced filling of the ventricles during diastole decreases the systolic stroke volume, and the cardiac output declines.

These derangements trigger compensatory mechanisms aimed at maintaining tissue perfusion, initially through activation of the sympathetic nervous system (e.g., elevation of the heart rate). Nonetheless, failure to evacuate the effusion leads to inadequate perfusion of vital organs, shock, and ultimately death.

Clinical Features

Cardiac tamponade should be suspected in any patient with known pericarditis, pericardial effusion, or chest trauma who develops signs and symptoms of systemic vascular congestion and decreased cardiac output (Table 14.5). The key physical findings include (1) jugular venous distention; (2) systemic hypotension; and (3) a "small, quiet heart" on physical examination, a result of the insulating effects of the effusion. Other signs include sinus tachycardia and pulsus paradoxus (described later). Dyspnea and tachypnea reflect pulmonary congestion and decreased oxygen delivery to peripheral tissues.

If tamponade develops suddenly, symptoms of profound hypotension are evident, including confusion and agitation. However, if the effusion

Table 14.5. Clinical Features of Cardiac Tamponade
Jugular venous distention
Hypotension with pulsus paradoxus
Quiet precordium on palpation
Sinus tachycardia

BOX 14.1 | Measurement of Pulsus Paradoxus at the Bedside

Pulsus paradoxus is an exaggeration of the normal decline in systolic blood pressure that occurs with inspiration. It can be measured at the bedside using a manual sphygmomanometer. First, inflate the sphygmomanometer to a level greater than the patient's systolic pressure. As the cuff is slowly deflated, carefully listen for the appearance of the first Korotkoff sounds. This level marks the maximum systolic pressure and occurs during expiration. If the pressure is held at that level (i.e., if you stop deflating the cuff) in a patient with pulsus paradoxus, the Korotkoff sounds will drift in and out, audible with expiration, and absent with inspiration. That is, the systolic pressure will fall during inspiration to a level below the cuff's pressure and no sound will be heard during that time. Next, slowly deflate the cuff and continue listening. When the cuff pressure falls to the level just below the patient's systolic pressure during inspiration, the Korotkoff sounds stop drifting in and out (i.e., they are audible during both inspiration and expiration). Pulsus paradoxus is calculated as the difference between the initial systolic pressure (when the intermittent Korotkoff sounds are first heard) and this pressure (when the sounds are first audible throughout the respiratory cycle). In the presence of cardiac tamponade, this pressure difference is >10 mm Hg.

---

develops more slowly, over a period of weeks, then fatigue (caused by low cardiac output) and peripheral edema (owing to right-sided heart failure) may be the presenting complaints.

Pulsus paradoxus is an important physical sign in cardiac tamponade that can be recognized at the bedside using a standard blood pressure cuff. It refers to a *decrease of systolic blood pressure (more than 10 mm Hg) during normal inspiration* (see Box 14.1).

Pulsus paradoxus is not really "paradoxical"; it is just an exaggeration of appropriate cardiac physiology. Normally, expansion of the thorax during inspiration causes the intrathoracic pressure to become more negative compared with the expiratory phase. This facilitates systemic venous return to the chest and augments filling of the right ventricle (RV). The transient increase in RV size shifts the interventricular septum toward the left, which diminishes left ventricular filling. As a result, in normal persons, LV stroke volume and systolic blood pressure decline slightly following inspiration.

In cardiac tamponade, this situation is exaggerated because both ventricles share a reduced, fixed volume as a result of external compression by the tense pericardial fluid. In this case, the inspiratory increase of right ventricular volume and bulging of the interventricular septum toward the left have a proportionally greater effect on the limitation of

LV filling. Thus, in tamponade there is a more substantial reduction of LV stroke volume (and therefore systolic blood pressure) following inspiration.

Pulsus paradoxus may also be manifested by other conditions in which inspiration is exaggerated, including severe asthma and chronic obstructive airway disease.

Diagnostic Studies

Echocardiography is the most useful noninvasive technique to evaluate whether pericardial effusion has led to cardiac tamponade physiology. An important indicator of high-pressure pericardial fluid is compression of the RV and right atrium during diastole (see Fig. 3.12). In addition, echocardiography can differentiate between cardiac tamponade and other causes of low cardiac output, such as ventricular contractile dysfunction. The definitive diagnostic procedure for cardiac tamponade is *cardiac catheterization* with measurement of intracardiac and intrapericardial pressures, usually combined with therapeutic *pericardiocentesis*, as described in the next section.

Treatment

Removal of the high-pressure pericardial fluid is the only intervention that reverses the life-threatening physiology of this condition. Pericardiocentesis is best performed in the cardiac catheterization laboratory, where the hemodynamic effect of fluid removal can be assessed. The patient is positioned head up at a 45° angle to promote pooling of the effusion, and a needle is inserted into the pericardial space through the skin, usually just below the xiphoid process (which is the safest location to avoid piercing a coronary artery). A catheter is then threaded into the pericardial space and connected to a transducer for pressure measurement. Another catheter is threaded through a systemic vein into the right side of the heart, and simultaneous recordings of intracardiac and intrapericardial pressures are compared. In tamponade, the pericardial pressure is elevated and is equal to the diastolic pressures within all of the cardiac chambers, reflecting the compressive force of the surrounding effusion.

In addition, the right atrial pressure tracing, which is equivalent to the jugular venous pulsation observed on physical examination, displays a characteristic abnormality (Fig. 14.6). During early diastole in a normal person, as the right ventricular pressure falls and the tricuspid valve opens, blood quickly flows from the right atrium into the RV, leading to a rapid decline in the right atrial pressure tracing (y descent). In tamponade, however, the pericardial fluid compresses the right ventricle and prevents its rapid expansion. Thus, the right atrium cannot empty quickly, and the y descent is blunted.

Following successful pericardiocentesis, the pericardial pressure falls to normal and is no longer equal to the diastolic pressures within the heart chambers, which also decline to their normal levels. After initial aspiration of fluid, the pericardial catheter may be left in place for 1 to 2 days to allow more complete drainage.

When pericardial fluid is obtained for diagnostic purposes, it should be stained and cultured for bacteria, fungi, and acid-fast bacilli (tuberculosis), and cytologic examination should be performed to evaluate for malignancy. Other common measurements of pericardial fluid include cell counts (e.g., white cell count is elevated in bacterial infections

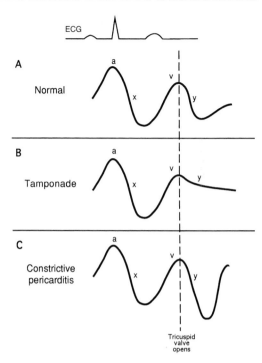

Figure 14.6. Schematic diagrams of right atrial (or jugular venous) pressure recordings. A. Normal. The initial *a* wave represents atrial contraction. The *v* wave reflects passive filling of the atrium during systole, when the tricuspid valve is closed. After the tricuspid valve opens, the right atrial pressure falls (*y* descent) as blood empties into the right ventricle. B. Cardiac tamponade. High-pressure pericardial fluid compresses the heart, impairing right ventricular filling, so that the *y* descent is blunted. C. Constrictive pericarditis. The *earliest* phase of diastolic filling is not impaired so that the *y* descent is not blunted. The *y* descent appears accentuated because it descends from a higher than normal right atrial pressure. The right atrial *c* wave (described in Chapter 2) is not shown.

and other inflammatory conditions) and protein and lactate dehydrogenase (LDH) levels. If the concentration ratio of pericardial protein to serum protein is >0.5, or that of pericardial LDH to serum LDH is >0.6, then the fluid is consistent with an exudate; otherwise, it is more likely a transudate. When tuberculosis is suspected, it is also useful to measure the level of adenosine deaminase in the pericardial fluid. Studies have indicated that an elevated level is highly sensitive and specific for tuberculosis.

If cardiac tamponade recurs following pericardiocentesis, the procedure can be repeated. In some cases, a more definitive surgical undertaking (removal of part or all of the pericardium) is required to prevent reaccumulation of the effusion.

CONSTRICTIVE PERICARDITIS

The other major potential complication of pericardial diseases is constrictive pericarditis. This is a condition not frequently encountered but is important to understand, because it can masquerade as other more common disorders. In addition, it is an affliction that may cause profound symptoms yet is often fully correctable if recognized.

Etiology and Pathogenesis

In the early part of the 20th century, tuberculosis was the major cause of constrictive pericarditis, but that is much less common today in industrialized societies. The most frequent cause now is "idiopathic" (i.e., months to years following presumed idiopathic or viral acute pericarditis). However, any etiology of pericarditis can lead to this complication.

Pathology

Following an episode of acute pericarditis, any pericardial effusion that has accumulated usually undergoes gradual resorption. However, in patients who later develop constrictive pericarditis, the fluid undergoes organization, with subsequent fusion of the pericardial layers, followed by fibrous scar formation. In some patients, calcification of the adherent layers ensues, further stiffening the pericardium.

Pathophysiology

The pathophysiologic abnormalities in constrictive pericarditis occur during diastole; systolic contraction of the ventricles is usually normal. In this condition, a rigid, scarred pericardium encircles the heart and *inhibits normal filling of the cardiac chambers*. For example, as blood passes from the right atrium into the right ventricle during diastole, the RV size expands and quickly reaches the limit imposed by the constricting pericardium. At that point, further filling is suddenly arrested, and venous return to the right heart ceases. Thus, systemic venous pressure rises, and signs of right-sided heart failure ensue. In addition, the impaired filling of the left ventricle causes a reduction in stroke volume and cardiac output, which leads to lower blood pressure.

Clinical Features

The symptoms and signs of constrictive pericarditis usually develop over months to years. They result from (1) reduced cardiac output (fatigue, hypotension, and reflex tachycardia) and (2) elevated systemic venous pressures (jugular venous distention, hepatomegaly with ascites, and peripheral edema). Because the most impressive physical findings are often the insidious development of hepatomegaly and ascites, patients may be mistakenly suspected of having hepatic cirrhosis or an intra-abdominal tumor. However, careful inspection of the elevated jugular veins can point to the correct diagnosis of constrictive pericarditis.

On cardiac examination, an early diastolic "knock" may follow the second heart in patients with severe calcific constriction. It represents the sudden cessation of ventricular diastolic filling imposed by the rigid pericardial sac.

In contrast to cardiac tamponade, pericardial constriction results in pulsus paradoxus less frequently. Recall that in tamponade, this finding reflects inspiratory augmentation of RV filling, at the expense of LV filling. However, in constrictive pericarditis, the negative intrathoracic pressure generated by inspiration is not easily transmitted through the rigid pericardial shell to the right-sided heart chambers; therefore, inspiratory augmentation of RV filling is more limited. Rather, when a patient with severe pericardial constriction inhales, the negative intrathoracic pressure draws blood toward the thorax, where it cannot be accommodated by the constricted right-sided cardiac chambers. As a result, the increased venous return accumulates in the intrathoracic systemic veins, causing the jugular veins to become more distended during inspiration (**Kussmaul sign**). This is the opposite of normal physiology, in which inspiration results in a *decline* in jugular venous pressure, as venous return is drawn into the heart. Thus, typical findings in pericardial disease can be summarized as follows:

	Constrictive Pericarditis	Cardiac Tamponade
Pulsus paradoxus	+	+++
Kussmaul sign	+++	−

Diagnostic Studies

The *chest radiograph* in constrictive pericarditis shows a normal or mildly enlarged cardiac silhouette. Calcification of the pericardium can be detected in some patients with severe chronic constriction. The ECG generally shows only nonspecific ST and T-wave abnormalities, although atrial arrhythmias are common.

Echocardiographic evidence of constriction is subtle. The pericardium, if well imaged, is thickened. The ventricular cavities are small and contract vigorously, but ventricular filling terminates abruptly in early diastole, as the chambers reach the limit imposed by the surrounding rigid shell. Aberrant diastolic motion of the interventricular septum and alterations of LV inflow velocities by Doppler also reflect the abnormal pattern of diastolic filling.

Computed tomography or *magnetic resonance imaging* is superior to echocardiography in the assessment of pericardial anatomy and thickness. The presence of normal pericardial thickness (<2 mm) by these modalities makes constrictive pericarditis a less likely diagnosis.

The diagnosis of constrictive pericarditis can be confirmed by *cardiac catheterization,* which reveals four key features:

1. Elevation and equalization of the diastolic pressures in each of the cardiac chambers.
2. An early diastolic "dip and plateau" configuration in the right and left ventricular tracings (Fig. 14.7). This pattern reflects blood flow into the ventricles at the very onset of diastole, just after the tricuspid and mitral valves open, followed by sudden cessation of filling as further expansion of the ventricles is arrested by the surrounding rigid pericardium.

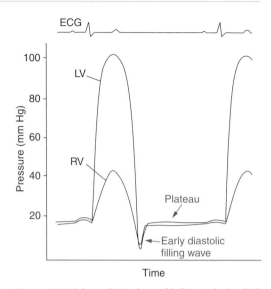

Figure 14.7. Schematic tracings of left ventricular (LV) and right ventricular (RV) pressures in constrictive pericarditis. Early diastolic ventricular filling abruptly halts as the volume in each ventricle quickly reaches the limit imposed by the constricting pericardium. Throughout most of diastole, the LV and RV pressures are abnormally elevated and equal.

3. A prominent *y* descent in the right atrial pressure tracing (see Fig. 14.6). After the tricuspid valve opens, the right atrium quickly empties into the RV (and its pressure rapidly falls) during the very brief period before filling is arrested. This is in contrast to cardiac tamponade, in which the external compressive force throughout the cardiac cycle *prevents* rapid ventricular filling, even in early diastole, such that the *y* descent is blunted.

4. During the respiratory cycle, there is discordance in the RV and LV *systolic* pressures (the RV systolic pressure rises with inspiration, while that of the LV declines). This is explained as follows: in normal persons, the negative intrathoracic pressure induced by inspiration causes the systolic pressure of both ventricles to decline slightly. In contrast, in constrictive pericarditis, the heart is isolated from the rest of the thorax by the surrounding rigid shell. In this circumstance, negative intrathoracic pressure induced by inspiration decreases the pressure in the pulmonary veins but not in the left-sided cardiac chambers. This causes a decline in the pressure gradient

Table 14.6. Differences Between Constrictive Pericarditis and Restrictive Cardiomyopathy

Feature	Constrictive Pericarditis	Restrictive Cardiomyopathy
Chest radiography		
• Pericardial calcifications	Yes (25–30% of patients)	Absent
CT or MRI		
• Thickened pericardium	Yes	No
Echocardiography		
• Thickened pericardium	Yes (but difficult to visualize)	No
• Respiratory cycle effect on transvalvular Doppler velocities	Exaggerated variations	Normal
Cardiac catheterization		
• Equalized LV and RV diastolic pressures	Yes	Often, LV > RV
• Elevated PA systolic pressure	Uncommon	Common
• Effect of inspiration on systolic pressures	Discordant : LV↓, RV↑	Concordant: LV↓, RV↓
Endomyocardial biopsy	Normal	Abnormal (e.g., amyloid)

CT, computed tomography; LV, left ventricle; MRI, magnetic resonance imaging; PA, pulmonary artery; RV, right ventricle.

driving blood back to the left side of the heart from the pulmonary veins, such that left ventricle filling is diminished. Less ventricular filling reduces the stroke volume and results in a *lower* LV systolic pressure (and is the likely mechanism of pulsus paradoxus in some patients with constrictive pericarditis). Simultaneously, because the two ventricles share a fixed space limited by the rigid pericardium, the reduced LV volume allows the interventricular septum to shift toward the left, which enlarges the RV (this reciprocal behavior is termed *ventricular interdependence*). The subsequent increase in RV filling *augments* systolic pressure during inspiration. During expiration, the situation is reversed, with the RV systolic pressure declining and that of the LV increasing.

The clinical and hemodynamic findings of constrictive pericarditis are often similar to those of restrictive cardiomyopathy (see Chapter 10), another uncommon condition. Distinguishing between these two syndromes is important because pericardial constriction is often correctable, whereas most cases of restrictive cardiomyopathy have very limited effective treatments (Table 14.6). An endomyocardial biopsy is sometimes necessary to distinguish between these (the biopsy results are normal in constriction but usually abnormal in restrictive cardiomyopathy; see Chapter 10).

Treatment

The only effective treatment of severe constrictive pericarditis is surgical removal of the pericardium. Symptoms and signs of constriction may not resolve immediately because of the associated stiffness of the neighboring outer walls of the heart, but subsequent clinical improvement is the rule in patients with otherwise intact cardiac function.

SUMMARY

1. Acute pericarditis is most often of idiopathic or viral cause and is usually a self-limited illness. More serious forms of pericarditis arise from the conditions listed in Table 14.1.

2. Common findings in acute pericarditis include (a) pleuritic chest pain; (b) fever; (c) pericardial friction rub; and (d) diffuse ST segment elevation on the ECG, often accompanied by PR segment depression.

3. Complications of pericarditis include cardiac tamponade (accumulation of pericardial fluid under high pressure, which compresses the cardiac chambers) and constrictive pericarditis (restricted filling of the heart because of surrounding rigid pericardium).

Acknowledgments

Contributors to the previous editions of this chapter were Yanerys Ramos, MD; Angela Fowler, MD; Kathy Glatter, MD; Thomas G. Roberts, MD; Alan Braverman, MD; and Leonard S. Lilly, MD.

Additional Reading

ESC Committee for Practice Guidelines. Guidelines on the diagnosis and management of pericardial diseases, executive summary. *Eur Heart J.* 2004;25:587–610.

Dal-Bianco JP, Sengupta PP, Mookadam F, et al. Role of echocardiography in the diagnosis of constrictive pericarditis. *J Am Soc Echocardiogr.* 2009;22:24–33.

Imazio M, Bobbio M, Cecchi E, et al. Colchicine in addition to conventional therapy for acute pericarditis: results of the COlchicine for acute Pericarditis (COPE) trial. *Circulation.* 2005;112:2012–2016.

Khandaker MH, Espinosa RE, Nishimura RA, et al. Pericardial disease: Diagnosis and management. *Mayo Clin Proc.* 2010;85:572–593.

Little WC, Freeman GL. Pericardial disease. *Circulation.* 2006;113:1622–1632.

Roy CL, Minor MA, Brookhart MA, et al. Does this patient with a pericardial effusion have cardiac tamponade? *N Engl J Med.* 2007;297:1810–1818.

Shabetai R. *The Pericardium.* Boston, MA: Kluwer Academic; 2003.

Spodick DH. Risk prediction in pericarditis: who to keep in hospital? *Heart.* 2008;94:398–399.

Diseases of the Peripheral Vasculature

Fan Liang
Mark A. Creager

DISEASES OF THE AORTA
Aortic Aneurysms
Aortic Dissection
PERIPHERAL ARTERY DISEASES
Peripheral Atherosclerotic Vascular Disease
Acute Arterial Occlusion
Vasculitic Syndromes

VASOSPASM: RAYNAUD PHENOMENON
VENOUS DISEASE
Varicose Veins
Venous Thrombosis

*P*eripheral vascular disease is an umbrella term that includes a number of diverse pathologic entities that affect arteries, veins, and lymphatics. Although this terminology makes a distinction between the "central" coronary and "peripheral" systemic vessels, the vasculature as a whole comprises a dynamic, integrated, and multifunctional organ system that does not naturally comply with this semantic division.

Blood vessels serve many critical functions. First, they regulate the differential distribution of blood and delivery of nutrients and oxygen to tissues. Second, blood vessels actively synthesize and secrete vasoactive substances that regulate vascular tone, and antithrombotic substances that maintain the fluidity of blood and vessel patency (see Chapters 6 and 7). Third, the vessels play an integral role in the transport and distribution of immune cells to traumatized or infected tissues.

Disease states of the peripheral vasculature interfere with these essential functions.

Peripheral vascular diseases result from processes that can be grouped into three categories: (1) *structural changes in the vessel wall* secondary to degenerative conditions, infection, or inflammation that lead to dilatation, aneurysm, dissection, or rupture; (2) *narrowing of the vascular lumen* caused by atherosclerosis, thrombosis, or inflammation; and (3) *spasm of* vascular smooth muscle. These processes can occur in isolation or in combination.

DISEASES OF THE AORTA

The aorta is the largest conductance vessel of the vascular system. In adults, its diameter is approximately 3 cm at its origin at the base of the heart. The **ascending aorta,** 5 to 6 cm in length, leads to the **aortic arch,** from which arise three major branches: the brachiocephalic (which bifurcates

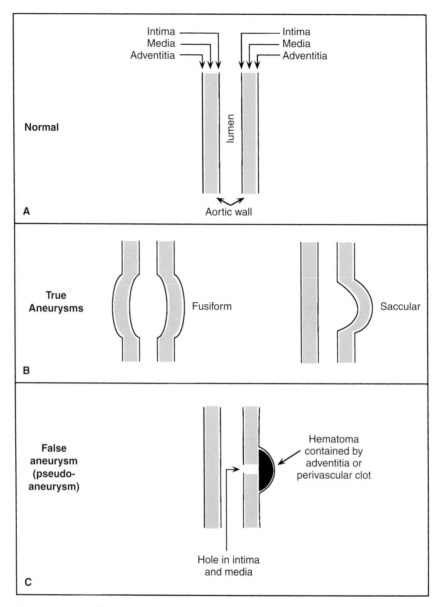

Figure 15.1. Classification of aortic aneurysms. A. The normal arterial wall consists of three layers: the intima, the media, and the adventitia. **B.** True aneurysms represent localized dilatation of all three layers of the arterial wall. Fusiform aneurysms involve the entire circumference of the aorta, whereas saccular aneurysms are a localized bulge of only a portion of the circumference. **C.** A false aneurysm (or pseudoaneurysm) is actually a hole in the intima and media, with hematoma contained by a thin layer of adventitia or perivascular clot.

into the right common carotid and subclavian arteries), the left common carotid, and the left subclavian arteries. As the **descending aorta** continues beyond the arch, its diameter narrows to approximately 2 to 2.5 cm in healthy adults. As the aorta pierces the diaphragm, it becomes the **abdominal aorta,** providing arteries to the abdominal viscera before bifurcating into the left and right common iliac arteries, which supply the pelvic organs and lower extremities.

The aorta, like other arteries, is composed of three layers (Fig. 15.1). At the luminal surface, the *intima* is composed of endothelial cells overlying the internal elastic lamina. The endothelial layer is a functional interface between the vasculature and circulating blood cells and plasma. The *media* is composed of smooth muscle cells and a matrix that includes collagen and elastic fibers. Collagen provides tensile strength that enables the vessels to withstand high-pressure loads. Elastin is capable of stretching to 250% of its original length and confers a distensible quality on vessels that allows them to recoil under pressure. The *adventitia* is primarily composed of collagen fibers, perivascular nerves, and vasa vasorum, a rich vascular network that supplies oxygenated blood to the aorta.

The aorta is subject to injury from mechanical trauma because it is continuously exposed to high pulsatile pressure and shear stress. The predominance of elastin in the media (2:1 over collagen) allows the aorta to expand during systole and recoil during diastole. The recoil of the aorta against the closed aortic valve contributes to the distal propagation of blood flow during the phase of left ventricular relaxation. With advancing age, the elastic component of the aorta and its branches degenerates, and as collagen becomes more prominent, the arteries stiffen. Systolic blood pressure, therefore, tends to rise with age because less energy is dissipated into the aorta during left ventricular contraction.

Diseases of the aorta most commonly appear as one of three clinical conditions: aneurysm, dissection, or obstruction.

Aortic Aneurysms

An aneurysm is an abnormal localized dilatation of an artery. In the aorta, aneurysms are distinguished from *diffuse ectasia*, which is a generalized yet lesser increase of the aortic diameter. Ectasia develops in older patients as elastic fiber fragments, smooth muscle cells decrease in number, and acid mucopolysaccharide ground substance accumulates within the vessel wall.

The term *aneurysm* is applied when the diameter of a portion of the aorta has increased by at least 50% compared with normal. A **true aneurysm** represents a dilatation of all three layers of the aorta, creating a large bulge of the vessel wall. True aneurysms are characterized as either fusiform or saccular, depending on the extent of the vessel's circumference within the aneurysm (see Fig. 15.1). A *fusiform* aneurysm, the more common type, is characterized by symmetrical dilation of the entire circumference of a segment of the aorta. A *saccular* aneurysm is a localized outpouching involving only a portion of the circumference.

In contrast, a **pseudoaneurysm,** or **false aneurysm,** is a contained *rupture* of the vessel wall that develops when blood leaks out of the vessel lumen through a hole in the intimal and medial layers and is contained by a layer of adventitia or perivascular organized thrombus (see Fig. 15.1). Pseudoaneurysms develop at sites of vessel injury caused by infection or trauma, such as puncture of the vessel during surgery or percutaneous catheterization. They are very unstable and are prone to rupture completely.

Aneurysms may be confined to the abdominal aorta (most common), the thoracic aorta, or involve both locations. They may also appear in peripheral and cerebral arteries.

Etiology and Pathogenesis of True Aortic Aneurysms

The etiology of aortic aneurysm formation varies depending on the location of the lesion. *Ascending thoracic aortic aneurysms* typically are characterized by **cystic medial degeneration** (also termed cystic medial necrosis), a condition of degeneration and fragmentation of elastic fibers, with subsequent accumulation of collagenous and mucoid material within the medial layer. Cystic medial necrosis occurs normally with aging, but is also associated with hypertension. Additionally, it develops in certain inherited disorders of connective tissue that affect the structural integrity of the aortic wall, including Marfan syndrome, Loeys–Dietz syndrome, and the vascular form of Ehlers–Danlos syndrome (type IV). *Marfan syndrome* is caused by missense mutations of the fibrillin-1 gene (FBN1), which impair formation of functional microfibrils in elastin. Abnormal fibrillin-1 also limits the binding and inactivation of transforming growth factor β (TGF-β), a signaling molecule that regulates cellular

341

proliferation and differentiation. *Loeys–Dietz syndrome* is an autosomal dominant disorder caused by genetic mutations of TGF-β receptors. While thoracic aortic aneursyms have been associated with both increased activity of TGF-β and mutations of its receptors, the mechanism by which aberrant TGF-β signaling alters vascular integrity is not yet known. *Ehlers–Danlos type IV* syndrome results from mutations encoding type III procollagen. Cystic medial necrosis also characterizes familial thoracic aortic aneurysms and those associated with bicuspid aortic valves.

Aneurysms of the *descending thoracic* and *abdominal aorta* are usually associated with **atherosclerosis** and its risk factors, including smoking, hypertension, dyslipidemia, male gender, and advanced age. However, it is unlikely that atherosclerosis alone is responsible for such aneurysm development. Rather, important contributions appear to derive from genetic predisposition (on a polygenetic basis), local vessel inflammation, and an imbalance between synthesis and degradation of extracellular matrix proteins. For example, the breakdown of elastin and collagen is contributed to by specific proteases (e.g., elastase, collagenase) and matrix metalloproteinases derived from inflammatory cells and vascular endothelial and smooth muscle cells. Aneurysm formation is also associated with markers of inflammation, including C-reactive protein (CRP) and cytokines such as interleukin 6 (IL-6). Levels of both CRP and IL-6 have been shown to correlate with the size of aneurysms, and inflammatory cells such as B and T lymphocytes and macrophages are frequently found on histologic examination. Angiotensin II, via its effect on inflammation and oxidative stress, has also been implicated in experimental models of abdominal aortic aneurysms.

Infrequent causes of aortic aneurysms (Table 15.1) include weakness of the media from infections of the vessel wall by *Salmonella* species, staphylococci, streptococci, tuberculosis, syphilis, or fungi. Inflammatory diseases such as Takayasu arteritis or giant cell arteritis (both described later in the chapter) may similarly weaken the vessel and result in aneurysm formation.

Table 15.1. Conditions Associated with True Aortic Aneurysms

1. Cystic medial necrosis (usually affects ascending thoracic aorta)
   - Marfan syndrome
   - Loeys–Dietz syndrome
   - Ehlers–Danlos syndrome (type IV)
   - Bicuspid aortic valve
2. Atherosclerosis/degenerative (usually affects descending thoracic and abdominal aorta)
3. Infections of arterial wall
4. Vasculitis
   - Takayasu arteritis
   - Giant cell arteritis

Clinical Presentation and Diagnosis

Most aneurysms are asymptomatic, though some patients, especially those with abdominal aortic aneurysms, may be aware of a pulsatile mass. Others present with symptoms related to compression of neighboring structures by an expanding aneurysm. Thoracic aortic aneurysms may compress the trachea or mainstem bronchus, resulting in cough, dyspnea, or pneumonia. Compression of the esophagus can result in dysphagia, and involvement of the recurrent laryngeal nerve may lead to hoarseness. Aneurysms of the ascending aorta may dilate the aortic ring, resulting in aortic regurgitation and symptoms of congestive heart failure. Abdominal aortic aneurysms may cause abdominal or back pain or nonspecific gastrointestinal symptoms.

Aortic aneurysms are often first suspected when dilatation of the vessel is observed on chest or abdominal radiographs, particularly if the wall is calcified. Aneurysms of the abdominal aorta or of the large peripheral arteries may also be discovered by careful palpation during physical examination. The diagnosis is confirmed by ultrasonography, contrast-enhanced computed tomography (CT), or magnetic resonance angiography (Fig. 15.2).

The most devastating consequence of an aortic aneurysm is rupture, which can be fatal. An aneurysm may leak slowly or burst suddenly, resulting in profound blood loss and hypotension. Thoracic aortic aneurysms may rupture into the pleural space,

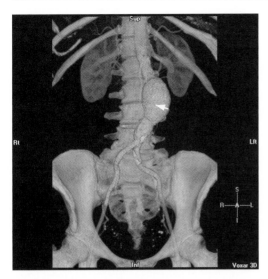

Figure 15.2. Abdominal aortic aneurysm. Computed tomographic angiogram (CTA) of an abdominal aortic aneurysm, indicated by the *arrow*. (Courtesy of Dr. Frank Rybicki, Brigham and Women's Hospital, Boston, MA.)

mediastinum, or bronchi. Abdominal aortic aneurysms may rupture into the retroperitoneal space or abdominal cavity or erode into the intestines, resulting in massive gastrointestinal bleeding.

Natural history studies have shown that the risk of rupture is related to the size of the aneurysm, as predicted by Laplace's relationship (i.e., wall tension is proportional to the product of pressure and radius). The mean rates of thoracic and abdominal aortic aneurysms expansion are 0.1 and 0.4 cm/year, respectively. Thoracic aneurysms rupture at an annual rate of 2% for aneurysms <5 cm in diameter, 3% for aneurysms 5 to 5.9 cm, and 7% for aneurysms >6 cm. Abdominal aneurysms <4 cm, 4 to 4.9 cm, and 5 to 5.9 cm have annual rates of rupture of 0.3%, 1.5%, and 6.5%, respectively. Abdominal aneurysms >6 cm have a markedly higher risk of rupture.

Treatment

Treatment of an aortic aneurysm is based on its size and the patient's overall medical condition. Once an aneurysm is identified, its dimensions should be closely monitored through repeated imaging every 6 to 12 months. In general, surgical treatment is considered for ascending aortic aneurysms >5.5 to 6.0 cm. Ascending aortic aneurysms in patients with Marfan syndrome (in whom the risk of complications is greater) should be considered for surgical repair if the diameter is >5 cm. Surgical repair is generally recommended for descending thoracic aortic aneurysms measuring 6.5 to 7.0 cm, for abdominal aortic aneurysms measuring 5.5 cm or more, and for smaller aneurysms that enlarge at a rate >1.0 cm/year.

The mortality associated with elective surgical repair of thoracic aortic aneurysms is 3% to 5%. Patients are maintained on cardiopulmonary bypass as the aneurysm is resected and replaced with a prosthetic Dacron graft. Patients with aneurysms involving multiple aortic segments have staged repairs, in which one segment is corrected at a time. Some patients may be candidates for minimally invasive repair, in which a transluminally placed endovascular stent graft is positioned across the aneurysm.

Surgical repair of abdominal aortic aneurysms involves placement of a prosthetic graft. The operative mortality for such procedures at high-volume institutions is 1% to 2%. Percutaneous endovascular repair of infrarenal abdominal aortic aneurysms with stent grafts can be performed in selected patients with less acute morbidity, and results appear to be similar to that of surgical repair.

Medical management, including risk-factor reduction (e.g., smoking cessation), is currently recommended for patients with small aneurysms. β-Blockers may reduce the expansion rate of thoracic aortic aneurysms in patients with Marfan syndrome; it is not clear whether they are effective for other causes or types of aneurysms. Angiotensin II receptor antagonists, which also inhibit TGF-β, are undergoing clinical trials in Marfan syndrome.

Aortic Dissection

Aortic dissection is a life-threatening condition in which blood from the vessel lumen passes through a tear in the intima into the medial layer and spreads along the artery. Other related acute syndromes include aortic intramural hematoma, penetrating aortic ulcer, and aortic rupture. Acute intramural hematoma is a variant of aortic dissection characterized by a hemorrhage in the wall of the aorta without evidence of an intimal tear. A penetrating atherosclerotic ulcer results from erosion of a plaque into the aortic wall. Aortic rupture may be a complication of aortic dissection, intramural hematoma, penetrating atherosclerotic ulcer, or result from trauma.

Etiology, Pathogenesis, and Classification

Aortic dissection is thought to arise from a circumferential or transverse tear in the intimal layer of the vessel wall that allows blood from the lumen, under the driving force of the systemic pressure, to enter into the media and propagate along the plane of the muscle layer. Another postulated origin of aortic dissection relates to rupture of vasa vasorum with hemorrhage into the media, forming a hematoma in the arterial wall that subsequently tears through the intima and into the vessel's lumen.

Any condition that interferes with the normal integrity of the elastic or muscular components of the medial layer can predispose to aortic dissection. Such degeneration may arise from chronic hypertension, aging, and/or cystic medial degeneration (which, as described earlier, is a feature of certain hereditary connective tissue disorders, such as Marfan syndrome and Ehlers–Danlos syndrome). In addition, traumatic insult to the aorta (e.g., blunt chest trauma or accidental vessel damage during intra-arterial catheterization or cardiac surgery) can also initiate dissection.

Aortic dissection is most common in the sixth and seventh decades and occurs more frequently in men. More than two thirds of patients have a history of hypertension. Dissection most commonly involves the ascending thoracic aorta (65%) and descending thoracic aorta (20%), while the aortic arch (10%) and abdominal aortic (5%) segments are less commonly affected.

Dissections are commonly classified into two categories (Stanford types A and B), depending on their location and extent (Fig. 15.3). In a

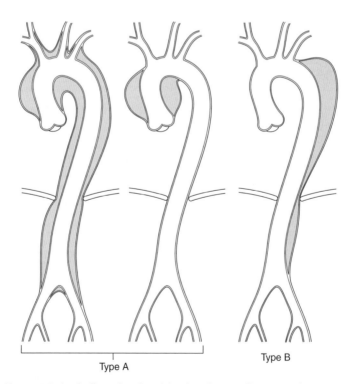

Figure 15.3. **Aortic dissection.** Type A involves the ascending aorta, whereas type B does not. (Modified with permission from Cotran RS, Kumar V, Robbins SL. *Robbin's Pathologic Basis of Disease*. Philadelphia: WB Saunders; 1989.)

type A dissection (proximal), the ascending aorta is involved, regardless of the site of the primary tear. A type B dissection (distal) does not involve the ascending aorta or arch and is, therefore, confined to the descending thoracic and abdominal aorta. This distinction is important because treatment strategies and prognoses are determined by location. Proximal aortic involvement tends to be more devastating because of the potential for extension into the coronary and arch vessels, the support structures of the aortic valve, or the pericardial space. Approximately two thirds of dissections are type A and one third are type B. Dissections may also be classified as acute or chronic, with acute dissections presenting with symptoms of less than 2 weeks' duration.

Clinical Presentation and Diagnosis

The most common symptom of aortic dissection is sudden, severe pain with a "tearing" or "ripping" quality in the anterior chest (typical of type A dissections) or between the scapulae (type B dissections). The pain travels as the dissection propagates along the aorta and can radiate anywhere in the thorax or abdomen. Painless dissection is possible but uncommon (6.4% of cases).

Other symptoms relate to the catastrophic complications that can occur at the time of presentation or thereafter (Table 15.2) and include (1) rupture through the adventitia anywhere along the aorta (often into the left pleural space or pericardium); (2) occlusion of major branches of the aorta by the propagating

Table 15.2. Complications of Aortic Dissection

Rupture
　Pericardial tamponade
　Hemomediastinum
　Hemothorax (usually left sided)

Occlusion of aortic branch vessels
　Carotid (stroke)
　Coronary (myocardial infarction)
　Splanchnic (visceral infarction)
　Renal (acute renal failure)
　Iliac, brachiocephalic, subclavian (limb ischemia)

Distortion of aortic annulus
　Aortic regurgitation

hematoma within the vessel wall, which compresses the lumen and can result in myocardial infarction (coronary artery involvement), stroke (carotid artery involvement), visceral ischemia, renal failure, or loss of pulse in an extremity; and (3) extension into the aortic root, with disruption of the aortic valve support apparatus causing aortic regurgitation.

Several important physical findings may be present. Hypertension is frequently detected, either as an underlying cause of dissection, a result of the sympathetic nervous system response to the severe pain, or because of diminished renal vascular flow, with activation of the renin–angiotensin system. If the dissection has occluded one of the subclavian arteries, a difference in systolic blood pressure between the arms is noted. Neurologic deficits may accompany dissection into the carotid vessels. If a type A dissection results in aortic regurgitation, an early diastolic murmur can be detected on auscultation. Leakage from a type A dissection into the pericardial sac may produce signs of cardiac tamponade (see Chapter 14).

The diagnosis of aortic dissection must not be delayed, because catastrophic complications or death may rapidly ensue. The confirmatory imaging techniques most useful in detecting dissection include contrast-enhanced CT, transesophageal echocardiography (TEE), magnetic resonance imaging, and contrast angiography. Each of these techniques has specific advantages and disadvantages, and the decision of which to employ is often guided by the hospital's local expertise. In emergency situations, CT scanning or TEE can generally be obtained rapidly and offer excellent sensitivity and specificity for the diagnosis.

Treatment

The goal of acute treatment is to arrest progression of the dissecting channel. Suspicion of acute aortic dissection warrants immediate medical therapy to reduce systolic blood pressure (aiming for a systolic pressure of 100 to 120 mm Hg) and to decrease the force of left ventricular contraction and thus minimize aortic wall shear stress. Useful pharmacologic agents in this regard include β-blockers (to reduce the force of contraction and heart rate as well as to lower blood pressure) and vasodilators such as sodium nitroprusside (to rapidly reduce blood pressure). In proximal (type A) dissections, early surgical correction has been shown to improve outcomes compared with medical therapy alone. Surgical therapy involves repairing the intimal tear, suturing the edges of the false channel, and if necessary, inserting a synthetic aortic graft.

In contrast, patients with uncomplicated type B dissections are initially managed with aggressive medical therapy alone; early surgical intervention does not improve the outcome in these patients. Surgery is indicated, however, if there is clinical evidence of propagation of the dissection, compromise of major branches of the aorta, impending rupture, or continued pain. Percutaneous catheter-based repair with endovascular stent grafts has been used successfully in selected stable patients with type B dissections. The graft seals the entry site of the dissection, resulting in thrombosis of the false lumen.

PERIPHERAL ARTERY DISEASES

Peripheral artery disease (PAD) is defined by the presence of a flow-limiting lesion in an artery that provides blood supply to the limbs. The major causes of such arterial stenosis or occlusion are atherosclerosis, thromboembolism, and vasculitis. The clinical presentation of these disorders results from decreased perfusion to the affected extremity.

Peripheral Atherosclerotic Vascular Disease

Etiology and Pathogenesis

The most common cause of PAD is atherosclerosis. It is a prevalent vascular disorder, affecting approximately 4% of persons over the age of 40 and 15% to 20% of those over the age of 70. The pathology of atherosclerotic PAD is identical to that of coronary artery disease (CAD), and the major coronary risk factors (e.g., cigarette smoking, diabetes mellitus, dyslipidemia, and hypertension) are also associated with PAD. Approximately 40% of patients with PAD actually have clinically significant CAD. As a consequence of the systemic nature of atherosclerosis, patients with PAD have a twofold to fivefold increased risk of cardiovascular death

compared with patients who do not have this condition. Thus, detection of PAD is useful in identifying patients at increased risk of adverse cardiovascular events.

The pathophysiology of atherosclerotic PAD is also similar to that of CAD. Ischemia of the affected region occurs when the balance between oxygen supply and demand is upset; exercise raises the demand for blood flow in the limbs' skeletal muscle, and a stenosed or obstructed artery cannot provide an adequate supply. Rest improves symptoms as the balance between oxygen supply and demand is restored.

Recall from Chapter 6 that the degree of blood flow reduction relates closely to the extent of vessel narrowing, the length of the stenosis, and blood viscosity. Poiseuille's equation describes this relationship:

$$Q = \frac{\Delta P \pi r^4}{8 \eta L}$$

in which Q = flow, ΔP = pressure drop across the stenosis, r = vessel radius, η = blood viscosity, and L = length of stenosis. Thus, the degree of vessel narrowing by the stenosis (i.e., the change in r) has the greatest impact on flow. For example, if the radius is reduced by one half, the flow will be reduced to 1/16th of its baseline. The equation also indicates that for stenoses of the same length and radius, higher flow rates correspond to greater pressure drops across the stenoses. That is, as the flow velocity increases across a stenotic vessel, the blood turbulence results in a loss of kinetic energy. The result is a decline in perfusion pressure distal to the stenosis.

During exercise, products of skeletal muscle metabolism (e.g., adenosine) act locally to dilate arterioles. The resulting decrease in vascular resistance serves to increase blood flow to the active muscle (recall that flow = pressure ÷ resistance). In turn, the increased flow stimulates healthy arterial endothelium to release vasodilating factors such as nitric oxide, thereby increasing the radii of upstream conduit vessels. However, in PAD, obstructed arteries cannot respond to the vasodilating stimuli, thereby limiting flow increases. In addition, dysfunctional atherosclerotic endothelium does not release normal amounts of vasodilating substances (see Chapter 6). Thus, the physical properties of a stenosis and the reduced vasodilator activity imposed by diseased endothelium prevent adequate blood flow from reaching distal tissues and contribute to ischemia.

Hemodynamic changes alone cannot account for the dramatic reductions in exercise capacity experienced by PAD patients; changes in muscle structure and function are also seen. One such change is the denervation and dropout of muscle fibers, which is thought to occur as an adaptation to intermittent ischemia. The loss of such fibers can explain the reduced muscle strength and atrophy that occur in PAD patients. Even viable muscle fibers in affected limbs may show abnormalities of mitochondrial oxidative metabolism.

In summary, atherosclerotic lesions produce stenoses in peripheral conduit vessels and limit blood flow to the affected extremity. Mechanisms normally in place to compensate for increased demand, such as endogenous release of vasodilators during exercise and recruitment of microvessels, fail in the face of endothelial dysfunction and diminished flow velocity. Thus, states of increased oxygen demand are not met with adequate supply, producing limb ischemia. Adaptations to ischemia include changes in muscle fiber metabolism and muscle fiber dropout. Together, these physical and biochemical changes result in weak lower limbs that suffer ischemic discomfort during exercise. *Severe* peripheral atherosclerosis may reduce limb blood flow to such an extent that it cannot satisfy *resting* metabolic requirements. This results in critical limb ischemia, which may progress to tissue necrosis and gangrene that may threaten viability of the extremity.

Clinical Presentation and Diagnosis

PAD may affect the aorta or the iliac, femoral, popliteal, and tibioperoneal arteries (Fig. 15.4). Patients with PAD may therefore develop buttock, thigh, or calf discomfort precipitated by walking and relieved by rest. This classic

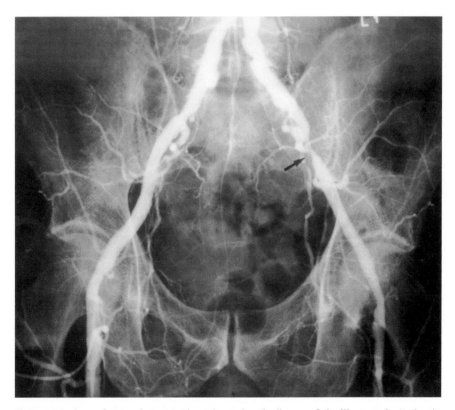

Figure 15.4. An angiogram demonstrating atherosclerotic disease of the iliac vessels. Notice the severe stenosis of the left external iliac artery *(arrow).*

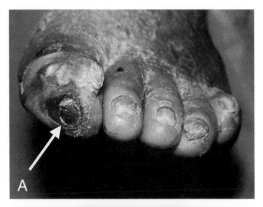

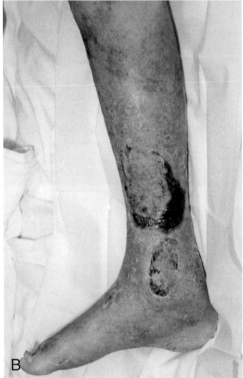

Figure 15.5. Ulcerations caused by vascular insufficiency.
A. Arterial insufficiency. Ulceration *(arrow)* affecting the great toe in a patient with severe peripheral artery disease. **B.** Venous insufficiency ulcer near the medial malleolus of the right leg. Notice the pigmentation of the surrounding skin.

Table 15.3. Relation of Stenotic Site to Claudication Symptoms	
Site	*Location of Claudication Symptoms*
Distal aorta or iliac arteries	Buttocks, hips, thighs, or calves
Femoral or popliteal arteries	Calves
Subclavian or axillary arteries	Arms

The location of claudication corresponds to the diseased artery, with the femoral and popliteal arteries being the most common sites (Table 15.3). The arteries of the upper extremities are less frequently affected, but brachiocephalic or subclavian artery disease can cause arm claudication.

Physical examination generally reveals loss of pulses distal to the stenotic segment. Bruits (swishing sounds auscultated over a region of turbulent blood flow) may be audible in the abdomen (because of stenoses within the mesenteric or renal arteries) or over iliac, femoral, or subclavian arterial stenoses. In patients with chronic severe ischemia, the lack of blood perfusion results in muscle atrophy, pallor, cyanotic discoloration, hair loss, and occasionally gangrene and necrosis of the foot and digits.

Ischemic ulcers resulting from PAD often begin as small traumatic wounds in areas of increased pressure or in regions prone to injury, such as the tips of toes and lateral malleolus (see Fig. 15.5A). These often painful ulcers fail to heal owing to the inadequate blood supply. Diabetic patients with peripheral sensory neuropathies are particularly susceptible to ulcers at sites of trauma or pressure from ill-fitting footwear. Ischemic ulcers can be distinguished from venous insufficiency ulcers, which develop more proximally and on the medial portion of the leg. Venous ulcers are also associated with reddish-brown pigmentation and varicose veins (see Fig. 15.5B).

In the evaluation of PAD, it is helpful to measure the ratio of blood pressure in the ankles to that in the arms (termed the *ankle-brachial index* [*ABI*]) using a blood pressure cuff and a Doppler instrument to detect blood

symptom of exertional limb fatigue and pain is known as **claudication.** In severe PAD, patients may experience pain at rest, usually affecting the feet or toes. The chronically reduced blood flow in this case predisposes the extremity to ulceration, infection, and skin necrosis (Fig. 15.5). Patients who smoke or have diabetes mellitus are at high risk of these complications.

flow. A normal ABI is ≥ 1.0 (i.e., the ankle pressure is equal to, or slightly greater than, that in the arms). An index <0.9 is diagnostic of PAD and may be associated with symptoms of claudication, whereas an index <0.5 is often observed in patients with rest pain and severe arterial compromise of the affected extremity. Other testing to assess peripheral perfusion includes limb *segmental systolic pressure measurements* (using pneumatic cuffs placed along the extremity) and *pulse volume recordings* (i.e., graphical measurement of volume changes in segments of the extremity with each pulse). *Duplex ultrasonography* is a commonly used noninvasive method to visualize and assess the extent of arterial stenoses and the corresponding reductions in blood flow. Other more advanced imaging studies (e.g., *magnetic resonance angiography, computed tomographic angiography,* or intra-arterial *contrast angiography*) are obtained when revascularization procedures are planned.

Treatment

For all patients with PAD, antiplatelet therapy and risk factor modification (including smoking cessation, lipid lowering, and control of diabetes and hypertension) are important in reducing the likelihood of *coronary* events. Platelet inhibitors such as aspirin have been shown to reduce cardiovascular morbidity and mortality in patients with PAD. It has not been established if antiplatelet agents reduce symptoms or prevent thrombotic complications of PAD itself.

Specific treatment of PAD includes supportive care of the feet to prevent trauma or restriction of blood flow. Exercise, particularly walking, improves endurance in part by increasing metabolic efficiency in the skeletal muscle of the legs. A formal exercise program is considered first-line therapy in the management of PAD.

Certain medical therapies are sometimes useful in the treatment of claudication. *Cilostazol* is a selective phosphodiesterase inhibitor that increases cyclic adenosine monophosphate and has vasodilator and platelet-inhibiting properties; it has been shown to improve exercise capacity in patients with PAD. *Pentoxifylline* is a drug purported to improve the deformability of red and white blood cells and may improve claudication symptoms in some patients. Conversely, most vasodilator drugs (see Chapter 17) are not helpful in relieving claudication.

More effective medical therapies for PAD are on the horizon. Advances in angiogenesis research and ongoing clinical trials provide hope that pharmacologic revascularization with angiogenic growth factors, such as vascular endothelial growth factor and basic fibroblast growth factor, may be possible.

Mechanical revascularization is indicated when medical therapy has failed for patients with disabling claudication and as first-line therapy in cases of severe limb ischemia. In advanced cases, therapy is directed at healing ischemic ulcerations and preventing limb loss. Catheter-based interventions, such as percutaneous transluminal angioplasty and stent implantation, can be performed on selected patients with low morbidity. Surgical procedures include bypass operations to circumvent the occluded arteries using saphenous vein or prosthetic grafts. However, amputation may be necessary if blood flow cannot be satisfactorily reestablished to maintain limb viability.

Acute Arterial Occlusion

Acute arterial occlusion is caused either by embolization from a cardiac or proximal vascular site or by thrombus formation in situ. The origin of arterial emboli is most often the heart, usually resulting from disorders involving intracardiac stasis of flow (Table 15.4). Emboli may also originate from thrombus or atheromatous material overlying a segment of the aorta. Rarely, arterial emboli originate from the *venous* circulation. If a venous clot travels to the right-heart chambers and is able to pass through an abnormal intracardiac communication (e.g., an atrial septal defect), it then enters the systemic arterial circulation (a condition known as a **paradoxical embolism**). Primary arterial thrombus formation may appear at sites of endothelial damage or atherosclerotic stenoses, or within bypass grafts.

The extent of tissue damage from thromboembolism depends on the site of the occluded artery, the duration of occlusion, and the degree of collateral circulation serving the tissue

Table 15.4. Origins of Arterial Emboli

Cardiac origin

Stagnant left atrial flow (e.g., atrial fibrillation, mitral stenosis)

Left ventricular mural thrombus (e.g., dilated cardiomyopathy, myocardial infarction, ventricular aneurysm)

Valvular lesions (endocarditis, thrombus on prosthetic valve)

Left atrial myxoma (mobile tumor in left atrium)

Aortic origin

Thrombus material overlying atherosclerotic segment

Venous origin

Paradoxical embolism travels through intracardiac shunt

beyond the obstruction. Common symptoms and signs that may develop from reduced blood supply include pain, pallor, paralysis, paresthesia, and pulselessness (termed the "five *P*s"). A sixth *P*, poikilothermia (coolness), is also often manifest.

Patients with a proven acute arterial occlusion should be treated with anticoagulant agents such as heparin (followed by warfarin) to prevent propagation of the clot and to reduce the likelihood of additional embolic events. A revascularization procedure (catheter-based thrombolysis or thrombectomy, surgical embolectomy, or bypass surgery) is indicated if limb viability is at risk.

Atheroembolism is the condition of peripheral arterial occlusion by atheromatous material (i.e., cholesterol, platelets, and fibrin) derived from more proximal vascular sites, such as atherosclerotic lesions or aneurysms. The emboli lodge distally, resulting in occlusion of small arteries in the muscle and skin. Patients typically present with acute pain and tenderness at the involved site. Occlusion of digital vessels may result in the "blue toe" syndrome, culminating in gangrene and necrosis. Other findings may include livedo reticularis (purplish mottling of involved skin), kidney failure (caused by renal atheroembolism), and intestinal ischemia. Although an estimated 50% to 60% of cases are spontaneous, atheroembolism may occur after intra-arterial procedures (e.g.,

cardiac catheterization) when atherosclerotic material is unintentionally dislodged from the proximal vasculature. Ischemia resulting from atheroemboli is difficult to manage because the heterogeneous composition and distribution of emboli often precludes surgical removal or thrombolytic therapy. Surgical intervention to remove or bypass the source of emboli may be necessary to prevent recurrences.

Vasculitic Syndromes

Vasculitis (vessel wall inflammation) results from immune complex deposition or cell-mediated immune reactions directed against the vessel wall. Immune complexes activate the complement cascade with subsequent release of chemoattractants and anaphylatoxins that direct neutrophil migration to the vessel wall and increase vascular permeability. Neutrophils injure the vessel by releasing lysosomal contents and producing toxic oxygen-derived free radicals. In cell-mediated immune reactions, T lymphocytes bind to vascular antigens and release lymphokines that attract additional lymphocytes and macrophages to the vessel wall. These inflammatory processes can cause end-organ ischemia through vascular necrosis or local thrombosis.

The cause of most of the vasculitic syndromes is unknown, but they often can be distinguished from one another by the pattern of involved vessels and by histologic characteristics (Table 15.5).

Takayasu arteritis is a chronic vasculitis of unknown etiology that targets the aorta and its major branches. The estimated annual incidence is 1.2 to 2.6 cases per million. Between 80% and 90% of affected persons are women, with onset typically between the ages of 10 and 40. Most reported cases have been from Asia and Africa, but it is a worldwide disease. Patients typically present with systemic complaints such as malaise and fever; focal symptoms are related to inflammation of the affected vessel and include cerebrovascular ischemia (brachiocephalic or carotid artery involvement), myocardial ischemia (coronary artery), arm claudication (brachiocephalic or subclavian artery), or hypertension (renal artery). The carotid and limb pulses are diminished or absent in nearly 85% of patients at the time of diagnosis; hence, this

Table 15.5. Vasculitic Syndromes

Type	Arteries Commonly Affected	Histology
Takayasu arteritis	Aorta and its branches	Granulomatous arteritis with fibrosis; significant luminal narrowing
Giant cell arteritis	Medium to large size (especially cranial vessels, as well as aortic arch and its branches)	Lymphocyte infiltration, intimal fibrosis, granuloma formation
Thromboangiitis obliterans (Buerger disease)	Small size (especially distal arteries of extremities)	Inflammation and thrombosis without necrosis

condition is often termed "pulseless" disease. Takayasu arteritis is also an uncommon cause of aortic aneurysm or aortic dissection. Histologic examination of affected vessels reveals continuous or patchy granulomatous inflammation with lymphocytes, histiocytes, and multinucleated giant cells, resulting in intimal proliferation, disruption of the elastic lamina, and fibrosis. Antiendothelial antibodies may also play a role in the disease. Steroid and cytotoxic drugs may reduce vascular inflammation and alleviate symptoms of Takayasu arteritis. Surgical bypass of obstructed vessels may be helpful in severe cases. The 5-year survival rate is 80% to 90%.

Giant cell arteritis (also termed **temporal arteritis**) is a chronic vasculitis of medium-sized to large arteries that most commonly involves the cranial vessels or the aortic arch and its branches. It is an uncommon disease, with an incidence of 24 per 100,000, and the typical onset is after age 50; 65% of patients are female. Giant cell arteritis may be associated with the inflammatory condition known as polymyalgia rheumatica. Histologic findings in affected vessels include lymphocyte and macrophage infiltration, intimal fibrosis, and focal necrosis, with granulomas containing multinucleated giant cells.

Symptoms and signs of giant cell arteritis depend on the distribution of affected arteries and may include diminished temporal pulses, prominent headache (temporal artery involvement), or facial pain and claudication of the jaw while chewing (facial artery involvement). Ophthalmic artery arteritis leads to impaired vision, with permanent partial or complete loss in 15% to 20% of patients. In giant cell arteritis, the erythrocyte sedimentation rate and CRP are invariably elevated as markers of inflammation. Ultrasound examination can support the diagnosis by demonstrating a hypoechoic halo around the involved arterial lumen with vessel stenosis and/or occlusion. The diagnosis can be confirmed by biopsy of an involved vessel, usually a temporal artery, but treatment should not wait for biopsy results. High-dose systemic steroids are effective in treating vasculitis and preventing visual complications. Giant cell arteritis usually has a self-limited course of 1 to 5 years.

Thromboangiitis obliterans (Buerger disease) is a segmental inflammatory disease of small and medium-sized arteries, veins, and nerves involving the distal vessels of the upper and lower extremities. It is most prevalent in the Far and Middle East and has a very strong association with cigarette smoking. It is most common in men younger than age 45; only 10% to 25% of patients are female. There is an increased incidence of human leukocyte antigen A9 (HLA-A9) and HLA-B5 in affected persons.

Thromboangiitis obliterans presents with a triad of symptoms and signs: distal arterial occlusion, Raynaud phenomenon (described in the next section), and migrating superficial vein thrombophlebitis. Arterial occlusion results in arm and foot claudication as well as ischemia of the digits. Traditional laboratory markers of inflammation and autoimmune disease are usually not detected. Arteriographic features of involved arteries include areas of stenosis interspersed with normal-appearing vessels with more severe disease distally, collateral vessels with a "corkscrew" appearance around the stenotic regions, and lack of atherosclerosis in proximal arteries. The diagnosis can be established by tissue

351

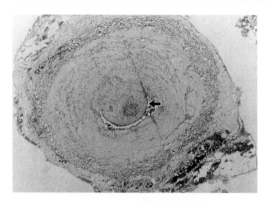

Figure 15.6. **Histologic section of an artery displaying thromboangiitis obliterans.** Endothelial cell and fibroblast proliferation appears in the vessel wall, and thrombus is present in the vessel lumen *(arrow)*.

biopsy, although this is rarely needed. Biopsy specimens of affected vessels reveal an occlusive, highly cellular, inflammatory thrombus, with limited involvement of the vessel wall and preservation of the internal elastic lamina (Fig. 15.6). The most important treatment for thromboangiitis obliterans is smoking cessation, which usually prevents progression of the disease and its complications. Debridement of necrotic tissue may be necessary in advanced cases. Revascularization is not usually an option because of the distal location of the arterial lesions.

VASOSPASM: RAYNAUD PHENOMENON

Raynaud phenomenon is a vasospastic disease of the digital arteries that occurs in susceptible people when exposed to cool temperatures or sometimes during emotional stress. Vasospasm is an extreme vasoconstrictor response that temporarily obliterates the vascular lumen, inhibiting blood flow. Typically, such episodes are characterized by a triphasic color response. First, the fingers and/or toes blanch to a distinct white as blood flow is interrupted (Fig. 15.7). The second phase is characterized by cyanosis, related to local accumulation of desaturated hemoglobin, followed by a third phase of ruddy color as blood flow resumes. The color response may be accompanied by numbness, paresthesias, or pain of the affected digits.

This condition may occur as an isolated disorder, termed *primary Raynaud phenomenon* or *Raynaud disease*. Patients are predomi-

nantly women between the ages of 20 and 40. Primary Raynaud phenomenon most often manifests in the fingers, but 40% of patients also have involvement of the toes. The prognosis of primary Raynaud phenomenon is relatively benign, with only a minority reporting a worsening of symptoms over time.

Secondary Raynaud phenomenon may appear as a component of other conditions. Common causes include connective tissue diseases (e.g., scleroderma and systemic lupus erythematosus) and arterial occlusive disorders. Other causes of secondary Raynaud phenomenon include carpal tunnel syndrome, thoracic outlet syndrome, blood dyscrasias, certain drugs, and thermal or vibration injury.

Even in healthy vessels, cold exposure normally produces a vasoconstrictor response. Cooling stimulates the sympathetic nervous system, resulting in local discharge of norepinephrine, which binds to vascular adrenergic receptors. In the fingers and toes, only vasoconstricting α-receptors are present; other regional circulations have both constrictor and dilator adrenergic responses. Thus, a modest vasoconstriction of the digits results when healthy people are exposed to cooling. In contrast, in Raynaud phenomenon, cold exposure induces *severe* vasoconstriction.

A variety of mechanisms have been proposed to explain the vasospastic response to cold and stress in patients with primary Raynaud phenomenon, including an exaggerated sympathetic discharge in response to cold, heightened vascular sensitivity to adrenergic stimuli, or excessive release of vasoconstrictor stimuli, such as serotonin, thromboxane, and endothelin. In patients with secondary Raynaud phenomenon caused by connective tissue diseases or arterial occlusive disease, the digital vascular lumen is largely obliterated by sclerosis or inflammation, resulting in lower intraluminal pressure and greater susceptibility to sympathetically mediated vasoconstriction.

Treatment of Raynaud phenomenon involves avoiding cold environments, dressing in warm clothes, and wearing insulated gloves or footwear. There has also been some success in preventing vasospasm with pharmacologic agents that relax vascular tone,

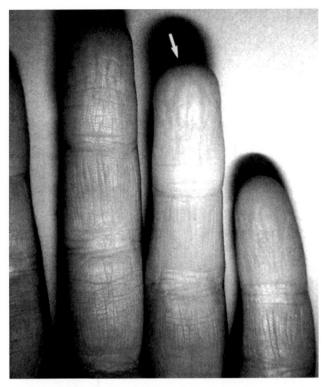

Figure 15.7. **Raynaud phenomenon.** The fourth digit *(arrow)* is blanched (phase 1 of the tricolor response).

including calcium-channel blockers and α-adrenergic blockers (see Chapter 17), but such therapies are reserved for severe cases.

VENOUS DISEASE

Veins are high-capacitance vessels that contain more than 70% of the total blood volume. In contrast to the muscular structure of arteries, the subendothelial layer of veins is thin, and the tunica media comprises fewer, smaller bundles of smooth muscle cells intermixed with reticular and elastic fibers. While veins of the extremities possess intrinsic vasomotor activity, transport of blood back to the heart relies greatly on external compression by the surrounding skeletal muscles and on a series of one-way endothelial valves.

Veins of the extremities are classified as either deep or superficial. In the lower extremities, where most peripheral venous disorders occur, the deep veins generally course along the arteries, whereas the superficial veins are located subcutaneously. The superficial vessels

drain into deeper veins through a series of perforating connectors, ultimately returning blood to the heart.

Varicose Veins

Varicose veins (Fig. 15.8) are dilated, tortuous superficial vessels that often develop in the lower extremities. Clinically apparent varicose veins occur in 10% to 20% of the general population. They affect women two to three times more frequently than men, and roughly half of patients have a family history of this condition. Varicosities can occur in any vein in the body but are most common in the saphenous veins of the leg and their tributaries. They may also develop in the anorectal area (hemorrhoids), in the lower esophageal veins (esophageal varices), and in the spermatic cord (varicocele).

Varicosity is thought to result from intrinsic weakness of the vessel wall, from increased intraluminal pressure, or from congenital defects in the structure and function of venous

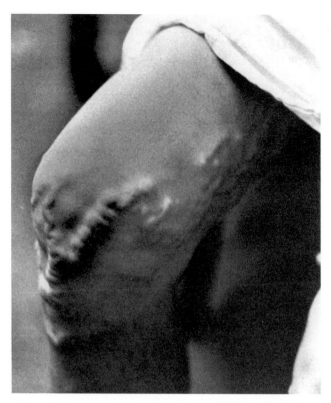

Figure 15.8. A patient with extensive venous varicosities of the right leg.

valves. Varicose veins in the lower extremities are classified as either primary or secondary. *Primary* varicose veins originate in the superficial system, and factors that lead to their development include pregnancy, prolonged standing, and obesity. During pregnancy or prolonged standing, the high venous pressure within the legs contributes to varicosities when there is underlying weakness of the vessel walls. In obese patients, the adipose tissue surrounding vessel walls offers less structural support to veins than lean mass. *Secondary* varicose veins occur when an abnormality in the deep venous system is the cause of superficial varicosities. These may develop in the setting of deep venous insufficiency or occlusion, or when the perforating veins are incompetent. In such cases, deep venous blood is shunted retrogradely through perforating channels into superficial veins, increasing intraluminal pressure and volume and causing dilatation and varicosity formation.

Many people with varicose veins are asymptomatic but seek treatment for cosmetic reasons. When symptoms do develop, they include a dull ache, "heaviness," or a pressure sensation in the legs after prolonged standing. Superficial venous insufficiency may result when venous valves are unable to function normally in the dilated veins. This can cause swelling and skin ulceration that is particularly severe near the ankle. Stasis of blood within varicose veins can promote superficial vein thrombosis, and varicosities can also rupture, causing a localized hematoma.

Varicose veins are usually treated conservatively. Patients should elevate their legs while supine, avoid prolonged standing, and wear external compression stockings that counterbalance the increased venous hydrostatic pressure. Small symptomatic varicosities are sometimes treated by injection of a sclerosing agent into the vein. Laser treatments can be used to improve the cosmetic appearance of small affected vessels. Endovenous laser therapy, radiofrequency ablation procedures, and surgical vein ligation and removal are used for patients who are very symptomatic, suffer recurrent superficial vein thrombosis, or develop skin ulcerations.

Venous Thrombosis

The term *venous thrombosis* or *thrombophlebitis* is used to describe thrombus formation within a superficial or deep vein and the inflammatory response in the vessel wall that it incites. Thrombi in the lower extremities are classified by location as either deep venous thrombi or superficial venous thrombi.

Initially, the venous thrombus is composed principally of platelets and fibrin. Later, red blood cells become interspersed within the fibrin, and the thrombus tends to propagate in the direction of blood flow. The changes in the vessel wall can be minimal or can include granulocyte infiltration, loss of endothelium, and edema. Thrombi may diminish or obstruct

vascular flow, or they may dislodge and form thromboemboli.

Deep Venous Thrombosis and Pulmonary Embolism

Epidemiology, Etiology, and Pathophysiology

Deep venous thrombosis (DVT) occurs most commonly in the veins of the calves but may also develop initially in more proximal veins such as the popliteal, femoral, and iliac vessels. If left untreated, 20% to 30% of DVTs that occur in the calves may propagate to these proximal veins. The two major consequences of DVT are pulmonary embolism (PE) (venous thromboembolism) and postphlebitic syndrome.

PE supervenes when a clot, most often from a DVT in the proximal veins of the lower extremities, dislodges and travels through the inferior vena cava and right-heart chambers, finally reaching and obstructing a portion of the pulmonary vasculature (Fig. 15.9). PE is

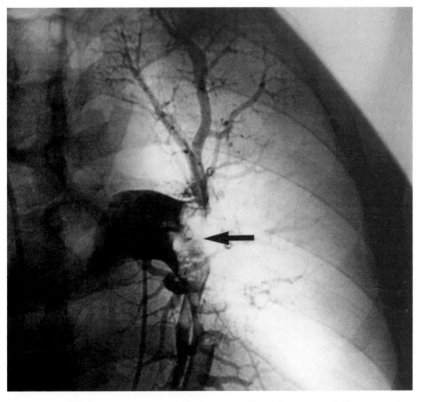

Figure 15.9. Pulmonary angiogram displaying a massive pulmonary embolism. There is a large filling defect in the left main pulmonary artery *(arrow)*, additional filling defects in the lower pulmonary artery branches, and a paucity of vessels in the left midlung region (a result of obstructed flow).

common (incidence of approximately 600,000 per year in the United States) and is often fatal, with an untreated mortality rate of 30% to 40%. In patients with PE, gas exchange is often impaired because of the associated anatomic dead space and ventilation–perfusion mismatches that ensue in the lungs. As a result, the alveolar–arterial oxygen gradient increases and hypoxemia may occur. Pulmonary vascular resistance may rise as a consequence of the mechanical obstruction, and because vasoactive and bronchoconstrictive mediators released by platelets within emboli induce constriction of the pulmonary vasculature and bronchospasm, respectively. The increased pulmonary vascular resistance may lead to elevation of right ventricular (RV) wall stress, dilatation, and contractile failure, compromising cardiac output.

Postphlebitic syndrome, or chronic deep venous insufficiency, results from venous valvular damage and/or persistent occlusion by DVT. This may lead to chronic leg swelling, stasis pigmentation, and skin ulcerations.

In 1856, Virchow described a triad of factors that predispose to venous thrombosis: (1) stasis of blood flow, (2) hypercoagulability, and (3) vascular damage. Stasis disrupts laminar flow and brings platelets into contact with the endothelium. This allows coagulation factors to accumulate and retards the influx of clotting inhibitors. Factors that slow venous flow and induce stasis include immobilization (e.g., prolonged bed rest after surgery, or sitting in a car or an airplane for a long trip), cardiac failure, and hyperviscosity syndromes (Table 15.6).

Various clinical disorders cause systemic hypercoagulability, including resistance of coagulation factor V to activated protein C, a prothrombin gene mutation, and inherited deficiencies of antithrombin, protein C, and protein S. Pancreatic, lung, stomach, breast, and genitourinary tract adenocarcinomas are associated with a high prevalence of venous thrombosis. This is thought to occur in part because necrotic tumor cells release thrombogenic factors. Other conditions that contribute to hypercoagulability are listed in Table 15.6.

Vascular damage, either by external injury or by intravenous catheters, can denude the

Table 15.6. Conditions that Predispose to DVT and Pulmonary Embolism

Stasis of blood flow
Prolonged inactivity (following surgery, prolonged travel)
Immobilized extremity (following bone fracture)
Heart failure (with systemic venous congestion)
Hyperviscosity syndromes (e.g., polycythemia vera)

Hypercoagulable states
Inherited disorders of coagulation
    Resistance to activated protein C (Factor V Leiden)
    Prothrombin gene mutation (PT G20210A)
    Antithrombin deficiency
    Deficiency of protein C or protein S
Antiphospholipid antibodies/lupus anticoagulant
Neoplastic disease (e.g., pancreatic, lung, stomach, or breast cancers)
Pregnancy and oral contraceptive use
Myeloproliferative diseases
Smoking

Vascular damage
Instrumentation (e.g., intravenous catheters)
Trauma

endothelium and expose subendothelial collagen. Exposed collagen acts as a substrate for the binding of von Willebrand factor and platelets and initiates the clotting cascade, leading to clot formation. Less severe damage can cause endothelial *dysfunction* that contributes to thrombosis by disrupting the production of vasodilating and antiplatelet substances (e.g., nitric oxide and prostacyclin) and antithrombotic molecules such as thrombomodulin and heparan sulfate.

The risk of venous thrombosis is particularly high after fractures of the spine, pelvis, and bones of the lower extremities. The risk following bone fracture may be related to stasis of blood flow, increased coagulability, and possibly traumatic endothelial damage. In addition, venous thrombosis occurs frequently in patients following surgical procedures, particularly major orthopedic operations.

Women have a several-fold increase in the incidence of venous thrombus formation during late pregnancy and the early postpartum period. In the third trimester, the fetus compresses the inferior vena cava and can cause stasis of blood flow, and high levels of circulating estrogen may induce a hypercoagulable state. Oral contraceptives and other pharmacologic estrogen products may also predispose to thrombus formation.

Clinical Presentation

Patients with DVT may be asymptomatic, or they may describe calf or thigh discomfort particularly when standing or walking, or report unilateral leg swelling. The physical signs of proximal DVT include edema of the involved leg and occasionally localized warmth and erythema. Tenderness may be present over the course of the phlebitic vein, and a deep venous cord (induration along the thrombosed vessel) is occasionally palpable. Calf pain produced by dorsiflexion of the foot (Homans' sign) is a nonspecific and unreliable sign of DVT.

Patients with PE may experience dyspnea, pleuritic chest pain (due to pleural irritation), hemoptysis, cough, or syncope (due to reduced cardiac output). Signs may include tachypnea, bronchospasm, and evidence of elevated pulmonary artery pressure, including an accentuated pulmonic component of the second heart sound and jugular venous distention.

Diagnosis

The primary laboratory tests for the diagnosis of DVT include measurement of the serum D-dimer level and venous compression ultrasonography. *D-dimer*, a byproduct of fibrin degradation that can be measured in a peripheral blood sample, is highly sensitive for the diagnosis of DVT and/or acute PE. Because D-dimer may also be elevated in many other conditions (such as cancer, inflammation, infection, and necrosis), a positive test result is *not specific* for DVT. Thus, a normal D-dimer value can help exclude the presence of DVT, but an elevated level does not confirm the diagnosis.

Venous compression duplex ultrasonography is a readily available noninvasive technique that is 95 % sensitive for the diagnosis of symptomatic DVT in a proximal vein but only

75 % sensitive for diagnosing symptomatic calf vein thrombi. This technique uses real-time ultrasound scanning to image the vein and pulsed Doppler ultrasound to assess blood flow within it (Fig. 15.10). Criteria used for diagnosis of DVT with duplex ultrasonography include the inability to compress the vein with direct pressure (suggesting the presence of an intraluminal thrombus), direct visualization of the thrombus, and absence of blood flow within the vessel.

Other diagnostic techniques are sometimes used. For example, *magnetic resonance venography* can aid in the diagnosis of proximal DVT, particularly pelvic vein thrombi, which are difficult to detect by ultrasound. *Contrast venography* is an invasive imaging technique that can provide a definitive diagnosis. Radiocontrast material is administered into a foot vein, and images are obtained as the contrast ascends through the venous system of the leg. DVT is diagnosed by the presence of a filling defect (see Fig. 15.10).

Additional tests are useful in the evaluation of suspected PE. The most common *electrocardiographic* abnormality in patients with PE is sinus tachycardia; there may be evidence of RV strain (e.g., inverted T waves in leads V_1–V_4, or an "S1–Q3–T3" pattern: a prominent S wave in lead I, Q wave in lead III, inverted T wave in lead III). RV strain may also cause elevated serum levels of cardiac-specific troponins or B-type natriuretic peptide (described in Chapters 7 and 9, respectively). *Arterial blood gas* analysis may show decreased arterial oxygenation, but is insensitive to the diagnosis of PE. The preferred test to confirm the diagnosis is *computed tomographic angiography* (CTA; see Fig. 3.20). For patients who cannot tolerate CTA, such as those with renal insufficiency or hypersensitivity to radioiodinated contrast agents, radionuclide *ventilation-perfusion (V/Q) lung scanning* is often obtained instead. Catheter-based *pulmonary angiography* is performed in selective cases to confirm the diagnosis.

Treatment

In patients with DVT, elevation of the affected extremity above the level of the heart helps reduce

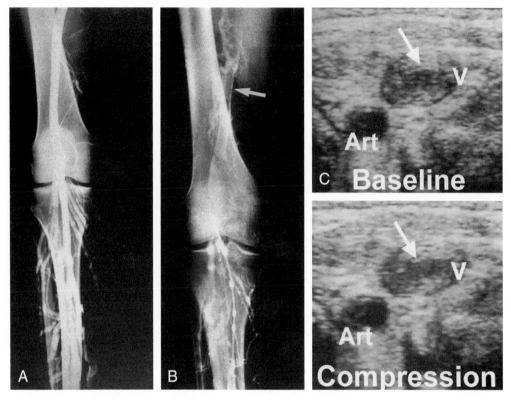

Figure 15.10. **Diagnostic imaging of deep venous thrombosis. A.** Normal venogram. Contrast material was injected into a foot vein and fills the leg veins in this radiograph. **B.** Venogram demonstrating extensive thrombosis of the deep calf veins, popliteal vein, and femoral vein. *Arrow* indicates a filling defect in the femoral vein due to the presence of thrombus. The deep calf veins are filled with thrombus and cannot be visualized. **C.** Ultrasound indicating deep venous thrombosis. The thrombus appears as an echogenic area *(arrow)* within the femoral vein (V). A healthy vein would be easily compressible by the ultrasound transducer. This vein, however, has the same diameter at baseline **(top panel)** and after compression **(bottom panel)**, confirming the presence of thrombus within it. Art, artery.

edema and tenderness, and anticoagulation prevents extension of the thrombus and PE. In patients with established PE, urgent anticoagulation is instituted to prevent recurrent embolism. Initial anticoagulation usually consists of subcutaneous *low molecular weight heparin (LMWH)*. Intravenous *unfractionated heparin* is a cost-effective alternative that has been used successfully for this purpose for many years, although some studies have shown superior outcomes with LMWH, which is also more convenient to administer (see Chapter 17). *Warfarin,* an oral anticoagulant, is prescribed for long-term management and is usually continued for 6 months or more, depending on the underlying cause of DVT. Catheter-based thrombolysis may be useful for selected patients with iliofemoral deep vein thrombosis.

In patients with proximal DVT or established PE who cannot be treated with anticoagulants (e.g., because of a bleeding disorder), an intravascular filter can be percutaneously inserted into the inferior vena cava to prevent emboli from reaching the lungs. Occasionally, systemic thrombolytic therapy or surgical pulmonary embolectomy is undertaken for patients with massive PE.

Treatment of patients with calf vein thrombosis (i.e., thrombus confined to below the knee) is more controversial because pulmonary emboli from that site are uncommon. Some physicians advocate serial noninvasive monitoring to determine if the thrombus propagates into proximal veins, whereas others treat such thrombosis with heparin (unfractionated or low molecular weight) followed by warfarin for 3 to 6 months.

Prophylaxis against DVT is mandatory in clinical situations in which the risk of developing the condition is high, such as during bed rest following surgery. Prophylactic measures include subcutaneous unfractionated heparin or LMWH, fondaparinux (see Chapter 17), low-dose oral warfarin, compression stockings, and/or intermittent external pneumatic compression of the legs to prevent venous stasis.

Superficial Thrombophlebitis

Superficial thrombophlebitis is a benign disorder associated with inflammation and thrombosis of a superficial vein, just below the skin. It may occur, for example, as a complication of an in-dwelling intravenous catheter. It is characterized by erythema, tenderness, and edema over the involved vein. Treatment consists of local heat and rest of the involved extremity. Aspirin or other anti-inflammatory medications may relieve the associated discomfort. Unlike DVT, superficial thrombophlebitis does not lead to PE.

SUMMARY

1. Aortic aneurysms are of two types: true aneurysms and false (pseudo) aneurysms. True aneurysms are caused by degenerative changes in the aortic wall. Cystic medial necrosis is associated with ascending thoracic aortic aneurysms, and atherosclerosis is commonly found in descending thoracic and abdominal aortic aneurysms. A false aneurysm represents a hole in the arterial intima and media contained by a layer of adventitia or perivascular clot.

2. Symptoms of aortic aneurysms relate to compression of adjacent structures (back pain, dysphagia, respiratory symptoms) or blood leakage. The most severe consequence is aneurysm rupture. An aneurysm can be repaired either with an open surgical procedure or by insertion of an endovascular graft.

3. An aortic dissection results from a tear in the intima that allows blood to enter into the medial layer, often in the setting of advanced age, hypertension, or other causes of medial degeneration (cystic medial necrosis). Type A (proximal) aortic dissections involve the ascending aorta, whereas type B dissections are confined to the descending aorta. The former are more common, more devastating, and require surgical treatment. Type B dissections are often managed by medical therapy alone.

4. PAD is a common atherosclerotic disease of large and medium-sized arteries, often resulting in claudication of the limbs. It is treated by risk factor modification, exercise, antiplatelet agents, and sometimes cilostazol, a selective phosphodiesterase inhibitor. Catheter-based or surgical revascularization procedures are implemented in patients with disabling symptoms or critical limb ischemia.

5. Acute arterial occlusion results from thrombus formation in situ or from arterial embolism. The latter arises from thrombus within the heart, from proximal arterial sites, or paradoxically from the systemic veins in the presence of an intracardiac shunt (e.g., atrial septal defect). Therapeutic options include anticoagulation, thrombolysis, and surgical or endovascular interventions.

6. Vasculitic syndromes are inflammatory diseases of blood vessels that impair arterial flow and result in localized and systemic symptoms. They are distinguished from one another by the pattern of vessel involvement and morphologic findings (see Table 15.5).

7. Raynaud phenomenon is an episodic vasospasm of arteries that supply the digits of the upper and lower extremities. It may be a primary condition (Raynaud disease) or may appear in association with other disorders such as connective tissue diseases or blood dyscrasias.

8. Varicose veins are dilated tortuous vessels that may present cosmetic problems. Occasionally, they cause discomfort, become thrombosed, or lead to venous insufficiency. Initial management is conservative, with periodic leg elevation and compression stockings. Severe symptomatic varicose veins can be treated with radiofrequency ablation, laser therapy, or surgical ligation and removal.

9. Venous thrombosis results from stasis of blood flow, hypercoagulability, and vascular damage. The major complication of DVT is PE. A chronic complication is venous insufficiency causing chronic leg swelling and skin ulceration.

10. D-dimer assay and venous compression ultrasonography are the primary tools used to diagnose DVT. Anticoagulation therapy with LMWH or unfractionated intravenous heparin (UFH), followed by oral warfarin, is the usual treatment.

11. PE can be confirmed by CT angiography or ventilation–perfusion scintigraphy. Anticoagulant therapy (LMWH or UFH) comprises standard therapy. If anticoagulants are contraindicated, an inferior vena cava filter can be inserted to prevent recurrent PE.

Acknowledgments

Contributors to the previous editions of this chapter were Arash Mostaghimi, MD; Mary Beth Gordon, MD; Geoffrey McDonough, MD; Michael Diminick, MD; Stuart Kaplan, MD; Jesse Salmeron, MD; and Mark A. Creager, MD.

Additional Reading

Creager MA, Dzau VJ, Loscalzo J, eds. *Vascular Medicine: A Companion to Braunwald's Heart Disease.* Philadelphia, PA: Elsevier Saunders; 2006.

Creager MA, Loscalzo J. Vascular diseases of the extremities. In: Longo DL, Fauci AS, Kasper D, et al., eds. *Harrison's Principles of Internal Medicine.* 18th ed. New York: McGraw-Hill; In press.

Creager MA, Loscalzo J. Diseases of the aorta. In: Longo DL, Fauci AS, Kasper D, et al., eds. *Harrison's Principles of Internal Medicine.* 18th ed. New York: McGraw-Hill. In press.

Elefteriades JA, Farkas EA. Thoracic aortic aneurysm. *J Am Coll Cardiol.* 2010;55:841–857.

Golledge J, Eagle KA. Acute aortic dissection. *Lancet.* 2008;372:55–66.

Gornik HL, Creager MA, Diseases of the aorta. In: Topol E, ed. *Textbook of Cardiovascular Medicine.* 3rd ed. Philadelphia, PA: Lippincott Williams & Wilkins; 2007:1473–1495.

Hirsch AT, Haskal ZJ, Hertzer NR, et al. ACC/AHA 2005 guidelines for the management of patients with peripheral arterial disease (lower extremity, renal, mesenteric, and abdominal aortic). *J Am Coll Cardiol.* 2006; 47:1239–1312.

Isselbacher, EM. Thoracic and abdominal aortic aneurysms. *Circulation.* 2005;111:816–828.

Kay NS, Kasthuri RS. Current treatment of venous thromboembolism. *Arterioscler Thromb Vasc Biol.* 2010;30:372–375.

Konstantinides, S. Clinical practice: acute pulmonary embolism. *N Engl J Med.* 2008;359: 2804–2813.

Norgren L, Hiatt WR, Dormandy JA, et al. Inter-society consensus for the management of peripheral arterial disease (TASC II). *J Vasc Surg.* 2007;45:S5–S67.

Raju S, Neglen P. Clinical practice. Chronic venous insufficiency and varicose veins. *N Engl J Med.* 2009;360:2319–2327.

Ramanath VS, Oh JK, Sundt TM III, et al. Acute aortic syndromes and thoracic aortic aneurysm. *Mayo Clin Proc.* 2009;84:465–481.

Congenital Heart Disease

David D. Berg
David W. Brown

Congenital heart diseases are the most common form of birth defects and are the leading cause of death from birth abnormalities in the first year of life. These conditions affect approximately 8 of 1,000 live births, and an estimated 1 million people in the United States have congenital heart lesions. Some abnormalities are severe and require immediate medical attention, whereas many are less pronounced and have minimal clinical consequences. Although congenital heart defects are present at birth, milder defects may remain inapparent for weeks, months, or years and, not infrequently, escape detection until adulthood.

The past half-century has witnessed tremendous growth in our understanding of the pathophysiology of congenital heart diseases and substantial improvements in the ability to evaluate and treat those afflicted. Research has shown that genetic mutations, environmental factors, maternal illness, or ingestion of toxins during pregnancy can contribute to cardiac malformations. However, specific etiologies remain unknown in most cases.

The survival of children with congenital heart disease has also improved dramatically in recent decades, largely because of better diagnostic and interventional techniques. However, the lifelong needs of affected patients include guidance regarding physical activity, pregnancy, and employment.

Formation of the cardiovascular system begins during the third week of embryonic development. Soon after, a unique circulation develops that allows the fetus to mature in the uterus, using the placenta as the primary organ of gas, nutrient, and waste exchange. At birth, the fetal lungs inflate and become functional, making the placenta unnecessary and dramatically altering circulation patterns to allow the neonate to adjust to life outside the womb. Given the remarkable complexity of these processes, it is easy to envision ways that cardiovascular malfunctions could develop.

This chapter begins with an overview of fetal cardiovascular development and then describes the most common forms of congenital heart disease.

NORMAL DEVELOPMENT OF THE CARDIOVASCULAR SYSTEM

By the third week of gestation, the nutrient and gas exchange needs of the rapidly growing embryo can no longer be met by diffusion alone, and the tissues begin to rely on the developing cardiovascular system to deliver these substances over long distances.

Development of the Heart Tube

In the middle of the third week of embryogenesis, mesodermal cells proliferate at the cranial end of the early embryonic disc. They eventually form two longitudinal cell clusters known as angioblastic cords. These cords canalize and become paired endothelial heart tubes (Fig. 16.1). Lateral embryonic folding gradually causes these two tubes to oppose one another and allows them to fuse in the ventral midline, forming a single endocardial tube by day 22. From inside to outside, the layers of this primitive heart tube are an endothelial lining that becomes the endocardium, a layer of gelatinous connective tissue (cardiac jelly), and a thick muscular layer that is derived from the splanchnic mesoderm and develops into the myocardium. The endocardial tube is continuous with the aortic arch system rostrally and with the venous system caudally. The primitive heart begins to beat around day 22 or 23, causing blood to circulate by the beginning of the fourth week. The space overlying the developing cardiac area eventually becomes the pericardial cavity, housing the future heart.

Formation of the Heart Loop

As the tubular heart grows and elongates, it develops a series of alternate constrictions and dilations, creating the first sign of the

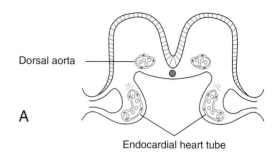
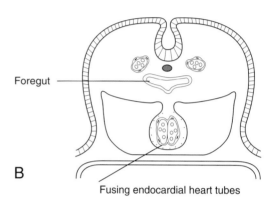
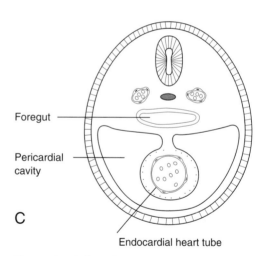

Figure 16.1. Embryonic transverse sections illustrating fusion of the two heart tubes into a single endocardial heart tube. A. 18 days. B. 21 days. C. 22 days.

primitive heart chambers—the truncus arteriosus, the bulbus cordis, the primitive ventricle, the primitive atrium, and the sinus venosus (Fig. 16.2). Continued growth and elongation within the confined pericardial cavity force the heart tube to bend on itself on day 23, eventually forming a U-shaped

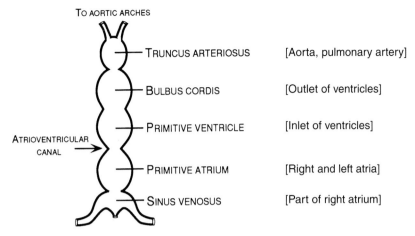

Figure 16.2. **The straight heart tube at approximately 22 days.** The structures that will ultimately form from each segment are listed in brackets.

loop with the round end pointing ventrally and to the right by day 28. The result of this looping is placement of the atrium and sinus venosus above and behind the truncus arteriosus, bulbus cordis, and ventricle (Fig. 16.3). At this point, neither definitive septa between the developing chambers nor definitive valvular tissue have formed. The connection between the primitive atrium and ventricle is termed the **atrioventricular (AV) canal**. In time, the AV canal becomes two separate canals, one housing the tricuspid valve and the other the mitral valve. The sinus venosus is eventually incorporated into the right atrium, forming both the coronary sinus and a portion of the right atrial wall. The bulbus cordis and truncus arteriosus contribute to the future ventricular outflow

tracts, forming parts of the proximal aorta and pulmonary artery.

Septation

Septation of the developing atrium, AV canal, and ventricle occurs between the fourth and sixth weeks. Although these events are described separately here, they actually occur simultaneously.

Septation of the Atria

The primary atrial septum, also known as the **septum primum**, begins as a ridge of tissue on the roof of the common atrium that grows downward into the atrial cavity (Fig. 16.4). As the septum primum advances, it leaves a

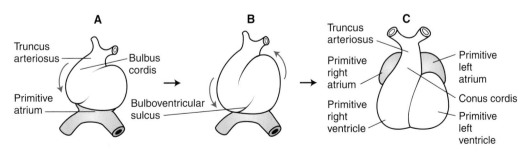

Figure 16.3. **Formation of the heart loop. A,B.** By day 24, continued growth and elongation within the confined pericardial space necessitate bending of the heart tube on itself, forming a U-shaped loop that points ventrally and to the right. **C.** Looping eventually places the atria above and behind the primitive ventricles.

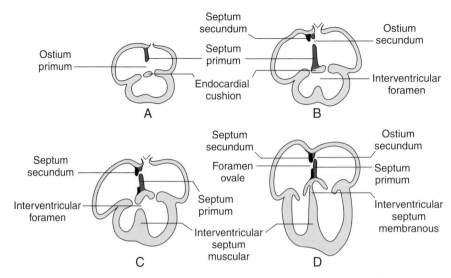

Figure 16.4. Atrial septal formation at 30 days (A), 33 days (B), and 37 days (C) of development as well as in the newborn (D). As the septum primum grows toward the ventricles, the opening between it and the AV canal is the ostium primum. Before the ostium primum completely closes, perforations within the upper portion of the septum primum form the ostium secundum. A second ridge of tissue, the septum secundum, grows downward to the right of the septum primum, partially covering the ostium secundum. The foramen ovale is an opening of the septum secundum that is covered by the "flap valve" of the lower septum primum. (Modified from Moss AJ, Adams FH. *Heart Disease in Infants, Children, and Adolescents.* Baltimore, MD: Williams & Wilkins; 1968:16.)

large opening known as the **ostium primum** between the crescent-shaped leading edge of the septum and the endocardial cushions surrounding the AV canal. The ostium primum allows passage of blood between the forming atria. Eventually, the septum primum fuses with the superior aspect of the endocardial cushions (described in more detail in the next section), obliterating the ostium primum. However, before closure of the ostium primum is complete, small perforations appear in the center of the septum primum that ultimately coalesce to form the **ostium secundum**, preserving a pathway for blood flow between the atria (see Fig. 16.4). Following closure of the ostium primum, a second, more muscular membrane, the **septum secundum**, begins to develop immediately to the right of the superior aspect of the septum primum. This septum grows downward and overlaps the ostium secundum. The septum secundum eventually fuses with the endocardial cushions, although only in a partial fashion, leaving an oval-shaped opening known as the **foramen ovale**. The superior edge of

the septum primum then gradually regresses, leaving the lower edge to act as a "flap-like" valve that allows only right-to-left flow through the foramen ovale (Fig. 16.5). During gestation, blood passes from the right atrium to the left atrium because the pressure in the fetal right atrium is greater than that in the left atrium. This pressure gradient changes direction postnatally, causing the valve to close, as described later.

Septation of the Atrioventricular Canal

Growth of the **endocardial cushions** contributes to atrial septation and, as described later, to the membranous portion of the interventricular septum. Endocardial cushions initially begin as swellings of the gelatinous connective tissue layer within the AV canal. They are then populated by migrating cells from the primitive endocardium and subsequently transform into mesenchymal tissue. Tissue growth occurs primarily in the horizontal plane, resulting in septation of the AV canal through the continued growth of the lateral, superior, and

A

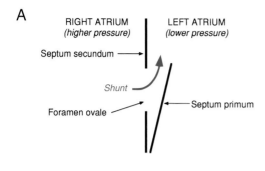

RIGHT ATRIUM
(higher pressure)

LEFT ATRIUM
(lower pressure)

Septum secundum →

Shunt

Foramen ovale →

← Septum primum

B

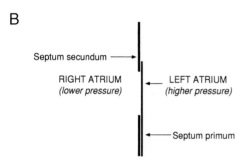

Septum secundum →

RIGHT ATRIUM
(lower pressure)

← LEFT ATRIUM
(higher pressure)

← Septum primum

Figure 16.5. Diagrammatic depiction of the flap-type valve of the foramen ovale. A. Before birth, the valve permits only right-to-left flow of blood from the higher-pressured right atrium (RA) to the lower-pressured left atrium (LA). **B.** Following birth, the pressure in the LA becomes greater than that in the RA, causing the septum primum to close firmly against the septum secundum. (Derived from Moore KL, Persaud TVN. *The Developing Human*. Philadelphia, PA: WB Saunders; 1993:318.)

inferior endocardial cushions (Fig. 16.6). Septation creates the right and left canals that later give rise to the tricuspid and mitral orifices, respectively.

Septation of the Ventricles and Ventricular Outflow Tracts

At the end of the fourth week, the primitive ventricle begins to grow, leaving a median muscular ridge, the primitive interventricular septum. Most of the early increase in height of the septum results from dilation of the two new ventricles forming on either side of it. Only later does new cell growth in the septum itself contribute to its size. The free edge of the muscular interventricular septum does not fuse with the endocardial cushions; the opening that remains and allows communication between the right and left ventricles is the **interventricular foramen** (Fig. 16.7). This remains open until the end of the seventh week of gestation, when the fusion of tissue from the right and left bulbar ridges and the endocardial cushions forms the membranous portion of the interventricular septum.

During the fifth week, neural crest-derived mesenchymal proliferation occurring in the bulbus cordis and truncus arteriosus creates a pair of protrusions known as the bulbar ridges (Fig. 16.8). These ridges fuse in the midline and undergo a 180° spiraling process, forming the aorticopulmonary septum. This septum divides the bulbus cordis and the truncus arteriosus into two arterial channels, the pulmonary artery and the aorta, the former continuous with the right ventricle (RV) and the latter with the left ventricle (LV).

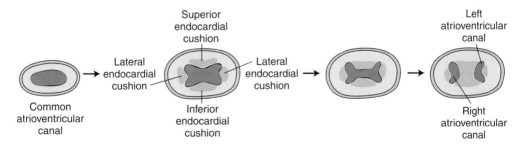

Figure 16.6. The progression of septal formation in the atrioventricular canal through successive stages. The septum forms through growth of the superior, inferior, and lateral endocardial cushions. The endocardial cushions are masses of mesenchymal tissue that surround the atrioventricular canal and aid in the formation of the orifices of the mitral and tricuspid valves, as well as the upper interventricular septum and lower interatrial septum.

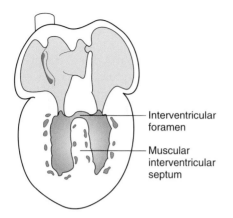

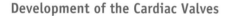

Figure 16.7. **The interventricular septum and the interventricular foramen.** (Derived from Moore KL, Persaud TVN. *The Developing Human.* Philadelphia, PA: WB Saunders; 1993:325.)

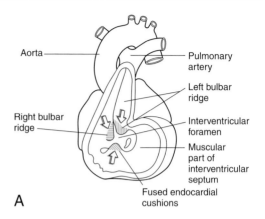

A

Development of the Cardiac Valves

Semilunar Valve Development (Aortic and Pulmonary Valves)

The semilunar valves start to develop just before the completion of the aorticopulmonary septum. The process begins when three outgrowths of subendocardial mesenchymal tissue form around both the aortic and pulmonary orifices. These growths are ultimately shaped and excavated by the joint action of programmed cell death and blood flow to create the three thin-walled cusps of both the aortic and pulmonary valves.

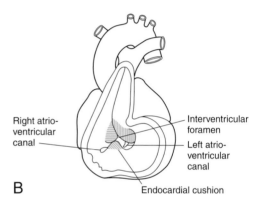

B

Atrioventricular Valve Development (Mitral and Tricuspid Valves)

After the endocardial cushions fuse to form the septa between the right and left AV canals, the surrounding subendocardial mesenchymal tissue proliferates and develops outgrowths similar to those of the semilunar valves. These are also sculpted by programmed cell death that occurs within the inferior surface of the nascent leaflets and in the ventricular wall. This process leaves behind only a few fine muscular strands to connect the valves to the ventricular wall (Fig. 16.9). The superior portions of these strands eventually degenerate and are replaced by strings of dense connective tissue, becoming the chordae tendineae.

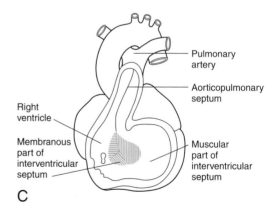

C

Figure 16.8. **Formation of the aorticopulmonary septum occurs via fusion of the bulbar ridges, resulting in division of the bulbus cordis and truncus arteriosus into the aorta and pulmonary artery (A, 5 weeks; B, 6 weeks; C, 7 weeks).** The bulbus cordis becomes the right ventricular outflow tract. Fusion of tissue from the endocardial cushions, the aorticopulmonary septum, and the muscular interventricular septum creates the membranous interventricular septum. (Derived from Moore KL, Persaud TVN. *The Developing Human.* Philadelphia, PA: WB Saunders; 1993:322.)

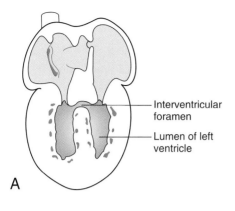

Interventricular foramen

Lumen of left ventricle

A

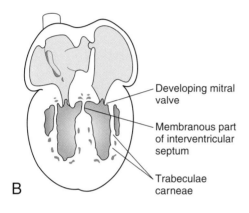

Developing mitral valve

Membranous part of interventricular septum

Trabeculae carneae

B

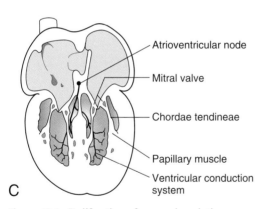

Atrioventricular node

Mitral valve

Chordae tendineae

Papillary muscle

Ventricular conduction system

C

Figure 16.9. Proliferation of mesenchymal tissue surrounding the atrioventricular canals forms the atrioventricular valves. A, B, C. Progression of the process, including degeneration of myocardium and replacement by connective tissue that forms the chordae tendineae; their muscular attachments to the ventricular wall are the papillary muscles. (Derived from Moore KL, Persaud TVN. *The Developing Human.* Philadelphia, PA: WB Saunders; 1993:325.)

FETAL AND TRANSITIONAL CIRCULATIONS

The fetal circulation elegantly serves the needs of in utero development. At birth, the circulation automatically undergoes modifications that establish the normal blood flow pattern of a newborn infant.

Fetal Circulation

In fetal life, oxygenated blood leaves the placenta through the umbilical vein (Fig. 16.10). Approximately half of this blood is shunted through the fetal **ductus venosus**, bypassing the hepatic vasculature and proceeding directly into the inferior vena cava (IVC). The remaining blood passes through the portal vein to the liver and then into the IVC through the hepatic veins. IVC blood is therefore a mixture of *well-oxygenated* umbilical venous blood and the blood of *low oxygen tension* returning from the systemic veins of the fetus. Because of this mixture, the oxygen tension of inferior vena caval blood is higher than that of blood returning to the fetal right atrium from the superior vena cava. This distinction is important because these two streams of blood are partially separated within the right atrium to follow different circulatory paths. The consequence of this separation is that the fetal brain and myocardium receive blood of relatively higher oxygen content, whereas the more poorly oxygenated blood is diverted to the placenta (via the descending aorta and umbilical arteries) for subsequent oxygenation.

Most IVC blood entering the right atrium is directed to the left atrium through the foramen ovale. This intracardiac shunt of relatively well-oxygenated blood is facilitated by the inferior border of the septum secundum, termed the crista dividens, which is positioned such that it overrides the opening of the IVC into the right atrium. This shunted blood then mixes with the small amount of poorly oxygenated blood returning to the left atrium through the fetal pulmonary veins (remember that the lungs are not ventilated in utero; the developing pulmonary tissues actually *remove* oxygen from the blood). From the left atrium, blood flows into the LV and is then pumped into the ascending aorta. This well-oxygenated blood is distributed primarily to three territories: (1) approximately 9% enters the coronary arteries and perfuses the myocardium, (2) 62% travels in the carotid and subclavian vessels to the upper body and brain, and (3) 29% passes

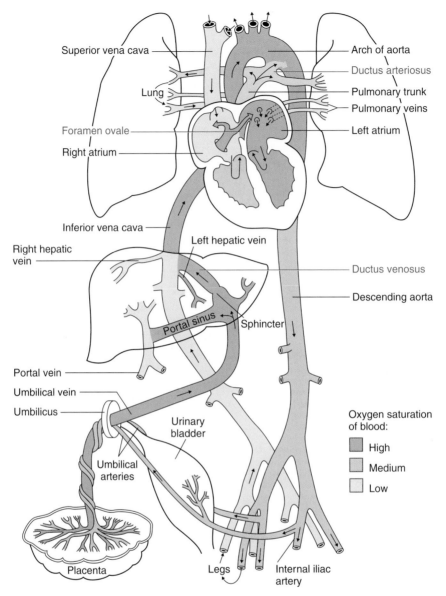

Superior vena cava

Arch of aorta

Ductus arteriosus

Lung

Pulmonary trunk

Pulmonary veins

Foramen ovale

Left atrium

Right atrium

Inferior vena cava

Left hepatic vein

Right hepatic vein

Ductus venosus

Descending aorta

Portal sinus

Sphincter

Portal vein

Umbilical vein

Umbilicus

Umbilical arteries

Urinary bladder

Oxygen saturation of blood:

High

Medium

Low

Placenta

Legs

Internal iliac artery

Figure 16.10. The fetal circulation. Arrows indicate the direction of blood flow. Three shunts (ductus venosus, foramen ovale, and ductus arteriosus) allow most of the blood to bypass the lungs and liver during fetal life but cease to function shortly after birth. (Modified from Moore KL, Persaud TVN. *The Developing Human*. Philadelphia, PA: WB Saunders; 1993:344.)

into the descending aorta to the rest of the fetal body.

The remaining well-oxygenated inferior vena caval blood entering the right atrium mixes with poorly oxygenated blood from the superior vena cava and passes to the RV. In the fetus, the RV is the actual "workhorse" of the heart, providing two thirds of the total cardiac output. This output flows into the pulmonary artery and from there either through the **ductus arteriosus** into the descending aorta (88% of RV output) or through the pulmonary arteries and into the lungs (12% of RV output). This unequal distribution of right ventricular outflow is actually quite efficient. Bypassing the lungs is desired because the fetal lungs are filled with amniotic fluid and are incapable of gas exchange. The low oxygen tension of this fluid causes constriction of the pulmonary vessels, which increases pulmonary vascular resistance and facilitates shunting of blood through the ductus arteriosus to the systemic circulation. From the descending aorta, blood is distributed to the lower body and to the umbilical arteries, leading back to the placenta for gas exchange.

Transitional Circulation

Immediately following birth, the neonate rapidly adjusts to life outside the womb. The newly functioning lungs replace the placenta as the organ of gas exchange, and the three shunts (ductus venosus, foramen ovale, and ductus arteriosus) that operated during gestation close. This shift in the site of gas exchange and the resulting changes in cardiovascular architecture allow the newborn to survive independently.

As the umbilical cord is clamped or constricts naturally, the low-resistance placental flow is removed from the arterial system, resulting in an increase in systemic vascular resistance. Simultaneously, pulmonary vascular resistance falls for two reasons: (1) the mechanical inflation of the lungs after birth stretches the lung tissues, causing pulmonary artery expansion and wall thinning, and (2) vasodilatation of the pulmonary vasculature occurs in response to the rise in blood oxygen tension accompanying aeration of the lungs. This reduction in pulmonary resistance results in a dramatic rise in pulmonary blood flow. It is most marked within the first day after birth but continues for the next several weeks until adult levels of pulmonary resistance are achieved.

As pulmonary resistance falls and more blood travels to the lungs through the pulmonary artery, venous return from the pulmonary veins to the left atrium also increases, causing left atrial pressure to rise. At the same time, cessation of umbilical venous flow and constriction of the ductus venosus cause a fall in IVC and right atrial pressures. As a result, the left atrial pressure becomes greater than that in the right atrium, and the valve of the foramen ovale is forced against the septum secun-

dum, eliminating the previous flow between the atria (see Fig. 16.5).

With oxygenation now occurring in the newborn lungs, the ductus arteriosus becomes superfluous and closes. During fetal life, a high circulating level of prostaglandin E_1 (PGE_1) is generated in response to relative hypoxia, which causes the smooth muscle of the ductus arteriosus to relax, keeping it patent. After birth, PGE_1 levels decline as the oxygen tension rises and the ductus therefore constricts. The responsiveness of the ductus to vasoactive substances depends on the gestational age of the fetus. The ductus often fails to constrict in premature infants, resulting in the congenital anomaly known as patent ductus arteriosus (described later in the chapter).

With the anatomic separation of the circulatory paths of the right and left sides of the heart now complete, the stroke volume of the LV increases and that of the RV decreases, equalizing the cardiac output from both ventricles. The augmented pressure and volume load placed on the LV induces the myocardial cells of that chamber to hypertrophy, while the decreased pressure and volume loads on the RV result in gradual regression of RV wall thickness.

COMMON CONGENITAL HEART LESIONS

Congenital heart defects are generally well tolerated before birth. The fetus benefits from shunting of blood through the ductus arteriosus and the foramen ovale, allowing the bypass of most defects. It is only after birth, when the neonate has been separated from the maternal circulation and the oxygenation it provides, and the fetal shunts have closed, that congenital heart defects usually become manifest.

Congenital heart lesions can be categorized as *cyanotic* or *acyanotic*. Cyanosis refers to a blue-purple discoloration of the skin and mucous membranes caused by an elevated blood concentration of deoxygenated hemoglobin (at least 4 g/dL, which usually corresponds to an arterial O_2 saturation of approximately 80% to 85%). In congenital heart disease, cyanosis results from defects that allow poorly oxygenated blood from the right side of the heart to be shunted to the left side, bypassing the lungs.

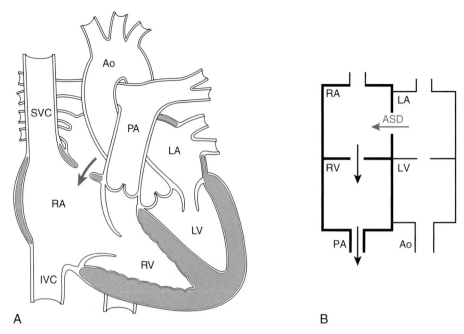

Figure 16.11. Atrial septal defect (ASD), ostium secundum type. A. The arrow indicates shunted flow from the left atrium (LA) toward the right atrium (RA). **B.** Schematic representation of blood flow through an uncomplicated ASD, resulting in enlargement of the RA, right ventricle (RV), and pulmonary artery (PA). Ao, aorta; IVC, inferior vena cava; LV, left ventricle; SVC, superior vena cava.

Acyanotic lesions include intracardiac or vascular stenoses, valvular regurgitation, and defects that result in *left-to-right* shunting of blood. Large left-to-right shunts at the atrial, ventricular, or great vessel level (all described in the following sections) cause the pulmonary artery volume and pressure to increase and can be associated with the later development of pulmonary arteriolar hypertrophy and increased resistance to flow. Over time, the elevated pulmonary resistance may force the direction of the original shunt to reverse, causing *right-to-left* flow to supervene, accompanied by the physical findings of hypoxemia and cyanosis. The development of pulmonary vascular disease as a result of a chronic large left-to-right shunt is known as *Eisenmenger syndrome* and is described later in the chapter.

Patients with congenital heart disease are susceptible to infective endocarditis. Chapter 8 describes the pathophysiology of endocarditis and summarizes the appropriate selection of patients for antibiotic prophylaxis prior to procedures that can result in bacteremia.

Acyanotic Lesions

Atrial Septal Defect

An atrial septal defect (ASD) is a persistent opening in the interatrial septum after birth that allows direct communication between the left and right atria. ASDs are relatively common, occurring with an incidence of 1 in 1,500 live births. They can occur anywhere along the atrial septum, but the most common site is at the region of the foramen ovale, termed an *ostium secundum* ASD (Fig. 16.11). This defect arises from inadequate formation of the septum secundum, excessive resorption of the septum primum, or a combination.

Less commonly, an ASD appears in the inferior portion of the interatrial septum, adjacent to the AV valves. Named as *ostium primum* defect, this abnormality results from the failure of the septum primum to fuse with the endocardial cushions.

A third type of atrial septal abnormality is termed a *sinus venosus defect* and is closely related to ASDs but is morphologically distinct. This condition represents an "unroofing" defect with absence of normal tissue between the right pulmonary vein(s) and the right atrium but is technically not a deficiency of the anatomic atrial septum (i.e., frequently the atrial septum itself is fully intact). As sinus venosus defects are often large and result in flow from the right pulmonary veins and left atrium into the right atrium, the pathophysiology is similar to that of a true ASD.

Another condition related to ASDs is *patent foramen ovale (PFO)*, which is thought to be present in ~20% of the general population. It too is not a true ASD (i.e., no atrial septal tissue is "missing"), but represents persistence of normal fetal anatomy. As described earlier, the foramen ovale typically functionally closes in the days after birth, and it permanently seals by the age of 6 months through fusion of the atrial septa. A PFO remains when this fusion fails to occur.

A PFO is usually clinically silent because the one-way valve, though not sealed, remains functionally closed since the left atrial pressure is higher than that in the right atrium. However, a PFO takes on significance if the right atrial pressure becomes elevated (e.g., in states of pulmonary hypertension or right-heart failure), resulting in pathologic *right-to-left* intracardiac shunting. In that case, deoxygenated blood passes directly into the arterial circulation. Occasionally, a PFO can be implicated in a patient who has suffered a systemic embolism (e.g., a stroke). This situation, termed *paradoxical embolism*, occurs when thrombus in a systemic vein breaks loose, travels to the right atrium, passes across the PFO to the left atrium (*if* right-heart pressures are elevated, at least transiently), and then into the systemic arterial circulation.

Pathophysiology

In the case of an uncomplicated ASD, oxygenated blood from the left atrium is shunted into the right atrium, but not vice versa. Flow through the defect is a function of its size and the filling properties (compliance) of the ventricles into which the atria pass their contents. Normally after birth, right ventricular compliance becomes greater than that of the LV owing to the regression of right ventricular wall thickness, facilitating a left-to-right directed shunt. The result is volume overload and enlargement of the right atrium and RV (see Fig. 16.11B). If right ventricular compliance decreases over time (because of the excessive load), the left-to-right shunt may lessen. Occasionally, if severe pulmonary vascular disease develops (e.g., Eisenmenger syndrome), the direction of the shunt may actually reverse (causing right-to-left flow), such that desaturated blood enters the systemic circulation, resulting in hypoxemia and cyanosis.

Symptoms

Most infants with ASDs are asymptomatic. The condition is typically detected by the presence of a murmur on routine physical examination during childhood or adolescence. If symptoms do occur, they include dyspnea on exertion, fatigue, and recurrent lower respiratory tract infections. The most common symptoms in adults are decreased stamina and palpitations due to atrial tachyarrhythmias resulting from right atrial enlargement.

Physical Examination

A prominent systolic impulse may be palpated along the lower-left sternal border, representing contraction of the dilated RV (termed an *RV heave*). The second heart sound (S$_2$) demonstrates a widened, fixed splitting pattern (see Chapter 2), because the normal respiratory variation in systemic venous return is countered by reciprocal changes in the volume of blood shunted across the ASD. The increased volume of blood flowing across the pulmonary valve often creates a systolic murmur at the upper-left sternal border. A mid-diastolic murmur may also be present at the lower-left sternal border owing to the increased flow across the tricuspid valve. Blood traversing the ASD itself does not produce a murmur because of the absence of a significant pressure gradient between the two atria.

Diagnostic Studies

On *chest radiographs*, the heart is usually enlarged because of right atrial and right ventricular dilatation, and the pulmonary artery is prominent with increased pulmonary vascular markings. The *electrocardiogram (ECG)* shows right ventricular hypertrophy, often with right atrial enlargement and incomplete or complete right bundle branch block. In patients with the ostium primum type of ASD, left axis deviation is common and is thought to be a result of displacement and hypoplasia of the left bundle branch's anterior fascicle. *Echocardiography* demonstrates right atrial and right ventricular enlargement; the ASD may be visualized directly, or its presence may be implied by the demonstration of a transatrial shunt by Doppler flow interrogation. The magnitude and direction of shunt flow and an estimation of right ventricular systolic pressure can be determined.

Given the high sensitivity of echocardiography, it is rarely necessary to perform *cardiac catheterization* to confirm the presence of an ASD. Catheterization may be useful to assess pulmonary vascular resistance and to diagnose concurrent coronary artery disease in older adults. In a normal person undergoing cardiac catheterization, the oxygen saturation measured in the right atrium is similar to that in the superior vena cava. However, an ASD with left-to-right shunting of well-oxygenated blood causes

the saturation in the right atrium to be much greater than that of the superior vena cava.

Treatment

Most patients with ASDs remain asymptomatic. However, if the volume of shunted blood is hemodynamically significant (even in the absence of symptoms), elective surgical repair is recommended to prevent the development of heart failure or pulmonary vascular disease. The defect is repaired by direct suture closure or with a pericardial or synthetic patch. In children and young adults, morphologic changes in the right heart often return to normal after repair. Percutaneous ASD repair, using a closure device deployed via an intravenous catheter, is a less invasive alternative to surgery in selected patients with secundum ASDs.

Ventricular Septal Defect

A ventricular septal defect (VSD) is an abnormal opening in the interventricular septum (Fig. 16.12). VSDs are relatively common, having an

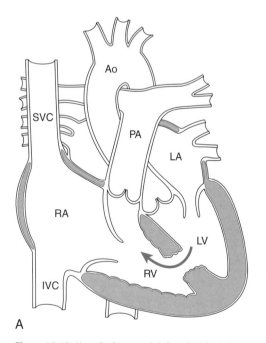
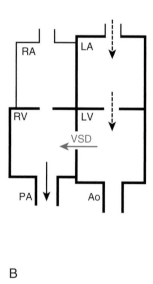

Figure 16.12. Ventricular septal defect (VSD). A. The arrow indicates shunted flow from the left ventricle (LV) toward the right ventricular (RV) outflow tract. **B.** Schematic representation of blood flow through an uncomplicated VSD. The dashed lines represent increased blood return to the left side of the heart as a result of the shunt, which causes enlargement primarily of the left atrium (LA) and LV. Ao, aorta; IVC, inferior vena cava; PA, pulmonary artery; RA, right atrium; SVC, superior vena cava.

incidence of 1.5 to 3.5 per 1,000 live births. They are most often located in the membranous (70%) and muscular (20%) portions of the septum. Rare VSDs occur just below the aortic valve or adjacent to the AV valves.

Pathophysiology

The hemodynamic changes that accompany VSDs depend on the size of the defect and the relative resistances of the pulmonary and systemic vasculatures. In small VSDs, the defect itself offers more resistance to flow than the pulmonary or systemic vasculature; thus, the magnitude of the shunt depends on the size of the hole. Conversely, with larger "nonrestrictive" defects, the volume of the shunt is determined by the relative pulmonary and systemic vascular resistances. In the perinatal period, the pulmonary vascular resistance approximates the systemic vascular resistance, and minimal shunting occurs between the two ventricles. After birth, however, as the pulmonary vascular resistance falls, an increasing left-to-right shunt through the defect develops. When this shunt is large, the RV, pulmonary circulation, left atrium, and LV experience a relative volume overload. Initially, the increased blood return to the LV augments stroke volume (via the Frank–Starling mechanism); but over time, the increased volume load can result in chamber dilatation, systolic dysfunction, and symptoms of heart failure. In addition, the augmented circulation through the pulmonary vasculature can cause pulmonary vascular disease as early as 2 years of age. As pulmonary vascular resistance increases, the intracardiac shunt may reverse its direction (Eisenmenger syndrome), leading to systemic hypoxemia and cyanosis.

Symptoms

Patients with small VSDs typically remain symptom free. Conversely, 10% of infants with VSDs have large defects and will develop early symptoms of congestive heart failure, including tachypnea, poor feeding, failure to thrive, and frequent lower respiratory tract infections. Patients with VSDs complicated by pulmonary vascular disease and reversed shunts may present with dyspnea and cyanosis. Bacterial endocarditis (see Chapter 8) can develop, regardless of the size of the VSD.

Physical Examination

The most common physical finding is a harsh holosystolic murmur that is best heard at the left sternal border. Smaller defects tend to have the loudest murmurs because of the great turbulence of flow that they cause. A systolic thrill can commonly be palpated over the region of the murmur. In addition, a mid-diastolic rumble can often be heard at the apex owing to the increased flow across the mitral valve. If pulmonary vascular disease develops, the holosystolic murmur diminishes as the pressure gradient across the defect decreases. In such patients, an RV heave, a loud pulmonic closure sound (P_2), and cyanosis may be evident.

Diagnostic Studies

On *chest radiographs,* the cardiac silhouette may be normal in patients with small defects, but in those with large shunts, cardiomegaly and prominent pulmonary vascular markings are present. If pulmonary vascular disease has developed, enlarged pulmonary arteries with peripheral tapering may be evident. The *ECG* shows left atrial enlargement and left ventricular hypertrophy in those with a large shunt, and right ventricular hypertrophy is usually evident if pulmonary vascular disease is present. *Echocardiography* with Doppler studies can accurately determine the location of the VSD, identify the direction and magnitude of the shunt, and provide an estimate of right ventricular systolic pressure. *Cardiac catheterization* demonstrates increased oxygen saturation in the RV compared with the right atrium, the result of shunting of highly oxygenated blood from the LV into the RV.

Treatment

By age 2, at least 50% of small and moderate-sized VSDs undergo sufficient partial or complete spontaneous closure to make intervention unnecessary. Surgical correction of the defect is recommended in the first few months of life for children with congestive heart failure or pulmonary vascular disease. Moderate-sized defects without pulmonary vascular disease but with significant left-to-right shunting can be corrected later in childhood. Less-invasive catheter-based treatments are also used in selected patients.

Patent Ductus Arteriosus

The ductus arteriosus is the vessel that connects the left pulmonary artery to the descending aorta during fetal life. Patent ductus arteriosus (PDA) results when the ductus fails to close after birth, resulting in a persistent connection between the great vessels (Fig. 16.13). It has an overall incidence of about 1 in 2,500 to 5,000 live term births. Risk factors for its presence include first trimester maternal rubella infection, prematurity, and birth at a high altitude.

Pathophysiology

As described earlier, the smooth muscle of the ductus arteriosus usually constricts after birth owing to the sudden rise in blood oxygen tension and a reduction in the level of circulating prostaglandins. Over the next several weeks, intimal proliferation and fibrosis result in permanent closure. Failure of the ductus to close results in a persistent shunt between the descending aorta and the left pulmonary artery. The magnitude of flow through the shunt depends on the cross-sectional area and length of the ductus itself as well as the relative resistances of the systemic and pulmonary vasculatures. Prenatally, when the pulmonary vascular resistance is high, blood is diverted away from the immature lungs to the aorta. As the pulmonary resistance drops postnatally, the shunt reverses direction and blood flows from the aorta into the pulmonary circulation instead. Because of this left-to-right shunt, the pulmonary circulation, left atrium, and LV become volume overloaded. This can lead to left ventricular dilatation and left-sided heart failure, whereas the right heart remains normal unless pulmonary vascular disease ensues. If the latter does develop, Eisenmenger syndrome results, with reversal of the shunt

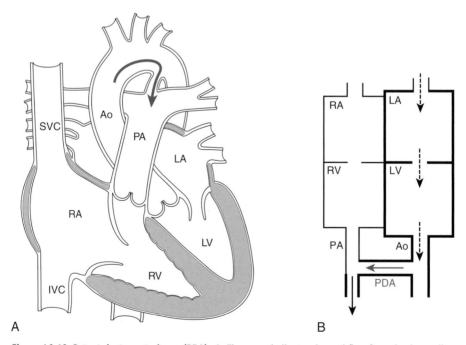

Figure 16.13. Patent ductus arteriosus (PDA). A. The arrow indicates shunted flow from the descending aorta (Ao) toward the pulmonary artery (PA). **B.** Schematic representation of blood flow through an uncomplicated PDA. The dashed lines represent increased blood return to the left side of the heart as a result of the shunt, which causes enlargement of the left atrium (LA), left ventricle (LV), and Ao. IVC, inferior vena cava; RA, right atrium; RV, right ventricle; SVC, superior vena cava.

causing blood to flow from the pulmonary artery, through the ductus, to the descending aorta. The resulting flow of desaturated blood to the lower extremities causes cyanosis of the feet; the upper extremities are not cyanotic, because they receive normally saturated blood from the proximal aorta.

Symptoms

Children with small PDAs are generally asymptomatic. Those with large left-to-right shunts develop early congestive heart failure with tachycardia, poor feeding, slow growth, and recurrent lower respiratory tract infections. Moderate-sized lesions can present with fatigue, dyspnea, and palpitations in adolescence and adult life. Atrial fibrillation may occur owing to left atrial dilatation. Turbulent blood flow across the defect can set the stage for endovascular infection, similar to endocarditis, but more accurately termed *endarteritis*.

Physical Examination

The most common finding in a patient with a left-to-right shunt through a PDA is a *continuous, machine-like* murmur (see Fig. 2.10), heard best at the left subclavicular region. The murmur is present throughout the cardiac cycle because a pressure gradient exists between the aorta and pulmonary artery in both systole and diastole. However, if pulmonary vascular disease develops, the gradient between the aorta and the pulmonary artery decreases, leading to diminished flow through the PDA, and the murmur becomes shorter (the diastolic component may disappear). If Eisenmenger syndrome develops, lower extremity cyanosis and clubbing may be present on examination as poorly oxygenated blood is shunted to the descending aorta.

Diagnostic Studies

With a large PDA, the *chest radiograph* shows an enlarged cardiac silhouette (left atrial and left ventricular enlargement) with prominent pulmonary vascular markings. In adults, calcification of the ductus may be visualized.

The *ECG* shows left atrial enlargement and left ventricular hypertrophy when a large shunt is present. *Echocardiography* with Doppler imaging can visualize the defect, demonstrate flow through it, and estimate right-sided systolic pressures. *Cardiac catheterization* is usually unnecessary for diagnostic purposes. When performed in patients with a left-to-right shunt, it demonstrates a step up in oxygen saturation in the pulmonary artery compared with the RV, and angiography shows the abnormal flow of blood through the PDA.

Treatment

In the absence of other congenital cardiac abnormalities or severe pulmonary vascular disease, a PDA should generally be therapeutically occluded. Although many spontaneously close during the first months after birth, this rarely occurs later. Given the constant risk of endarteritis and the minimal complications of corrective procedures, even a small asymptomatic PDA is commonly referred for closure. For neonates and premature infants with congestive heart failure, a trial of prostaglandin synthesis inhibitors (e.g., indomethacin) can be administered in an attempt to constrict the ductus. Definitive closure can be accomplished by surgical division or ligation of the ductus or by transcatheter techniques in which an occluding device is placed.

Congenital Aortic Stenosis

Congenital aortic stenosis (AS) is most often caused by abnormal structural development of the valve leaflets (Fig. 16.14). It occurs in 5 of 10,000 live births and is four times as common in males as in females. Twenty percent of patients have an additional abnormality, most commonly coarctation of the aorta (discussed later). The aortic valve in congenital AS usually has a **bicuspid** leaflet structure instead of the normal three-leaflet configuration, causing an eccentric stenotic opening through which blood is ejected. Most bicuspid aortic valves are actually nonobstructive at birth and therefore only rarely result in congenital AS. More often, bicuspid valves become progressively stenotic over a great many

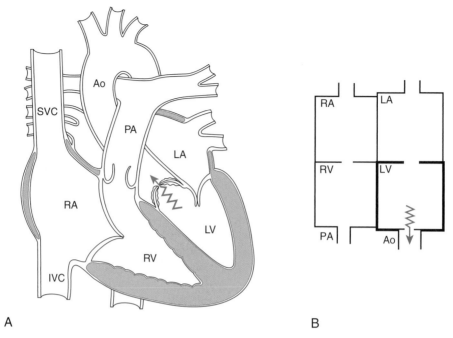

Figure 16.14. Congenital aortic valve stenosis. A. The jagged arrow traverses the narrowed aortic valve. **B.** Schematic representation of obstructed flow through the narrowed aortic valve *(jagged arrow)*. Left ventricular (LV) hypertrophy results from the chronically increased pressure load. Poststenotic dilatation of the aorta (Ao) is common. IVC, inferior vena cava; LA, left atrium; PA, pulmonary artery; RA, right atrium; RV, right ventricle; SVC, superior vena cava.

years, as the leaflets progressively fibrose and calcify, and represent a common cause of AS in adults (see Chapter 8).

Pathophysiology

Because the valvular orifice is significantly narrowed, left ventricular systolic pressure must increase to pump blood across the valve into the aorta. In response to this increased pressure load, the LV hypertrophies. The high-velocity jet of blood that passes through the stenotic valve may impact the proximal aortic wall and contribute to dilatation of that vessel.

Symptoms

The clinical picture of AS depends on the severity of the lesion. Fewer than 10% of infants experience symptoms of heart failure before age 1, but if they do, they manifest tachycardia, tachypnea, failure to thrive, and poor feeding. Most older children with congenital AS are asymptomatic and develop normally. When symptoms do occur, they are similar to those of adult AS and include fatigue, exertional dyspnea, angina pectoris, and syncope (see Chapter 8).

Physical Examination

Auscultation reveals a harsh crescendo–decrescendo systolic murmur, loudest at the base of the heart with radiation to the neck. It is often preceded by a systolic ejection click (see Chapter 2), especially when a bicuspid valve is present. Unlike the murmurs of ASD, VSD, or PDA, the murmur of congenital AS is characteristically present from birth because it does not depend on the postnatal decline in pulmonary vascular resistance. With advanced disease, the ejection time becomes longer, causing the peak of the murmur to occur later in systole. In severe disease, the significantly prolonged ejection time causes a delay in closure of the aortic valve such that A_2 occurs *after* P_2—a phenomenon known as reversed splitting of S_2 (see Chapter 2).

Diagnostic Studies

The *chest radiograph* of an infant with AS may show an enlarged LV and a dilated ascending aorta. The *ECG* often shows left ventricular hypertrophy. *Echocardiography* identifies the abnormal structure of the aortic valve and the degree of left ventricular hypertrophy. Doppler assessment can accurately measure the pressure gradient across the stenotic valve and allow calculation of the valve area. *Cardiac catheterization* confirms the pressure gradient across the valve.

Treatment

In its milder forms, congenital AS does not need to be corrected but should be followed closely as the degree of stenosis may worsen over time. Severe obstruction of the aortic valve during infancy may mandate immediate repair. Transcatheter balloon valvuloplasty is the first line of intervention, but surgical repair may be necessary if valvuloplasty fails to relieve the obstruction or if significant aortic regurgitation results from balloon dilation. Often, valvuloplasty in infancy is only palliative, and repeat catheter balloon dilation or surgical revision is needed later.

Pulmonic Stenosis

Obstruction to right ventricular outflow may occur at the level of the pulmonic valve (e.g., from congenitally fused valve commissures), within the body of the RV (in the RV outflow tract), or in the pulmonary artery. *Valvular* pulmonic stenosis is the most frequent form (Fig. 16.15).

Pathophysiology

The consequence of pulmonic stenosis is impairment of right ventricular outflow, which leads to increased RV pressures and chamber hypertrophy. The clinical course is determined by the severity of the obstruction. Although mild pulmonic stenosis rarely progresses and

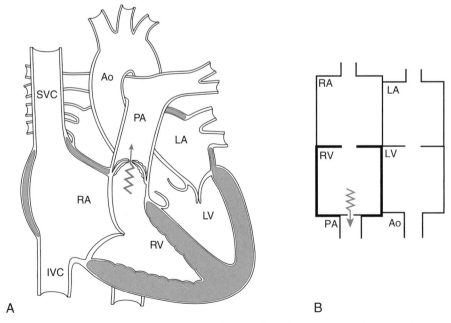

Figure 16.15. Congenital pulmonary valve stenosis. A. The jagged arrow traverses the narrowed pulmonary valve. **B.** Schematic representation of obstructed flow through the narrowed pulmonary valve (*jagged arrow*). Right ventricular hypertrophy results from the chronically increased pressure load. Ao, aorta; IVC, inferior vena cava; LA, left atrium; LV, left ventricle; PA, pulmonary artery; RA, right atrium; RV, right ventricle; SVC, superior vena cava.

Chapter 16

is unlikely to affect RV function, untreated severe pulmonic stenosis typically results in findings of right-sided heart failure.

Symptoms

Children with mild or moderate pulmonary stenosis are asymptomatic. The diagnosis is often first made on discovery of a murmur during a routine physical examination. Severe stenosis may cause manifestations such as dyspnea with exertion, exercise intolerance, and with decompensation, symptoms of right-sided heart failure such as abdominal fullness and pedal edema.

Physical Examination

The physical findings in pulmonic stenosis depend on the severity of the obstruction. If the stenosis is severe with accompanying right ventricular hypertrophy, a prominent jugular venous *a* wave can be observed (see Chapter 2) and an RV heave is palpated over the sternum. A loud, late-peaking, crescendo–decrescendo systolic ejection murmur is heard at the upper-left sternal border, often associated with a palpable thrill. Widened splitting of the S_2 with a soft P_2 component is caused by the delayed closure of the stenotic pulmonary valve.

In more moderate stenosis, a pulmonic ejection sound (a high-pitched "click") follows S_1 and precedes the systolic murmur. It occurs during the early phase of right ventricular contraction as the stenotic valve leaflets suddenly reach their maximum level of ascent into the pulmonary artery, just before blood ejection. Unlike other sounds and murmurs produced by the right side of the heart, the pulmonic ejection sound *diminishes* in intensity during inspiration. This occurs because with inspiration, the augmented right-sided filling elevates the leaflets into the pulmonary artery prior to RV contraction, preempting the rapid tensing in early systole that is thought to produce the sound.

Diagnostic Studies

The *chest radiograph* may demonstrate an enlarged right atrium and ventricle with

poststenotic pulmonary artery dilation (caused by the impact of the high-velocity jet of blood against the wall of the pulmonary artery). The *ECG* shows right ventricular hypertrophy and right axis deviation. *Echocardiography* with Doppler imaging assesses the pulmonary valve morphology, determines the presence of right ventricular hypertrophy, and accurately measures the pressure gradient across the obstruction.

Treatment

Mild pulmonic stenosis usually does not progress or require treatment. Moderate or severe valvular obstruction at the valvular level can be relieved by dilating the stenotic valve by means of transcatheter balloon valvuloplasty. Long-term results of this procedure have been uniformly excellent, and right ventricular hypertrophy usually regresses subsequently.

Coarctation of the Aorta

Coarctation of the aorta typically consists of a discrete narrowing of the aortic lumen (Fig. 16.16). This anomaly has an incidence of 1 in 6,000 live births and the most common associated cardiac abnormality is a bicuspid aortic valve. Aortic coarctation often occurs in patients with Turner syndrome (45, XO).

In the past, coarctations were described as either "preductal" (infantile) or "postductal"

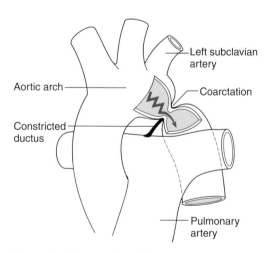

Figure 16.16. **Coarctation of the aorta.** A pressure gradient is present through the narrowed lumen of the aorta.

378

(adult-type) based on the location of the aortic narrowing in relation to the ductus arteriosus. These terms have been largely abandoned because the vast majority of coarctations are actually juxtaductal (i.e., "next to" the ductus) and etiologic differences between the preductal and postductal categories have not been substantiated.

While the actual pathogenesis of aortic coarctation has not been defined, one theory contends that reduced antegrade blood flow through the left side of the heart and ascending aorta during fetal life leads to hypoplastic development of the aorta ("no flow, no grow"). Another theory is that ectopic muscular ductus arteriosus tissue extends into the aorta during fetal life and constricts following birth at the same time the ductus is caused to close. More recent evidence suggests that aortic coarctation may be just one manifestation of a more diffuse aortic disease.

Pathophysiology

Because of the impedance of aortic narrowing in coarctation, the LV faces an increased afterload. Blood flow to the head and upper extremities is preserved because the vessels supplying these areas usually branch off the aorta proximal to the obstruction, but flow to the descending aorta and lower extremities may be diminished. If coarctation is not corrected, compensatory alterations include (1) development of left ventricular hypertrophy and (2) dilatation of collateral blood vessels from the intercostal arteries that bypass the coarctation and provide blood to the more distal descending aorta. Eventually, these collateral vessels enlarge and can erode the undersurface of the ribs.

Symptoms

Patients with severe coarctation usually present very shortly after birth with symptoms of heart failure. Infants may also exhibit *differential cyanosis* if the ductus arteriosus fails to constrict and remains patent. The upper half of the body, supplied by the LV and the ascending aorta, is perfused with well-oxygenated blood; however, the lower half appears cyanotic because it is largely supplied by right-to-left flow of poorly oxygenated blood from the pulmonary artery, across the PDA, and into the descending aorta.

When the coarctation is less severe, a patient may be asymptomatic or experience only mild weakness or pain in the lower extremities following exercise (i.e., *claudication*). In asymptomatic cases, coarctation may be suspected by the finding of upper extremity hypertension later in life (see Chapter 13).

Physical Examination

On examination, the femoral pulses are weak and delayed. An elevated blood pressure in the upper body is the most common finding. If the coarctation occurs *distal* to the takeoff of the left subclavian artery, the systolic pressure in the arms is greater than that in the legs. If the coarctation occurs *proximal* to the takeoff of the left subclavian artery, the systolic pressure in the right arm may exceed that in the left arm. A systolic pressure in the right arm that is 15 to 20 mm Hg greater than that in a leg is sufficient to suspect coarctation, because normally the systolic pressure in the legs is *higher* than that in the arms. A midsystolic ejection murmur (caused by flow through the coarctation) may be audible over the chest and/or back. A prominent tortuous collateral arterial circulation may create continuous murmurs over the chest in adults.

Diagnostic Studies

In adults with uncorrected coarctation of the aorta, *chest radiography* generally reveals notching of the inferior surface of the posterior ribs owing to enlarged intercostal vessels supplying collateral circulation to the descending aorta. An indented aorta at the site of coarctation may also be visualized. The *ECG* shows left ventricular hypertrophy resulting from the pressure load placed on that chamber. *Doppler echocardiography* confirms the diagnosis of coarctation and assesses the pressure gradient across the lesion. *Magnetic resonance imaging* demonstrates in detail the length and severity of coarctation (see Fig. 16.17). Diagnostic *catheterization* and angiography are rarely necessary.

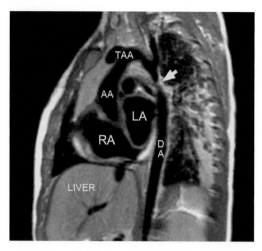

Figure 16.17. Magnetic resonance imaging of coarctation of the aorta. This lateral view demonstrates coarctation, manifest as a focal aortic narrowing (*white arrow*). AA, ascending aorta; DA, descending aorta; LA, left atrium; RA, right atrium; TAA, transverse aortic arch.

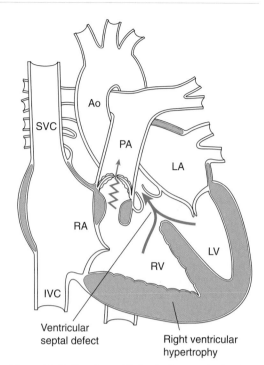

Figure 16.18. Tetralogy of Fallot is characterized by four associated anomalies. (1) A ventricular septal defect, (2) obstruction to right ventricular outflow (*jagged arrow*), (3) an overriding aorta that receives blood from both ventricles, and (4) right ventricular hypertrophy. Ao, aorta; IVC, inferior vena cava; LA, left atrium; LV, left ventricle; PA, pulmonary artery; RA, right atrium; RV, right ventricle; SVC, superior vena cava.

Treatment

In neonates with severe obstruction, prostaglandin infusion is administered to keep the ductus arteriosus patent, thus maintaining blood flow to the descending aorta before surgery is undertaken. In children, elective repair is usually performed to prevent systemic hypertension. Several effective surgical procedures are available, including excision of the narrowed aortic segment with end-to-end reanastomosis and direct repair of the coarctation, sometimes using synthetic patch material. For older children, adults, and patients with recurrent coarctation after previous repair, transcatheter interventions (balloon dilatation with or without stent placement) are usually successful.

Cyanotic Lesions

Tetralogy of Fallot

Tetralogy of Fallot results from a single developmental defect: an abnormal anterior and cephalad displacement of the infundibular (outflow tract) portion of the interventricular septum. As a consequence, four anomalies arise that characterize this condition, as shown in Figure 16.18: (1) a VSD caused by anterior

malalignment of the interventricular septum, (2) subvalvular pulmonic stenosis because of obstruction from the displaced infundibular septum (often with valvular pulmonic stenosis), (3) an overriding aorta that receives blood from both ventricles, and (4) right ventricular hypertrophy owing to the high-pressure load placed on the RV by the pulmonic stenosis. Tetralogy of Fallot is the most common form of cyanotic congenital heart disease after infancy, occurring in 5 of 10,000 live births and is often associated with other cardiac defects, including a right-sided aortic arch (25% of patients), ASD (10% of patients), and less often, anomalous origin of the left coronary artery. A microdeletion in chromosome 22 (22q11) has been identified in patients with a syndrome that includes tetralogy of Fallot as one of the cardiovascular manifestations (see Box 16.1).

BOX 16.1	Genetic Abnormalities in Congenital Heart Disease

Progress in the understanding of genetic influences on cardiac development and congenital heart disease is proceeding at a brisk pace, aided by the Human Genome Project. Although nearly all cardiac congenital anomalies can occur as isolated findings, the clustering of certain forms with heritable syndromes and known genetic abnormalities provides clues to the underlying basis of certain defects.

Among infants with **Down syndrome** (trisomy 21), the incidence of congenital heart defects is nearly 40%. Many of these are common abnormalities such as ASDs, VSDs, and PDAs. There is also a high incidence of a rarer condition known as common atrioventricular canal, which consists of a large primum ASD and VSD and a common (undivided) atrioventricular valve. These central heart structures are usually formed by the endocardial cushions and cells of neural crest origin, which are known to have abnormal migration patterns in patients with trisomy 21.

Turner syndrome (45, XO) is another heritable condition associated with congenital heart disease. Left-sided obstructive congenital heart lesions are common in patients with this syndrome, including bicuspid aortic valve, coarctation of the aorta, and occasionally hypoplastic left heart syndrome (underdevelopment of the left ventricle and aorta). The specific genes responsible for these abnormalities have not yet been elucidated.

In contrast, discrete gene abnormalities *have* been identified in other syndrome-associated forms of congenital heart disease. Many patients with **Williams syndrome** (characterized by mental retardation, hypercalcemia, renovascular hypertension, facial abnormalities, and short stature) have supravalvular aortic stenosis, and some have a more diffuse arteriopathy of the aorta as well as pulmonary artery obstruction. The genetic abnormality in Williams syndrome is a deletion on chromosome 7 (7q11.23), a region that includes the elastin gene. Abnormalities in the production of elastin, a critical component of the arterial wall, may be responsible for the observed arteriopathy.

DiGeorge syndrome (characterized by pharyngeal defects, hypocalcemia due to absent parathyroid glands, and T-cell dysfunction secondary to hypoplasia of the thymus) is associated with congenital abnormalities of the cardiac outflow tracts, including tetralogy of Fallot, truncus arteriosus (a large VSD over which a single large outflow vessel arises), and interrupted aortic arch. Most patients with DiGeorge syndrome have a microdeletion within chromosome 22 (22q11), a region that contains the *TBX1* gene. This gene encodes a transcription factor that appears to play a critical role in developmental patterning of the cardiac outflow tracts.

Several other transcription factors involved in heart development likely contribute to congenital heart disease. Some families with heritable forms of ASDs have mutations in the transcription factor gene *Nkx2.5*. An associated transcription factor gene *GATA4* appears to collaborate with *Nkx2.5* and has also been implicated in familial septal defect syndromes. Mutations in *TBX5*, yet another transcription factor gene, are responsible for **Holt–Oram syndrome** (also known as the heart–hand syndrome), an autosomal dominant disorder whose characteristic cardiac defects include secundum ASDs and VSDs.

Further deciphering of the genome will undoubtedly improve understanding of cardiac development and the molecular defects that lead to congenital heart abnormalities.

Pathophysiology

Increased resistance by the subvalvular pulmonic stenosis causes deoxygenated blood returning from the systemic veins to be diverted from the RV, through the VSD, to the LV, and into the systemic circulation, resulting in systemic hypoxemia and cyanosis. The magnitude of shunt flow across the VSD is primarily a function of the severity of the pulmonary stenosis, but acute changes in systemic and pulmonary vascular resistances can affect it as well.

Symptoms

Children with tetralogy of Fallot often experience dyspnea on exertion. "Spells" may occur following exertion, feeding, or crying when systemic vasodilatation results in an increased right-to-left shunt. Manifestations of such spells include irritability, cyanosis, hyperventilation, and occasionally syncope or convulsions. Children learn to alleviate their symptoms by squatting down, which is thought to increase systemic vascular resistance by "kinking" the femoral arteries, thereby decreasing the right-to-left shunt and directing more blood from the RV to the lungs.

Physical Examination

Children with tetralogy of Fallot and moderate pulmonary stenosis often have mild cyanosis, most notably of the lips, mucous membranes, and digits. Infants with severe pulmonary stenosis may present with profound cyanosis in the first few days of life. Chronic hypoxemia caused by the right-to-left shunt commonly results in clubbing of the fingers and toes. Right ventricular hypertrophy may be appreciated on physical examination as a palpable heave along the left sternal border. The S_2 is single, composed of a normal aortic component; the pulmonary component is soft and usually inaudible. A systolic ejection murmur heard best at the upper-left sternal border is created by turbulent blood flow through the stenotic right ventricular outflow tract. There is usually no distinct murmur related to the VSD, because it is typically large and thus generates little turbulence.

Diagnostic Studies

Chest radiography demonstrates prominence of the RV and decreased size of the main pulmonary artery segment, giving the appearance of a "boot-shaped" heart. Pulmonary vascular markings are typically diminished because of decreased flow through the pulmonary circulation. The *ECG* shows right ventricular hypertrophy with right axis deviation. *Echocardiography* details the right ventricular outflow tract anatomy, the malaligned VSD, right ventricular hypertrophy, and other associated defects, as does *cardiac catheterization.*

Treatment

Before definitive surgical correction of tetralogy of Fallot was developed, several forms of palliative therapy were undertaken. These involved creating anatomic communications between the aorta (or one of its major branches) to the pulmonary artery, establishing a left-to-right shunt to increase pulmonary blood flow. Such procedures are occasionally used today in infants for whom definitive repair is planned at an older age. Complete surgical correction of tetralogy of Fallot involves closure of the VSD and enlargement of the subpulmonary infundibulum with the use of a pericardial patch. Elective repair is usually recommended at 6 to 12 months of age to decrease the likelihood of future complications. Most patients who have undergone successful repair grow to become asymptomatic adults. However, antibiotic prophylaxis to prevent endocarditis is required in some patients (see Chapter 8).

Transposition of the Great Arteries

In transposition of the great arteries (TGA), each great vessel inappropriately arises from the opposite ventricle; that is, the aorta originates from the RV and the pulmonary artery originates from the LV (Fig. 16.19). This anomaly accounts for approximately 7% of congenital heart defects, affecting 40 of 100,000 live births.

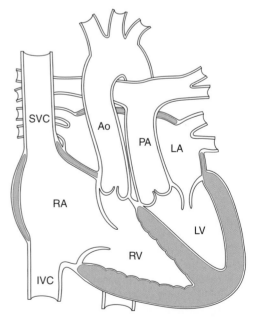

Figure 16.19. Transposition of the great arteries. The aorta (Ao) and pulmonary artery (PA) arise abnormally from the right ventricle (RV) and left ventricle (LV), respectively. IVC, inferior vena cava; LA, left atrium; RA, right atrium; SVC, superior vena cava.

Whereas tetralogy of Fallot is the most common etiology of cyanosis after infancy, TGA is the most common cause of cyanosis in the neonatal period.

The precise cause of transposition remains unknown. Historically, failure of the aortico-pulmonary septum to spiral in a normal fashion during fetal development was considered the underlying problem. It has also been suggested that the defect may be the result of abnormal growth and absorption of the subpulmonary and subaortic infundibuli during the division of the truncus arteriosus. Normally, reabsorption of the subaortic infundibulum places the forming aortic valve posterior and inferior to the pulmonary valve and in continuity with the LV. In TGA, the process of infundibular reabsorption may be reversed, placing the pulmonary valve over the LV instead.

Pathophysiology

TGA separates the pulmonary and systemic circulations by placing the two circuits in parallel rather than in series. This arrangement forces desaturated blood from the systemic venous system to pass through the RV and then return to the systemic circulation through the aorta without undergoing normal oxygenation in the lungs. Similarly, oxygenated pulmonary venous return passes through the LV and then back through the pulmonary artery to the lungs without imparting oxygen to the systemic circulation. The result is an extremely hypoxic, cyanotic neonate. Without intervention to create mixing between the two circulations, TGA is a lethal condition.

TGA is compatible with life in utero because flow through the ductus arteriosus and foramen ovale allows communication between the two circulations. Oxygenated fetal blood flows from the placenta through the umbilical vein to the right atrium, and then most of it travels into the left atrium through the foramen ovale. The oxygenated blood in the left atrium passes into the LV and is pumped out the pulmonary artery. Most of the pulmonary artery flow travels through the ductus arteriosus into the aorta, instead of the high-resistance pulmonary vessels, such that oxygen is provided to the developing tissues.

After birth, normal physiologic closure of the ductus and the foramen ovale eliminates the shunt between the parallel circulations and, without intervention, would result in death because oxygenated blood does not reach the systemic tissues. However, if the ductus arteriosus and foramen ovale remain patent (either naturally or with exogenous prostaglandins or surgical intervention), communication between the parallel circuits is maintained, and sufficiently oxygenated blood may be provided to the brain and other vital organs.

Symptoms and Physical Examination

Infants with transposition appear blue, with the intensity of the cyanosis dependent on the degree of intermixing between the parallel circuits. In most cases, generalized cyanosis is apparent on the first day of life and progresses rapidly as the ductus arteriosus closes. Palpation of the chest reveals a right ventricular impulse at the lower sternal border as the RV faces systemic pressures. Auscultation may reveal an accentuated S_2, which reflects closure of the anteriorly placed aortic valve just under the chest wall. Prominent murmurs are uncommon and may signal an additional defect.

Diagnostic Studies

Chest radiography is usually normal, although the base of the heart may be narrow owing to the more anterior–posterior orientation of the aorta and pulmonary artery. The *ECG* demonstrates right ventricular hypertrophy, reflecting the fact that the RV is the systemic "high-pressure" pumping chamber. The definitive diagnosis of transposition can be made by *echocardiography*, which demonstrates the abnormal orientation of the great vessels.

Treatment

TGA is a medical emergency. Initial treatment includes maintenance of the ductus arteriosus by prostaglandin infusion and creation of an interatrial communication using a balloon catheter (termed the Rashkind procedure). Such intervention allows adequate mixing of the two circulations until definitive corrective surgery can be performed. The current corrective procedure of choice is the "arterial switch" operation (Jatene procedure), which involves transection of the great vessels above the semilunar valves and origin of the coronary arteries. The great vessels are then reversed to the natural configuration, so the aorta arises from the LV and the pulmonary artery arises from the RV. The coronary arteries are then relocated to the new aorta.

EISENMENGER SYNDROME

Eisenmenger syndrome is the condition of severe pulmonary vascular obstruction that results from chronic left-to-right shunting through a congenital cardiac defect. The elevated pulmonary vascular resistance causes reversal of the original shunt (to the right-to-left direction) and systemic cyanosis.

The mechanism by which increased pulmonary flow causes this condition is unknown. Histologically, the pulmonary arteriolar media hypertrophies and the intima proliferates, reducing the cross-sectional area of the pulmonary vascular bed. Over time, the vessels become thrombosed, and the resistance of the pulmonary vasculature rises, causing the original left-to-right shunt to decrease. Eventually, if the resistance of the pulmonary circulation exceeds that of the systemic vasculature, the direction of shunt flow reverses.

With reversal of the shunt to the right-to-left direction, symptoms arise from hypoxemia, including exertional dyspnea and fatigue. Reduced hemoglobin saturation stimulates the bone marrow to produce more red blood cells (erythrocytosis), which can lead to hyperviscosity, symptoms of which include fatigue, headaches, and stroke (caused by cerebrovascular occlusion). Infarction or rupture of the pulmonary vessels can result in hemoptysis.

On examination, a patient with Eisenmenger syndrome appears cyanotic with digital clubbing. A prominent *a* wave in the jugular venous pulsation reflects elevated right-sided pressure during atrial contraction. A loud P_2 is common. The murmur of the inciting left-to-right shunt is usually *absent*, because the original pressure gradient across

the lesion is negated by the elevated right-heart pressures.

Chest radiography in Eisenmenger syndrome is notable for proximal pulmonary artery dilatation with peripheral tapering. Calcification of the pulmonary vasculature may be seen. The *ECG* demonstrates right ventricular hypertrophy and right atrial enlargement. *Echocardiography* with Doppler studies can usually identify the underlying cardiac defect and quantitate the pulmonary artery systolic pressure.

Treatment includes the avoidance of activities that can exacerbate the right-to-left shunt. These include strenuous physical activity, high altitude, and the use of peripheral vasodilator drugs. Pregnancy is especially dangerous; the rate of spontaneous abortion is 20% to 40% and the incidence of maternal mortality is ~45%. Supportive measures for Eisenmenger syndrome include prompt treatment of infections, management of rhythm disturbances, and phlebotomy for patients with symptomatic erythrocytosis.

Although there are no remedies that reverse the disease process in Eisenmenger syndrome, pulmonary vasodilator therapy can provide symptomatic relief and improve the patient's quality of life. Effective agents include endothelin receptor antagonists, prostacyclin analogs, and phosphodiesterase inhibitors. The only effective long-term strategy for severely affected patients is lung or heart–lung transplantation. Fortunately, with the dramatic advances that have been made in the detection and early correction of severe congenital heart defects, Eisenmenger syndrome has become less common.

SUMMARY

1. The significance of congenital heart lesions can be predicted from an understanding of cardiovascular embryonic development and the transition to postnatal circulatory pathways.

2. Cardiac malformations occur in 0.8% of live births. Such lesions can be grouped into cyanotic or acyanotic defects, depending on whether the abnormality results in

pulmonary-to-systemic (right-to-left) shunting of blood.

3. Acyanotic defects often result in either volume overload (ASD, VSD, PDA) or pressure overload (AS, pulmonic stenosis, coarctation of the aorta). Chronic volume overload resulting from a large left-to-right shunt can ultimately result in increased pulmonary vascular resistance, reversal of the direction of shunt flow, and subsequent cyanosis (Eisenmenger syndrome).

4. Among the most common cyanotic defects are tetralogy of Fallot and TGA.

Acknowledgments

Contributors to the previous editions of this chapter were Vijay G. Sankaran, MD; Yi-Bin Chen, MD; Douglas W. Green, MD; Lakshmi Halasyamani, MD; Andrew Karson, MD; Raymond Tabibiazar, MD; Michael D. Freed, MD; Richard Liberthson, MD; and David W. Brown, MD.

Additional Reading

Allen HD, Driscoll DJ, Shaddy RE, et al., eds. *Moss and Adams' Heart Disease in Infants, Children, and Adolescents*. 7th ed. Baltimore, MD: Lippincott Williams & Wilkins; 2007.

Bruneau BG. The developmental genetics of congenital heart disease. *Nature*. 2008;451:943–948.

Dhanantwari P, Lee E, Krishnan A, et al. Human cardiac development in the first trimester. *Circulation*. 2009;120:343–351.

Keane JF, Lock JE, Fyler DC, et al., eds. *Nadas' Pediatric Cardiology*. 2nd ed. Philadelphia, PA: WB Saunders; 2006.

Moore KL, Persaud TVN. *The Developing Human: Clinically Oriented Embryology*. 8th ed. Philadelphia, PA: WB Saunders; 2007.

Park MK. *Pediatric Cardiology for Practitioners*. 5th ed. St. Louis, MO: Mosby; 2008.

Perloff JK. *The Clinical Recognition of Congenital Heart Disease*. 5th ed. Philadelphia, PA: WB Saunders; 2003.

Pierpont ME, Basson CT, Benson DW Jr, et al. Genetic basis for congenital heart defects: current knowledge: a scientific statement from the American Heart Association Congenital Cardiac Defects Committee, Council on Cardiovascular Disease in the Young: endorsed by the American Academy of Pediatrics. *Circulation*. 2007;115:3015–3038.

Rudolph AM. *Congenital Diseases of the Heart: Clinical-Physiological Considerations*. 3rd ed. Chichester, UK: Wiley-Blackwell; 2009.

Sadler TW. *Langman's Medical Embryology*. 11th ed. Philadelphia, PA: Lippincott Williams & Wilkins; 2009.

Warnes CA, Williams RG, Bashore TM, et al. ACC/AHA 2008 Guidelines for the management of adults with congenital heart disease: executive summary. *J Am Coll Cardiol*. 2008;52:1890–1947.

Cardiovascular Drugs

Cyrus K. Yamin
Christopher A. Miller
Elliott M. Antman
Gary R. Strichartz
Leonard S. Lilly

This chapter reviews the physiologic basis and clinical use of cardiovascular drugs. Although a multitude of drugs are available to treat cardiac disorders, these agents can be grouped by their pharmacologic actions into a small number of categories. Additionally, many drugs are useful in more than one form of heart disease.

INOTROPIC DRUGS AND VASOPRESSORS

Inotropic drugs are used to increase the force of ventricular contraction when myocardial systolic function is impaired. The pharmacologic agents in this category include the cardiac glycosides, sympathomimetic amines, and phosphodiesterase-3 inhibitors. Although they work through different mechanisms, they are all thought to enhance cardiac contraction by increasing the intracellular calcium concentration, thus augmenting actin and myosin interactions. The hemodynamic effect is to shift a depressed ventricular performance curve (Frank–Starling curve) in an upward direction (Fig. 17.1), so that for a given ventricular filling pressure, stroke volume and cardiac output are increased.

Cardiac Glycosides (Digitalis)

The cardiac glycosides are called "digitalis" because the drugs of this class are based on extracts of the foxglove plant, *Digitalis purpurea*. The most commonly used member of this group is **digoxin**.

Mechanism of Action

The two desired effects of digoxin are (1) to improve contractility of the failing heart (mechanical effect) and (2) to prolong the refractory period of the atrioventricular (AV) node in patients with supraventricular arrhythmias (electrical effect).

Mechanical Effect

The action by which digoxin improves contractility appears to be inhibition of the sarcolemmal Na^+K^+-ATPase "pump," normally responsible for maintaining transmembrane Na^+ and K^+ gradients. By binding to and inhibiting this pump, digitalis causes the intracellular $[Na^+]$ to rise. As shown in Figure 17.2, an increase in intracellular sodium content reduces Ca^{++} extrusion from the cell by the Na^+–Ca^{++} exchanger. Consequently, more Ca^{++} is pumped into the sarcoplasmic reticulum, and when subsequent action potentials excite the cell, a greater-than-normal amount of Ca^{++} is released to the myofilaments, thereby enhancing the force of contraction. The magnitude of the positive inotropic effect correlates with the degree of Na^+K^+-ATPase inhibition.

Electrical Effect

The major therapeutic electrical effect of digoxin occurs at the AV node, where it slows conduction velocity and increases refractoriness (Table 17.1). Digoxin has modest direct effects on the electrical properties of cardiac tissue directly, but more importantly,

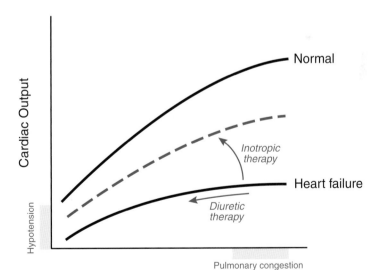

Figure 17.1. Ventricular performance (Frank–Starling) curve. In heart failure, the curve is displaced downward, so that at a given left ventricular end-diastolic pressure (LVEDP), the cardiac output is lower than in a normal heart. Diuretics reduce LVEDP but do not change the position of the curve; thus, pulmonary congestion improves but cardiac output may fall. Inotropic drugs shift the curve upward, toward normal, so that at any LVEDP, the cardiac output is greater.

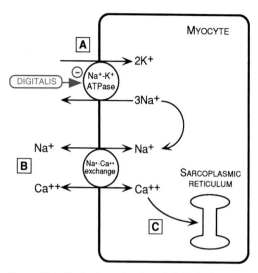

Figure 17.2. Mechanism of action of digitalis (inotropic effect). A. Digitalis inhibits the sarcolemmal Na$^+$K$^+$-ATPase, causing intracellular [Na$^+$] to rise. **B.** Increased cytosolic [Na$^+$] reduces the transmembrane Na$^+$ gradient; thus, the Na$^+$–Ca$^+$ exchanger drives less Ca^{++} out of the cell. **C.** The increased [Ca^{++}] is stored in the sarcoplasmic reticulum, such that with subsequent action potentials, greater-than-normal Ca^{++} is released to the contractile elements in the cytoplasm, intensifying the force of contraction.

it modifies autonomic nervous system output by enhancing vagal tone and reducing sympathetic activity. As a result, digitalis decreases the frequency of transmission of atrial impulses through the AV node to the ventricles. This is beneficial in reducing the rate of ventricular stimulation in patients with rapid supraventricular tachycardias such as atrial fibrillation or atrial flutter. In addition, by enhancing the refractoriness of the AV node, digoxin may convert supraventricular reentrant arrhythmias to normal rhythm.

However, if digoxin concentrations rise into the toxic range, further enhancement of vagal tone and more extreme inhibition of the Na$^+$K$^+$-ATPase pump can result in adverse electrophysiologic effects. For example, in atrial and ventricular Purkinje fibers, a high digoxin concentration has three important actions that may lead to dangerous arrhythmias (Fig. 17.3):

1. *Less negative resting potential.* Inhibition of the Na$^+$K$^+$-ATPase causes the resting potential to become less negative. Since the Na$^+$K$^+$-ATPase normally removes three Na$^+$ ions from the cell in exchange for two in-

wardly moving K$^+$ ions, inhibition of the pump results in a decrease of this outward current and a resulting depolarization of the cell. Consequently, there is a voltage-dependent partial inactivation of the fast Na$^+$ channels, which leads to a slower rise of phase 0 depolarization and reduction in conduction velocity (see Fig. 1.17). The slowed conduction, if present heterogeneously among neighboring cells, enhances the possibility of reentrant arrhythmias.

2. *Decreased action potential duration.* At high digitalis concentrations, the cardiac action potential shortens. This relates in part to the digitalis-induced elevated intracellular [Ca^{++}], which increases the activity of a Ca^{++}-dependent K$^+$ channel. The opening of this channel promotes K$^+$ efflux and more rapid *repolarization*. In addition, high intracellular [Ca^{++}] inactivates the Ca^{++} channels, decreasing the inward *depolarizing* Ca^{++} current. The decrease in action potential duration and the associated shortened refractory period increase the time during which cardiac fibers are responsive to external stimulation, allowing greater opportunity for propagation of arrhythmic impulses.

3. *Enhanced automaticity.* Digoxin enhances cellular automaticity and may generate ectopic rhythms by two mechanisms:

   a. The less negative membrane resting potential may induce phase 4 gradual depolarization, even in nonpacemaker cells (see Chapter 11), and an action potential is triggered each time the threshold voltage is reached.

   b. The digoxin-induced increase in intracellular [Ca^{++}] may trigger delayed afterdepolarizations (see Fig. 17.3). If an afterdepolarization reaches the threshold voltage, an action potential (ectopic beat) is generated. Ectopic beats may lead to additional afterdepolarizations and self-sustaining arrhythmias such as ventricular tachycardia.

In addition, the augmented direct and indirect vagal effects of toxic doses of digitalis slow conduction through the AV node, such that high degrees of AV block, including complete heart block, can occur. Thus, digoxin in

Table 17.1. Electrophysiologic Effects of Digitalis

Region	Mechanism of Action	Effect
Therapeutic effects		
AV node	Vagal effect ↓ Conduction velocity ↑ Effective refractory period	• ↓ Rate of transmission of atrial impulses to the ventricles in supraventricular tachyarrhythmias • ↓ Conduction velocity and ↑ refractory period may interrupt reentrant circuits passing through the AV node
Toxic effects		
Sinoatrial node	↑ Vagal effect and direct suppression	• Sinus bradycardia • Sinoatrial block (impulse not transmitted from SA node to atrium)
Atrium	Delayed afterdepolarizations (triggered activity), ↑ slope of phase 4 depolarization (↑ automaticity)	• Atrial premature beats • Nonreentrant SVT (ectopic rhythm)
	Variable effects on conduction velocity and ↑ refractory period (can fragment conduction and lead to reentry)	• Reentrant PSVT
AV node	Direct and vagal-mediated conduction block	• AV block (first, second, or third degree)
AV junction (between AV node and His bundle)	Delayed afterdepolarizations (triggered activity), ↑ slope of phase 4 depolarization (↑ automaticity)	• Accelerated junctional rhythm
Purkinje fibers and ventricular muscle	Delayed afterdepolarizations (triggered activity), ↓ conduction velocity and ↑ refractory period (can lead to reentry)	• Ventricular premature beats
	↑ Slope of phase 4 depolarization (↑ automaticity)	• Ventricular tachycardia

AV, atrioventricular; PSVT, paroxysmal supraventricular tachycardia.

toxic concentrations may lead to several types of rhythm disorders (see Table 17.1).

Clinical Uses

The most common use of digoxin historically has been as an inotropic agent to treat heart failure caused by decreased ventricular contractility (see Chapter 9). Digoxin increases the force of contraction and augments cardiac output, thereby improving left ventricular emptying, reducing left ventricular size, and decreasing the elevated ventricular filling pressures typical of patients with systolic dysfunction. It is *not* beneficial in forms of heart failure associated with normal ventricular contractility (i.e., heart failure with preserved ejection fraction).

Once the mainstay of therapy in congestive heart failure (CHF), the use of digitalis has waned in the face of newer, more effective therapies (as discussed later in this chapter; see also Chapter 9). Nonetheless, digitalis continues to be useful in treating patients with CHF complicated by atrial fibrillation (it has the added benefit of slowing the ventricular heart rate), or when symptoms do not respond adequately to angiotensin-converting enzyme (ACE) inhibitors, β-blockers, and diuretics.

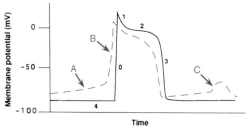

Figure 17.3. Direct effects of digitalis on the Purkinje cell action potential. The solid tracing represents depolarization and repolarization of a normal cell; the dashed tracing demonstrates the effects of digitalis. **A.** The maximum diastolic potential is less negative, and there is an increase in the slope of phase 4 depolarization, endowing the cell with intrinsic automaticity, and the potential for ectopic rhythms. **B.** Because depolarization of the cell occurs at a more positive voltage, there is partial inactivation of fast sodium channels, the rate of rise of phase 0 is decreased, and conduction velocity is slowed, which, if present heterogeneously among neighboring cells, produces conditions for reentry. **C.** Delayed afterdepolarizations may develop at high concentrations of digitalis in association with the increased intracellular calcium concentration and can result in triggered tachyarrhythmias.

Unlike ACE inhibitors and β-blockers, digoxin does not prolong the life expectancy of patients with chronic heart failure, though it may improve their quality of life.

The second most common use of digoxin is as an antiarrhythmic agent in the treatment of atrial fibrillation, atrial flutter, and paroxysmal supraventricular tachycardia (PSVT). In atrial fibrillation and flutter, digitalis reduces the number of impulses transmitted across the AV node, thereby slowing the ventricular rate. Digitalis may terminate reentrant supraventricular tachycardias, likely through enhancement of vagal tone, which slows impulse conduction, prolongs the effective refractory period, and can therefore interrupt reentrant circuits that pass through the AV node.

The use of digoxin as an antiarrhythmic has become less common because other agents such as β-blockers, calcium channel blockers (CCBs), and amiodarone are often more effective.

Pharmacokinetics and Toxicity

Digoxin is excreted unchanged by the kidney. A series of loading doses is necessary to raise the drug's concentration into the therapeutic range. If a loading dose is not given, the steady-state concentration is established in approximately 7 days. The maintenance dosage depends on the patient's ability to excrete the drug (i.e., renal function).

The potential for digitalis toxicity is significant because of a low toxic-to-therapeutic drug concentration ratio. Although many side effects are minor, life-threatening arrhythmias may result. Extracardiac signs of acute digitalis toxicity are often gastrointestinal (e.g., nausea, vomiting, anorexia), thought to be mediated by the action of digoxin on the area postrema of the brain stem. Cardiac toxicity includes several types of arrhythmias (see Table 17.1) that may precede extracardiac warning symptoms. The most frequently encountered rhythm disturbance is the development of ventricular extrasystoles. As described above, various degrees of AV block may occur because of the direct and vagal effects on AV nodal conduction. Digitalis toxicity is also a cause of nonreentrant types of supraventricular tachycardia (i.e., those caused by enhanced automaticity or delayed afterdepolarizations).

Many factors contribute to digitalis intoxication, the most common of which is hypokalemia, often caused by the concurrent administration of diuretics. Hypokalemia exacerbates digitalis toxicity because it further inhibits the Na^+K^+-ATPase pump. Other conditions that promote digitalis toxicity include hypomagnesemia and hypercalcemia. In addition, the concurrent administration of other drugs (e.g., amiodarone) may raise the serum digoxin concentration by altering its clearance or volume of distribution.

The treatment of digitalis-induced tachyarrhythmias includes administration of potassium (if hypokalemia is present) and often intravenous lidocaine (discussed later in the chapter). High-grade AV block may require temporary pacemaker therapy. In patients with severe intoxication, administration of digoxin-specific antibodies may be life saving.

Sympathomimetic Amines

Sympathomimetic amines are inotropic drugs that bind to cardiac $β_1$-receptors. Stimulation of these receptors increases the activity of adenylate cyclase, causing increased formation of cyclic adenosine monophosphate (cAMP; Fig. 17.4). Increased cAMP activates protein

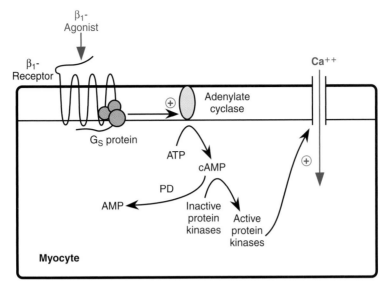

Figure 17.4. Mechanism by which β-adrenergic stimulation increases intracellular Ca++. $β_1$-Receptor stimulation acts through G proteins (guanine nucleotide regulatory proteins) to activate adenylate cyclase. The latter increases cyclic adenosine monophosphate (cAMP) production, which mediates protein kinase phosphorylation of cellular proteins, including ion channels. Phosphorylation of the slow Ca++ channel increases calcium influx. cAMP is degraded by phosphodiesterase (PD).

kinases, which promote intracellular calcium influx by phosphorylating L-type calcium channels. The increased calcium entry triggers a corresponding rise in Ca++ release from the sarcoplasmic reticulum, which enhances the force of contraction. Intravenous dopamine and dobutamine are commonly used sympathomimetic amines in the treatment of acute heart failure. Norepinephrine, epinephrine, and isoproterenol are prescribed in special circumstances, as described in the following paragraphs. Table 17.2 summarizes the receptor actions and major hemodynamic effects of these agents.

Dopamine is an endogenous catecholamine and the precursor of norepinephrine. It possesses an unusual combination of actions that makes it attractive in the treatment of heart failure associated with hypotension and poor renal perfusion. There are various types of receptors with different affinities for dopamine. At *low dosages*, <2 μg/kg/min, dopamine interacts primarily with dopaminergic receptors distributed in the renal and mesenteric vascular beds. Stimulation of these receptors causes local vasodilation and increases renal blood flow and glomerular filtration, facilitating diuresis.

Table 17.2. Sympathomimetic Drug Effects

| Drug | *Receptor Stimulation* | | | |
	D_1 (↑ *Renal Perfusion*)	$α$ (*Vasoconstriction*)	$β_1$ (↑ *Contractility*)	$β_2$ (*Vasodilation*)
Dopamine	+[a]	++++[b]	++++	++
Dobutamine	0	+	++++	+
Norepinephrine	0	++++	++++	0
Epinephrine	0	++++[b]	++++	++
Isoproterenol	0	0	++++	++++

[a] low dose
[b] high dose

Medium dosages of dopamine, 2 to 10 μg/kg/min, increase inotropy by stimulation of cardiac β_1-receptors directly and indirectly by promoting release of norepinephrine from sympathetic nerve terminals. This action increases heart rate, cardiac contractility, and stroke volume, all of which augment cardiac output.

At *high dosages*, >10 μg/kg/min, dopamine also stimulates systemic α-receptors, thereby causing vasoconstriction and elevating systemic resistance. High-dose dopamine is indicated in hypotensive states such as shock. However, these doses are inappropriate in most patients with cardiac failure because the peripheral vasoconstriction increases the resistance against which the heart must contract (i.e., higher afterload), further impairing left ventricular output.

The major toxicity of dopamine arises in patients who are treated with high-dose therapy. The most important side effects are acceleration of the heart rate and tachyarrhythmias.

Dobutamine is a synthetic analog of dopamine that stimulates β_1-, β_2-, and α-receptors. It increases cardiac contractility by virtue of the β_1 effect but does not increase peripheral resistance because of the balance between α-mediated vasoconstriction and β_2-mediated vasodilation. Thus, it is useful in the treatment of heart failure not accompanied by hypotension. Unlike dopamine, dobutamine does not stimulate dopaminergic receptors (i.e., no renal vasodilating effect), nor does it facilitate the release of norepinephrine from peripheral nerve endings. Like dopamine, it is useful for short-term therapy (<1 week), after which time it loses its efficacy, presumably because of downregulation of adrenergic receptors. The major adverse effect is the provocation of tachyarrhythmias.

Norepinephrine is an endogenous catecholamine synthesized from dopamine in adrenergic postganglionic nerves and in adrenal medullary cells (where it is both a final product and the precursor of epinephrine). Through its β_1 activity, norepinephrine has positive inotropic and chronotropic effects. Acting at peripheral α-receptors, it is also a potent vasoconstrictor. The increase in total peripheral resistance causes the mean arterial blood pressure to rise.

With this combination of effects, norepinephrine is useful in patients suffering from "warm shock," in which the combination of cardiac contractile dysfunction and peripheral vasodilation lowers blood pressure. However, the intense vasoconstriction elicited by this drug makes it less attractive than others in treating most other cases of shock. Norepinephrine's side effects include precipitation of myocardial ischemia (because of the augmented force of contraction and increased afterload) and tachyarrhythmias.

Epinephrine, the predominant endogenous catecholamine produced in the adrenal medulla, is formed by the decarboxylation of norepinephrine. As indicated in Table 17.2, epinephrine is an agonist of α-, β_1-, and β_2-receptors. Administered as an intravenous infusion at low dosages, its stimulation of the β_1-receptor increases ventricular contractility and speeds impulse generation. As a result, stroke volume, heart rate, and cardiac output increase. However, at this dosage range, β_2-mediated vasodilation may reduce total peripheral resistance and blood pressure.

At higher dosages, epinephrine is a potent vasopressor because α-mediated constriction dominates over β_2-mediated vasodilation. In this case, the effects of positive inotropy, positive chronotropy, and vasoconstriction act together to raise the arterial blood pressure.

Epinephrine is therefore used most often when the combination of inotropic and chronotropic stimulation is desired, such as in the setting of cardiac arrest. The α-associated vasoconstriction may also help support blood pressure in that setting. The most common toxic effect is the precipitation of tachyarrhythmias. Epinephrine should be avoided in patients receiving β-blocker therapy, because unopposed α-mediated vasoconstriction could produce significant hypertension.

Isoproterenol is a synthetic epinephrine analog. Unlike norepinephrine and epinephrine, it is a "pure" β-agonist, having activity almost exclusively at β_1- and β_2-receptors, with almost no α-receptor effect. In the heart, isoproterenol has positive inotropic and chronotropic effects, thereby increasing cardiac output. In peripheral vessels, stimulation of β_2-receptors results in vasodilation and reduced peripheral resistance, which may cause blood pressure to fall.

Isoproterenol is sometimes used in emergency circumstances to increase the heart rate in patients with bradycardia or heart block (e.g., as a temporizing measure before pacemaker implantation). It may also be useful in patients with systolic dysfunction and slow heart rates with high systemic vascular resistance (a situation sometimes encountered after cardiac surgery in patients who had previously been receiving β-blocker therapy). Isoproterenol should be avoided in patients with myocardial ischemia, in whom the increased heart rate and inotropic stimulation would further increase myocardial oxygen consumption.

Phosphodiesterase-3 Inhibitors

Milrinone is an example of a nondigitalis, noncatecholamine inotropic agent. It exerts its positive inotropic actions by inhibiting phosphodiesterase type 3 in cardiac myocytes (see Fig. 17.4). This inhibition reduces the breakdown of intracellular cAMP, the ultimate result of which is enhanced Ca^{++} entry into the cell and increased force of contraction. Additionally, in vascular smooth muscle, phosphodiesterase-induced augmentation of cAMP results in beneficial vasodilation (in vascular tissue, cAMP inhibits myosin light chain kinase and cross-bridge formation between myosin heads and actin filaments).

Milrinone is sometimes used in the treatment of acute heart failure when there has been insufficient improvement with conventional vasodilators, inotropic agents, and diuretics. It has the potential for serious adverse effects, including provocation of ventricular arrhythmias, and chronic milrinone therapy is associated with *increased* mortality. Its use is therefore limited to hospitalized patients for short-term therapy.

Table 17.3 summarizes the actions and toxicities of commonly used inotropic drugs.

Vasopressin

Vasopressin, the endogenous antidiuretic hormone secreted by the posterior pituitary, primarily functions to maintain water balance (see Chapter 9). It also acts as a potent nonadrenergic vasoconstrictor when administered intravenously at higher-than-natural doses, by directly stimulating vascular smooth muscle V_1 receptors. It has proved useful for maintaining blood pressure in patients with vasodilatory shock, as may occur in septic states. It may also be beneficial during cardiac arrest advanced life support because it increases coronary perfusion pressure, augments blood flow to vital organs, and improves the likelihood of successful resuscitation in patients with ventricular fibrillation.

VASODILATOR DRUGS

Vasodilator drugs play a central role in the treatment of heart failure and hypertension. As described in Chapter 9, the fall in cardiac output in heart failure triggers important compensatory pathways, including the adrenergic nervous system and the renin–angiotensin–aldosterone system (see Fig. 9.9). As a result of activating these pathways, two potent natural vasoconstrictors are released into the circulation: norepinephrine and angiotensin II (AII). These hormones bind to receptors in arterioles and veins, where they cause vascular smooth muscle contraction. Initially, such vasoconstriction is beneficial in heart failure because it maximizes left ventricular preload (increased venous tone enhances venous return) and helps to maintain systemic blood pressure (because of arterial constriction).

However, venous constriction may ultimately cause excessive venous return to the heart, with a rise in the pulmonary capillary hydrostatic pressure and development of pulmonary congestion. In addition, excessive arteriolar constriction increases the resistance against which the left ventricle must contract and therefore ultimately impedes forward cardiac output. Vasodilator therapy is directed at modulating the excessive constriction of veins and arterioles, thus reducing pulmonary

Table 17.3. Commonly Used Inotropic Drugs

Drug	Mechanism of Action	Major Adverse Effects
Cardiac glycosides		
Digoxin	Inhibition of sarcolemmal Na$^+$K$^+$-ATPase Enhanced vagal tone	**Gastrointestinal:** nausea, vomiting **Cardiac:** atrial, nodal, and ventricular tachyarrhythmias; high-degree AV block
Sympathomimetic amines		
Dopamine	Low dosage (<2 μg/kg/min): D$_1$ receptor stimulation results in mesenteric and renal arterial dilatation (facilitates diuresis) Medium dosage (2–10 μg/kg/min): β$_1$-receptor stimulation and release of norepinephrine from sympathetic nerve terminals (inotropic effect) High dosage (>10 μg/kg/min): α-receptor stimulation (peripheral vasoconstriction)	Tachycardia, arrhythmias, hypertension
Dobutamine	β$_1$-, β$_2$-, and α-receptor stimulation	Tachyarrhythmias
Phosphodiesterase inhibitors		
Milrinone	Increased intracellular cAMP due to inhibition of its breakdown by phosphodiesterase	**Gastrointestinal:** nausea, vomiting **Cardiac:** arrhythmias

AV, atrioventricular; cAMP, cyclic adenosine monophosphate; D$_1$, dopamine 1.

congestion and augmenting forward cardiac output (see Fig. 9.10).

Vasodilators are also useful antihypertensive drugs. Recall from Chapter 13 that blood pressure is the product of cardiac output and total peripheral resistance (BP = CO × TPR). Vasodilator drugs decrease arteriolar resistance and therefore lower elevated blood pressure.

Individual vasodilator drug classes act at specific vascular sites (Fig. 17.5). Nitrates, for example, are primarily venodilators, whereas hydralazine is a pure arteriolar dilator. Some drugs, such as the ACE inhibitors, α-blockers, sodium nitroprusside, and nesiritide, are balanced vasodilators that act on both sides of the circulation.

Angiotensin-Converting Enzyme Inhibitors

The renin–angiotensin system plays a critical role in cardiovascular homeostasis. The major effector of this pathway (Fig. 17.6) is AII, which

is formed by the cleavage of angiotensin I by ACE. All the actions of AII known to affect blood pressure control are mediated by its binding to AII receptors of the angiotensin II type 1 (AT$_1$) subtype (see Fig. 13.6). Interaction with this receptor generates a series of intracellular reactions that causes, among other effects, vasoconstriction and the adrenal release of aldosterone, which promotes Na$^+$ reabsorption from the distal nephron. As a result of these actions on vascular tone and sodium homeostasis, AII plays a major role in blood pressure and blood volume regulation. By blocking the formation of AII, ACE inhibitors decrease the systemic arterial pressure, facilitate natriuresis (e.g., by decreasing aldosterone production and reducing Na$^+$ reabsorption from the distal nephron), and reduce adverse ventricular remodeling (see Chapter 9).

Another action of ACE inhibitors, which likely contributes to their hemodynamic

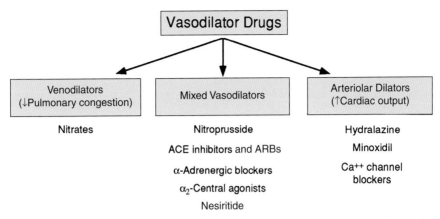

Figure 17.5. **Examples of vasodilator drugs and their sites of action: the venous bed, the arteriolar bed, or both.** ACE, angiotensin-converting enzyme; ARB, angiotensin receptor blocker.

effects, is related to bradykinin (BK) metabolism (Fig. 17.6). The natural vasodilator BK is normally degraded to inactive metabolites by ACE. Because ACE inhibitors impede that degradation, BK accumulates and contributes to the antihypertensive effect, likely by stimulating the endothelial release of nitric oxide and biosynthesis of vasodilating prostaglandins.

Clinical Uses

Hypertension

In hypertensive patients, ACE inhibitors lower blood pressure with little change in cardiac output or heart rate. One might assume that because this class of drug interferes with the renin–angiotensin system, it would be effective only

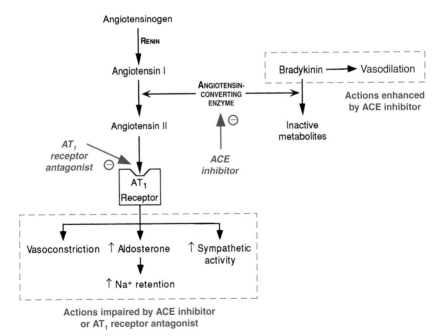

Figure 17.6. **The renin–angiotensin system.** Angiotensin-converting enzyme (ACE) generates angiotensin II, which results in actions that include vasoconstriction, sodium retention, and increased sympathetic activity. ACE inhibitors and angiotensin II type 1 (AT_1) receptor antagonists impair these effects. ACE also promotes the degradation of the natural vasodilator bradykinin; thus, ACE inhibition—but not AT_1 receptor inhibition—results in accumulation of bradykinin and enhanced vasodilation.

in patients with "high-renin" hypertension, but that is not the case. Rather, they are effective in most hypertensive patients, regardless of serum renin levels. The reason for this is not clear but may relate to the additional antihypertensive effects of BK and vasodilatory prostaglandins previously described. In addition, renin–angiotensin activity has been demonstrated within tissues outside the circulation, including the walls of the vasculature, where ACE inhibitors may exert a vasodilatory effect independent of the circulating renin concentration.

ACE inhibitors increase renal blood flow, usually without altering the glomerular filtration rate (GFR), because of dilation of both the afferent and efferent glomerular arterioles. Used alone, ACE inhibitors show similar antihypertensive efficacy as diuretics and β-blockers, but unlike the latter drugs, they do not adversely affect serum glucose or lipid concentrations. ACE inhibitors are often recommended therapy in diabetic hypertensive patients, because the drugs slow the development of diabetic nephropathy (a syndrome of progressive renal deterioration, proteinuria, and hypertension) through favorable effects on intraglomerular pressure.

Heart Failure

In heart failure, ACE inhibitors reduce peripheral vascular resistance (decrease afterload), reduce cardiac filling pressures (decrease preload), and increase cardiac output. The rise in cardiac output usually matches the fall in peripheral resistance such that blood pressure tends not to fall (remember, BP = CO × TPR), except in patients with intravascular volume depletion as might result from overly vigorous diuretic therapy. The augmented cardiac output reduces the drive for compensatory neurohormonal stimulation in CHF (see Chapter 9), such that elevated levels of norepinephrine fall. In addition, clinical trials have shown that ACE inhibitors significantly improve survival in patients with chronic heart failure and following myocardial infarction. Some studies have shown that ACE inhibition also reduces the risk of myocardial infarction and death in patients with chronic vascular disease, including coronary artery disease (CAD), even if left ventricular function is not impaired.

Table 17.4. Drugs That Interfere with the Renin–Angiotensin System

Drug	Major Elimination Pathway
ACE inhibitors	
Benazepril	Renal
Captopril	Renal
Enalapril	Renal
Fosinopril	Hepatic/renal
Lisinopril	Renal
Moexipril	Hepatic/renal
Perindopril	Renal
Quinapril	Renal
Ramipril	Renal
Trandolapril	Hepatic/renal
Angiotensin II receptor antagonists	
Candesartan	Hepatic/renal
Eprosartan	Hepatic/renal
Irbesartan	Hepatic/renal
Losartan	Hepatic/renal
Olmesartan	Hepatic/renal
Telmisartan	Hepatic
Valsartan	Hepatic/renal

The available ACE inhibitors are listed in Table 17.4. The primary excretory pathway of most of these agents is through the kidney, so their dosages should generally be reduced in patients with renal dysfunction.

Adverse Effects

Hypotension

This is a rare side effect when ACE inhibitors are used to treat hypertension. It is more likely to occur in heart failure patients in whom intravascular volume depletion has resulted from vigorous diuretic use. Such patients have significant activation of the renin–angiotensin system; therefore, blood pressure is largely maintained by the vasoconstricting actions of circulating AII. The administration of an ACE inhibitor in that setting may result in hypotension because of the sudden reduction of AII levels. This side effect is avoided by temporarily reducing the diuretic regimen and starting the ACE inhibitor at a low dosage.

Hyperkalemia

Because ACE inhibitors indirectly reduce the serum aldosterone concentration, the serum potassium concentration may rise, but only rarely into the clinically important hyperkalemic range. Conditions that can further increase serum potassium levels and *may* result in dangerous hyperkalemia during ACE inhibitor use include renal insufficiency, diabetes (owing to hyporeninemic hypoaldosteronism, a condition often present in elderly diabetics), and concomitant use of potassium-sparing diuretics.

Renal Insufficiency

Administration of an ACE inhibitor to patients with intravascular volume depletion may result in hypotension, decreased renal perfusion, and azotemia. Correction of volume depletion, or reduction of the ACE inhibitor dosage, usually corrects this complication.

ACE inhibitor therapy can also precipitate renal failure in patients with *bilateral renal artery stenosis* because such patients rely on high efferent glomerular arteriolar resistance (which is highly dependent on AII) to maintain intraglomerular pressure and filtration. Administering an ACE inhibitor abruptly decreases efferent arteriolar tone and glomerular hydrostatic pressure and may therefore worsen GFR in this setting.

Cough

Irritation of the upper airways resulting in a dry cough is reported in up to 20% of patients receiving ACE inhibitor therapy. Its mechanism has not been established but may relate to the increased BK concentration provoked by ACE inhibitors. This side effect may last weeks after the drug is discontinued.

Other Effects

Very rare adverse reactions to ACE inhibitors include angioedema and agranulocytosis. ACE inhibitors should not be used in pregnancy because they have been shown to cause fetal injury.

Angiotensin II Type 1 Receptor Antagonists

AT_1 receptor antagonists, also termed angiotensin receptor blockers (ARBs), are a second group of drugs that interfere with the renin–angiotensin system. There are at least two distinct types of AII receptors: AT_1 and AT_2. All the actions of AII known to affect blood pressure control (e.g., vasoconstriction, aldosterone release, renal Na^+ reabsorption, and sympathetic nervous system stimulation) are mediated by its binding to receptors of the AT_1 subtype. The AT_2 receptor subtype is abundant during fetal development and has been located in some adult tissues, but its precise actions are unknown.

ARBs compete with AII for AT_1 receptors and therefore inhibit AII-mediated effects (see Fig. 17.6), thus lowering the blood pressure of hypertensive patients. ARBs provide a more substantial blockade of the renin–angiotensin system than ACE inhibitors, because the latter do not completely block formation of AII (some AI is converted to AII by circulating enzymes other than ACE). Unlike ACE inhibitors, the AT_1 receptor antagonists do not affect serum BK levels.

The available ARBs are listed in Table 17.4. Each of these is excreted primarily in the bile but most are also partly excreted in the urine. Trials have demonstrated that ARBs are as effective as ACE inhibitors in treating hypertension, and they are among the best tolerated antihypertensive drugs. As with ACE inhibitors, the blood pressure–lowering effect of ARBs is enhanced by concurrent use of a thiazide diuretic. Also like ACE inhibitors, ARBs have the potential side effects of hypotension and hyperkalemia (owing to reduced aldosterone levels). Unlike ACE inhibitors, ARBs typically do not cause cough.

In the setting of moderate to severe heart failure, ARBs display hemodynamic benefits similar to those of ACE inhibitors (see Chapter 9). Thus, ARBs are generally recommended in heart failure for patients who are intolerant of ACE inhibitors (e.g., because of ACE inhibitor–induced cough). Studies in patients with type 2 diabetes have demonstrated that ARBs slow the progression of kidney disease, an effect that also has been demonstrated with ACE inhibitors.

Table 17.5. Direct Vasodilators

Drug	Clinical Use	Route of Administration	Major Adverse Effects
Hydralazine	• Hypertension (chronic and acute therapy) • CHF	Oral, intravenous bolus, intramuscular	• Hypotension, tachycardia • Headache, flushing • Angina • Drug-induced lupus
Minoxidil	• Chronic therapy of hypertension	Oral	• Reflex tachycardia • Na^+ retention • Hypertrichosis
Nitroprusside	• Hypertensive emergencies • Acute CHF	Intravenous infusion	• Hypotension • Cyanide and thiocyanate toxicity
Fenoldopam	• Hypertensive emergencies	Intravenous infusion	• Hypotension • Increased intraocular pressure

CHF, congestive heart failure.

In addition to ACE inhibitors and ARBs, other antagonists of the renin–angiotensin system in the treatment of hypertension include the direct renin inhibitor aliskiren (see Chapter 13) and aldosterone receptor antagonists (described later in this chapter).

Direct-Acting Vasodilators

Hydralazine, minoxidil, sodium nitroprusside, and fenoldopam are examples of direct-acting vasodilators (Table 17.5). Hydralazine and minoxidil are used primarily as long-term oral vasodilators, whereas nitroprusside and fenoldopam are administered intravenously in more acute settings.

Hydralazine is a potent and direct arteriolar dilator that acts at the level of the precapillary arterioles and has no effect on systemic veins. The cellular mechanism of its effect is unknown. The fall in blood pressure following arteriolar dilation results in a baroreceptor-mediated increase in sympathetic outflow and cardiac stimulation (e.g., reflex tachycardia), which could precipitate myocardial ischemia in patients with underlying CAD. Therefore, hydralazine is often combined with a β-blocker to blunt this undesired response.

As newer drugs have emerged, hydralazine is now used only occasionally as an antihypertensive, often in combination with other drugs.

It is sometimes prescribed concurrently with the venodilator isosorbide dinitrate to treat heart failure in patients with systolic dysfunction. This combination improves symptoms in patients with mild-to-moderate heart failure and has been shown to reduce morbidity and mortality rates (see Chapter 9).

Hydralazine possesses low bioavailability because of extensive first-pass hepatic metabolism. However, such metabolism depends on whether the patient displays fast or slow hepatic acetylation; on average, 50% of Americans are fast and 50% are slow acetylators. Slow acetylators show less hepatic degradation, higher bioavailability, and increased antihypertensive effects, whereas fast acetylators demonstrate the opposite responses. Hydralazine has a short half-life (2 to 4 hours) in the circulation, but its effect persists as long as 12 hours because the drug binds avidly to vascular tissues.

The most common side effects of hydralazine include headache (increased cerebral vasodilation), palpitations (reflex tachycardia), flushing (increased systemic vasodilation), nausea, and anorexia. In addition, a syndrome similar to systemic lupus (characterized by arthralgias, myalgia, skin rashes, and fever) may develop, especially in patients who are slow acetylators.

Minoxidil also results in arteriolar vasodilation without significant venodilation. Its mechanism of action involves an increase in potassium channel permeability, which results in smooth muscle cell hyperpolarization and relaxation. Like other agents that selectively cause arteriolar dilation, reflex adrenergic stimulation leads to increased heart rate and contractility, an undesired effect that can be blunted by coadministration of a β-blocker. In addition, decreased renal perfusion often results in fluid retention, so that a diuretic usually must be administered concurrently.

Minoxidil's primary clinical indication is in the treatment of severe or intractable hypertension. It is especially useful in patients with renal failure who are often refractory to other antihypertensive regimens. It is well absorbed from the gastrointestinal tract and is metabolized primarily by hepatic glucuronidation, but approximately one fifth is excreted unchanged by the kidney. Although it has a short half-life, its pharmacologic effects persist even after serum drug concentration falls, probably because, like hydralazine, the drug binds avidly to vascular tissues.

Side effects of minoxidil, in addition to reflex sympathetic stimulation and fluid retention, include hypertrichosis (excessive hair growth) and occasional pericardial effusion (unknown mechanism).

Sodium nitroprusside, a potent dilator of *both* arterioles and veins, is administered intravenously to treat hypertensive emergencies and, in intensive care settings, for blood pressure control. It is also prescribed for preload and afterload modulation in severe CHF. Sodium nitroprusside is a complex of iron, cyanide groups, and a nitroso moiety, and its metabolism by red blood cells results in the liberation of nitric oxide (Fig. 17.7). Nitric oxide causes vasodilation through activation of guanylate cyclase in vascular smooth muscle (as described later in this chapter; see also Chapter 6).

Sodium nitroprusside's hemodynamic effects result from its ability to decrease arterial resistance and to increase venous capacitance. In patients with normal left ventricular function, it can actually decrease cardiac output because of the reduction in venous return (see Fig. 9.10). However, in a patient with impaired left ventricular contractile function, the decreased systemic resistance induced by sodium nitroprusside (i.e., decreased afterload) augments forward cardiac output, while venous dilation reduces return of blood to the heart. The latter decreases pulmonary capillary hydrostatic pressure and improves symptoms of pulmonary congestion.

Sodium nitroprusside is often the treatment of choice for hypertensive emergencies because of its great potency and rapid action. A β-blocker is often administered concurrently to counteract the reflex increase in sympathetic outflow that may occur with this drug.

Sodium nitroprusside is administered by continuous intravenous infusion. Its onset of action begins within 30 seconds, and its peak effect is achieved in 2 minutes. Its effectiveness dissipates within minutes of its discontinuation. After sodium nitroprusside is metabolized into nitric oxide and cyanide, the liver, in the presence of a sulfhydryl donor, transforms cyanide into thiocyanate; the thiocyanate, in turn, is excreted by the kidney. *Thiocyanate accumulation and toxicity*, manifested by blurred vision, tinnitus, disorientation, and/or nausea, may occur with continued use, especially in the setting of renal impairment. Thus, it is important

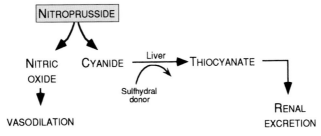

Figure 17.7. Sodium nitroprusside is a complex of iron, cyanide (CN), and a nitroso group. Erythrocyte metabolism liberates CN and the active vasodilator nitric oxide. The CN is metabolized in the liver to thiocyanate, which is eliminated by the kidneys.

to monitor serum levels of thiocyanate if sodium nitroprusside is administered for more than 24 hours. In addition, excessive infusion rates of sodium nitroprusside, or a deficiency in hepatic thiosulfate stores, can result in lethal *cyanide toxicity*, the early signs of which include metabolic acidosis, headache, and nausea, followed by loss of consciousness.

Fenoldopam is a rapidly acting potent arteriolar vasodilator administered intravenously to treat severe hypertension. It is a selective agonist of peripheral dopamine 1 (D_1) receptors, the activation of which results in arteriolar vasodilation through a cAMP-dependent mechanism. Unlike other intravenous antihypertensive agents, it beneficially maintains or enhances renal perfusion, and its activation of renal tubular D_1 receptors facilitates natriuresis. Unlike dopamine, fenoldopam does not stimulate α- or β-adrenergic receptors.

Fenoldopam is administered by continuous intravenous infusion. Its onset of action is rapid, achieving 50% of maximal effect within 15 minutes and steady state in 30 to 60 minutes. It is metabolized by the liver to inactive substances that are excreted through the kidney. It has a rapid offset of action after discontinuation (an elimination half-life of <10 minutes), which is a desirable effect that minimizes the risk of excessive blood pressure reduction during the treatment of hypertensive emergencies. These pharmacologic properties also make fenoldopam useful for controlling hypertension in the postoperative setting. However, nitroprusside works even faster and remains more popular for this purpose. Unlike nitroprusside, fenoldopam does not cause thiocyanate toxicity. The most common side effects are headache, dizziness, and tachycardia. Fenoldopam also increases intraocular pressure (probably by slowing aqueous humor drainage) and should therefore be avoided in patients with glaucoma.

Calcium Channel Blockers

The CCBs are discussed here as a group, but differences exist among the drugs of this class. The common property of CCBs is their ability to impede the influx of Ca^{++} through membrane channels in cardiac and smooth muscle cells. Two principal types of voltage-gated

Ca^{++} channels have been identified in cardiac tissue, termed L and T. The L-type channel is responsible for the Ca^{++} entry that maintains phase 2 of the action potential (the "plateau" in Fig. 1.14). The T-type Ca^{++} channel likely plays a role in the initial depolarization of nodal tissues. It is the L-type channel that is antagonized by currently available CCBs.

Mechanisms of Action

The cellular mechanism of CCBs has been partly delineated. Increased concentrations of intracellular Ca^{++} lead to augmented contractile force in both myocardium and vascular smooth muscle. At both sites, the net effect of Ca^{++} channel blockade is to decrease the amount of Ca^{++} available to the contractile proteins within these cells, which translates into vasodilation of vascular smooth muscle and a negative inotropic effect in cardiac muscle.

Vascular Smooth Muscle

Contraction of vascular smooth muscle depends on the cytoplasmic Ca^{++} concentration, which is regulated by the transmembrane flow of Ca^{++} through voltage-gated channels during depolarization. Intracellular Ca^{++} interacts with calmodulin to form a Ca^{++}–calmodulin complex. This complex stimulates myosin light chain kinase, which phosphorylates myosin light chains and leads to cross-bridge formation between myosin heads and actin, causing smooth muscle contraction. CCBs promote relaxation of vascular smooth muscle by inhibiting Ca^{++} entry through the voltage-gated channels. Other organs possessing smooth muscle (including gastrointestinal, uterine, and bronchiolar tissues) are also susceptible to this relaxing effect.

Cardiac Cells

As described in Chapter 1, cardiac muscle also depends on Ca^{++} influx during depolarization for contractile protein interactions, but by a different mechanism than that in vascular smooth muscle. Ca^{++} entry into the cardiac cell during depolarization triggers additional intracellular Ca^{++} release from the sarcoplasmic reticulum, leading to contraction. By

Table 17.6. Calcium Channel Blockers

Drug	Vasodilation	Negative Inotropic Effect	Suppress AV Node Conduction	Major Adverse Effects
Verapamil	+	+++	+++	• Hypotension • Bradycardia, AV block • Constipation
Diltiazem	++	++	++	• Hypotension • Peripheral edema • Bradycardia

Dihydropyridines
  Amlodipine
  Felodipine
  Isradipine
  Nicardipine
  Nifedipine
  Nisoldipine
	+++	0 to +	0	• Hypotension
				• Headache, flushing
				• Peripheral edema

AV, atrioventricular

blocking Ca^{++} entry, CCBs interfere with excitation–contraction coupling and decrease the force of contraction. Because the pacemaker tissues of the heart (e.g., sinoatrial [SA] and AV node) are the most dependent on the inward Ca^{++} current for depolarization, one would expect that CCBs would reduce the rate of sinus firing and AV nodal conduction. Some, but not all, CCBs have this property (Table 17.6). The effect on cardiac conduction appears to depend not only on whether the specific CCB reduces the inward Ca^{++} current, but also on whether it delays recovery of the Ca^{++} channel to its preactivated state. **Verapamil** and **diltiazem** have this property,

whereas **nifedipine** and the other dihydropyridine CCBs do not.

Clinical Uses

As a result of their actions on vascular smooth muscle and cardiac cells, CCBs are useful in several cardiovascular disorders through the mechanisms summarized in Table 17.7. In angina pectoris, they exert beneficial effects by reducing myocardial oxygen consumption as well as by potentially increasing oxygen supply through coronary dilatation. The latter effect is also useful in the management of coronary artery vasospasm.

Table 17.7. Clinical Effects of Calcium Channel Blockers

Condition	Mechanism

Angina pectoris	↓ Myocardial oxygen consumption
	  ↓ Blood pressure (↓ afterload)
	  ↓ Contractility
	  ↓ Heart rate (verapamil and diltiazem)
	
	↑ Myocardial oxygen supply
	  ↑ Coronary dilatation

Coronary artery spasm	Coronary artery vasodilation
Hypertension	Arteriolar smooth muscle relaxation
Supraventricular arrhythmias	(Verapamil and diltiazem): decrease conduction velocity and increase refractoriness of atrioventricular node

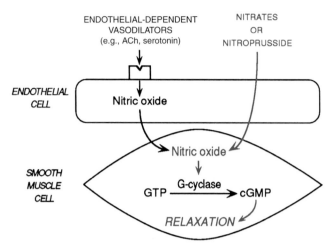

Figure 17.8. Organic nitrates incite vascular smooth muscle (SM) relaxation by conversion to nitric oxide (NO) at or near the cell membrane. Nitroprusside and endothelial-dependent vasodilators also promote NO delivery to vascular smooth muscle and cause relaxation. In the SM, NO stimulates formation of cyclic guanosine monophosphate (cGMP), which mediates relaxation.

CCBs are often used to treat hypertension. More so than β-blockers or ACE inhibitors, CCBs are particularly effective in elderly patients. Nifedipine and the other dihydropyridines are the most potent vasodilators of this class.

CCBs are usually administered orally, and once-a-day formulations are available for these agents. Routes of excretion vary. For example, nifedipine and verapamil are eliminated primarily in the urine, whereas diltiazem is excreted through the liver. Common side effects (see Table 17.6) include hypotension (owing to excessive vasodilation) and ankle edema (caused by local vasodilation of peripheral vascular beds). Since verapamil and diltiazem may result in bradyarrhythmias, they should be used with caution in patients already receiving β-blocker therapy.

The safety of *short-acting* CCBs has been called into question. In several observational studies, a higher incidence of myocardial infarction or death has been reported in patients with hypertension or coronary disease taking such agents. In contrast, these adverse outcomes have not been demonstrated with long-acting CCBs (i.e., formulations meant for once-a-day ingestion). Thus, the long-acting versions should generally be prescribed for extended use. Also, recall from Chapter 6 that β-blockers and/or nitrates are preferred over CCBs for initial therapy in patients with CAD.

Organic Nitrates

The nitrates constitute one of the oldest treatments of angina pectoris. They are also used in acute ischemic syndromes and in heart failure. The main physiologic action of the nitrates is vasodilation, particularly of the systemic veins.

Mechanism of Action

Nitrates produce vascular smooth muscle relaxation. The proposed mechanism involves the conversion of the administered drug to nitric oxide at or near the plasma membrane of vascular smooth muscle cells (Fig. 17.8). Nitric oxide, in turn, activates guanylate cyclase to produce cyclic guanosine monophosphate (cGMP), and the intracellular accumulation of cGMP leads to smooth muscle relaxation. This mechanism of vascular smooth muscle relaxation is similar to that associated with nitroprusside and endogenous endothelial-derived nitric oxide.

Hemodynamic Effects and Clinical Uses

At low doses, nitroglycerin, the prototypical organic nitrate, produces greater dilation of veins than of arterioles. The venodilation results in venous pooling, diminished venous return, and hence decreased right and left ventricular filling. Systemic arterial resistance is generally unaffected, but cardiac output may fall because of the diminished preload, especially in patients with intravascular volume depletion (see Fig. 9.10). *Arterial* dilation occurs to some extent in the coronary arteries and may also occur in the facial vessels and the meningeal arterioles, giving rise to the side effects of flushing and headache, respectively.

At *high* doses, nitrates can result in widespread arteriolar dilation, which may result in systemic hypotension and reflex tachycardia. However, the increase in heart rate is not typically manifest in patients with heart failure, because decreasing afterload in that situation may actually improve cardiac output and reduce the sympathetic drive.

The major use of nitrates is in the treatment of angina pectoris through venodilation leading to reduced left ventricular preload. The smaller left ventricular size lowers ventricular wall stress and myocardial oxygen consumption, which alleviates the oxygen imbalance in ischemic states. Nitrates are also useful in patients with coronary artery spasm (Prinzmetal variant angina) by dilating the coronary arterioles.

Agents and Pharmacokinetics

Many formulations of nitrates are available. When the relief of acute angina is the objective, rapid onset of action is essential. However, in the long-term prevention of anginal attacks in a patient with chronic CAD, duration of action and predictability of effect are more crucial than the speed of drug effect.

Sublingual **nitroglycerin tablets** or **sprays** are used in the treatment of acute angina attacks. The peak action of these agents occurs within 3 minutes, because they are rapidly absorbed into the bloodstream via the oral mucosa; their effect, however, diminishes rapidly, falling off within 15 to 30 minutes, as the drug is deactivated in the liver. These forms of nitroglycerin are also effective when taken prophylactically, immediately before situations known by the patient to produce angina (e.g., before walking up a hill).

Long-acting nitrates are used to prevent chest discomfort in the chronic management of CAD and must be given in sufficient dosage to saturate the liver's deactivating capacity. For this purpose, oral doses of **sustained-release nitroglycerin, isosorbide dinitrate,** or **isosorbide mononitrate** are used. These agents have a duration of action of 2 to 14 hours. **Transdermal nitroglycerin patches** or **nitroglycerin paste** applied to the skin also deliver a sustained release of nitroglycerin. Of note, the efficacy of long-acting nitrate therapy is attenuated by the rapid development of drug tolerance with continuous use. For this reason, it is important that the dosing regimens allow a drug-free interval of several hours each day to maintain efficacy.

Intravenous nitroglycerin is administered by continuous infusion. This form is most useful in the treatment of hospitalized patients with unstable angina or acute heart failure.

Adverse Effects

The most common adverse effects of the nitrates include hypotension, reflex tachycardia, headache, and flushing.

Natriuretic Peptides

As described in Chapter 9, natriuretic peptides are secreted from atrial and ventricular myocardium in patients with heart failure. Among their beneficial physiologic effects, these peptides promote vasodilation and result in sodium and water excretion. The pharmacologic agent **nesiritide** (human recombinant B-type natriuretic peptide) replicates these effects and is available for intravenous administration to hospitalized patients with decompensated heart failure. It results in vasodilation, augmented cardiac output, and reduction of the undesired activation of the renin–angiotensin and sympathetic nervous systems that are typical in heart failure. In some patients, it promotes diuresis.

Nesiritide binds to G protein–coupled receptors in multiple tissues, including the blood vessels (resulting in vasodilation), kidneys, and adrenals. In the kidney, natriuresis is a consequence of several effects of the drug. An augmented GFR results from dilation of the afferent renal arterioles and constriction of the efferent renal arterioles, thereby increasing the filtered load of sodium. In the proximal tubule, AII-mediated sodium uptake is inhibited. Because the proximal tubule is where the vast majority of sodium is reabsorbed (as described later in the chapter), this interruption in uptake results in sodium excretion. In the distal tubule, natriuretic peptides appear to further reduce sodium reabsorption through epithelial sodium channels. In the adrenal zona glomerulosa, the drug inhibits aldosterone synthesis, which leads to enhanced sodium excretion in the distal nephron.

Despite these benefits, the clinical role of nesiritide is still being defined, because its use has not been shown to improve survival in heart failure patients and in one study was actually associated with increased mortality.

Phosphodiesterase-5 Inhibitor— Sildenafil

Sildenafil, a phosphodiesterase type 5 inhibitor used to treat erectile dysfunction, has been shown to decrease pulmonary vascular resistance in patients with primary pulmonary hypertension (PPH). It inhibits the breakdown of cGMP in the pulmonary vasculature, which enhances vasodilation and oxygenation. Other phosphodiesterase inhibitors have not been shown to be effective in PPH. When combined with nitrates, sildenafil can cause severe hypotension; therefore, these groups of drugs should not be prescribed concurrently.

ANTIADRENERGIC DRUGS

Drugs that interfere with the sympathetic nervous system act at various sites, including the central nervous system (CNS), postganglionic sympathetic nerve endings, and peripheral α- and β-receptors (Fig. 17.9).

Normally, when a sympathetic nerve is stimulated, norepinephrine is released, which traverses the synapse and stimulates postsynaptic α- and β-receptors. Norepinephrine within the synapse can also bind to *presynaptic* β- and α_2-receptors, providing a feedback mechanism that modulates further release of the hormone. The β-receptor increases, and the α_2-receptor inhibits further, norepinephrine release.

The consequences of receptor stimulation depend on the organ involved (Table 17.8). The effect of α_1-receptor stimulation on vascular smooth muscle is vasoconstriction, whereas β_2 stimulation causes vasodilation. In the CNS, α_2 stimulation *inhibits* sympathetic outflow to the periphery, thereby contributing to vasodilation.

Central Adrenergic Inhibitors (CNS α_2-Agonists)

α_2-Receptors are located in the presynaptic neurons of the CNS. When stimulated by an α_2-agonist, they lead to *diminished* sympathetic outflow from the medulla. This action reduces peripheral vascular resistance and decreases cardiac stimulation, resulting in a fall in blood pressure and heart rate. CNS α_2-agonists were once among the most commonly used antihypertensive drugs but have largely given way to better tolerated agents. They are not sufficiently potent to serve as vasodilators in the treatment of heart failure.

The drugs in this group are listed in Figure 17.9. They are all available as oral preparations, and clonidine can also be prescribed as a skin patch that is applied and left in place for 1 week at a time, facilitating drug compliance. Side effects of CNS α_2-agonists include sedation, dry mouth, bradycardia, and, if the drug is stopped suddenly, the possibility of a sudden, paradoxical rise in blood pressure.

Sympathetic Nerve-Ending Antagonists

Reserpine was the first drug found to interfere with the sympathetic nervous system. It inhibits the uptake of norepinephrine into storage vesicles in postganglionic and central neurons, leading to norepinephrine degradation. The antihypertensive effect results from the depletion of catecholamines, which causes the force of myocardial contraction and total peripheral resistance to decrease.

Reserpine's CNS toxicity represents its chief drawback. It often produces sedation and can impair concentration. The most serious potential toxicity is psychotic depression. Newer, better tolerated antihypertensive agents have largely supplanted the use of reserpine and other sympathetic nerve-ending antagonists.

Peripheral α-Adrenergic Receptor Antagonists

Peripheral α-antagonists (Table 17.9) are divided into those that act on both α_1- and α_2-receptors,

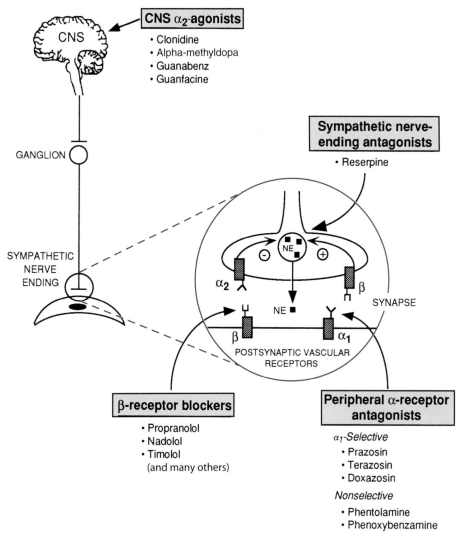

CNS α₂-agonists
- Clonidine
- Alpha-methyldopa
- Guanabenz
- Guanfacine

CNS

GANGLION

SYMPATHETIC
NERVE
ENDING

Sympathetic nerve-ending antagonists
- Reserpine

α_2

β

NE

SYNAPSE

NE

β

α_1

POSTSYNAPTIC VASCULAR
RECEPTORS

β-receptor blockers
- Propranolol
- Nadolol
- Timolol
(and many others)

Peripheral α-receptor antagonists

α_1-Selective
- Prazosin
- Terazosin
- Doxazosin

Nonselective
- Phentolamine
- Phenoxybenzamine

Figure 17.9. Sites of action of the antiadrenergic drugs. Note that receptors at the sympathetic nerve-ending bind norepinephrine (NE) and provide feedback: the β-receptor stimulates, and the α_2-receptor inhibits, further NE release. CNS, central nervous system.

and those that inhibit α_1 alone. α_1-Selective receptor antagonists (**prazosin, terazosin, doxazosin**) are occasionally prescribed in the treatment of hypertension. Their selectivity for the α_1-receptor explains their ability to produce less reflex tachycardia than nonselective agents. Normally, drug-induced vasodilation results in baroreceptor-mediated stimulation of the sympathetic nervous system and an undesired increase in heart rate. This effect is amplified by drugs that block the presynaptic α_2-receptor, because feedback inhibition of norepinephrine release is prevented. However, α_1-selective agents do not block the negative feedback on the α_2-receptor.

Thus, further norepinephrine release and reflex sympathetic side effects are blunted.

Historically, the principal indication for α_1-antagonists has been in the treatment of hypertension. However, in a large prospective, randomized trial, patients treated with the α_1-antagonist doxazosin experienced more adverse cardiac outcomes than those treated with a thiazide diuretic. Thus, α_1-antagonists have fallen out of favor in the management of hypertension. Terazosin and doxazosin are mainly used today to treat the symptoms of benign prostatic hyperplasia, because the drugs also beneficially relax prostatic smooth muscle tone.

Table 17.8. Responses to Adrenergic Receptor Stimulation

Receptor Type	Distribution	Response
α_1	Vascular smooth muscle (arterioles and veins)	Vasoconstriction
α_2	Presynaptic adrenergic nerve terminals	Inhibition of NE release
	Vascular smooth muscle (coronary and renal arterioles)	Vasoconstriction
β_1	Heart	Increases heart rate
		Increases contractility
		Speeds AV node conduction
	Kidney (JG cells)	Increases renin release
	Presynaptic adrenergic nerve terminals	Increases NE release
	Adipose tissue	Stimulates lipolysis
β_2	Vascular smooth muscle (arterioles, except skin and cerebral)	Vasodilation
	Bronchial smooth muscle	Bronchodilation
	Liver	Stimulates glycogenolysis

AV, atrioventricular; NE, norepinephrine.

Table 17.9. α-Receptor Antagonists

Mechanism/Drug	Indications	Major Adverse Effects
Selective peripheral α_1-blockade		
Prazosin	• Hypertension	• Postural hypotension
Terazosin	• Benign prostatic hyperplasia	• Headache, dizziness
Doxazosin		
Nonselective α-blockade		
Phentolamine	• Pheochromocytoma	• Postural hypotension
Phenoxybenzamine		• Reflex tachycardia
		• Arrhythmias

Phentolamine and **phenoxybenzamine** are nonselective α-blockers. They are used in the treatment of pheochromocytoma, a tumor that abnormally secretes catecholamines into the circulation (see Chapter 13). Otherwise, these drugs are rarely used because the α_2-blockade impairs the normal feedback inhibition of norepinephrine release, an undesired effect, as indicated earlier.

β-Adrenergic Receptor Antagonists

The β-adrenergic antagonists are used for a number of cardiovascular conditions, including ischemic heart disease, hypertension, heart failure, and tachyarrhythmias.

Because catecholamines increase inotropy, chronotropy, and conduction velocity in the heart, it follows that β-receptor antagonists decrease inotropy, slow the heart rate, and decrease conduction velocity. When stimulation of the β-receptors is low, as in a normal resting person, the effect of blocking agents is likewise mild. However, when the sympathetic nervous system is activated (e.g., during exercise), these antagonists can substantially diminish catecholamine-mediated effects.

The β-blockers can be distinguished from one another by specific properties (Table 17.10): (1) the relative affinity of the drug for β_1- and β_2-receptors, (2) whether partial β-*agonist* activity is present, (3) whether the drug also has vasodilator properties (e.g., via α_1-receptor blockade), and (4) differences in pharmacokinetic properties. The goal of β_1-*selective* agents is to achieve myocardial receptor blockade, with less effect on

Table 17.10. β-Adrenergic Blockers

Activity	Nonselective β-Blockers	β₁-Selective β-Blockers
No β-agonist activity	Carvedilol[a]	Atenolol
	Labetalol[a]	Betaxolol
	Propranolol	Bisoprolol
	Nadolol	Esmolol[b]
	Timolol	Metoprolol
		Nebivolol[c]
β-Agonist activity	Carteolol	Acebutolol
	Penbutolol	
	Pindolol	

[a]Also has α_1-adrenergic–blocking properties.

[b]Administered intravenously only.

[c]Also has vasodilating properties, likely mediated by nitric oxide.

bronchial and vascular smooth muscle (tissues that exhibit β_2-receptors), thus producing less bronchospasm and vasoconstriction in susceptible patients. Agents with partial β-agonist effects (also termed *intrinsic sympathomimetic activity*) tend to slow the heart rate less than other β-blockers.

During short-term use, nonselective β-antagonists tend to reduce cardiac output because they decrease heart rate and contractility as well as slightly increase peripheral resistance (via β_2-receptor blockade). β-Antagonists that have partial agonist activity (such as pindolol) or those that possess some α-blocking activity (such as labetalol) can actually lower peripheral resistance by interacting with their respective β_2- and α-receptors.

Clinical Uses

Ischemic Heart Disease

The beneficial effects of β-blockers in ischemic heart disease are related to their ability to decrease myocardial oxygen demand. They reduce the heart rate, blood pressure (afterload), and contractility. The negative inotropic effect is directly related to blockade of the cardiac β-receptor, which results in decreased calcium influx into the myocyte (see Fig. 17.4). β-Blockers also improve survival following acute myocardial infarction. Agents with intrinsic sympathomimetic activity are less beneficial in this regard than β-blockers without it.

Hypertension

β-Blockers are effective antihypertensive agents. Despite their widespread use in this capacity, the mechanisms responsible for blood pressure lowering are not completely understood. With initial use, the antihypertensive action is thought to result from a decrease in cardiac output, in association with slowing of the heart rate and mild decrease in contractility. However, with chronic administration, other mechanisms are likely at work, including reduced renal secretion of renin and possibly CNS effects.

Heart Failure

The negative inotropic effect of β-blockade would be expected to worsen heart failure symptoms in patients with underlying left ventricular systolic dysfunction. However, trials in patients with all classes of clinically stable heart failure have actually shown a survival *benefit* with chronic β-blocker administration using carvedilol, metoprolol, or bisoprolol (see Chapter 9). The mechanism may relate to blunting of the cardiotoxic effects of excessive circulating catecholamines. Because of the potential risk of transiently *worsening* heart failure in tenuous patients, β-blocker therapy should be started at low dosage, augmented slowly, and carefully monitored.

Other conditions that benefit from β-blocker therapy include tachyarrhythmias (as discussed later in the chapter) and hypertrophic cardio-myopathy (see Chapter 10).

Adverse Effects

Fatigue may occur during β-blocker therapy and is most likely a CNS side effect. β-Blockers with less lipid solubility (e.g., nadolol) do not penetrate the blood–brain barrier and may have fewer CNS adverse effects than more lipid-soluble drugs, such as propranolol. Other potential adverse effects relate to the predictable consequences of β-blockade:

1. $β_2$-Blockade associated with use of nonselective agents (or large doses of $β_1$-selective blockers) can exacerbate *bronchospasm*, worsening preexisting asthma or chronic obstructive lung disease.
2. The impairment of AV nodal conduction by $β_1$-blockade can cause conduction blocks.
3. $β_2$-Blockade can precipitate arterial *vasospasm*, which can result in Raynaud phenomenon or worsen symptoms of peripheral vascular disease.
4. Abrupt withdrawal of a β-antagonist after chronic use could precipitate myocardial ischemia in patients with CAD.
5. Undesirable reduction of high-density lipoprotein (HDL) cholesterol and elevation of triglycerides can occur through an unknown mechanism. This effect appears to be less pronounced with β-blockers that have partial β-agonist activity or combined β- and α-blocking properties.
6. $β_2$-Blockade may impair recovery from hypoglycemia in diabetics suffering an insulin reaction. In addition, β-blockers may mask the sympathetic warning signs of hypoglycemia, such as tachycardia. If β-blockers are used in diabetics, $β_1$-selective agents are generally preferred.

Other potential side effects include insomnia, depression, and impotence. Finally, β-antagonists should be used with caution in combination with nondihydropyridine CCBs (verapamil or diltiazem), because both types of drugs can impair myocardial contractility and AV nodal conduction, possibly precipitating heart failure or AV conduction blocks.

ANTIARRHYTHMIC DRUGS

Drug therapy is a common approach to treat cardiac tachyarrhythmias. However, antiarrhythmic drugs are among the most dangerous pharmacologic agents because of potential serious adverse effects. Therefore, a thorough understanding of their mechanisms of action, indications, and toxicities is of particular importance.

Although a number of classification systems for these agents exist, antiarrhythmic drugs are commonly separated into four groups based on their primary electrophysiologic mechanisms of action (Table 17.11):

1. *Class I* drugs block the fast sodium channel responsible for phase 0 depolarization of the action potential. They are further divided into three subtypes based on the degree of sodium channel blockade and the effect of the drug on the cell's action potential duration.
2. *Class II* drugs are β-adrenergic receptor antagonists (β-blockers).
3. *Class III* drugs block potassium channels responsible for repolarization, thereby prolonging the action potential with little effect on the rise of phase 0 depolarization.
4. *Class IV* drugs block the L-type calcium channel.

Drugs that do not conveniently fit into these classes (and are discussed separately) include adenosine and the digitalis glycosides.

Regardless of the class, the goal of antiarrhythmic therapy is to abolish the mechanisms by which tachyarrhythmias occur (see Chapter 11). These mechanisms are (1) increased automaticity of pacemaker or non-pacemaker cells, (2) reentrant pathways, and (3) triggered activity.

In the case of arrhythmias caused by *increased automaticity*, treatment is aimed at lowering the maximum frequency at which cardiac action potentials can occur by (1) reducing the slope of spontaneous phase 4 diastolic depolarization and/or (2) prolonging the effective refractory period. These actions reduce or extinguish abnormally high rates of firing.

Antiarrhythmic drugs inhibit *reentrant* rhythms by a different mechanism. The initiation of a reentrant circuit relies on a region

Table 17.11. Classification of Antiarrhythmic Drugs

Class	General Mechanism	Examples
I	**Na⁺ channel blockade**	
IA	Moderate block ($\downarrow\downarrow$ phase 0 upstroke rate; prolonged AP duration)	Quinidine Procainamide Disopyramide
IB	Mild block ($\downarrow$phase 0 upstroke rate; shortened AP duration)	Lidocaine Mexiletine
IC	Marked block ($\downarrow\downarrow\downarrow$ phase 0 upstroke rate; no change in AP duration)	Flecainide Propafenone
II	**β-Adrenergic receptor blockade**	Propranolol Esmolol Metoprolol
III	**K⁺ channel blockade** (prolongation of action potential duration)	Amiodarone Dronedarone Sotalol Ibutilide Dofetilide
IV	**Ca⁺⁺ channel antagonists**	Verapamil Diltiazem

AP, action potential.

of unidirectional block and slowed conduction (Fig. 17.10). For a reentrant rhythm to sustain itself, the length of time it takes for an impulse to propagate around the circuit must exceed the effective refractory period of the tissue. If an impulse returns to an area of myocardium that was depolarized moments earlier but has not yet recovered excitability, it cannot restimulate that tissue. Thus, one strategy to stop reentry is to lengthen the tissue's refractory period. When the refractory period is pharmacologically prolonged, a propagating impulse confronts inactive sodium channels, cannot conduct further, and is extinguished.

A second means to interrupt reentrant circuits is to *additionally impair* impulse propagation within the already slowed retrograde limb. This is accomplished via pharmacologic blockade of the Na⁺ channels responsible for phase 0 depolarization. Such blockade fully abolishes the compromised impulse conduction within the retrograde limb and breaks the self-sustaining loop.

The elimination of the third type of tachyarrhythmia, *triggered activity*, requires suppression of early and delayed after depolarizations.

An ideal pharmacologic agent would suppress ectopic foci and interrupt reentrant loops without affecting normal conduction pathways. Unfortunately, when the concentrations of antiarrhythmic drugs exceed their narrow therapeutic ranges, even normal electrical activity may become suppressed. In addition, most antiarrhythmic drugs have the potential to aggravate rhythm disturbances (termed

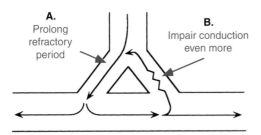

Figure 17.10. Two strategies to interrupt reentry. **A.** Prolonging the tissue refractory period causes returning impulses to find the tissue unexcitable. **B.** Further impairing conduction causes the impulse to "die out" in the slow retrograde limb of the circuit.

proarrhythmic effect). For example, this may occur when an antiarrhythmic drug prolongs the action potential and induces early afterdepolarizations, resulting in a triggered-type of arrhythmia, such as torsades de pointes (see Chapter 12). Drug-induced proarrhythmia occurs most often in patients with left ventricular dysfunction or in those with an increased QT interval (a sign that the action potential is already prolonged).

Class IA Antiarrhythmics

Mechanisms of Action

Effect on Reentrant Arrhythmias

Class IA agents produce moderate blockade of the fast sodium channels, thus slowing the rate of phase 0 depolarization and reducing tissue conduction velocities. If impaired sufficiently within a reentrant circuit, the impulse will die out within the already slowed retrograde limb, aborting the rhythm. In addition, class IA agents prolong the cell's action potential and the refractory period (largely via blockade of potassium channels responsible for repolarization). Thus, an impulse traveling in the reentrant loop encounters unexcitable tissue and is extinguished.

Effect on Arrhythmias Caused by Increased Automaticity

As shown in Figure 17.11, class IA agents raise the threshold value and, perhaps by inhibition of pacemaker channels, they depress the slope of phase 4 depolarization. As a result, it takes longer to reach threshold and fire the action potential. These effects are most pronounced at Purkinje fibers and abnormal ectopic pacemakers.

Effect on the Electrocardiogram

Because the conduction velocity is decreased and the action potential duration and repolarization are prolonged, the effect of class IA agents is to mildly prolong the QRS and QT intervals (Table 17.12). At higher dosages, the drugs may substantially lengthen these intervals, potentially setting the stage for afterdepolarizations and drug-induced arrhythmias.

Clinical Uses

Class IA drugs are effective in treating reentrant and ectopic supraventricular and ventricular tachycardias (Table 17.13). However, their use has declined because of the development of more effective and less proarrhythmic strategies, as discussed later in the chapter.

Specific Class IA Drugs

Quinidine displays the electrophysiologic effects inherent to class IA agents but also has anticholinergic properties that may *augment* conduction at the AV node, thus antagonizing its direct suppressant effect. Because quinidine is metabolized primarily by the liver, its dosage must be reduced in patients with hepatic dysfunction.

Noncardiac and cardiac side effects occur frequently during quinidine therapy. The most common are related to the gastrointestinal tract, including nausea, vomiting, and diarrhea. *Cinchonism* refers to CNS toxicity by quinidine manifested by tinnitus, confusion, hearing loss, and visual disturbances. Quinidine can cause excessive prolongation of the QT interval, which may lead to the life-threatening ventricular tachyarrhythmia torsades de pointes, described in Chapter 12.

The electrophysiologic effects of **procainamide** are similar to those of quinidine, though it does not prolong the action potential (and therefore QT interval) as much. Procainamide has mild ganglionic blocking effects that may cause peripheral vasodilation and a negative cardiac inotropic effect.

Procainamide is available for oral or parenteral administration and is primarily used when IV delivery of a class IA drug is desired. More than 50% of the drug is excreted unchanged in the urine; the remainder undergoes acetylation by the liver to form *N*-acetyl procainamide (NAPA), which is subsequently excreted by the kidneys. In renal failure, or in patients who are rapid acetylators, high serum levels of NAPA may accumulate. NAPA shares procainamide's ability to prolong the action potential and refractory period, but it does not alter the

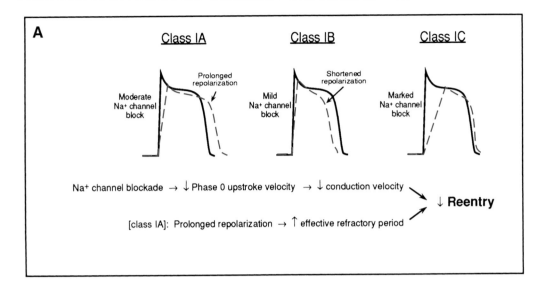

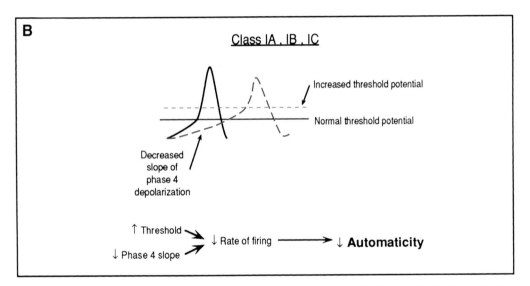

Figure 17.11. **Electrophysiologic effects of the class I antiarrhythmic drugs. A.** Effect on the Purkinje cell action potential. **B.** Effect on pacemaker cell action potential.

Table 17.12. **Effect of Antiarrhythmic Drugs on Electrocardiographic Intervals**

Class	PR	QRS	QT
IA	0	↑	↑
IB	0	0	0 or ↓
IC	↑	↑	0 or ↑
II	0 or ↑	0	0
III	0 or ↑	0 or ↑	↑
IV	↑	0	0

rate of phase 4 depolarization or the slope of phase 0 upstroke of the action potential.

Noncardiac side effects of procainamide are common and include fever and rash. Approximately one third of patients develop a systemic lupus–like syndrome after 6 months of therapy, manifested by arthralgias, rash, and connective tissue inflammation. It most often occurs among patients who are slow acetylators and is reversible on cessation of drug therapy. As a result of

Class	Use
IA	• Atrial fibrillation and flutter • PSVT • Ventricular tachycardia
IB	• Ventricular tachycardia • Digitalis-induced arrhythmias
IC	• Atrial fibrillation and PSVT
II	• Atrial or ventricular premature beats • PSVT • Atrial fibrillation and flutter • Ventricular tachycardia
III	• Ventricular tachycardia (amiodarone and sotalol) • Atrial fibrillation and flutter • Bypass tract–mediated PSVT
IV	• PSVT • Atrial fibrillation and flutter (↓ VR) • Multifocal atrial tachycardia (↓ VR)

Table 17.13. Common Clinical Uses of Antiarrhythmic Drugs

PSVT, paroxysmal supraventricular tachycardia (e.g., AV nodal reentrant tachycardia); VR, ventricular rate.

these side effects, procainamide is generally reserved for short-term use.

Disopyramide's electrophysiologic and antiarrhythmic effects are similar to those of quinidine. However, disopyramide has a greater anticholinergic effect, so that common side effects include constipation, urinary retention, and exacerbation of glaucoma. More so than quinidine or procainamide, disopyramide has a pronounced negative inotropic effect and must be used with caution in patients with left ventricular systolic dysfunction. However, its negative inotropic property renders it a useful antiarrhythmic agent for patients who have hypertrophic cardiomyopathy with dynamic outflow tract obstruction (see Chapter 10).

Disopyramide is administered orally. The primary excretory pathway is via the kidneys, and toxic levels may accumulate in patients with renal insufficiency. QT prolongation and precipitation of ventricular arrhythmias (including torsades de pointes) can occur.

Class IB Antiarrhythmics

Class IB drugs inhibit the fast sodium channel, but unlike IA agents, they typically *shorten* the action potential duration and the refractory period. Such shortening is attributed to blockade of small sodium currents that normally continue through phase 2 of the action potential.

Class IB drugs at therapeutic concentrations do not substantially alter the electrical activity of normal tissue; rather, they preferentially act on diseased or ischemic cells. Conditions present during ischemia—such as acidosis, faster rates of cell stimulation, and increased extracellular potassium concentration (and consequently a less negative diastolic membrane potential)—increase the ability of class IB drugs to block the sodium channel. This blockade promotes conduction block in ischemic cells by reducing the slope of phase 0 depolarization and slowing the conduction velocity, thus inhibiting reentrant arrhythmias (see Fig. 17.11). The automaticity of ectopic pacemakers is also suppressed by decreasing phase 4 spontaneous depolarization and (in the case of some drugs of this class) by raising the threshold potential. In addition, intravenous lidocaine, a member of this class, suppresses delayed afterdepolarizations.

The most common use of class IB drugs is in the suppression of ventricular arrhythmias, especially those that appear in association with ischemia or digitalis toxicity. Conversely, they have little effect on *atrial* tissue at therapeutic concentrations because of the shorter action potential duration of atrial cells, which allows less time for the drug to bind and block the Na$^+$ channel. Thus, these agents are ineffective in atrial fibrillation, atrial flutter, and supraventricular tachycardias.

Because the QT interval is not prolonged by class IB drugs, early afterdepolarizations do not occur, and torsades de pointes is not an expected complication.

Specific Class IB Drugs

Lidocaine is used to suppress some ventricular arrhythmias in hospitalized patients. It is administered intravenously only, because oral administration results in unpredictable plasma levels.

As a result of rapid distribution and hepatic metabolism, lidocaine must be administered as a continuous infusion following two or three loading boluses. The half-life of the drug depends greatly on hepatic blood flow. Reduced flow (as in heart failure or in older individuals) or intrinsic liver disease can greatly increase serum lidocaine concentrations and toxic effects; therefore, the infusion rate should be lowered in such patients.

The most common side effects of lidocaine are not cardiac; rather, they are related to the CNS and include confusion, paresthesias, dizziness, and seizures. These effects are dosage related and can be prevented by monitoring serum levels of the drug or preemptively reducing the infusion rate when liver disease or decreased hepatic blood flow is suspected.

Mexiletine is structurally similar to lidocaine and shares its electrophysiologic properties, but mexiletine is administered orally. Ninety percent of mexiletine is metabolized in the liver to inactive products, and the dosage of the drug should be reduced in patients with hepatic dysfunction. Dose-related side effects of mexiletine are common, especially of the CNS (dizziness, tremor, slurred speech) and the gastrointestinal tract (nausea, vomiting).

Class IC Antiarrhythmics

The class IC drugs are the most potent sodium channel blockers. They markedly decrease the upstroke of the action potential and conduction velocity in atrial, ventricular, and Purkinje fibers (see Fig. 17.11). Although they have little effect on the duration of the action potential or refractory period of Purkinje fibers, they significantly prolong the refractory period within the AV node and in accessory bypass tracts.

The group IC agents were originally developed to treat ventricular arrhythmias. However, that use has diminished because studies have shown an *increased* mortality rate in patients taking class IC drugs for ventricular ectopy following myocardial infarction and in those who have survived cardiac arrest. In patients with underlying left ventricular dysfunction, class IC drugs can precipitate heart failure. Thus, drugs of this subclass should be avoided in patients who have other underlying heart abnormalities, such as CAD or ventricular dysfunction. Class IC drugs *have* been shown to be beneficial (and generally safe) in the treatment of supraventricular arrhythmias in patients who have otherwise structurally normal hearts (see Table 17.13).

Flecainide is well absorbed after oral administration. Approximately 40% of the drug is excreted unchanged in the urine, and the remainder is converted to inactive metabolites by the liver. Cardiac toxicities include the aggravation of ventricular arrhythmias and precipitation of CHF in patients with underlying left ventricular dysfunction. Noncardiac side effects are referable to the CNS and include confusion, dizziness, and blurred vision.

The electrophysiologic properties of **propafenone** are similar to those of flecainide, but additionally it exhibits weak β-adrenergic blocking activity. Propafenone is metabolized by the liver, but because the level of genetic variation is high, a patient's dosage must be titrated by observing the drug's effect. Extracardiac side effects are not common and include dizziness and disturbances of taste.

Class II Antiarrhythmics

The class II drugs are β-adrenergic receptor antagonists, which are used in the management of both supraventricular and ventricular arrhythmias. Most of their antiarrhythmic properties can be attributed to inhibition of cardiac sympathetic activity. Additional actions of some β-blockers, such as β_1-cardioselectivity or a membrane-stabilizing effect, seem to make no contribution to antiarrhythmic activity.

Chapter 11 describes how β-adrenergic stimulation results in a more rapid upslope of phase 4 depolarization and an increased firing rate of the SA node. β-Adrenergic antagonists inhibit these effects, thus reducing automaticity (Fig. 17.12). This action extends to the cardiac Purkinje fibers, where arrhythmias due to enhanced automaticity are inhibited. In addition, because afterdepolarizations may be caused by excessive catecholamines, β-blockers may prevent triggered arrhythmias induced by that mechanism. β-Blockers also increase the effective refractory period of the AV node.

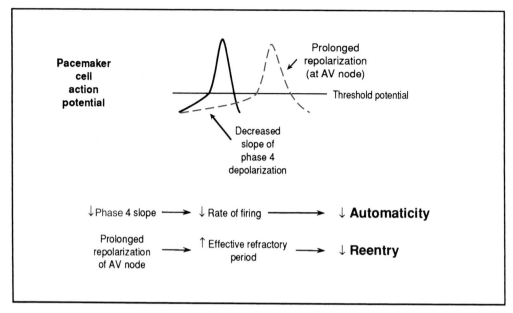

Figure 17.12. Electrophysiologic effects of the class II antiarrhythmic drugs on the pacemaker cell action potential.

β-Blockers may also have a beneficial antiarrhythmic effect by decreasing myocardial oxygen demand, thus reducing myocardial ischemia. Several drugs from this group have been shown to reduce mortality following myocardial infarction (see Chapter 7), which may in part relate to their antiarrhythmic effect. Since the AV nodal conduction time is prolonged by β-blockers, the PR interval on the ECG may become prolonged (see Table 17.12). The QRS and QT intervals are usually unaffected.

Clinical Uses

β-Blockers are most useful in suppressing tachyarrhythmias induced by excessive catecholamines (e.g., during exercise or emotional stimulation). They are also frequently used to slow the ventricular rate in atrial flutter and fibrillation by impairing conduction and increasing the refractoriness of the AV node. In addition, β-blockers may terminate reentrant supraventricular arrhythmias in which the AV node constitutes one limb of the reentrant pathway.

β-Blockers are effective in suppressing ventricular premature beats and other ventricular arrhythmias, especially when induced by exercise. They are also effective in treating ventricular arrhythmias related to prolongation of the QT interval because, unlike group IA agents, they do not lengthen that interval.

Class III Antiarrhythmics

Class III drugs are structurally dissimilar from one another but share the property of significantly prolonging the action potential of Purkinje and ventricular muscle fibers (Fig. 17.13), predominantly by blocking the outward K^+ current of phase 3 repolarization. Unlike class I agents, class III antiarrhythmics generally have little effect on phase 0 depolarization or conduction velocity.

Amiodarone is a powerful antiarrhythmic with many potential adverse reactions. Its major therapeutic effect is to prolong the action potential duration and refractoriness of all cardiac regions. However, it also shares actions with each of the other antiarrhythmic classes. The slope of phase 0 depolarization may be depressed through sodium channel blockade (class I effect), it exerts a β-blocking effect (class II), and also demonstrates weak calcium channel blockade (class IV). As a result, the electrophysiologic effects of amiodarone are to decrease the sinus node firing rate, suppress automaticity, interrupt reentrant circuits, and prolong the PR, QRS, and QT intervals on the ECG.

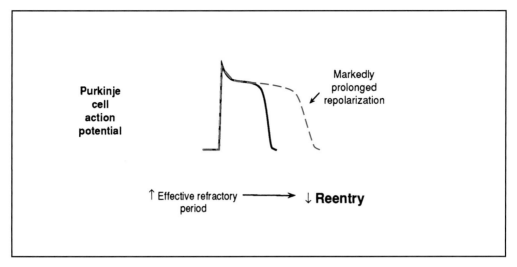

Figure 17.13. Electrophysiologic effects of the class III antiarrhythmic drugs on the Purkinje cell action potential.

In addition, amiodarone is a vasodilator (because of α-receptor and calcium channel blocking effects) and a negative inotrope (β-blocker and CCB effects). The resulting vasodilation is more prominent than the negative inotropic effect, so that cardiac output does not usually suffer in patients treated with this drug.

Amiodarone is more effective than most other antiarrhythmic drugs for a wide spectrum of ventricular and supraventricular tachyarrhythmias. These include atrial fibrillation, atrial flutter, ventricular tachycardia, ventricular flutter, and supraventricular tachycardias, including those involving bypass tracts. It is a first-line agent for the emergency treatment of ventricular arrhythmias during cardiac resuscitation (including ventricular fibrillation and ventricular tachycardia refractory to electrical shocks) and is more effective than lidocaine for this purpose. It is commonly used to treat arrhythmias in patients with ventricular systolic dysfunction because it causes fewer proarrhythmic complications in that population than other agents. In addition, low-dose amiodarone is effective for long-term suppression of atrial fibrillation and flutter.

Amiodarone is absorbed slowly from the gastrointestinal tract, requiring 5 to 6 hours to reach peak plasma concentrations. It is highly lipophilic, is extensively sequestered in tissues, and undergoes very slow hepatic metabolism.

Its elimination half-life is long and variable, averaging 25 to 60 *days*. The drug is excreted by the biliary tract, lacrimal glands, and skin but not by the kidney; thus, its dosage does not need to be adjusted in patients with renal failure. However, because the drug's action has a delayed onset and very long duration, its effects cannot be altered quickly if side effects ensue.

There are numerous potential adverse reactions of amiodarone. The most serious is pulmonary toxicity, manifest by pneumonitis leading to pulmonary fibrosis. Its origin is unclear but may represent a hypersensitivity reaction and, if recognized early, is reversible.

Other life-threatening side effects of amiodarone relate to cardiac toxicity: symptomatic bradycardia and aggravation of ventricular arrhythmia each occur in approximately 2% of patients. Because amiodarone significantly prolongs the QT interval, early afterdepolarizations and torsades de pointes can occur, but this happens only rarely. Intravenously administered amiodarone occasionally causes pronounced hypotension.

Abnormalities of thyroid function are common during amiodarone treatment, because the drug contains a significant iodine load and because it inhibits the peripheral conversion of T_4 to T_3. During the first few weeks of therapy, it is common to observe transient abnormalities of thyroid biochemical tests without clinical findings of thyroid disease: serum TSH and T_4 rise, and serum T_3 falls. Over time, some patients develop overt hypothyroidism (owing mostly to the antithyroid effects of iodine) or hyperthyroidism (because of either an iodine effect in iodine-deficient communities or a direct thyroid inflammatory process incited by amiodarone in susceptible patients).

Gastrointestinal side effects of amiodarone include anorexia, nausea, and elevation of liver function tests, all of which improve with lower doses of the drug. Neurologic side effects include proximal muscle weakness, peripheral neuropathy, ataxia, tremors, and sleep disturbances. Corneal microdeposits can be detected in patients receiving chronic amiodarone therapy, but these rarely affect vision.

As a result of these potential adverse effects, ECGs, thyroid and liver function blood tests, chest radiographs, and sometimes pulmonary function studies are performed on a regular basis in patients receiving chronic therapy. Amiodarone interacts with, and increases the activity of, certain drugs including warfarin and digoxin, such that the dosages of those agents must be adjusted. Because amiodarone prolongs the QT interval, other drugs that do the same should be used with caution.

Dronedarone, a noniodinated analog of amiodarone, is a recently introduced agent for the treatment of atrial fibrillation and flutter. While it is not as potent an antiarrhythmic drug, it lacks amiodarone's pulmonary, thyroid, and liver toxicities. Similar to amiodarone, it blocks potassium, sodium, and L-type calcium channels, and inhibits β- and α-adrenergic receptors. It is administered orally and reaches a steady state in 4 to 8 days, much faster than oral amiodarone. Dronedarone can increase the QT interval but only rarely results in torsades de pointes. The major side effects are gastrointestinal: nausea, vomiting, and diarrhea. Dronedarone is contraindicated in patients with advanced heart failure (NYHA class IV) and those with moderate heart failure (NYHA class II to III) and recent decompensation, as increased mortality has been demonstrated with the drug's use in such patients.

Sotalol is a nonselective β-blocker, but it is used in practice as an oral antiarrhythmic drug because of its additional class III properties. It prolongs the duration of the action potential, increases the refractory period of atrial and ventricular tissue, and inhibits conduction in accessory bypass tracts. The phase 0 upstroke velocity is not altered in the usual dosage range. It is effective in the treatment of both supraventricular and ventricular arrhythmias.

Because sotalol is excreted exclusively by the kidneys, its dosage should be adjusted in the presence of renal disease. Potential side effects include those of the β-blockers described earlier. Because the drug prolongs the QT interval, the most serious potential adverse effect is provoking torsades de pointes. This complication occurs in approximately 2% of patients and is more common in patients with a history of heart failure and in women (for unknown reasons).

Dofetilide is another oral class III agent that blocks the outward potassium current, causing prolongation of the action potential duration and an increase in the effective refractory period. It is used in the management of atrial fibrillation and atrial flutter. QT prolongation complicated by torsades de pointes is the major potential adverse effect. Dofetilide is excreted by the kidney, and its dose must be adjusted in patients with renal failure.

Ibutilide is a class III drug used intravenously for the acute conversion of atrial fibrillation or atrial flutter of recent onset. This agent prolongs the action potential duration and increases atrial and ventricular refractoriness. Unlike other class III drugs, its major mechanism relates to activation of a slow inward sodium current that prolongs the plateau (phase 2) of the action potential. In clinical trials, the success rate for conversion of atrial flutter is approximately 60%, but only 30% for those in atrial fibrillation.

Because ibutilide prolongs the QT interval, torsades de pointes can be precipitated, especially in patients with underlying ventricular dysfunction. Therefore, careful electrocardiographic monitoring is necessary for several hours after drug administration.

Class IV Antiarrhythmics

Class IV drugs exert their electrophysiologic effects by selective blockade of L-type cardiac calcium channels and include **verapamil** and

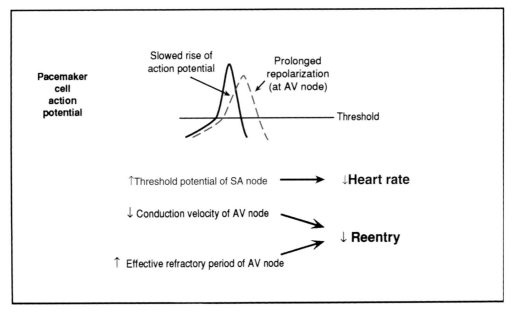

Figure 17.14. **Electrophysiologic effects of the class IV antiarrhythmic drugs on the pacemaker cell action potential.**

diltiazem, but not nifedipine or the other dihydropyridine CCBs. They are most potent in tissues in which the action potential depends on calcium currents, such as the SA and AV nodes. Within nodal tissue, calcium channel blockade decreases the rate of rise of phase 0 depolarization and conduction velocity, and lengthens the refractory period of the AV node (Fig. 17.14). These agents also raise the threshold potential at the SA node. The resulting clinical effects are: (1) the heart rate slows; (2) transmission of rapid atrial impulses through the AV node to the ventricles decreases, thus slowing the ventricular rate in atrial fibrillation and atrial flutter; and (3) reentrant rhythms traveling through the AV node may terminate.

A primary use of class IV drugs is for the treatment of reentrant supraventricular tachycardias (e.g., AV nodal reentrant tachycardia). At one time, intravenous verapamil was the treatment of choice for acute episodes of such rhythms, but intravenous adenosine (described in the next section) has assumed that role.

The pharmacology and toxicities of CCBs were presented earlier in this chapter. The most important side effect of verapamil and diltiazem, when administered intravenously, is hypotension. In addition, these agents should be avoided, or used cautiously, in patients receiving β-blocker therapy, because the combined negative inotropic and chronotropic effects may precipitate heart failure and/or significant bradycardia.

Adenosine

Adenosine is an endogenous nucleoside with a very short half-life. Administered intravenously, it is the most effective drug for the rapid termination of reentrant SVT, such as AV nodal reentrant tachycardia.

Adenosine has substantial electrophysiologic effects on specialized conduction tissues, especially the SA and AV nodes. By binding to specific adenosine receptors, it activates potassium channels (Fig. 17.15). The resultant increase in the outward potassium current hyperpolarizes the membrane, which suppresses spontaneous depolarization of the SA node and slows conduction through the AV node. In addition, adenosine decreases the intracellular cAMP concentration by inhibiting adenylate cyclase. The result is a decrease in the inward pacemaker current (I_f) and the inward calcium current (see Fig. 17.15). Thus, the net effect of adenosine is to slow the SA node firing rate and to decrease AV nodal conduction. By

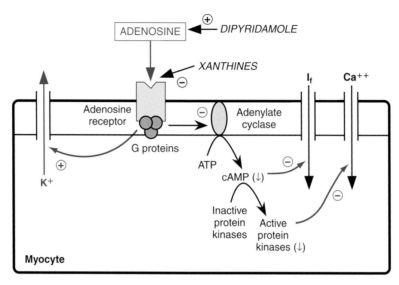

Figure 17.15. Mechanism of antiarrhythmic action of adenosine. Stimulation of the myocyte adenosine receptor activates potassium channels, and the resultant outward K$^+$ current hyperpolarizes the membrane, resulting in decreased automaticity. Adenosine also inhibits membrane adenylate cyclase activity. The subsequent decline in cAMP has two pertinent effects: the inward pacemaker current (I_f) is diminished and the production of active protein kinases is lessened, leading to a reduction of the inward Ca^{++} current. These effects contribute to decreased automaticity and slowed conduction through the AV node. Xanthines compete for the receptor, blocking adenosine's effects. Conversely, dipyridamole interferes with cellular uptake and degradation of adenosine and therefore amplifies its effect.

inducing transient AV nodal block, adenosine terminates reentrant pathways that include the AV node as part of the circuit. Ventricular myocytes are relatively immune to these effects, in part because the specific potassium channels responsive to adenosine are not present in those cells.

With a half-life of only 10 seconds, adenosine has very transient side effects (headache, chest pain, flushing, bronchoconstriction). Because methylxanthines (caffeine, theophylline) competitively antagonize the adenosine receptor, higher doses of adenosine may be necessary in patients using those substances. Conversely, dipyridamole inhibits the breakdown of adenosine and amplifies its effect.

DIURETICS

Diuretics are most often used to treat heart failure and hypertension. In heart failure, enhanced renal reabsorption of sodium and water, with subsequent expansion of the extracellular volume, contributes to peripheral edema and pulmonary congestion. Diuretics eliminate excess sodium and water through renal excretion and are therefore a cornerstone of therapy (see Chapter 9). In the treatment of hypertension, diuretics similarly reduce intravascular volume and in some cases promote vascular dilatation. To better understand these intended functions of diuretics, the section begins with a brief review of normal renal transport of sodium and water.

In the kidney, the rate of glomerular filtration typically averages 135 to 180 L/day in normal adults. Most of the filtered Na$^+$ is reabsorbed by the renal tubules, leaving only a small quantity in the final urine (Fig. 17.16). Approximately 65% to 70% of the filtered Na$^+$ is reabsorbed isosmotically in the proximal tubule by active transport. In the thick ascending limb of the loop of Henle, an additional 25% of the filtered sodium is reabsorbed, through a Na$^+$–K$^+$ cotransport system coupled to the uptake of two Cl$^-$ ions. Because this region is impermeable to the reabsorption of water, it is the site of hypotonic tubular fluid formation, and the surrounding interstitium becomes hypertonic. In the distal convoluted tubule, an additional small fraction of NaCl is reabsorbed (approximately 5%). In the cortical collecting

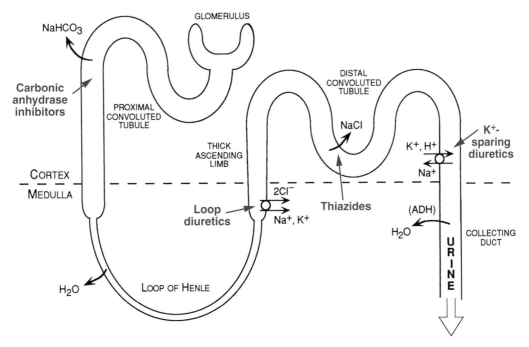

Figure 17.16. Schematic diagram of the renal tubules. Approximately 70% of filtered sodium is reabsorbed in the proximal convoluted tubule, 25% in the thick ascending limb of the loop of Henle, 5% in the distal convoluted tubule, and 1% to 2% in the cortical collecting tubule (mediated by the action of aldosterone). Antidiuretic hormone (ADH) increases the permeability of the distal nephron for water. Diuretics are secreted into the proximal convoluted tubule and act at the sites shown.

duct, Na^+ permeability is modulated by an aldosterone-sensitive mechanism, such that Na^+ is reabsorbed into the tubular cells in the presence of aldosterone, creating a lumen-negative potential difference that enhances K^+ and H^+ excretion. Approximately 1% to 2% of sodium reabsorption takes place at this location.

Most of the distal tubule is impermeable to water. In the collecting tubule, however, water permeability and reabsorption are promoted by antidiuretic hormone and driven by the osmotic gradient between the tubule and the hypertonic interstitium. Therefore, substances that interfere with antidiuretic hormone, such as ethanol, have diuretic actions.

The three most commonly used groups of diuretics are loop diuretics, thiazide diuretics, and potassium-sparing diuretics (Table 17.14 and Fig. 17.16). These classes are distinguished by the site of the kidney tubule where they act and by their potency. Loop diuretics impair absorption in the thick ascending limb of the loop of Henle, thiazide diuretics act on the distal tubule and collecting segment, and potassium-sparing

diuretics act on the aldosterone-sensitive region of the cortical collecting tubule. Members of a fourth group, the carbonic anhydrase inhibitors, are weak diuretics rarely used in the treatment of hypertension or heart failure. They act at the proximal convoluted tubule, resulting in a loss of bicarbonate (and sodium) in the urine.

Loop Diuretics

These agents are so named because they act principally on the thick ascending limb of the loop of Henle. They are powerful diuretics that result in the excretion of 20% to 25% of the filtered Na^+ load through inhibition of the Na^+–$2Cl^-$–K^+ cotransport system. Because inhibition at this site impairs the generation of a hypertonic interstitium, the gradient for passive water movement out of the collecting duct is diminished and water diuresis results.

Loop diuretics are of great importance in the acute management of pulmonary edema (administered intravenously) and in the treatment of chronic heart failure or peripheral edema

Table 17.14. Commonly Used Diuretics

Diuretic	Method of Administration	Onset of Action (Hours)	Duration of Action (Hours)	Potential Adverse Effects
Thiazides				
Chlorothiazide	PO	1	6–12	Hypokalemia,
	IV	0.25	2	hypomagnesemia,
Hydrochlorothiazide	PO	2	12	hyponatremia,
Chlorthalidone	PO	2	24	hypercalcemia,
Metolazone	PO	1	12–24	hyperglycemia,
Indapamide	PO	1–2	16–36	hyperuricemia, hypercholesterolemia, hypertriglyceridemia, metabolic alkalosis
Loop diuretics				
Furosemide	PO	1	6	Hypotension,
	IV	5 minutes	2	hypokalemia,
Bumetanide	PO	0.5–1	4–6	hypomagnesemia,
	IV	0.25	0.5–1	hyperglycemia,
Torsemide	PO	<1	6–8	hyperuricemia,
	IV	10 minutes	6–8	metabolic alkalosis
Ethacrynic acid	IV	0.25	3	
K$^+$-sparing diuretics				
Spironolactone	PO	>24	2–3 days	Hyperkalemia,
Eplerenone	PO	>24	24	GI disturbances;
Triamterene	PO	2	12–16	gynecomastia
Amiloride	PO	2	24	(spironolactone only)

GI, gastrointestinal; IV, intravenous; PO, by mouth.

(taken orally). Unlike other diuretics, they tend to be effective in the setting of impaired renal function. In addition to the diuretic effect, and even preceding it, drugs of this class may induce venous vasodilation, which is also beneficial in reducing venous return to the heart and pulmonary congestion (see Chapter 9). The mechanism of venous vasodilation appears to involve drug-induced prostaglandin and nitric oxide generation from endothelial cells, which act to relax vascular smooth muscle (see Chapter 6).

The most common side effects of the loop diuretics are intravascular volume depletion, hypokalemia, and metabolic alkalosis. *Hypokalemia* arises because (1) these agents impair the reabsorption of sodium in the loop of Henle, such that an increased amount of Na$^+$ is delivered to the distal tubule, where it prompts greater-than-normal exchange for potassium (and therefore more K$^+$ excretion

into the urine) and (2) diuretic-induced intravascular volume depletion activates the renin–angiotensin system. The subsequent rise in aldosterone promotes additional Na$^+$-K$^+$ exchange.

Metabolic alkalosis during loop diuretic therapy results from two mechanisms: (1) increased H$^+$ secretion into the distal tubule (and therefore into the urine) due to the secondary hyperaldosteronism described earlier and (2) contraction alkalosis, in which reduced intravascular volume promotes increased sodium bicarbonate reabsorption by the proximal tubule (see Fig. 17.16).

Additional side effects may also occur during continued loop diuretic therapy. *Hypomagnesemia* may result, because magnesium reabsorption depends on NaCl transport in the thick ascending limb of the loop of Henle, the action blocked by these drugs. *Ototoxicity* (cranial nerve VIII toxicity) occasionally develops, impairing hearing and vestibular function. It is thought to arise from electrolyte disturbances of the endolymphatic system, most likely because of Na^+–$2Cl^-$–K^+ cotransport inhibition by the diuretic at that site.

The most commonly used loop diuretic is **furosemide**, the oral form of which demonstrates reliable gastrointestinal absorption but a short duration of action (4 to 6 hours) that limits its usefulness in the chronic treatment of hypertension. **Bumetanide** is similar to furosemide and shares its actions and adverse effects but has greater potency and bioavailability. It also appears to have a lower incidence of ototoxicity than the other drugs of this class. Bumetanide is sometimes useful in heart failure patients when edema is refractory to other agents and in some patients allergic to furosemide. **Torsemide** is also similar to furosemide, with more complete bioavailability. **Ethacrynic acid** is the only nonsulfonamide loop diuretic, so it can be prescribed to patients with sulfonamide intolerance. It is otherwise not widely used because of its high incidence of ototoxicity.

Thiazide Diuretics

Thiazides and related compounds (chlorthalidone, indapamide, and metolazone) are commonly used diuretics because they demonstrate excellent gastrointestinal absorption when administered orally and are usually well tolerated. Though less potent than the loop diuretics, their sustained action makes them useful in chronic conditions such as hypertension and mild CHF.

Thiazides act at the distal tubule, where they block the reabsorption of approximately 3% to 5% of the filtered sodium (see Fig. 17.16). Na^+ reabsorption at this site is mediated through a Na^+–Cl^- cotransporter on the luminal membrane. The thiazides inhibit this carrier by a mechanism that has not been elucidated but may involve competition for the Cl^- site. The antihypertensive effect is initially associated with a decrease in cardiac output due to reduced intravascular volume with unchanged peripheral resistance. With long-term thiazide use, however, cardiac output often returns to normal as vasodilation leads to a reduction in vascular resistance. **Indapamide** is unique among this class in that it displays a particularly prominent vasodilating effect.

Thiazides are typically administered orally. Diuresis occurs after 1 to 2 hours, but the full antihypertensive effect of continued therapy may not emerge for up to 12 weeks (possibly related to the vasodilator mechanism alluded to in the previous paragraph). **Chlorothiazide**, the parent compound, has low lipid solubility and hence low bioavailability: higher doses are therefore required to achieve therapeutic levels compared with the more commonly used **hydrochlorothiazide**. **Chlorthalidone** is slowly absorbed and hence has a long duration of action. **Metolazone**, unlike other drugs of this class, is sometimes effective in patients with reduced renal function.

Clinically, the thiazides differ from the loop diuretics in that they are less potent, have a longer duration of action, and (with the exception of metolazone) demonstrate poor diuretic efficacy in the setting of impaired renal function: generally, they are not effective when the GFR is <25 mL/min.

Thiazides serve as a cornerstone of antihypertensive therapy because of their low cost, effectiveness, and proven benefits in reducing the risk of stroke and cardiac events. They are sometimes used in heart failure, generally for patients with mild chronic congestive symptoms. In addition, they can be added to loop diuretic therapy for patients who have become refractory to the diuretic effect of the latter. Since they act on sequential segments of the renal tubule, the combination produces a more profound natriuretic effect than either agent used alone.

Among the most important potential adverse effects of thiazides are (1) *hypokalemia* and *metabolic alkalosis*, which result from increased Na^+ delivery to the distal tubule, where exchange for K^+ and H^+ takes place, and from volume contraction and secondary hyperaldosteronism, as previously described for the loop diuretics; (2) *hyponatremia*, during prolonged treatment because of continued Na^+ excretion in the setting of chronic free water consumption; (3) *hyperuricemia* (and possible precipitation of gout) owing to decreased clearance of uric acid; (4) *hyperglycemia*, because of either impaired pancreatic insulin release or decreased peripheral glucose utilization; (5) *alterations in serum lipids* (*at least transiently*), characterized by increased low-density lipoprotein (LDL) cholesterol and triglycerides; and (6) *weakness, fatigability*, and *paresthesias*, which can occur with long-term use because of volume depletion and hypokalemia. In addition, serum calcium levels often rise slightly during thiazide therapy, but this is rarely clinically significant.

Potassium-Sparing Diuretics

These are relatively weak diuretics that antagonize physiologic Na^+ reabsorption at the distal convoluted tubule and cortical collecting tubule. Potassium-sparing agents reduce K^+ excretion; thus, unlike other diuretics, hypokalemia is not a side effect. They are used when maintenance of serum potassium levels is crucial and in states characterized by aldosterone excess (e.g., primary or secondary hyperaldosteronism). Two types of drugs make up this group: (1) aldosterone antagonists (e.g., spironolactone and eplerenone) and (2) direct inhibitors of Na^+ permeability in the collecting duct, which act independently of aldosterone (e.g., triamterene and amiloride).

Na^+ and K^+ exchange in the collecting tubules accounts for only a small percentage of sodium reuptake, so diuretic effectiveness is modest when these agents are used alone. They are often used in combination with the loop or thiazide classes for additive diuretic effect and to prevent hypokalemia.

Spironolactone is a synthetic steroid that competes for the cytoplasmic aldosterone receptor, thereby inhibiting the aldosterone-sensitive Na^+ channel in the kidney. Because Na^+ reabsorption through the sodium channel is inhibited, no lumen-negative potential exists to drive K^+ and H^+ ion excretion at the distal nephron sites; thus, K^+ and H^+ ions are retained in the circulation. Spironolactone also displays beneficial cardiac antiremodeling effects in patients with heart failure (see Chapter 9). In a trial of patients with severe heart failure, spironolactone (added to an ACE inhibitor and a loop diuretic) improved heart failure symptoms and reduced mortality rates.

The most serious potential complication of spironolactone is hyperkalemia, resulting from the impaired excretion of that ion. Thus, caution should be observed when administering K^+ supplements, ACE inhibitors, or ARBs concurrently with potassium-sparing diuretics because they could contribute to this complication. Spironolactone also displays antiandrogenic activity that may produce gynecomastia in men and menstrual irregularities in women.

Eplerenone is a more specific inhibitor of the aldosterone receptor that does not have the systemic antiandrogenic effects of spironolactone. Like spironolactone, it is used in the treatment of hypertension and chronic systolic heart failure. In patients with clinical evidence of heart failure following a myocardial infarction, eplerenone has also been shown to improve survival when added to usual care.

Triamterene and **amiloride** are structurally related potassium-sparing diuretics that act independently of aldosterone. At the distal tubules, they inhibit the reabsorption of Na^+, which subsequently diminishes the excretion of K^+ and H^+. Triamterene is metabolized by the liver, and its active product is secreted into the proximal tubule by the organic cation transport system. Amiloride is secreted directly into the proximal tubule and appears unchanged in the urine. As with spironolactone, the most important potential adverse effect of these drugs is hyperkalemia.

ANTITHROMBOTIC DRUGS

Platelets and the coagulation proteins play a key role in the pathogenesis of many cardiovascular disorders, including acute coronary syndromes, deep venous thrombosis, and thrombi that may complicate atrial fibrillation, dilated cardiomyopathy, or mechanical prosthetic heart valves. Therefore, the modulation of platelet function and of the coagulation pathway is often critically important in cardiovascular therapeutics.

The formation of a thrombus, whether in normal hemostasis or in pathologic clot formation, requires three events: (1) exposure of circulating blood elements to thrombogenic material (e.g., unmasking of subendothelial collagen after atherosclerotic plaque rupture); (2) activation and aggregation of platelets; and (3) triggering of the coagulation cascade, ultimately resulting in a fibrin clot. Hemostasis effected by platelets and the coagulation system is closely interlinked: activated platelets accelerate the coagulation pathway, and certain coagulation proteins (e.g., thrombin) contribute to platelet aggregation.

This section focuses first on drugs that interfere with platelet function and then on those that inhibit the coagulation cascade. Fibrinolytic agents, which dissolve clots that have already formed, are described in Chapter 7.

Platelet Inhibitors

Platelets are responsible for primary hemostasis by a three-part process: (1) adhesion to the site of injury, (2) release reaction (secretion of platelet products and activation of key surface receptors), and (3) aggregation. For example, following blood vessel injury, platelets quickly adhere to exposed subendothelial collagen by means of membrane glycoprotein (GP) receptors, a process that depends on von Willebrand factor. Following adhesion to the vessel wall, platelets release the preformed contents of their granules in response to agonists (including collagen and thrombin) that bind to platelet receptors. Among these prepackaged substances are adenosine diphosphate (ADP), serotonin, fibrinogen, growth factors, and procoagulants. Concurrently within the activated platelet, there is de novo synthesis and secretion of thromboxane A_2 (TXA_2), a powerful vasoconstrictor (Fig. 17.17).

Certain agonists, including ADP, thrombin, and TXA_2, stimulate platelets to aggregate and form the primary hemostatic plug as additional platelets are recruited from the circulation. During this process, the platelet membrane GP IIb/IIIa receptors undergo a critical conformational change. This alteration allows the previously inactive GP IIb/IIIa receptor to bind fibrinogen molecules, an

action that tightly links platelets to one another and constitutes the final common pathway of platelet aggregation. The developing clump of platelets is stabilized and tethered to the site of injury by a mesh of fibrin, which is produced by the simultaneous activation of the coagulation protein cascade.

Platelet activation is regulated to a great extent by release of stored Ca^{++} from the platelet-dense tubular system. This action results in an increase in cytosolic calcium concentration, with activation of protein kinases and phosphorylation of intraplatelet regulatory proteins. The augmented cytosolic Ca^{++} also stimulates phospholipase A_2 (PLA_2), causing the release of arachidonic acid, the precursor of TXA_2 (see Fig. 17.17).

The critical release of calcium is modulated by several factors. Acting at their respective platelet membrane receptors, thrombin and other agonists generate intermediaries that *stimulate* the release of calcium from the dense tubules. TXA_2 increases the intracellular Ca^{++} by binding to its platelet receptor, which inhibits the activity of adenylate cyclase and thereby reduces cAMP formation, an action that augments the release of Ca^{++} from the dense tubules (see Fig. 17.17). Conversely, endothelial cell-derived prostacyclin (PGI_2) *stimulates* adenylate cyclase activity and increases platelet cAMP concentration, which *inhibits* Ca^{++} release from the dense tubular system.

Antiplatelet drugs interfere with platelet function at various points along the sequence of activation and aggregation (see Fig. 17.17). The most commonly used antiplatelet drug is aspirin, but the roles of newer antiplatelet drugs, especially the thienopyridines and GP IIb/IIIa receptor antagonists, have rapidly expanded.

Aspirin

As described in the previous section, TXA_2 is an important mediator of platelet activation and clot formation. Aspirin (acetylsalicylic acid) acts by irreversibly acetylating (and thus blocking the action of) cyclooxygenase, an enzyme essential to TXA_2 production from arachidonic acid (see Fig. 17.17). The form of the enzyme found in platelets is

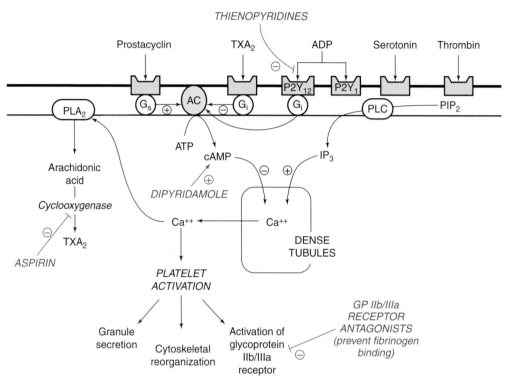

Figure 17.17. Platelet activation is mediated by cytosolic Ca++. Factors that promote and inhibit calcium release from the platelet-dense tubules are shown. Thrombin and serotonin, acting at their specific receptors, stimulate the formation of inositol triphosphate (IP_3) from phosphatidylinositol diphosphate (PIP_2) by phospholipase C (PLC). IP_3 subsequently enhances the intracellular release of calcium. Thromboxane A_2 (TXA_2) also facilitates calcium release. It inhibits adenyl cyclase (AC) and reduces cyclic adenosine monophosphate (cAMP) formation. Because cAMP normally *prevents* Ca^{++} release from the dense tubules, the reduction of this effect by TXA_2 *increases* Ca^{++} release into the cytosol. Conversely, endothelial-derived prostacyclin has the opposite effect. It reduces intraplatelet calcium release because it *stimulates* AC activity and cAMP formation. ADP also stimulates calcium release via its two receptors (see text for details). Calcium promotes the action of phospholipase A_2 (PLA_2), which generates the precursors of TXA_2 from the cell membrane. Platelet activation modulated by [Ca^{++}] ultimately results in granule secretion, cytoskeletal reorganization, and the critical conformational change in glycoprotein IIb/IIIa receptors that is necessary for platelet aggregation. The sites of action of commonly used antiplatelet drugs are shown in color.

cyclooxygenase 1 (COX-1), which is effectively inhibited by the nonselective action of aspirin (but it is *not* inhibited by selective COX-2 antagonists, such as celecoxib). Because platelets lack nuclei and therefore cannot synthesize new proteins (including cyclooxygenase), aspirin *permanently* disables TXA_2 production in exposed cells.

The prostaglandin PGI_2, a major antagonist of TXA_2 that is produced by endothelial cells, shares a dependency on cyclooxygenase activity for its formation, and aspirin, at high doses, impairs its synthesis as well. Unlike platelets, however, endothelial cells *are* able to generate new cyclooxygenase to replace what has been deactivated by acetylation. Thus, when used at low doses, aspirin effectively inhibits platelet TXA_2 synthesis without significantly interfering with the presence and beneficial actions of PGI_2.

Because the antiplatelet effect of aspirin is limited to inhibition of TXA_2 formation, platelet aggregation induced by other factors (e.g., ADP) is not significantly impeded. Thus, aspirin is not a "complete" antithrombotic agent.

Clinical Uses

Aspirin has many proven clinical benefits in patients with cardiovascular disease (Table 17.15). In individuals with unstable angina, acute myocardial infarction, or a history of myocardial infarction, aspirin reduces the incidence of future fatal and nonfatal coronary events. Similarly, in

Table 17.15. Cardiovascular Uses of Antithrombotic Drugs

Drug	Chronic Angina	Unstable Angina/ NSTEMI	STEMI	DVT	Mechanical Heart Valve	Atrial Fibrillation	PCI	HIT
Platelet inhibitors								
Aspirin	+	+	+		(1)	(2)	+	
Thienopyridines		+	+				(3)	
GP IIb/IIIa antagonists		+	(4)				+	
Dipyridamole					(5)			
Anticoagulants								
UFH		+	+	+	(6)	(6)	+	
LMWH		+	+	+				
Direct thrombin inhibitors		(7)					+	+
Fondaparinux		(8)		+				
Warfarin			(9)	+	+	+		

(1) Sometimes used in combination with warfarin.

(2) If patient has a low risk of stroke, or if warfarin is contraindicated.

(3) When intracoronary stent is implanted.

(4) If PCI undertaken.

(5) Sometimes used in combination with warfarin for recurrent embolism.

(6) For hospitalized patients unable to take warfarin.

(7) If undergoing PCI.

(8) Emerging use.

(9) For 3–6 months after MI if large akinetic segment is present.

DVT, deep venous thrombosis; HIT, heparin-induced thrombocytopenia; LMWH, low molecular weight heparin; NSTEMI, non–ST elevation myocardial infarction (MI); PCI, percutaneous coronary intervention; STEMI, ST-elevation MI; UFH, unfractionated heparin.

patients with chronic stable angina without a history of myocardial infarction, aspirin lessens the occurrence of subsequent myocardial infarction and mortality. In patients who have suffered a minor stroke or transient cerebral ischemic attack, aspirin reduces the rate of future stroke and cardiovascular events. Additionally, aspirin lowers the likelihood of graft occlusion in patients who have undergone coronary artery bypass surgery.

Less clear is the benefit of aspirin for *primary* prevention (i.e., in individuals without a history of cardiovascular events or symptoms). When tested in a large cohort of healthy American middle-aged men, aspirin was associated with a reduced incidence of nonfatal myocardial infarction but an increased rate of nonfatal hemorrhagic stroke and gastrointestinal bleeding; there was no effect on total vascular mortality. Subsequent meta-analyses

of clinical trials have similarly concluded that aspirin is effective for primary prevention of myocardial infarction in patients with coronary risk factors, but it also increases the risk of hemorrhagic stroke. In the prospective, primary prevention trial known as the Women's Health Initiative, aspirin lowered the risk of ischemic stroke in women but did not reduce the incidence of MI or death from cardiovascular disease. Thus, whereas aspirin plays an extremely important role in patients with known cardiovascular disease, it is not evident that otherwise healthy people should routinely take aspirin for "cardiovascular protection."

Current recommendations are that aspirin (at a dosage of 75 to 325 mg/day) be administered to patients with clinical manifestations of coronary disease in the absence of contraindications (i.e., aspirin allergy or complications described in the next section). It should not be prescribed routinely for primary prevention purposes in completely healthy individuals. However, pending the results of ongoing research, many physicians believe it is appropriate to recommend aspirin use in men and women older than age 50 who have at least one major atherosclerosis risk factor (see Chapter 5). In addition, the American Diabetes Association recommends that all diabetics with at least one other coronary risk factor take aspirin for cardiovascular protection. Finally, aspirin is not as beneficial as warfarin (described later in the chapter) for the prevention of stroke in high-risk patients with atrial fibrillation.

Adverse Effects

The most common adverse effects of aspirin are related to the gastrointestinal system, including dyspepsia and nausea, which often can be ameliorated by lowering the dosage and/or using enteric-coated or buffered tablets. More serious potential side effects include gastrointestinal bleeding, hemorrhagic strokes, allergic reactions, and asthma exacerbation in aspirin-sensitive patients. Because aspirin is excreted by the kidneys and competes with uric acid for the renal proximal tubule organic anion transporter, it may also occasionally exacerbate gout.

Thienopyridines

The thienopyridines inhibit ADP-mediated activation of platelets (see Fig. 17.17). Normally, extracellular ADP activates platelets by binding to two types of surface purinoceptors. The first (termed $P2Y_1$) acts through phospholipase C to increase intraplatelet $[Ca^{++}]$, which potentiates platelet activation. The second purinoceptor ($P2Y_{12}$) is linked to an inhibitory G protein and reduces cAMP production when activated, thus also raising intraplatelet $[Ca^{++}]$ (see Fig. 17.17). ADP-induced platelet aggregation requires that ADP simultaneously activate *both* $P2Y_1$ and $P2Y_{12}$ purinoceptors. The thienopyridines, after conversion to active metabolites in the liver, irreversibly block $P2Y_{12}$ by binding directly to it or to a nearby membrane protein. As a result, platelet aggregation is inhibited.

Clopidogrel, **ticlopidine**, and **prasugrel** are the thienopyridines approved for clinical use. All are well absorbed orally and have good bioavailability. Meta-analyses of the use of ticlopidine or clopidogrel in patients at risk for coronary syndromes have concluded that these drugs are modestly superior to aspirin in reducing the risk of myocardial infarction, stroke, or vascular deaths, but at an increased risk of side effects and at a higher economic cost. Studies evaluating the combination of aspirin *plus* clopidogrel in patients with unstable angina, non–ST elevation myocardial infarction (NSTEMI) and ST-elevation myocardial infarction (STEMI) have demonstrated a significant benefit in cardiovascular outcomes compared with aspirin alone, though at an increased bleeding risk.

Thienopyridines are currently used as antiplatelet substitutes in patients allergic to aspirin and to prevent thrombotic complications following percutaneous coronary stenting (see Chapter 6). The combination of clopidogrel plus aspirin is also approved for patients with unstable angina, NSTEMI, or STEMI to reduce the rate of recurrent cardiac events (see Chapter 7).

Side effects of the thienopyridines include bleeding, dyspepsia, and diarrhea. In addition, the use of ticlopidine has been limited by potentially life-threatening adverse reactions: severe neutropenia (occurring in 0.8% to 2.5% of patients) and thrombotic thrombocytopenic purpura (in approximately 0.02% of treated patients). These hematologic effects are much rarer with clopidogrel, which is currently the preferred agent of this class.

Clopidogrel is a prodrug that requires cytochrome P450-mediated biotransformation to the active metabolite, which contributes to the drug's delayed onset of action and to variability in its antiplatelet effect. For example, patients with common reduced-function polymorphisms of the cytochrome P450 2C19 (CYP2C19) gene demonstrate weakened platelet inhibition and less clinical benefit. In addition, studies have implicated proton pump inhibitors (e.g., omeprazole) as drugs that can interfere with hepatic CYP2C19 activation of clopidogrel and its cardiovascular benefit.

Newer drugs address these shortcomings. For example, prasugrel, another thienopyridine, is metabolized to an active form more readily than clopidogrel and has a more potent antiplatelet effect. Compared to clopidogrel, it has been shown to further reduce the risk of future myocardial infarction in patients with ACS who undergo percutaneous coronary intervention. This benefit comes with an increased risk of bleeding, a complication that is more likely to occur in patients who are elderly, those with prior cerebrovascular disease, and individuals with a low body weight.

A limitation of the thienopyridines, including clopidogrel and prasugrel, is that they are *irreversible* platelet inhibitors. If a thienopyridine-treated patient with an ACS requires coronary artery bypass surgery, a waiting period of several days is necessary to allow adequate return of platelet function to prevent perioperative bleeding complications. As a result, a newer generation of *reversible* platelet $P2Y_{12}$ ADP receptor blockers is in active development.

Glycoprotein IIb/IIIa Receptor Antagonists

The GP IIb/IIIa receptor antagonists constitute one of the most potent classes of antiplatelet agents. This group reversibly inhibits the critical and final common pathway of platelet aggregation—the binding of activated platelet GP IIb/IIIa receptors to fibrinogen and von Willebrand factor. As a result, platelets are inhibited from "sticking" to one another, impairing the formation of a hemostatic plug. Three types of GP IIb/IIIa receptor antagonists have been developed: (1) monoclonal antibodies (e.g., **abciximab**, which is the Fab fragment of a chimeric human–mouse monoclonal antibody); (2) synthetic peptide antagonists (e.g., **eptifibatide**); and (3) synthetic nonpeptide antagonists (e.g., **tirofiban**). As described in Chapters 6 and 7, the GP IIb/IIIa antagonists significantly improve outcomes of patients undergoing percutaneous coronary interventions and in high-risk acute coronary syndromes.

All the GP IIb/IIIa receptor inhibitors in current use must be given intravenously. Oral GP IIb/IIIa receptor inhibitors have been developed but have not demonstrated beneficial outcomes in clinical trials.

The major side effects of the GP IIb/IIIa receptor inhibitors are bleeding (in 1% to 10%

of patients) and thrombocytopenia (in approximately 2% of patients treated with abciximab and less commonly with the other agents). Abciximab has a short plasma half-life (30 minutes); thus, its effects can be reversed by discontinuing the drug or by administering a platelet transfusion. Because the other GP IIb/IIIa receptor antagonists have longer half-lives, they may continue to inactivate transfused platelets. Nonetheless, bleeding complications are infrequent using current protocols and careful dosing.

Dipyridamole

The antiplatelet drug **dipyridamole** is occasionally prescribed to patients who are intolerant to aspirin, but it is not as effective. Its mechanism of antiplatelet action is unclear, but it may act in part by increasing platelet cAMP levels, either by inhibiting the enzyme phosphodiesterase or by blocking cellular uptake and destruction of endogenous adenosine. As a result, cytosolic $[Ca^{++}]$ falls, which inhibits platelet aggregation (see Fig. 17.17). By itself, dipyridamole has no proven cardiac benefits. It is sometimes prescribed in combination with warfarin for an augmented antithrombotic effect in patients with recurrent thromboembolism from prosthetic heart valves, but the pairing of aspirin plus warfarin is more effective. The combination of dipyridamole plus aspirin *is* effective at prevention of recurrent strokes in patients with prior cerebrovascular symptomatology and is approved for that purpose.

Anticoagulant Drugs

Anticoagulant drugs (see Table 17.15) interfere with the coagulation cascade and impair secondary hemostasis. Because the final step in both the intrinsic and extrinsic coagulation pathways is the formation of a fibrin clot by the action of thrombin, major goals of anticoagulant therapy are to inhibit the activation of thrombin by factor Xa (e.g., using unfractionated heparin [UFH], low molecular weight forms of heparin, or fondaparinux), to inhibit thrombin itself (e.g., UFH or direct thrombin inhibitors), or to decrease the production of functional prothrombin (e.g., warfarin).

Unfractionated Heparin

UFH is a heterogeneous mixture of glycosamin-oglycans. Although it has little anticoagulant action by itself, it associates with antithrombin (AT) in the circulation, greatly increasing its effect. AT is a natural protein that inhibits the action of thrombin and other clotting factors. When UFH complexes with AT, the affinity of AT for thrombin increases 1,000-fold, markedly reducing thrombin's ability to generate fibrin from fibrinogen. The UFH–AT complex also inhibits activated factor X, additionally contributing to the anticoagulant action. Furthermore, UFH has antiplatelet properties by binding to, and blocking the action of, von Willebrand factor.

UFH is administered parenterally because it is not absorbed from the gastrointestinal tract. For most acute indications, an intravenous bolus is followed by a continuous infusion of the drug. The bioavailability of UFH varies from patient to patient because it is a heterogeneous collection of molecules that bind to plasma proteins, macrophages, and endothelial cells. The dosage–effect relationship is often not predictable; thus, frequent blood samples are required to monitor the degree of anticoagulation (most commonly, measurement of the activated partial thromboplastin time), so that the infusion rate can be adjusted accordingly.

The usual cardiovascular settings in which intravenous UFH is indicated include (1) *unstable angina* and *NSTEMI* (see Chapter 6), (2) *acute myocardial infarction* after fibrinolytic therapy or if an extensive wall motion abnormality is present (see Chapter 7), and (3) *pulmonary embolism* or *deep venous thrombosis* (see Chapter 15). Among hospitalized or bed-ridden patients not receiving intravenous heparin, fixed low dosages of *subcutaneous* UFH are often administered to prevent deep venous thrombosis.

The most important side effect of heparin is *bleeding*. An overdose of UFH can be treated with intravenous **protamine sulfate**, which forms a stable complex with UFH and immediately reverses the anticoagulation effect.

Heparin-induced thrombocytopenia (*HIT*) is another potential major adverse effect and can occur in two forms. The more common type, thought to result from direct heparin-induced platelet aggregation, occurs in up to 15% of patients and is usually asymptomatic, dose dependent, and self-limited. This mild HIT rarely causes severe reductions in platelet counts and usually does not require cessation of heparin.

The less common, much more dangerous form of HIT is immune-mediated, a condition that affects 3% of UFH-treated patients. It can lead to life-threatening bleeding and, paradoxically, to thrombosis. Thrombosis is caused by the formation of antibodies directed against heparin–platelet complexes, resulting in platelet activation, aggregation, and clot production. In the immune-mediated form of HIT, the platelet count can fall markedly and is not dependent on the dose of heparin. Therapy requires immediate cessation of heparin and substitution by alternate antithrombotic therapy to prevent further clotting (e.g., a direct thrombin inhibitor, described later in the chapter).

Patients receiving long-term UFH therapy are also prone to a dose-dependent form of osteoporosis through an unclear mechanism.

Low Molecular Weight Heparins

Some of the shortcomings of UFH (e.g., short half-life and unpredictable bioavailability) have been addressed by the development of low molecular weight heparins (LMWHs), examples of which are **enoxaparin**, **dalteparin**, and **tinzaparin**. As the name implies, LMWH molecules are smaller than UFH (approximately one third the size). These agents also interact with AT, but unlike UFH, the LMWH–AT complex preferentially inhibits factor Xa more than thrombin (thrombin inhibition requires heparin molecules larger than those in LMWHs). Selectively inhibiting factor Xa upstream in the coagulation cascade has a multiplier effect in preventing downstream formation of thrombin.

Advantages of LMWHs over UFH include (1) inhibition of platelet-bound factor Xa, contributing to a more prominent anticoagulant effect; (2) less binding to plasma proteins and endothelial cells, resulting in more predictable bioavailability and a longer half-life; (3) fewer bleeding complications; and (4) a lower incidence of immune-mediated HIT.

From a practical standpoint, the major advantages of LMWH formulations are the ease of use and more consistent level of anticoagulation. They can be administered as subcutaneous injections once or twice a day in fixed doses, without the frequent blood monitoring required for UFH. In rare cases in which monitoring the anticoagulant effect *is* necessary (e.g., in patients with renal dysfunction, because LMWHs are cleared via the kidneys), a factor Xa inhibition assay is used.

In clinical trials, LMWH therapy is at least as effective as UFH in preventing deep venous thrombosis and treating unstable angina. It also has a better safety profile than UFH, with lower rates of bleeding, thrombocytopenia, and osteoporosis. LMWHs should not, however, be used in patients with a history of HIT, and unlike UFH, the effects of LMWHs cannot be completely reversed by protamine. Current clinical indications for LMWH therapy are (1) prophylaxis against deep venous thrombosis following hip, knee, or abdominal surgery; (2) treatment of deep venous thrombosis (with or without pulmonary embolism); and (3) management of acute coronary syndromes.

Direct Thrombin Inhibitors

The anticoagulation effects of UFH and LMWH are limited because their activity depends, at least in part, on AT, and they inhibit only *circulating* thrombin. The large heparin–AT complex cannot inactivate thrombin that is already bound to fibrin within a clot. In contrast, the direct thrombin inhibitors (**lepirudin**, **bivalirudin**, **argatroban**, and others) inhibit thrombin activity independently of AT and are effective against both circulating and clot-bound thrombin. They do not cause thrombocytopenia and are used to maintain anticoagulation and prevent thrombosis in patients with HIT. Bivalirudin is approved for use as an anticoagulant in patients with unstable angina undergoing percutaneous coronary intervention. All direct thrombin inhibitors are potent anticoagulants and the major adverse effect is bleeding.

Fondaparinux

The anticoagulant fondaparinux is a synthetic pentasaccharide that specifically inhibits factor Xa, thereby reducing thrombin activation. Like heparin, fondaparinux binds to AT with high affinity, greatly increasing AT's ability to inactivate factor Xa. Unlike UFH, fondaparinux does not inactivate formed thrombin, nor does it interfere with platelet actions or cause HIT. It is administered by subcutaneous injection, and its half-life is sufficiently long (17 to 21 hours) that it can be prescribed just once a day. There are no known antidotes to its anticoagulant effect.

Fondaparinux is currently approved for prevention of deep venous thrombosis after certain surgical procedures and as treatment for deep venous thrombosis and pulmonary embolism.

Warfarin

Warfarin is an oral agent prescribed for long-term anticoagulation. It acts by antagonizing an enzyme (vitamin K epoxide reductase) that is required for usual vitamin K metabolism. Normally, the reduced form of vitamin K promotes the carboxylation of a glutamic acid residue within specific coagulation factors (factors II, VII, IX, and X), an action that is necessary for the factors to subsequently bind calcium, become functional, and participate in coagulation (Fig. 17.18). By interfering with the formation of reduced vitamin K, warfarin indirectly inhibits carboxylation of the coagulation factors, rendering them inactive. Because certain natural coagulation *inhibitors* (protein C and protein S) are also vitamin K dependent, warfarin impairs their functions as well, which in some cases may counteract the drug's anticoagulant effect.

Warfarin's action has a delayed onset of 2 to 7 days; thus, if immediate anticoagulation is needed, UFH or LMWH must be prescribed concurrently at first (known as anticoagulant "bridging"). The half-life of warfarin is long (37 hours), and the drug's dosage must be individualized to achieve a therapeutic effect while minimizing the risk of bleeding complications. The extent of anticoagulation is monitored by measuring the prothrombin time in blood samples, reported as an international normalized ratio (INR). There are two target ranges of anticoagulant intensity.

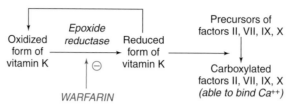

Figure 17.18. Mechanism of action of warfarin. Normally, coagulation factors II, VII, IX, and X are converted to functional forms by carboxylation in the liver, in the presence of reduced vitamin K. During this reaction, vitamin K undergoes oxidation and must be regenerated back to the reduced state for the sustained synthesis of functional clotting factors. Warfarin inhibits the formation of reduced vitamin K by antagonizing the enzyme epoxide reductase, such that the conversion of the coagulation factors does not occur and they remain nonfunctional.

For patients at greatest risk of pathologic thrombosis (e.g., those with certain types of mechanical heart valves), the desired INR is 2.5 to 3.5. For others (e.g., those with uncomplicated atrial fibrillation), the target INR is usually 2.0 to 3.0.

Many factors influence the anticoagulation effect of warfarin and require alterations in its dosage. For example, liver disease and heart failure each reduce the warfarin requirement, whereas a high dietary ingestion of foods containing vitamin K (e.g., green leafy vegetables) increases the re-

quired dose. Similarly, many pharmaceuticals alter warfarin's anticoagulation effect (Table 17.16). Finally, the combined use of warfarin with aspirin or other antiplatelet agents increases the risk of a bleeding complication.

If serious bleeding arises during warfarin therapy, the drug's effect can be reversed within hours by the administration of vitamin K (or even more quickly by transfusing fresh-frozen plasma, which directly replenishes functional circulating clotting factors). In patients with mechanical heart

Table 17.16. Drugs That Alter the Anticoagulation Effect of Warfarin	
Reduced Anticoagulation Effect	*Increased Anticoagulation Effect*
Hepatic enzyme induction	**Hepatic enzyme inhibition**
Barbiturates	Amiodarone
Rifampin	Cephalosporins
Carbamazepine	Cimetidine
Nafcillin	Erythromycin
Warfarin malabsorption	Fluconazole
Cholestyramine	Isoniazid
Sucralfate	Ketoconazole
	Metronidazole
	Propafenone
	Trimethoprim–sulfamethoxazole
	Displacement from protein-binding sites
	Allopurinol
	Gemfibrozil
	Phenytoin
	Altered vitamin K production by gut flora
	Ciprofloxacin
	Piperacillin

valves, vitamin K should be avoided unless life-threatening bleeding occurs, because of the possibility of rebound valve thrombosis. Warfarin is teratogenic and should not be taken during pregnancy, especially during the first trimester.

Given the many limitations and inconvenience of warfarin use, much current effort is directed toward the development of new anticoagulants (including oral direct thrombin inhibitors and factor Xa antagonists) endowed with more predictable pharmacologic properties.

LIPID-REGULATING DRUGS

As described in Chapter 5, abnormal serum lipid levels play a critical role in the pathogenesis of atherosclerosis. Drugs that improve lipid abnormalities are cardioprotective; they inhibit the progression (and may induce regression) of atherosclerosis, improve cardiovascular outcomes, and, in high-risk patients, reduce mortality rates.

HMG CoA Reductase Inhibitors

The HMG CoA reductase inhibitors, commonly known as "statins," are the most effective drugs for reducing LDL cholesterol. By virtue of their potency, excellent tolerability, and mortality benefits, they are widely prescribed. The available agents of this group, in increasing order of potency, are **fluvastatin, lovastatin, pravastatin, simvastatin, atorvastatin,** and **rosuvastatin** (Table 17.17).

Statins are competitive inhibitors of the enzyme HMG CoA reductase, a rate-controlling factor in cholesterol biosynthesis (Fig. 17.19). By inhibiting cholesterol production in the liver, statins lower serum LDL cholesterol through three mechanisms: (1) the reduced intrahepatic cholesterol content induces increased expression of the LDL receptor gene, causing a greater number of LDL receptors to appear on the surface of the hepatocyte, which facilitates the binding and clearance of LDL from the circulation; (2) circulating LDL precursors (known as very low density

Class	LDL Effect (%)	HDL Effect (%)	Triglyceride Effect (%)	Adverse Effects
HMG CoA reductase inhibitors (in increasing order of potency) Fluvastatin Lovastatin Pravastatin Simvastatin Atorvastatin Rosuvastatin	↓ 20–55	↑ 5–15	↓ 7–30	Transaminitis, myopathy
Bile acid–binding agents Cholestyramine Colestipol Colesevelam	↓ 15–30	↑ 3–5	May ↑	Constipation, bloating
Cholesterol absorption inhibitor Ezetimibe	↓ 15–20	↑ 1–2	↓ 0–5	Rare allergic reaction
Niacin	↓ 5–25	↑ 15–35	↓ 20–50	Flushing, hepatotoxicity, hyperglycemia, hyperuricemia, exacerbation of peptic ulcer disease
Fibric acid derivatives Fenofibrate Gemfibrozil	↓ 0–20 *or* ↑ 0–10	↑ 10–20	↓ 20–50	Nausea, gallstones

Table 17.17. Lipid-Regulating Drugs

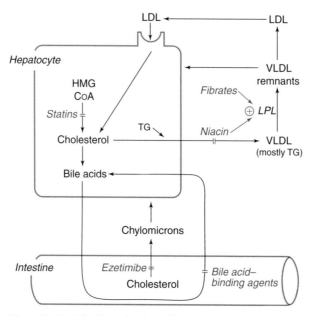

Figure 17.19. Major sites of action of lipid-regulating drugs. The *statins* inhibit cholesterol biosynthesis in the liver by competing with the enzyme HMG CoA reductase. This action depletes intrahepatic cholesterol stores, which results in increased expression of surface low-density lipoprotein (LDL) receptors. The latter enhance clearance of LDL and very low density lipoprotein (VLDL) remnants from the circulation. The lower intrahepatic cholesterol content leads to reduction in VLDL synthesis. *Ezetimibe* selectively inhibits cholesterol uptake in the small intestine, thereby reducing chylomicron production and cholesterol delivery to the liver. *Bile acid–binding agents* interrupt the enterohepatic circulation of bile acids in the intestine, causing more hepatic cholesterol to be diverted to new bile acid production. In response to reduced availability of intrahepatic cholesterol, LDL receptor expression and LDL clearance increase. Among its effects, *niacin* inhibits VLDL production. It also increases lipoprotein lipase (LPL) activity, thus promoting triglyceride (TG) clearance from circulating VLDL particles. Niacin raises circulating high-density lipoprotein (HDL) by impairing hepatic uptake of apo AI, a major HDL apoprotein (not shown). *Fibrates* enhance VLDL catabolism by increasing the synthesis of lipoprotein lipase via peroxisome proliferator–activated receptor α (PPAR-α), a nuclear transcription factor. They also raise HDL by stimulating the production of HDL-associated apoproteins (not shown).

lipoprotein [VLDL] remnants and intermediate-density lipoprotein particles) are cleared more rapidly from the circulation because of their cross-recognition with the hepatic LDL receptor; and (3) hepatic VLDL production falls due to the reduced availability of intracellular cholesterol for lipoprotein assembly. Because the catabolism of VLDL in the circulation ultimately forms LDL, lowering VLDL production also decreases circulating LDL levels. The reduced production of VLDL is also likely responsible for the triglyceride-lowering effect of statins, because this lipoprotein is the major carrier of triglycerides in the circulation.

The overall effect is that statins reduce serum LDL levels by 20% to 55%, depending on which agent is used. Statins also decrease plasma triglyceride levels by 7% to 30%, and by an unclear mechanism, HDL levels increase by 5% to 15%.

The lowering of LDL reduces the lipid content of atherosclerotic lesions and promotes plaque stability. This lessens the vulnerability of plaque to rupture, thus decreasing the likelihood of thrombus formation and vascular occlusion. In addition to their lipid-modulating properties, statins have other potentially cardioprotective effects. They improve endothelial function as evidenced by enhanced synthesis of nitric oxide. They further promote plaque stability by inhibiting monocyte penetration into the arterial wall and reducing macrophage secretion of metalloproteinases, enzymes that degrade and weaken the fibrous caps of plaques. Statins also diminish the vulnerability of lipoproteins to oxidation, thus inhibiting the unregulated uptake of modified LDL cholesterol by macrophages (see Chapter 5). Finally, they appear to suppress inflammation, a key component of atherogenesis.

Statins are widely prescribed for patients with CAD, because major trials have shown that they substantially reduce mortality, cardiac events, and strokes in this population, whether LDL cholesterol is elevated or even in the "normal" range. In studies of patients not known to have CAD, statin therapy has been shown to reduce coronary events in high-risk individuals—those with elevated LDL cholesterol levels or those with average total cholesterol but low HDL values.

Statins are well-tolerated drugs. Mild gastrointestinal upset occasionally occurs. The most significant potential adverse effects are hepatotoxicity and myopathy (skeletal muscle toxicity), and these are rare. *Hepatotoxicity* is dose related and occurs in fewer than 1% of patients. Those affected may experience fatigue, anorexia, and weight loss. More commonly, the patient is asymptomatic, but routine laboratory studies show an increase in transaminase levels (ALT, AST). Symptoms disappear almost immediately after the drug is discontinued, but transaminase levels may remain elevated for weeks. The risk of statin-associated hepatic toxicity is higher in patients who drink excessive amounts of alcohol.

Myopathy, typically involving the proximal leg or arm muscles symmetrically, can range from vague aches to intense myalgias and muscle weakness, and rarely may lead to rhabdomyolysis (destruction of muscle) with myoglobinuria and renal failure. While benign muscle aches are reported in 2% to 10% of patients on statins, significant myositis (defined as an elevated serum level of muscle-derived creatine kinase >10 times the upper limit of normal) develops in <0.5%. However, the incidence of muscle injury is increased by concomitant therapy with certain other drugs, including other lipid-lowering agents (i.e., niacin and the fibric acid derivatives) and drugs that inhibit the 3A4 isoform of cytochrome P-450, which is responsible for the hepatic metabolism of many statins. Such agents include macrolide antibiotics (e.g., erythromycin, clarithromycin), azole antifungal drugs (e.g., ketoconazole, itraconazole), and many HIV protease inhibitors. Notably, pravastatin, rosuvastatin, and fluvastatin are not substantially dependent on the cytochrome P-450 3A4 isoform for their metabolism and may be less likely to cause myopathy in combination with these other drugs.

Bile Acid–Binding Agents

This group includes the resins **cholestyramine** and **colestipol** and the hydrophilic polymer **colesevelam**. These drugs are large, highly positively charged molecules that bind bile acids (which are negatively charged) in the intestine and prevent their normal reabsorption to the liver through the enterohepatic circulation (see Fig. 17.19). To make up for the loss, more hepatic cholesterol is converted into newly produced bile acids. This action depletes intrahepatic cholesterol stores, thus stimulating the production of LDL receptors. Similar to the effect of the statins, an increased number of hepatic LDL receptors bind a greater amount of circulating LDL, reducing the circulating concentration of the lipoprotein. However, unlike statins, *new* hepatic cholesterol production is also stimulated by the reduced intrahepatic cholesterol content. The boost in cholesterol synthesis augments VLDL production, which likely explains the commonly observed rise in serum triglyceride levels during therapy with a bile acid–binding agent.

In one of the first drug trials of patients with hypercholesterolemia, cholestyramine significantly reduced the risk of fatal and nonfatal myocardial infarctions. However, drugs of this class are difficult for patients to take (e.g., cholestyramine and colestipol are unappealing gritty powders that must be mixed with liquids) and their potency is inferior to that of statins. Thus, the bile acid–binding agents are only occasionally used today, mainly as second-line lipid-regulating drugs, in combination with statin therapy. Because they can cause elevations of the serum triglyceride level, they should be avoided in patients with hypertriglyceridemia.

The bile acid–binding agents interfere with the absorption of fat-soluble vitamins and certain drugs (e.g., warfarin, digoxin, propranolol, and thyroid hormones). Thus, other medications should be consumed 1 hour before or 3 to 4 hours after these agents. The main side effects are gastrointestinal: bloating, constipation, and nausea. Because bile acid–binding agents are not absorbed into the circulation, they do not cause systemic side effects.

Cholesterol Absorption Inhibitors

Ezetimibe, the first member of this class of agents, is a selective inhibitor of cholesterol uptake at the brush border of epithelial cells in the small intestine. It acts by competitively inhibiting a transporter known as the Niemann–Pick C1–like 1 protein. Normally, a portion of dietary and biliary cholesterol taken up in this manner is esterified and incorporated into chylomicrons, which then enter into the circulation and are transported to the liver (see Box 5.1). By inhibiting cholesterol uptake (see Fig. 17.19), ezetimibe results in reduced chylomicron production and therefore less cholesterol delivery to the liver. The reduced cholesterol content stimulates compensatory hepatic production of LDL receptors, which augment clearance of circulating LDL particles. The net result is lowering of circulating LDL (and therefore serum cholesterol levels).

Used alone at standard dosage, ezetimibe reduces LDL cholesterol by about 18%. When combined with statin therapy, more potent LDL lowering ensues. Ongoing trials are assessing whether LDL reduction by ezetimibe translates into improved clinical outcomes.

Unlike bile acid–binding agents, side effects from ezetimibe therapy are rare. When combined with a statin, the incidence of transaminase elevation is only slightly greater than that of statin therapy alone. The addition of ezetimibe to a statin regime does not appear to significantly increase the risk of statin-associated myopathy.

Niacin

Niacin is one of the oldest lipid-regulating drugs and has favorable effects on all the circulating lipid fractions. It is the most effective agent available for raising HDL cholesterol (by 15% to 35%), and it reduces LDL cholesterol (by 5% to 25%) and triglyceride levels (by 20% to 50%). Furthermore, unlike most other lipid-lowering drugs, niacin substantially reduces the circulating level of lipoprotein(a), an LDL-like lipoprotein that carries an independent risk of cardiovascular disease (see Chapter 5).

Niacin modifies lipid levels through multiple mechanisms. It inhibits the release of fatty acids from adipose tissue. As a result, fewer fatty acids are transported to the liver and hepatic triglyceride synthesis declines. Impaired triglyceride production by the liver reduces VLDL secretion into the circulation; consequently, less LDL is formed (see Fig. 17.19). Niacin also enhances the clearance of triglycerides from circulating VLDL by promoting the activity of lipoprotein lipase at adipose and muscle cells. The net effect of these actions is a reduction in serum triglyceride and LDL levels. Niacin is thought to raise circulating HDL cholesterol levels by decreasing the hepatic uptake of its apoprotein, apo AI, thus reducing clearance of HDL particles from the circulation. This mechanism does not disturb hepatic retrieval (and disposal) of cholesterol from the HDL particles.

In a major study of niacin in men who had experienced a prior myocardial infarction (the Coronary Drug Project), niacin reduced the risk of future cardiac events and lowered the mortality rate in long-term follow-up. That study was performed before the better tolerated and more effective statin drugs were available. Niacin is now mainly used to treat patients with low serum HDL levels and/or elevated serum triglycerides.

Niacin has several common side effects. Transient cutaneous flushing episodes occur in most patients. These episodes are prostaglandin mediated and can be minimized by taking aspirin prior to the niacin dose. Gastrointestinal side effects include nausea and exacerbation of peptic ulcer disease. Hepatotoxicity can occur, manifested by fatigue, weakness, and elevated serum transaminases (ALT, AST). Niacin should be used cautiously in diabetic patients because it can contribute to insulin resistance and hyperglycemia. It also raises serum uric acid levels and can precipitate gout in susceptible patients. Rare cases of myopathy have been reported with niacin therapy. The incidence is increased when niacin is prescribed concurrently with a statin.

Fibrates

The fibric acid derivatives, or fibrates, include **gemfibrozil** and **fenofibrate**. They are the most powerful agents to reduce serum triglyceride levels (by up to 50%), and they raise HDL cholesterol levels (by up to 20%). However, their effect on LDL cholesterol is more variable and less beneficial than other lipid-altering drugs (see Table 17.17).

A large study of men with hypercholesterolemia, but no known coronary disease, showed that gemfibrozil reduced the number of subsequent myocardial infarctions, without benefiting the total death rate. In another study of men with known CAD, normal LDL levels, and low HDL levels, the rate of coronary events was decreased, but again total mortality was not significantly affected. In a 5-year study of patients with type 2 diabetes, fenofibrate reduced the incidence of nonfatal myocardial infarction but not the total cardiovascular mortality.

Fibrates are thought to exert their antilipid effects through interactions with peroxisome proliferator–activated receptor α (PPAR-α), a nuclear transcription factor. Activation of PPAR-α leads to a decrease in triglycerides, at least in part by augmenting fatty acid oxidation and increasing the synthesis of lipoprotein lipase (see Fig. 17.19). The latter results in increased VLDL catabolism, which may actually *raise* the circulating LDL level, especially in patients with baseline hypertriglyceridemia. Fibrates are believed to augment HDL cholesterol levels via PPAR-α activation of the gene for apoprotein AI, a key constituent of HDL particles.

Fibrates are primarily used to lower triglyceride levels and raise HDL cholesterol levels. They are metabolized by hepatic glucuronida-

tion with subsequent renal excretion. Thus, they should be avoided or prescribed at lower dosages for patients with impaired liver or kidney function.

Fibrates are generally well tolerated. Potential side effects include dyspepsia, gallstones, and myalgias. When used in combination with a statin, the risk of rhabdomyolysis is increased. Therefore, if these drugs are prescribed concurrently, it is recommended that the serum creatine kinase (a marker of muscle inflammation or necrosis) be monitored every several months. Fibrates augment the effect of warfarin by displacing it from albumin-binding sites, possibly necessitating a decrease in the anticoagulant dosage. They also enhance the effects of oral hypoglycemic drugs.

Table 17.17 summarizes the expected results and potential side effects of the commonly used lipid-altering drugs.

SUMMARY

This chapter has presented an overview of the most commonly used cardiovascular drugs. These agents are covered in greater detail in the references listed in the section "Additional Reading." It is hoped that the tables, figures, and brief explanations presented here will be useful to the reader now, and again when considering the basic pathophysiology of heart disease while caring for patients.

Acknowledgments

Contributors to the previous editions of this chapter were Martin W. Schoen, MD; Mark Friedberg, MD; Andrew C. Hecht, MD; Steven N. Kalkanis, MD; Steven P. Leon, MD; Chiadi E. Ndumele, MD; David Sloane, MD; Ralph A. Kelly, MD; Gary R. Strichartz, MD; Elliott M. Antman MD; and Leonard S. Lilly, MD.

Additional Reading

Antman EM. *Cardiovascular Therapeutics: A Companion to Braunwald's Heart Disease*. 3rd ed. Philadelphia, PA: Elsevier Saunders; 2006.

Bangalore S, Messerli FH, Kostis JB, et al. Cardiovascular protection using beta-blockers: a critical review of the evidence. *J Am Coll Cardiol*. 2007; 50:563–572.

Berger JS, Roncaglioni MC, Avanzini F, et al. Aspirin for the primary prevention of cardiovascular events in women and men. *JAMA*. 2006;295:306–313.

Cattaneo M. New P2Y$_{12}$ inhibitors. *Circulation*. 2010; 121:171–179.

DeBacker D, Biston P, Devriendt J, et al. Comparison of dopamine and norepinephrine in the treatment of shock. *N Engl J Med*. 2010;362:779–789.

Ernst ME, Moser M. Use of diuretics in patients with hypertension. *N Engl J Med*. 2009;361: 2153–2164.

Ho PM, Maddox TM, Wang L, et al. Risk of adverse outcomes associated with concomitant use of clopidogrel and proton pump inhibitors following acute coronary syndrome. *JAMA*. 2009;301:937–944.

Joy TR, Hegele RA. Narrative review: statin-related myopathy. *Ann Intern Med*. 2009;150:858–868.

Lafuente-Lafuente C, Mouly S, Longas-Tejero MA, et al. Antiarrhythmic drugs for maintaining sinus rhythm after cardioversion of atrial fibrillation. *Arch Intern Med*. 2006;166:719–728.

Marin F, Gonzalex-Conejero R, Capranzano P, et al. Pharmacogenetics in cardiovascular antithrombotic therapy. *J Am Coll Cardiol*. 2009;54: 1041–1057.

Maron BA, Leopold JA. Aldosterone receptor antagonists: effective but often forgotten. *Circulation*. 2010;121:934–939.

Mega JL, Close SL, Wiviott SD, et al. Cytochrome P-450 polymorphisms and response to clopidogrel. *N Engl J Med*. 2009;360:354–362.

Opie LH, Gersh BJ, eds. *Drugs for the Heart*. 7th ed. Philadelphia, PA: W.B. Saunders; 2009.

Patel C, Yan G-X, Kowey PR. Dronedarone. *Circulation*. 2009;120:636–644.

Ram CVS. Angiotensin receptor blockers: current status and future prospects. *Am J Med*. 2008; 121:656–663.

Index

Page numbers in italics denote figures; those followed by "t" denote tables; those followed by "b" denote boxes.

Terazosin, 405, 406t
Terminal cisternae, 11
Tetralogy of Fallot, 380–382
TFPI (*see* Tissue factor pathway inhibitor (TFPI))
Thallium-201 (^{201}Tl)
  imaging, 62, 65
Thermodilution method, 60–61
Thiazide diuretics, 237
Thienopyridines, 178
Third-degree atrioventricular block, 283–284, *284*
Third heart sound, 35–36
Three-dimensional (3-D) echocardiography, 53
    (*see also* Echocardiography)
Thrombin, 163, 165
Thromboembolism, 187
Thrombogenic potential, 123, 124, 125
Thrombolysis in Myocardial Infarction (TIMI) risk
    score, 179–180
Thrombolytic therapy, 178–179, 182 (*see also*
    Fibrinolytic therapy)
Thrombomodulin, 163
Thrombophlebitis, superficial, 359
Thrombosis
  antithrombotic agents, 162–164
  consequences of, *166*
  formation of, 165–166
  partially occlusive, 162
  pathogenesis of, 164–166, *166*
  significance of, 165–166, *166*
Thromboxane (TXA$_2$), 178, 423
Ticlopidine, 426
TIMI risk score (*see* Thrombolysis in Myocardial
    Infarction (TIMI) risk score)
Tirofiban, 427
Tissue factor pathway inhibitor (TFPI), 162
Tissue plasminogen activator (tPA), 163, 180,
    181, 182
Titin, 23
TNF-α (*see* Tumor necrosis factor-α (TNF-α))
Torsades de pointes, 295, *298*, 298–299
Torsemide, 420t, 421
Total peripheral resistance (TPR), 227
TPA (*see* Tissue plasminogen activator (tPA))
TPR (*see* Total peripheral resistance (TPR))
Trabeculae carneae, 4
Transesophageal echocardiography (TEE), 51–53,
    52, 213
Transmural infarcts, 167, 170t
Transposition of the great arteries,
    382–384
Transthoracic echocardiography (TTE), *50*,
    50–51, 212
Traube sign, 206t
Triamterene, 422
Tricuspid regurgitation, 39, 234
Tricuspid regurgitation (TR), 207–208
Tricuspid stenosis (TS), 207
Tricuspid valve
  anatomy of, 4
  development of, 366
  insufficiency of, 64t

opening of, 35
stenosis of, 58, 207
Triggered activity
  description of, 268–269
  treatment of, 409–410
Triglycerides, 120b
Tropomyosin, 23
Troponins (Tn), 23
  defined, 175
  I, 175
  myocardial necrosis detection by, 176
  myocardial necrosis diagnosed by, 175–176
  T, 175
Truncus arteriosus, 363
TS (*see* Tricuspid stenosis (TS))
TTE (*see* Transthoracic echocardiography (TTE))
T tubules, 11
Tuberculous pericarditis, 325
Tumor necrosis factor-α (TNF-α), 115
Turner syndrome, 378, 381b
Two-dimensional (2-D) echocardiography
  apical views, *50*, 51
  description of, 49–50, *50*
  indications
    coronary artery disease, 55
    pericardial disease, 55–60
    ventricular assessments, *53*, 53–54
  parasternal view, *50*, 51
  subcostal view, *50*, 51

U

Unfractionated heparin, 178, 428 (*see also* Heparin)
Unidirectional block, 270–272
Unstable angina
  characteristics of, 146
  clinical features of, 174t
  clinical presentation of, 171–172
  complications of, 183
  definition of, 136t
  diagnosis of, 174
  pathophysiologic findings, *145*
  treatment of
    anti-ischemic agents, 177–178
    antithrombotic agents, 178–179
    β-blockers, 177–178
    calcium channel blockers, 178
    clopidogrel, 178
    conservative *vs.* early invasive approaches,
      179–180
    heparin, 179
    nitrates, 178
Uremic pericarditis, 326

V

Valsalva maneuver, 254–255 (*see also* Hypertrophic
    cardiomyopathy (HCM))
Valvular heart disease
  mitral valve prolapse, 201–202
  pulmonic regurgitation, 40, 208